Urologic Surgery in Infants and Children

Urologic Surgery in Infants and Children

Lowell R. King, M.D.

Professor of Urology,
Associate Professor of Pediatrics
Duke University School of Medicine
Durham, North Carolina

Head, Section of Pediatric Urology
Department of Surgery
Duke University Medical Center
School of Medicine
Durham, North Carolina

W.B. SAUNDERS COMPANY
A Division of Harcourt Brace & Company
Philadelphia London Toronto Montreal Sydney Tokyo

W.B. SAUNDERS COMPANY
A Division of Harcourt Brace & Company

The Curtis Center
Independence Square West
Philadelphia, Pennsylvania 19106

Library of Congress Cataloging-in-Publication Data

Urologic surgery in infants and children / [edited by] Lowell R. King—1st ed.

p. cm.

ISBN 0–7216–6857–7

1. Genitourinary organs—Surgery. 2. Children—Surgery. 3. Pediatric urology. I. King, Lowell R. [DNLM: 1. Urologic Diseases—in infancy & childhood. 2. Urologic Diseases—surgery. WS 320 U7748 1998]
RD571.U753 1998

617.4′61′0083—dc21

DNLM/DLC 97-4118

UROLOGIC SURGERY IN INFANTS AND CHILDREN ISBN 0–7216–6857–7

Printed in the United States of America.

Last digit is the print number: 9 8 7 6 5 4 3 2 1

To my children,
Erica and Drew,
who are now adults,
and who grew up
and turned out great
in spite of
a very busy father.

Contributors

Laurence S. Baskin, M.D. Assistant Professor of Urology and Pediatrics, University of California San Francisco, School of Medicine, San Francisco, California. *Urethral Anomalies and Obstruction*

Stuart Bauer, M.D. Associate Professor of Urology, Harvard Medical School, Boston, Massachusetts; Senior Associate in Urology, Children's Hospital, Boston, Massachusetts. *The Surgical Correction of Incontinence in Myelodysplastic Children*

Jacob Ben-Chaim, M.D. Fellow in Pediatric Urology, Johns Hopkins University School of Medicine, Baltimore, Maryland; Fellow in Pediatric Urology, Johns Hopkins Hospital, Baltimore, Maryland. *Exstrophy and Epispadias*

John W. Brock III, M.D. Associate Professor of Urologic Surgery and Associate Professor of Pediatrics, Vanderbilt University Medical Center, Nashville, Tennessee; Director of Pediatric Urology, Vanderbilt Children's Hospital, Nashville, Tennessee. *Diagnosis and Management of Testicular Torsion*

Douglas Canning, M.D. Assistant Professor of Surgery, University of Pennsylvania, Philadelphia, Pennsylvania; Staff Urologist, Children's Hospital of Philadelphia, Philadelphia, Pennsylvania. *Continent Urinary Diversion*

Anthony J. Casale, M.D. Associate Professor, Department of Urology, Indiana University School of Medicine, Indianapolis, Indiana; Staff Urologist, Riley Hospital for Children, Indianapolis, Indiana. *Genitourinary Trauma in Children*

Bartley G. Cilento, Jr., M.A., M.D. Head, Pediatric Urology, Naval Medical Center San Diego, San Diego, California. *Ureteropelvic Junction Obstruction*

Gregor K. Emmert, Jr., M.D. Medical College Hospital, Toledo, Ohio; Attending Staff, Toledo Hospital, St. Vincent's Hospital, Flower Hospital, Toledo, Ohio. *Multicystic Kidney*

Israel Franco, M. D., F.A.C.S., F.A.A.P. Assistant Professor of Urology and Pediatrics, New York Medical College, Valhalla, New York; Director of Pediatric Urology, Nyack Hospital, Nyack, New York. *Ectopic Ureter and Incontinence*

John P. Gearhart, M.D. Professor of Pediatric Urology and Professor of Pediatrics, Johns Hopkins University School of Medicine, Baltimore, Maryland; Chief of Pediatric Urology, Johns Hopkins Hospital, Baltimore, Maryland. *Exstrophy and Epispadias*

Bhagwant Gill, M.D., F.R.C.S., F.A.A.P. Clinical Associate Professor of Urology, Albert Einstein College of Medicine, Bronx, New York; Attending, Pediatric Urology, Albert Einstein Hospital and Montefiore Medical Center, Bronx, New York. *Cryptorchidism*

Edmond T. Gonzales, Jr., M.D. Professor of Urology, Baylor College of Medicine, Houston, Texas; Head, Department of Surgery and Chief, Urology Service, Texas Children's Hospital, Houston, Texas. *Ureteroceles*

Terry W. Hensle, M.D. Professor of Urology, College of Physicians and Surgeons, Columbia University, New York, New York; Director of Pediatric Urology, Babies and Children's Hospital of New York, Columbia Presbyterian Medical Center, New York, New York. *The Pediatric Varicocele*

Edward F. Ikeguchi, M.D. Chief Resident in Urology, College of Physicians and Surgeons, Columbia University, New York, New York; Chief Resident in Urology, Columbia Presbyterian Medical Center, New York, New York. *The Pediatric Varicocele*

Martin Kaefer, M.D. National Kidney Foundation Scholar, Harvard Medical School, Boston, Massachusetts; Fellow in Pediatric Urology, Department of Urology, Children's Hospital, Boston, Massachusetts. *The Surgical Correction of Incontinence in Myelodysplastic Children*

George W. Kaplan, M.S., M.D. Clinical Professor of Surgery and Pediatrics and Chief, Pediatric Urology, University of California at San Diego School of Medicine,

San Diego, California; Chief of Urology, Children's Hospital, San Diego, California. *Ureteropelvic Junction Obstruction*

Robert Kay, M.D. Head, Section of Pediatric Urology, Cleveland Clinic Foundation, Cleveland, Ohio. *Testis Tumors*

Lowell R. King, M.D. Professor of Urology, Associate Professor of Pediatrics, Duke University School of Medicine, Durham, North Carolina; Head, Section of Pediatric Urology, Department of Surgery, Duke University Medical Center, Durham, North Carolina. *Hypospadias*

Barry A. Kogan, M.D. Professor of Urology and Pediatrics, University of California, San Francisco, School of Medicine, San Francisco, California. *Urethral Anomalies and Obstruction*

Stanley J. Kogan, M.D. Clinical Professor of Urology, New York Medical College, Valhalla, New York, and New York Hospital/Cornell University School of Medicine, New York, New York; Attending Pediatric Urologist, Westchester County Medical Center, Valhalla, New York, New York Hospital, New York, New York, and Montefiore Medical Center, Bronx, New York. *Cryptorchidism*

Chi K. Lee, M.D. Fellow in Pediatric Urology, Schneider Children's Hospital/LIJ, Queens, New York. *Ectopic Ureter and Incontinence*

Selwyn Levitt, M.D., F.A.C.S., F.A.A.P. Clinical Professor of Urology, New York Medical College, Valhalla, New York; Adjunct Clinical Professor of Urology, Cornell Medical School, New York, New York; Attending Pediatric Urologist, Schneider Childrens Hospital/LIJ, Queens, New York, and Westchester County Medical Center, Valhalla, New York. *Ectopic Ureter and Incontinence*

Kevin P. McLaughlin, M.D. Assistant Professor, Loma Linda University School of Medicine, Loma Linda, California. *Bladder and Prostate Rhabdomyosarcoma*

Hrair-George O. Mesrobian, M.D. Associate Professor of Surgery (Urology) and Pediatrics and Chief, Division of Pediatric Urology, Medical College of Wisconsin, Milwaukee, Wisconsin; Medical Director, Section of Urology, Children's Hospital of Wisconsin, Milwaukee, Wisconsin. *Prune-Belly Syndrome*

Alan D. Perlmutter, M.D. Professor of Urology, Emeritus, Wayne State University School of Medicine, Detroit, Michigan; Chief of Pediatric Urology, Emeritus, Children's Hospital of Michigan, Detroit, Michigan. *Intersex*

Alan B. Retik, M.D. Professor of Surgery (Urology), Harvard Medical School, Boston, Massachusetts; Chief, Department of Urology, Children's Hospital, Boston, Massachusetts. *Comments on Ureteroileocecal Sigmoidostomy—An Alternative Method of Urinary Diversion*

Michael L. Ritchey, M.D. Associate Professor, Department of Surgery and Pediatrics, University of Texas, Medical School at Houston, Houston, Texas; Chief of Pediatric Urology, Hermann Children's Hospital, Houston, Texas. *The Management of Wilms' Tumor*

Richard C. Rink, M.D. Associate Professor of Urology, Indiana University School of Medicine, Indianapolis, Indiana; Chief, Pediatric Urology, James W. Riley Hospital for Children, Indiana University Medical Center, Indianapolis, Indiana. *Bladder and Prostate Rhabdomyosarcoma*

Jonathan H. Ross, M.D. Section of Pediatric Urology, Cleveland Clinic Foundation, Cleveland, Ohio. *Testis Tumors*

R. Dixon Walker, M.D. Professor of Surgery and Pediatrics, University of Florida College of Medicine, Gainesville, Florida; Chief, Pediatric Urology, Shands Children's Hospital, Gainesville, Florida. *Vesicoureteral Reflux*

John R. Woodard, M.D. Clinical Professor of Surgery (Urology) and Director of Pediatric Urology, Emory University School of Medicine, Atlanta, Georgia; Chief of Urology, Egleston Children's Hospital, Atlanta, Georgia. *Megaloureter*

Elizabeth B. Yerkes, M.D. Resident, Department of Urologic Surgery, Vanderbilt University Medical Center, Nashville, Tennessee. *Diagnosis and Management of Testicular Torsion*

Preface

In 1976, in the Preface to the first edition of *Clinical Pediatric Urology,* we stated that "almost all aspects of pediatric urology have advanced rapidly in the last decade, and really significant clinical progress continues to be made at a rapid pace . . . ." That is still true. Also, although much more laboratory research is now being done in pediatric urology, clinical advances seem to be continuing to change and to dominate the field. In 1988, I edited *Urologic Surgery in Neonates and Young Infants,* a one-volume text that was brought out between editions of *Clinical Pediatric Urology.* This volume emphasized the value of prenatal sonography in making the presumptive diagnosis of several serious urologic conditions before birth so that the baby could be evaluated and treated immediately after birth if necessary. Just putting newborns on antibacterial prophylaxis when vesicoureteral reflux is presumed has reduced dramatically the incidence of multiple renal scars, nephropathy, and renal failure. The purpose of the present volume, *Urologic Surgery in Infants and Children,* is to present the best methods of patient management as clearly and as succinctly as possible.

In many areas, such as ureterocele, prune belly syndrome, urethral valves, and others, consensus in treatment has developed fairly recently so that the management of such patients, when their conditions are uncomplicated, is now relatively straightforward. Hypospadias surgery continues to evolve, with emphasis now on using an "extra layer" of subcutaneous tissue to buttress urethroplasties that already seem secure. The management of vesicoureteral reflux, neurogenic bladder, trauma, cryptorchidism, and tumors is presented in a straightforward manner, stressing diagnosis and surgical management. The descriptions of operative technique are generally detailed and illustrated. The text emphasizes how to avoid common complications as well as how to manage them if they occur.

At this writing the diagnosis and management of ureteropelvic and ureterovesical obstruction, generally detected by fetal ultrasonography are still subjects of intense debate. It is clear that such obstructions sometimes take longer than expected to cause renal damage. We view this as an advantage, since preservation of renal function is the urologist's job, and we feel that *when obstruction can be diagnosed* it should be repaired promptly. The debate surrounding this issue is very interesting but is largely beyond the scope of this book.

We are emphasizing advances in pediatric urology and trying to present them in a useful way. We presume that the reader has a general knowledge of urology and wants to know mainstream thought on pediatric urologic problems, presented in a concise manner with emphasis on case management. Most readers will not be doing intersex surgery, exstrophy, or pediatric renal transplants, but these conditions occur relatively frequently and a detailed description of them seems warranted. Conversely, cloacal exstrophy, hydrocolpos, and various rare congenital conditions are not included because their management must truly be individualized and varies from case to case.

We trust that the reader will find this book friendly and easy to use. It is not intended to compete with *Clinical Pediatric Urology* and lacks its wealth of detail. Its virtue is simplicity.

LOWELL R. KING, M.D.

Acknowledgments

I want to thank all of my colleagues who contributed to this book and who did most of the work and made it possible. I think it is a timely endeavor. This volume should be very helpful to urologists who wish to "brush up" on pediatric urology and to residents in training; it should also serve as an easy reference for review in preparation for performing various surgical procedures.

Ms. Karla Chaucer and Ms. Kathy Morris helped tremendously in the preparation of the manuscript. Janet Abernathy, as usual, kept me focused and helped immeasurably in staying in contact with other contributors and in keeping things on track. Sandra Valkhoff and Stephanie Donley at the W.B. Saunders Company have been great editors to work with. Any errors are mine. You all deserve the credit.

DRUG NOTICE

Contents

PART I

Intersex

1

ALAN D. PERLMUTTER

Intersex

Intersex is a term widely used to categorize individuals with morphologic ambiguity or contradictions of genital development. Sexual differentiation is influenced by a variety of underlying genetic, gonadal, and endocrine abnormalities. This chapter begins with a brief overview of normal and disordered sexual differentiation followed by the evaluation and diagnosis of infants with genital ambiguity and then—the main emphasis of the chapter—surgical reconstruction and management, including complications, follow-up, and outcome.

One of the first and most meaningful events at the birth of a healthy infant is the glance at the infant's external genitals by parents and those in attendance to determine and announce the sex of the newborn. This simple happening is accurate for the vast majority of births. However, in those rare instances of genital ambiguity, the emotional impact on the parents is overwhelming. It is all too easy for someone responsible to make a hasty, often incorrect gender assignment to satisfy the pressures of the moment; yet the most appropriate, and kindest, response is to indicate in an empathic fashion that the infant's genitals are incompletely developed and that further studies are needed to determine the sex.

The birth of an infant with genital ambiguity constitutes an urgent medical and social problem that requires a careful and thorough assessment to make an appropriate gender assignment as soon as feasible. This chapter provides developmental and clinical information intended to be helpful in that endeavor.

SEXUAL DIFFERENTIATION

Normal sexual differentiation involves orderly, exquisitely timed, sequential processes. Disturbances in the timing and control of these events may result in genital ambiguity. A brief summary of normal sexual differentiation, which follows, is essential to an understanding of disordered sexual development.

The bilateral bipotential gonadal ridge develops into an ovary or testis based on the chromosomal sex. Testicular development requires a signal or signals located on the short arm of the Y chromosome. A gene has been identified, named *SRY* (sex-determining region of the Y chromosome), and is responsible for this induction. More details are available in a 1995 review.[1]

All embryos, female and male, initially have a pair of primordial ducts on each side (paramesonephric and mesonephric) along the dorsal coelom, capable of evolving into female or male internal reproductive structures. In the female, the internal and external sex structures develop autonomously; the paramesonephric ducts evolve into the fallopian tubes, uterus, and upper portion of the vagina.

In the male, development of reproductive structures requires induction. Testosterone from the normal fetal testis acts locally to induce differentiation of the ipsilateral mesonephric duct into the epididymis, vas deferens, ejaculatory duct, and seminal vesicle. A second hormone called müllerian inhibiting substance (MIS), a nonsteroidal glycoprotein from Sertoli's cells in the fetal testis, acts to cause regression of the paramesonephric ducts.

Initially, the external genital primordia are bipotential (Fig. 1–1). The genital tubercle becomes the glans clitoris or enlarges to become the glans penis; the urethral folds become the labia minora or fuse to become the anterior urethra. The genital swellings become the labia majora or fuse and migrate posteriorly to become the scrotum. The pathway of male external genital development requires the presence of local dihydrotestosterone (DHT). Testosterone is converted by the enzyme 5α-reductase to DHT, which binds to an intracellular androgen receptor in the urogenital sinus and external genital tissues to induce penile lengthening, ventral closure of the urogenital sinus with outward fusion of the urethral folds to enclose the future male urethra, and fusion and posterior migration of the future scrotum. Incomplete fusion and labioscrotal migration result in varying degrees of hypospadias or genital ambiguity.

Abnormal sexual differentiation (ambiguous sexual development) results from three general causes: chromosomal abnormalities producing incomplete or anomalous testicular differentiation, deficiencies in genetic males in androgen production or in its action (androgen receptor defect or a deficiency in the 5α-reductase enzyme required to convert testosterone to DHT), and excess androgen in genetic females.[1]

In summary, genital ambiguity may be attributed to

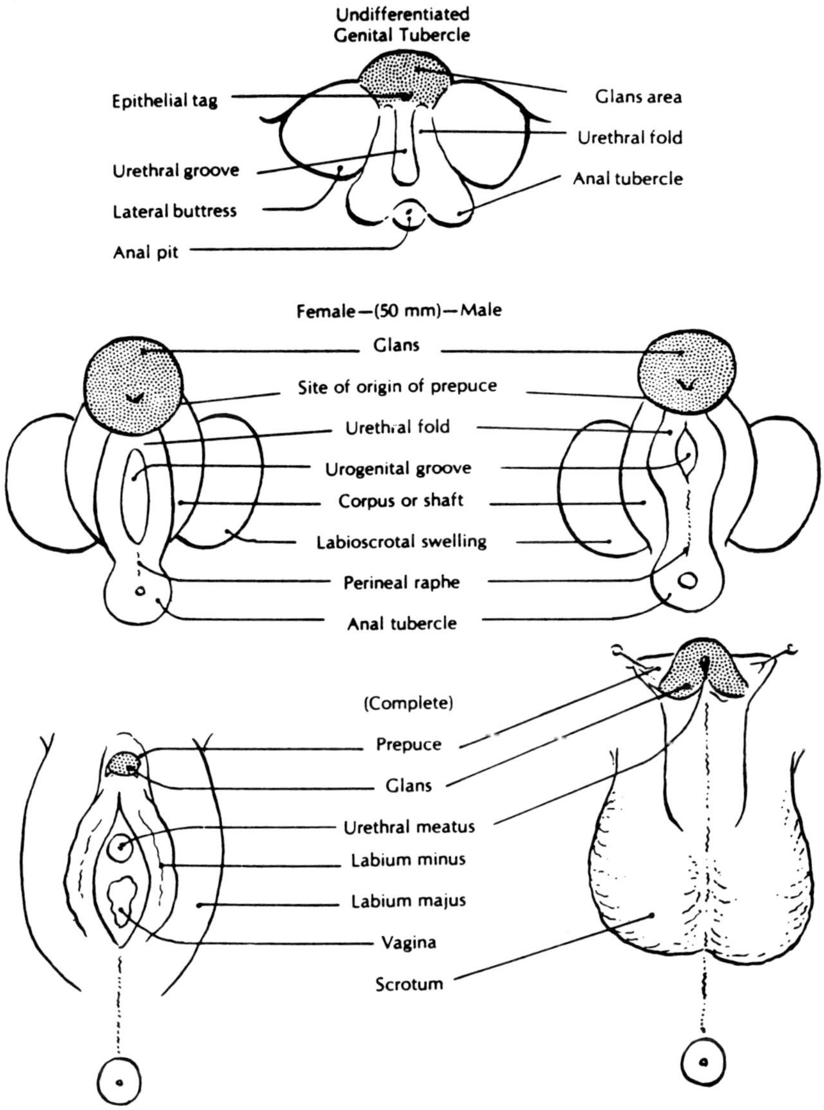

Figure 1–1 Normal external genital differentiation from bipotential primordia. From Perlmutter AD, Reitelman C. Surgical management of intersexuality. In Walsh PC, Retik, AB, Stamey TA, Vaughan ED Jr (eds), Campbell's Urology, 6th ed. Philadelphia: WB Saunders, 1992, pp 1951–1966. Used with permission.

incomplete virilization of a genetic male fetus or of a fetus with testicular tissue or partial virilization of a genetic female fetus. Delayed onset and decreased levels of fetal testosterone then will result in incomplete differentiation of the mesonephric duct derivatives and of the external genitalia. Delayed or incomplete stimulation of the external genital precursors results in variable phallic enlargement, persistence of fetal chordee, and variable fusion of the urogenital sinus, from a perineal cleft to an anterior urethra with a hypospadiac meatus. If the testis (testes) is (are) abnormal or dysgenetic, MIS may be diminished or absent, with decreased or absent inhibition of paramesonephric (müllerian) derivatives. For genetic females there is no MIS production because there is no testicular tissue, so the internal genital ducts will persist and differentiate regardless of the degree of external virilization.

Chromosomal Causes of Intersex

The most commonly encountered chromosomal defect causing genital ambiguity is a mosaic, 45,X/46,XY, known as *mixed gonadal dysgenesis* (MGD). The most typical gonadal findings are a testis on one side, usually intra-abdominal, and a streak gonad on the other. The testis and streak are or rapidly become dysgenetic and prone to become malignant; early gonadectomy for the streak and the intra-abdominal testis is advised. Paramesonephric structures are present—fallopian tubes, uterus, and cervix or, on the side of the streak, a fallopian tube and hemiuterus; on the side of the testis there may be variable development of mesonephric structures. The external genitalia are ambiguous to a varying degree; a urogenital sinus opening or an identifiable vaginal opening is generally apparent, and phallic size varies from mild clitorimegaly to, occasionally, a near-normal-sized, hypospadiac penis. The single testis in some cases is in the hemiscrotum. Testosterone and MIS in mixed gonadal dysgenesis appear to be inadequate to virilize the external genitalia fully and to cause complete müllerian regression. Delay in onset in the action of these hormones may also play a role.

Most of these children are destined to possess short stature as adults, and most are assigned a female gender, although successful hypospadias reconstructions with excision of discordant müllerian structures have been done.

Bilateral gonadal dysgenesis with similar genital findings can occur in the absence of mosaicism, with an apparently normal 46,XY karyotype; the pathophysiology is not yet understood.

True hermaphroditism is defined as genital ambiguity in the presence of both ovarian and testicular tissue. The gonadal tissue may be distributed in a variety of ways: the lateral type with a testis on one side and an ovary on the other, the unilateral type with an ovotestis on one side and an ovary or testis on the other, and the bilateral type with an ovotestis on each side. In most cases, a hemiuterus or uterus is present because the internal genital ducts tend to develop concordant with the ipsilateral gonadal tissue (i.e., a vas deferens on the side of a testis and fallopian tube on the side of an ovary).

Eighty percent of true hermaphrodites have a 46,XX karyotype in which *SRY* has not been detected, so the explanation for development of this syndrome is not yet understood[1]; the remainder demonstrate a variety of mosaic patterns. On physical examination, gonadal tissue may be palpable in one or both groins or labioscrotal folds. The degree of virilization—phallic size and urogenital sinus fusion—is variable and may be quite marked; both male and female gender assignments have been made. Fertility in true hermaphrodites, although unusual, has been reported in both female and male roles.

Androgen-Related Causes of Intersex

Genetic males with intersex (male pseudohermaphroditism) may have deficient testosterone biosynthesis or defective androgen action, the latter resulting from an androgen receptor defect or from a 5α-reductase deficiency. The biosynthesis of testosterone from cholesterol requires five enzymes, and a deficiency of any of these in an autosomal recessive disorder will result in androgen insufficiency and attendant external genital ambiguity; MIS is present and normal suppression of paramesonephric development occurs.

Defective androgen action from an androgen receptor defect results in partial or complete loss of response to testosterone and DHT. When complete, the condition is known as *testis feminizing syndrome,* which involves a morphologically normal female appearance but no paramesonephros-derived structures because of normal MIS action. Complete testicular feminization is not an intersex state because there is no phenotypic ambiguity. With partial testicular feminization, such as in Reifenstein's syndrome, varying degrees of virilization are present, and sex assignment should be based on the severity of the ambiguity and the reconstructive and functional genital potential.

A 5α-reductase deficiency is associated with pseudovaginal perineoscrotal hypospadias, in which deficiency in local DHT results in incomplete virilization of the external genital structures.

Females With Excessive Androgen Activity

Genetic female fetuses with excessive endogenous or exogenous androgen will demonstrate ambiguous genitalia (female pseudohermaphroditism); virilization from exogenous sources of fetal androgen is now rarely encountered. The most common cause of genital ambiguity in genetic females is the syndrome of congenital adrenal hyperplasia (CAH), present in more than one half of all infants with genital ambiguity. Girls with CAH have a 46,XX karyotype but a deficiency in one of several enzymes required for cortisol biosynthesis. Consequently, corticotropin production is elevated, resulting in adrenocortical hyperplasia and increased production of cortisol precursors with androgenic action. The degree of virilization varies from minimal clitorimegaly with a normal or minimally foreshortened vestibule to a completely developed but empty scrotum and a normal male phallus enclosing a normal anterior urethra. Despite the degree of virilization, normal ovaries, tubes, uterus, and upper vagina are always present (Fig. 1–2).

With lesser degrees of virilization, the lower vagina, which develops from the urogenital sinus, is variably narrowed, particularly at its entrance into the urogenital sinus. Whether or not the vaginal orifice is visible on examination, it terminates distal to the external urinary sphincter zone. In severely virilized cases, with urethralization of the urogenital sinus into a phallic urethra, the distal vagina is strikingly hypoplastic and enters the urogenital sinus ("posterior urethra") intra- or suprasphincterically (see Fig. 1–2). The suprasphincteric vaginal orifice terminates in the middle of a verumontanum-like structure; with this severe virilization, prostatic tissue, which also derives from the urogenital sinus, has been identified. Depending on the particular enzyme defect, the specific clinical manifestations will vary; these are described in detail elsewhere.[2] The particular enzyme defects in CAH are 21-hydroxylase, 11-hydroxylase, or 3β-OL deficiency; 21-hydroxylase deficiency is the cause in more than 90% of cases. There are two forms of 21-hydroxylase deficiency: mild and severe. The mild form has a reduced enzyme activity; some cortisol synthesis is

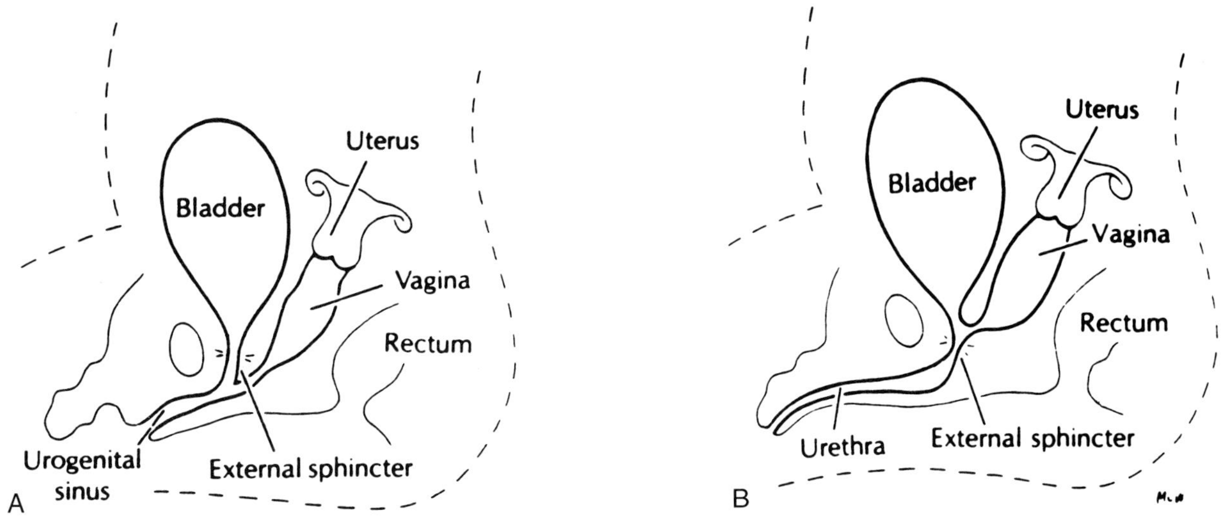

Figure 1–2 Diagram of anatomic variations in the urogenital anatomy of genetic females with congenital adrenal hyperplasia (CAH). Note presence of normally developed paramesonephric duct derivatives (fallopian tubes, uterus, upper vagina), regardless of severity of virilization. *A*, Typical form of CAH from 21-hydroxylase deficiency. *B*, Severe virilization with salt-losing form of CAH and suprasphincteric entry of vagina into posterior urethra at location of verumontanum. From Perlmutter AD, Reitelman C. Surgical management of intersexuality. In Walsh PC, Retik AB, Stamey TA, Vaughn ED Jr (eds), Campbell's Urology, 6th ed. Philadelphia: WB Saunders, 1992, pp 1951–1966. Used with permission.

present. The severe form, with its greater degrees of cortisol and aldosterone deficiency, is associated with greater virilization and salt wasting. Untreated within the first 1 to 2 weeks after birth, signs and symptoms of adrenal insufficiency may appear: anorexia, vomiting, dehydration, and finally vascular collapse. These symptoms, although not dissimilar to those of pyloric stenosis, tend to appear 2 to 3 weeks earlier.

The 11β-hydroxylase deficiency is associated with salt and water retention, which can result in hypertension. The 3β-OL deficiency is rare and has had a high neonatal mortality rate, but recent improvements in early diagnosis and management have resulted in survivors who become candidates for genital reconstruction.

CLASSIFICATION

The long-standing classification of genital ambiguity remains widely accepted, with four broad categories listed as follows in order of relative frequency: female pseudohermaphroditism, mixed gonadal dysgenesis, male pseudohermaphroditism, and true hermaphroditism. These categories have been incorporated earlier in the prior discussion of abnormal sexual differentiation. In addition to this standard listing, genital anomalies can be encountered sporadically in association with a number of rare and unusual syndromes as part of groups of abnormal physical findings.

EVALUATION AND GENDER ASSIGNMENT

Genital ambiguity in the neonate presents the clinician with an urgent medical and social problem to be resolved with skill and sensitivity. In addition to the issues involved in establishing an appropriate, early gender assignment, immediate medical therapy for infants with CAH may be life saving. The psychological impact on the family with an affected infant requires recognition and proper support. When confronted by a newborn with abnormal, ambiguous, or discordant genitals, it is critical to avoid guessing about or making a tentative sex assignment. On the other hand, it is essential to begin a thorough evaluation without delay. As mentioned, the parents should immediately be told, as kindly as possible, that the external sexual organs are incompletely developed or formed and that additional testing is necessary to establish the infant's sex and to determine the direction for future development. Dealing with these complex issues usually requires an experienced team, which should include at least some of the following professionals: a pediatrician, neonatologist, or pediatric endocrinologist or a combination; a pediatric reconstructive surgeon (i.e., urologist or surgeon); and a pediatric psychiatrist, psychologist, or social worker.

A family history is essential to rule out unexplained deaths among siblings and close relatives and to reveal family members with infertility, amenorrhea, genital anomalies, and the like. Maternal illness or exposure to androgenic substances in early pregnancy should be ruled out.

Physical Examination

A small phallus, urogenital sinus, and rugated labioscrotal folds with or without genital skin pigmentation are clearly hallmarks of genital ambiguity. However, findings are not always "typical." A hypospadiac phallus and bifid-appearing scrotum or even a fully formed penis may be present, with the only clue in a genetic female to suggest ambiguity being an empty scrotum with no palpable gonads.

When gonads are palpable, symmetric findings (i.e., gonads similarly above or below the inguinal ring) suggest a hormonal defect. When the gonadal findings are asymmetric (i.e., a palpable inguinal or scrotal gonad on one side), the cause may be genetic, such as mixed gonadal dysgenesis. A gonad palpated beyond the inguinal canal suggests the presence of testicular tissue, such as a testis or ovotestis, because an ovary does not descend below the inguinal ring.

A palpable infantile uterus and cervix on rectal examination are consistent with CAH, MGD, or true hermaphroditism. These structures are more readily palpable because of stimulation from fetal estrogen in response to placental human chorionic gonadotropin (hCG).

Imaging Studies

Pelvic and perineal ultrasonography in the hands of an expert pediatric imager should demonstrate a cervix and uterus. To define the local anatomy further, and the site of confluence of the vagina and urogenital sinus (low vs. high insertion), a urogenital sinogram should be obtained. Contrast material instilled through a blunt-nosed syringe pressed against the urogenital sinus or a catheter placed just within it should outline the urethra, bladder base, and vagina, even when the vaginal connection is narrow (Fig. 1–3). A voiding cystourethrogram will sometimes document the vaginal confluence but is less reliable than a retrograde sinogram at filling a vagina with a narrow opening. At times, a sinogram will not fill a suprasphincteric vagina which has a tiny opening into it. In this setting, cystourethroscopy and contrast study after cannulation of the vaginal opening with a ureteral catheter may be needed to define the anatomy further.

Laboratory Studies

Of the various conditions underlying genital ambiguity, CAH is the one that, left untreated, can be life threatening from adrenal insufficiency. Blood measurements of electrolytes, 17-hydroxyprogesterone, and karyotype are essential. In addition, measurement of levels of gonadotropins, testosterone, and DHT before and after hCG stimulation and MIS can be useful, and genomic deoxyribonucleic acid–messenger ribonucleic acid probes for androgen receptor and 5α-reductase and other molecular studies are becoming available.[1] Elevation of serum 17-hydroxyprogesterone is diagnostic for female pseudohermaphrodites with CAH, and appropriate glucocorticoid and mineralocorticoid replacement should be initiated by the pediatric endocrinologist. Endocrine management is a lifelong commitment.

Endoscopic Studies

Endoscopic examination of the urogenital sinus, posterior urethra, and vagina can help to sort out the anatomic details and to plan future reconstruction, particularly in cases of ambiguity with more severe degrees of virilization. When the vaginal opening is too small to accept a pediatric endoscope, or if the vaginal cavity cannot be assessed adequately, one should place a ureteral catheter and obtain a contrast vaginogram.

Laparoscopy is helpful in defining the gonadal and internal ductal patterns in cases involving true hermaphroditism or mosaicism, as an alternative to laparotomy when definitive gonadectomy and hysterectomy are not planned simultaneously. Neither urethroscopy nor laparoscopy are needed for evaluating typical CAH because the findings are predictable; however, with severe virilization, urethroscopy is helpful in assessing a high vaginal insertion and the degree of lower vaginal development when planning the definitive reconstruction strategy and for placing a Fogarty balloon catheter into the vagina to assist with the dissection during reconstruction.

GENDER ASSIGNMENT

Although most intersex patients will be infertile on the basis of the underlying cause of the condition, female pseudohermaphrodites—typically those with CAH—are potentially fertile regardless of the severity of their virilization, and these patients should always be reared as females. For male pseudohermaphrodites and infants with a genetic cause of intersex such as MGD and true hermaphroditism, the decisions are more difficult. As a guiding principle, functional anatomic potential should be the principal factor in the choice of sex; an inadequate phallus in male pseudohermaphroditism is unsuitable for a male assignment. Unfortunately, phallic inadequacy is often hard to establish with certainty because the responsiveness of the external genitalia to exogenous testosterone, which can be used in this setting as a diagnostic trial before gender assignment, is influenced by the cause of the ambiguity; patients with partial androgen resistance will respond less effectively than those with hypogonadism and normal androgen receptor activity.

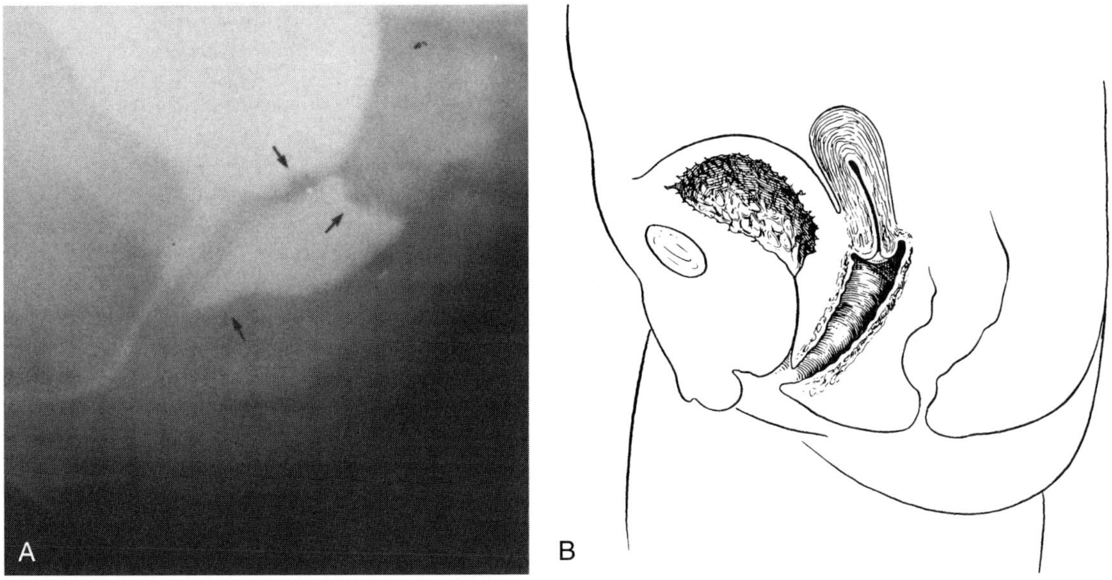

Figure 1–3 Urogenital sinogram. Infant girl with typical form of congenital adrenal hyperplasia (CAH). *A, Arrows* depict interureteric ridge, cervix, and narrow distal vagina. *B,* Line drawing to show relationship among urethra, narrow distal vagina, and urogenital sinus. From Perlmutter AD. Management of intersexuality. In Harrison JH, Gittes RF, Perlmutter AD, et al (eds), Campbell's Urology, 4th ed. Philadelphia: WB Saunders, 1979, pp 1535–1548.

At term the mean phallic length is 3.5 ± 0.5 and the mean width is 1.1 ± 0.2 cm. Data for normal ranges of sizes as related to degrees of fetal maturity have been established and are available on a useful nomogram.[3] A phallic length of 2 cm or less at term is cause for concern about functional potential; some use a length of 1.5 cm or less and a width of 0.7 cm as minimums.[1] Standardized measurement of phallic length involves stretching the phallus and measuring the dorsal shaft from the bony penopubic angle to the tip of the glans. With severe chordee, this measurement becomes difficult and inaccurate. Use of a flexible paper or cloth tape measure is helpful in this setting.

The criteria for the use of exogenous androgen as a diagnostic measure before gender assignment are not well established. The decision to do so generally is based on a diagnosis of male pseudohermaphroditism, and often needs to be initiated before the results of other studies are available. Because the genital response to testosterone in the absence of androgen resistance can be dramatic, testosterone administration is often used in the presence of an initially inadequate phallus[4, 5]; this may postpone sex assignment for up to 2 months. The dose is 25 mg of intramuscular (depository) testosterone enanthate or cypionate in oil, repeated in 1 month if necessary. For some responders, evidence of a change is apparent within 2 weeks and by 1 month in others. The first changes are genital hyperemia, most marked of the glans, and a palpable thickening of the corpora, even before a measurable increase in length has occurred. If an adequate response to androgen occurs, a male assignment can be made and a third monthly testosterone dose administered if necessary to enhance penile size further. Then, in preparation for hypospadias repair, an additional two or three monthly doses of androgen can be administered if needed near the end of the first year of life without concern for advancement of bone age.

In cases of mixed gonadal dysgenesis, a female sex assignment is preferable because of the need for a surgically induced agonadal state (to treat a dysgenetic testis and streak), the probability of short adult stature, and the presence of a reconstructible vagina. However, the degree of virilization is quite variable, and a reasonably sized, hypospadiac penis and a descended, solitary testis may be present. Some of these children have been raised effectively as males, especially when diagnosis has been delayed. At some point in the reconstructive process discordant structures should be excised; specifically, the patient should undergo abdominal hysterosalpingectomy, subtotal vaginectomy, and gonadectomies. If a small periurethral vaginal remnant causes later difficulties, such as entrapment of infected urine or calculus formation, endoscopic fulguration of the lining can successfully obliterate the lumen.[6] A descended, scrotal testis may be less likely than an intra-abdominal testis to undergo malignant change, and in this setting some surgeons leave the scrotal testis in place and monitor the patient, although this is controversial.

The external genital findings in true hermaphroditism, as in MGD, have a spectrum of virilization ranging from minimal to marked and most typically a uterus and fallopian tube or tubes. Sex assignment may be based on functional and reconstructive criteria. Here, too, discordant tissues should be removed. Because the gonadal tissue in true hermaphroditism is not dysgenetic and not at high risk for malignant transformation, the gonad or the portion of the gonadal tissue from an ovotestis or ovotestes compatible with the sex of assignment should be retained.

SURGICAL MANAGEMENT

The prototype of feminizing reconstructive surgery for genital ambiguity is that for CAH, and the techniques described are applicable to all causes of ambiguous genitalia. Masculinizing reconstructive surgery for genital ambiguity falls under repair of severe hypospadias and is not included in this chapter.

Timing of Surgery

Among those with a major commitment to correction of genital ambiguity, there is no agreement regarding the optimal timing for feminizing genitoplasty, although there is a general consensus that "early" surgery is desirable to preclude the child's awareness of being different and to reduce the family's anxiety and allow members to come to closure regarding their child's phenotype, which reinforces acceptance of gender assignment and role. This translates into surgery before 3 years of age, when sexual awareness is increasing.[7]

The goals of feminizing genitoplasty are both functional and cosmetic. For each time period, there are both advantages and disadvantages to be considered. Some investigators favor surgery in the neonatal period to reduce parental stress. In addition to the technical challenges of a precise and meticulous procedure at that time with its greater risks of vaginal injury or stricture formation, a neonatal clitoroplasty will need to be done before taking surgical advantage of a degree of physiologic regression of clitorimegaly, which gradually occurs in the first 4 to 6 weeks after initiating replacement glucocorticoid therapy. For surgery planned late in the first year of life, physiologic obesity, when marked, can compromise the cosmetic details of the reconstruction by interfering with determination of spatial relationships. However, when anatomic conditions are appropriate in the latter months of the first year, there is no contraindication to performing the reconstruction.

My preference, and that of some others, is to plan the surgery for about 1 year of age and by 15 to 18 months if the earlier time is not feasible. At these age ranges conscious sexual awareness has not evolved, and technical considerations are not generally an issue. In selected circumstances, namely milder degrees of virilization and marked parental anxiety, the reconstruction can be completed at about 6 months of age.

Planning Surgical Strategy

The goals of feminizing genitoplasty involve establishing a normal-appearing vestibule with a vaginal opening adequate for later sexual intercourse and a cosmetically acceptable clitoris with preserved erotic sensation. It is my preference to complete the reconstruction in one encounter; planning and accomplishing the entire reconstruction as a single procedure is the best assurance of an acceptable cosmetic as well as functional outcome, namely an appropriately sized vulva for age, with the glans clitoris positioned in proper relationship to the vagina and the remainder of the vestibule.

In the older literature, proponents of delaying vaginoplasty until after puberty emphasized that the procedure is technically easier after pubertal genital growth has occurred, when postoperative introital stenosis is less likely to occur and, if present, easy to treat; therefore, they advised that only the clitoroplasty should be done in infancy. A contrary argument is that the resultant initial lack of complete surgical feminization with this staged approach may create later body image problems and greater difficulty in establishing the appropriate positioning of the vestibular structures at the initial procedure. Contemporary, delicate surgical instruments and precise surgical technique help to make early, complete reconstruction feasible.

Endocrine management of patients with CAH includes communication from the treating endocrinologist that the patient's CAH is being regulated optimally, plus instructions for proper glucocorticoid and mineralocorticoid dosing intraoperatively and immediately postoperatively.

Surgical Techniques

Feminizing genitoplasty involves three steps: vulvoplasty, flap vaginoplasty, and clitoroplasty. The first step involves exteriorization of the urogenital sinus, which will be the basis of the future vulva. The next step is to exteriorize the vagina and to create an adequate lumen by interposing a perineal skin flap into an incision in the narrow, urogenital sinus–derived lower vagina. If vaginoplasty for any reason is being postponed, such as for male pseudohermaphroditism without a vagina present, completion of the initial vulvoplasty will create a cosmetically acceptable superficial vulva into which a vaginal substitution can be placed at later surgery. The third and final step in the reconstruction is reduction and recession of the enlarged clitoris with preservation of the neurovascular supply to the glans clitoris and completion of the vulvoplasty.

Vulvoplasty and Flap Vaginoplasty

Place the patient supine, with thighs at greater than 90 degrees of flexion and mildly abducted. Be careful not to flex the thighs extremely because this can stretch the sciatic nerves or cauda equina. In children, padded calf and foot holders can secure the lower extremities while avoiding pressure points. In infants, the lower extremities can be suspended straight legged from a high anesthesia screen mounted at the bottom end of the operating table, using longitudinal adhesive strips along the legs and thighs.

Using a skin marker, outline a broad-based, rounded skin flap with the apex directed upward (ventrally) (Fig. 1–4). The base should be as broad as possible, ending at the level of and just within the palpable ischial tuberosities. Avoid creating too long a flap; in infants a 2½-cm length is generally sufficient to lay the flap easily into an incision in the narrow lower vaginal segment; the flap is elastic and will hinge over the perineal body when inlaid. From the apex of the flap, outline a midline incision ventrally to the opening of the urogenital sinus. In infrequent instances of minimal urogenital sinus fusion and a visible but slightly narrow vaginal opening, a flap is not needed; here a simple, short, midline episiotomy with trimming of any underlying fibrodysplastic tissue is sufficient, followed by a Heineke-Mikulicz type of approximation to complete the vulval reconstruction.

The initial incision is to begin to develop the perineum-based flap. A thick layer of subcutaneous fat should be preserved, particularly at the base of the flap, to ensure an adequate blood supply. A traction suture or sutures near the flap apex, with a hemostat attached, will keep the flap folded inferiorly, out of the way during the continuing dissection.

With a Robnel or similar catheter in the urogenital sinus, make the midline incision using a fine-tipped electrocautery for dissection to enhance hemostasis and carry through all tissue layers to the catheter. Depending on the degree of virilization, a layer of corpus spongiosum of varied thickness surrounds the urogenital sinus, anatomically equivalent to the male bulbous urethra. This portion of the procedure tends to be bloody; hemostasis here can be accomplished with fine electrocoagulation and delicate figure-eight hemostatic sutures as necessary along the cut edge of the spongiosum, incorporating a bit of urothelium. This portion of the dissection effectively defines the future vulva; the urothelium of the roof of the urogenital sinus will become the midline, subclitoral, mucosal strip of the vulva, and its length can be shortened if necessary during the clitoroplasty. During this midline dissection, traction sutures on the edges of the genital skin, corpus spongiosum, and urothelium as necessary can be clamped and draped over bilaterally placed drape clamps, which act as pulleys to provide lateral traction for exposure and tissue stability (see Fig. 1–4).

The dissection to this point generally exposes the urethral meatus and the adjacent, narrow vaginal opening surrounded by a rim of hypoplastic hymen, with the more severe degrees of virilization, the vaginal opening may be somewhat more proximal, or "hypospadiac," requiring a further midline cutback of the urogenital sinus to exteriorize it.

The next step in preparation for the inlay of the perineal skin flap is to expose the narrow segment of lower vagina. With a probe, hemostat, or small catheter through the vaginal opening, dissect free the dorsal vaginal wall. To minimize blood loss, keep the dissection close to the midline, incising and debriding as necessary any perivaginal fibrous tissue and gently wiping and bluntly dissecting the perivaginal musculature cephalad to expose and mobilize the dorsal vaginal wall further until a normal vaginal barrel is encountered. Then incise the vagina in the dorsal midline through the hypoplastic, narrow area until the more proximal, normal-sized vaginal lumen is reached. Symmetric traction sutures can be placed in the cut vaginal wall during this process to stabilize and help exteriorize this area.

The midline perineal U flap can now be laid into this vaginal split to augment the circumference of the vaginal barrel and begin the reconstruction, using fine absorbable suture such as 5-0 chromic, Dexon, or Vicryl. At the outer vaginal rim, the base of the flap can be sutured to adjacent perineal skin. If the adjacent skin consists of redundant labioscrotal tissue, then this portion of the closure should be left open until the clitoroplasty is completed and the fashioning of the minor labial folds is being done. The original "episiotomy" incision, which exteriorized the urogenital sinus and converted the roof of the urogenital sinus (bulbous urethra) into the future midline mucosal strip, also created an incision on each side between the mucosal strip and the adjacent labioscrotal skin. The labioscrotal skin should be further mobilized, and these bilateral incisions should be extended to the base of the phallus to create a bed to place the future labia minora. At that time, any redundancy of the labia majora can be trimmed down during the final portion of the reconstruction.

For the most severely virilized infants with a suprasphincteric vaginal opening, the technique for exposure is somewhat different and is only summarized here; the details of reconstruction are beyond the intent of this chapter. These patients should be referred to a children's medical center with experience in treating this most severe deformity.[1, 8] In this scenario, the entire vagina tends to be short, and the distal vagina is unusually small and hypoplastic, with a very narrow, high, fistula-like insertion into the suprasphincteric posterior urethra. A Fogarty balloon catheter should be placed endoscopically to aid in the identification and dissection of the lower vaginal attachment to the urethra. The vagina must be detached and separated from the posterior urethra, and mobilized sufficiently to pull down toward the perineum where local flaps can be attached.

Clitoroplasty

The objectives of clitoroplasty are to achieve a more feminine position and appearance of the enlarged clitoris

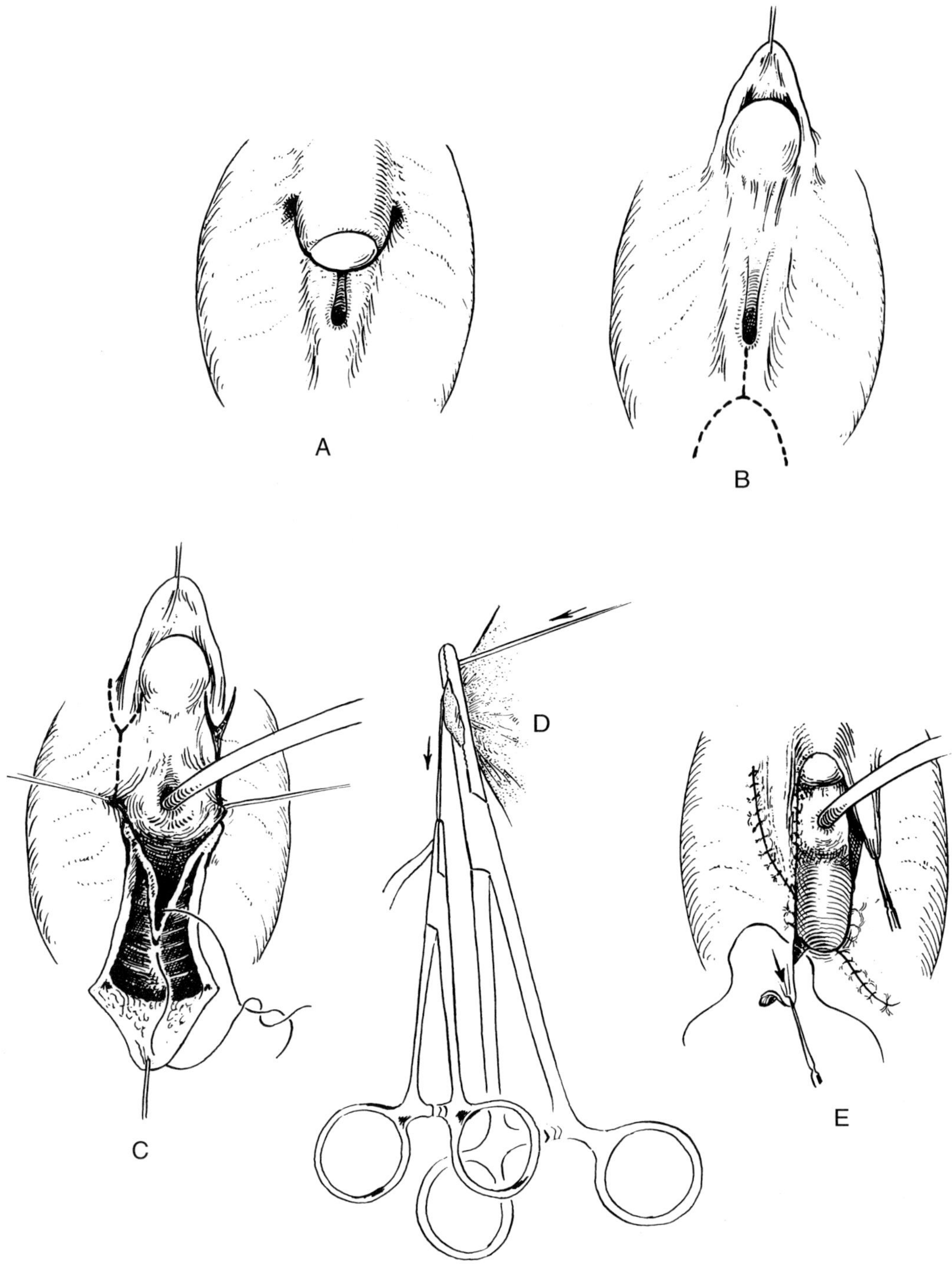

Figure 1–4 Technique of flap vaginoplasty. *A,* Preoperative appearance of genitalia. *B,* Outline of skin incisions to open midline planes and to develop short, broad-based U flap. C, Posterior wall of congenitally narrow lower vagina has been exposed. At times, it is surrounded by corpus spongiosum that, after division, requires hemostasis by cautery or by oversewing with fine catgut suture. A midline incision has been made in the narrow vaginal segment, which should be carried into the wider, thicker müllerian-derived portion of the vagina, after blunt dissection and exposure of the posterior wall in the midline. This diagram also shows the incision around the ventral preputial folds, which will be drawn posteriorly to create labia minora. *D,* A heavy clamp on the perineal drape, lateral to the genitalia, is shown as a hook over which sutures can be placed to provide lateral traction for symmetric exposure during dissection and repair. *E,* Details of labial advancement and vaginal flap suturing. If labioscrotal skin is redundant, this tissue can be pulled downward as diagrammed and trimmed if necessary to flatten the rugae and to give the labia majora a more appropriate appearance. From Perlmutter AD, Reitelman C. Surgical management of intersexuality. In Walsh PC, Retik AB, Stamey TA, Vaughan ED Jr (eds), Campbell's Urology, 6th ed. Philadelphia: WB Saunders, 1992, pp 1951–1966. Used with permission.

and to preserve clitoral sensation. Clitoroplasty involves reducing the size of the clitoris and relocating the glans and shaft. There are several options for clitoroplasty, depending on the size of the phallus and the surgeon's preference. Clitoridectomy, once a preferred solution to severe clitorimegaly in the early years of developing reconstructive approaches, is no longer an acceptable option because of the loss of clitoral sensation.

Recession of the clitoris alone is suitable only for the mildly enlarged phallus that does not lengthen and bulge excessively with erection (Fig. 1–5). In most instances, recession of the shaft alone by concealing it under the mons pubis is insufficient and should be combined with a reduction glans plasty (Fig. 1–6), with or without a corporal plication (Fig. 1–7).

The choice of technique for clitoroplasty should not be decided until the degree of regression in clitoral size has been assessed after a few months of appropriate steroid replacement. For minimal clitoral hypertrophy, approximation of the mons pubis and upper labia majora over the clitoral shaft[9] is a simple solution (see Fig. 1–5). Unfortunately, in my experience, this procedure is applicable to very few patients. Multiple corporal plication[10] has been my preferred approach to reduce a mildly prominent clitoral shaft by limiting length, bulk, and bulging during erections (see Fig. 1–7). The plicating sutures limit phallic length and partially obliterate the corporal space, limiting erectile bulk. A moderately heavy nonabsorbable suture, such as a braided or monofilament 3-0 material, is suitable. Care should be taken to avoid the dorsal neurovascular bundles during placement; the knots should be placed ventrally. To prevent shaft protrusion, it also may be necessary to place a few sutures between the outer ventral shaft and the crura or proximal ventral shaft to maintain flexion. To expose the shaft initially, make a circumcising incision close to the glans and deglove the shaft (Fig. 1–8). Dissect the midline mucosa with its underlying fibrodysplastic plate of chordee cleanly off the ventral shaft, keeping it intact. During closure, this midline strip and plate can be shortened sufficiently to establish age-appropriate dimensions of the vulva.

For any of the approaches to clitoroplasty, a reduction in the size of the glans will likely be needed to complete the reconstruction (see Fig. 1–6). A variety of methods exist to accomplish this, and these may be combined as necessary. I have found excision of a ventral wedge to be the most useful way to narrow the glans. This also provides an epithelial edge and a raw bed when reattaching

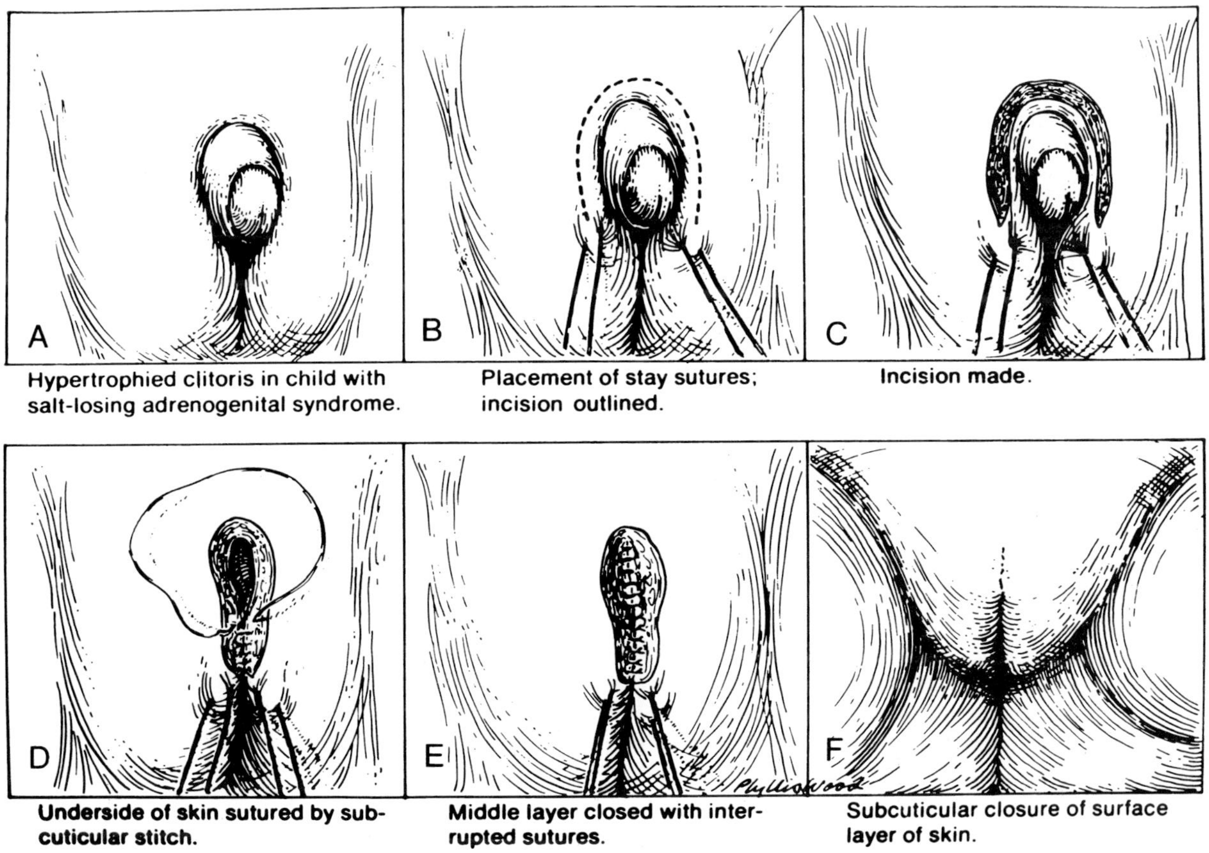

Figure 1–5 *A–F,* Technique for simple clitoral recession (concealment). From Ansell JS, Rajfer J. A new and simplified approach to concealing the hypertrophied clitoris. J Pediatr Surg 16:681, 1981. Used with permission.

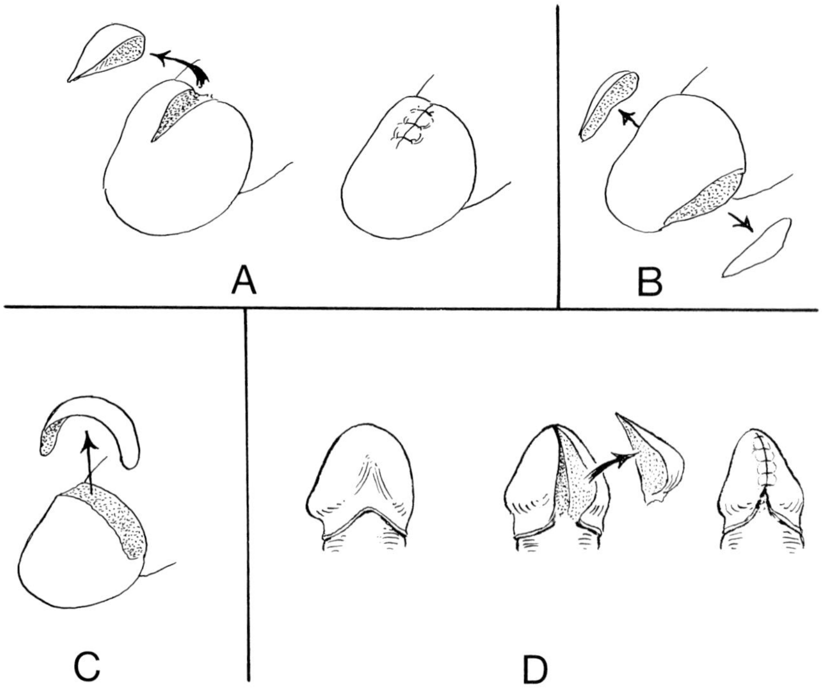

Figure 1–6 *A–D,* Options for glans reduction. From Perlmutter AD, Reitelman C. Surgical management of intersexuality. In Walsh PC, Retik AB, Stamey TA, Vaughan ED Jr (eds), Campbell's Urology, 6th ed. Philadelphia: WB Saunders, 1992, pp 1951–1966. Used with permission.

the ventral margin of the glans to the midline mucosal strip after partial closure of the glans. To shorten the apparent glans length, the coronal margin and adjacent coronal epithelial skirt can be shaved away, leaving spongy glans tissue onto which the prepuce can be reattached, establishing a cosmetically acceptable clitoral hood to partially conceal the now diminished glans.

For moderate to marked phallic enlargement with substantial corporal bulk and length, corporal reduction by subtunical excision of a segment of the erectile bodies[11] has been my procedure of choice, using a modification of the published technique (Fig. 1–9). The advantage of segmental, subtunical resection of the erectile bodies over a full-thickness en bloc resection of a segment of the phallic shaft is the protection of the dorsal neurovascular bundle and the glans, which preservation of the dorsal tunica albuginea affords. After completing the vaginoplasty, place a traction suture in the glans clitoris, and deglove the clitoral shaft. The dissection under the midline mucosa and chordee should extend proximally sufficient to ensure that resection of the erectile bodies will remove all excessive phallic length.

Incise along the midlateral axis of the phallus on each side through the tunica albuginea to the erectile

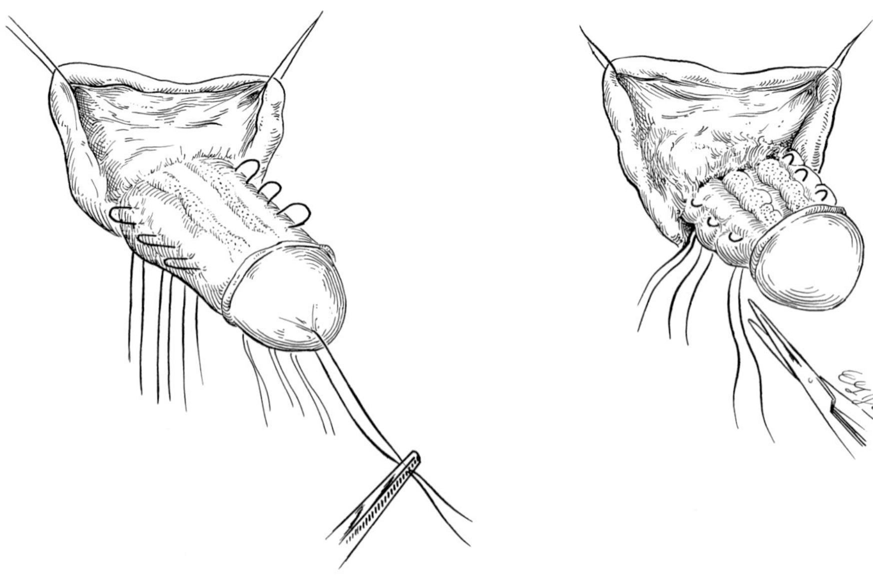

Figure 1–7 Corporal plication, as described by Stefan. From Perlmutter AD, Reitelman C. Surgical management of intersexuality. In Walsh PC, Retik AB, Stamey, TA, Vaughan ED Jr (eds), Campbell's Urology, 6th ed. Philadelphia: WB Saunders, 1992, pp 1951–1966. Used with permission.

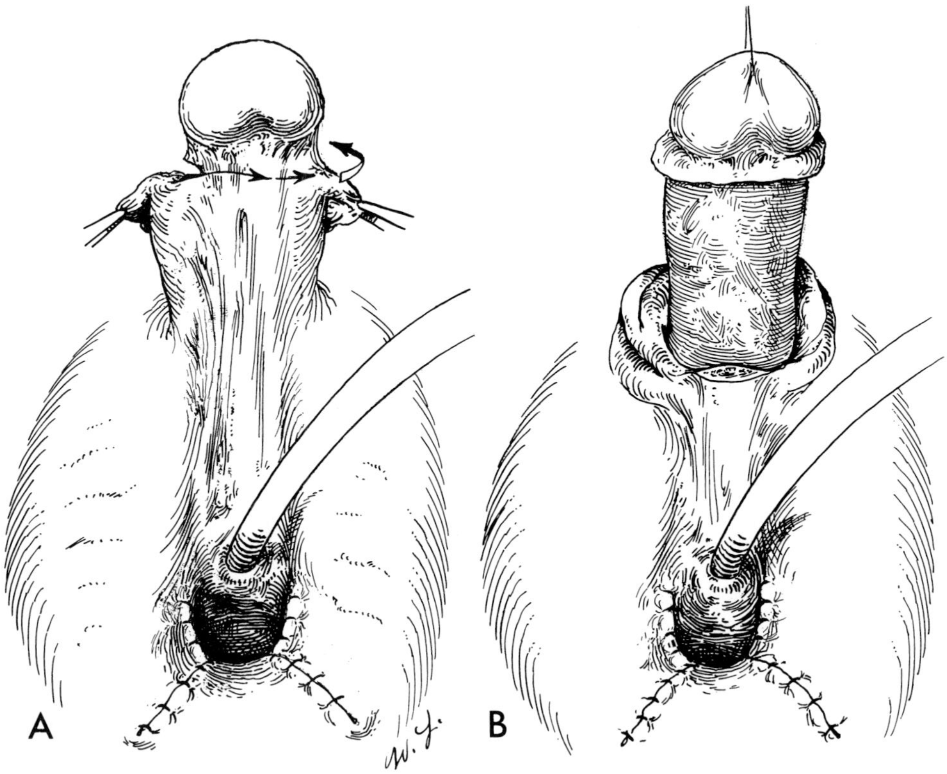

Figure 1–8 *A* and *B*, Degloving of phallus.

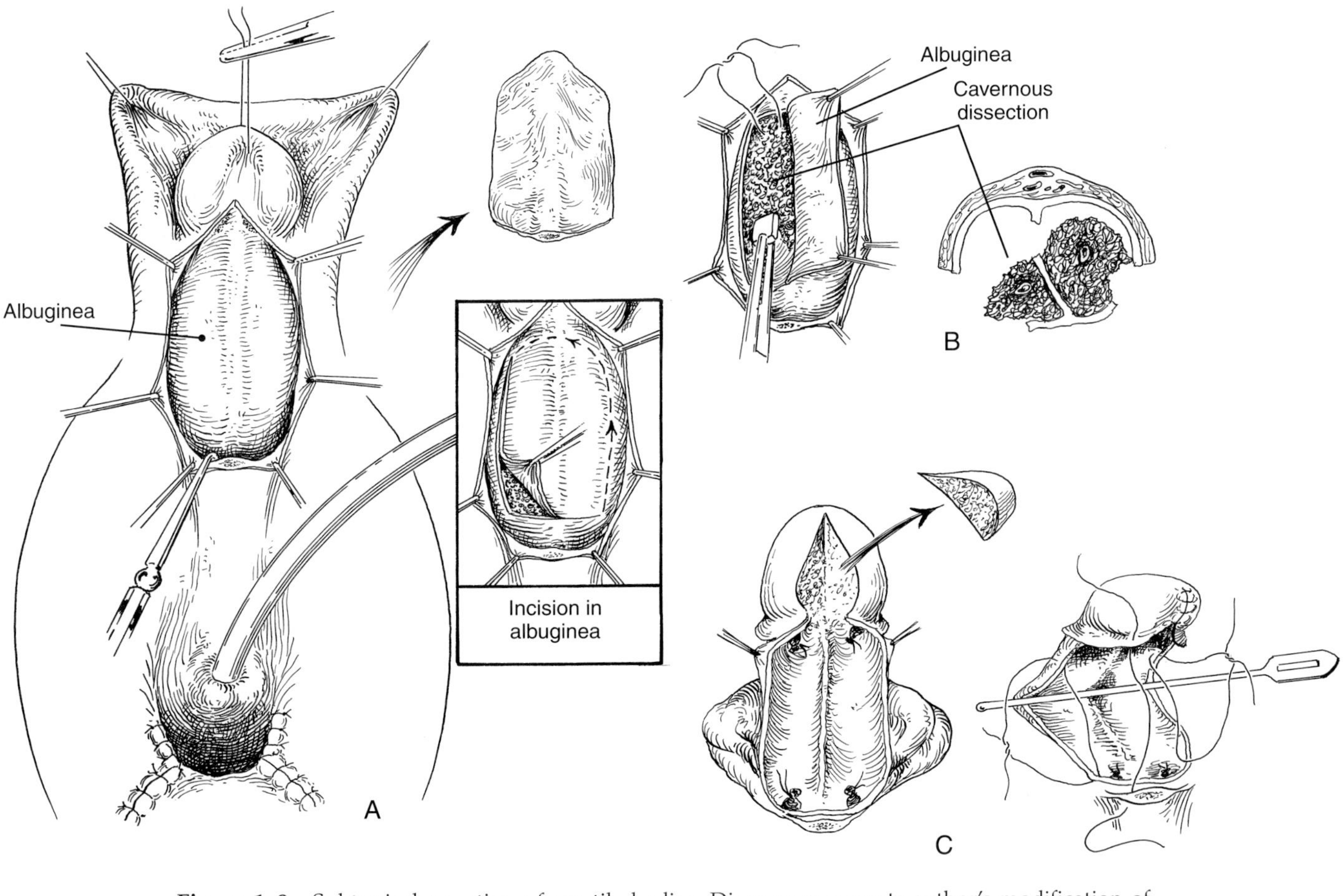

Figure 1–9 Subtunical resection of erectile bodies. Diagram represents author's modification of the technique of Kogan and colleagues (see text). From Perlmutter AD, Reitelman C. Surgical management of intersexuality. In Walsh PC, Retik AB, Stamey TA, Vaughan ED Jr (eds), Campbell's Urology, 6th ed. Philadelphia: WB Saunders, 1992, pp 1951–1966. Used with permission.

bodies and connect these two incisions ventrally at the phallic base and distally at the base of the glans. My modification includes removal of the two erectile bodies in continuity with the attached septum. With meticulous technique using miniature wipes and fine dissection, separate the erectile bodies from their sheath of dorsal and lateral tunica albuginea. The fine dorsal strands and vessels attaching the septum to the tunica albuginea are easily identified during this dissection and can be obliterated precisely by point coagulation, using a low-heat eye cautery or fine-needle electrocautery with a low current setting.

Place a circumferential, occluding, absorbable suture at the proximal and distal ends of each erectile body to control central arterial and venous bleeding. The proximal sutures can pass through the intact ventral tunica albuginea to minimize their slipping or cutting through the soft, erectile bodies. If the inner surface of the dorsal tunica albuginea also is included in the sutures, take care to include as little tunica as possible to avoid accidentally incorporating the neurovascular bundles, which are on the outer surface of the tunica albuginea.

Reconstruction involves shortening the midline mucosal strip and its underlying plate of fibrous spongiosum to a length judged to be appropriate for age. Position this plate and anchor it with absorbable sutures to the underlying proximal, intact tunica albuginea to stabilize the length and position of the plate. Then attach the glans to the mucosal strip and plate, suturing the epithelial edge of the ventral glans to the leading edge of the cut mucosal strip and plate. Hinge the tunica albuginea on itself, and, once the glans has been secured, suture the lateral margins together on each side to obliterate the dead space. If the folded envelope of the enucleated tunica albuginea is unusually long, then the suspensory ligament can be divided and a pocket dissected along the anterior pubic periosteum so that the envelope can be fitted neatly into this prepubic space and sutured laterally as necessary on each side to the periosteum. Perform any reduction and reconfiguration of the glans at this time before completing the closure.

To complete the reconstruction, first reconfigure the degloved, hooded prepuce and shaft skin to fashion an appropriately sized clitoral hood with lateral flaps to serve as labia minora. Make a dorsal slit in the midline of the redundant skin to develop two flaps. Leave sufficient dorsal skin intact to serve as a hood to partially cover the glans. The epithelial edges of the central V split can be rounded off before suturing them with fine, absorbable, interrupted sutures, such as 4-0 or 5-0 interrupted chromic catgut, to the epithelial edge of the reconfigured dorsal glans, taking care not to narrow the lateral flaps excessively, which could compromise their blood supply. To unfurl each flap as a V and advance them inferiorly as labia minora, it is generally necessary to make a counter incision laterally in the sulcus between the labia majora and the shaft skin (see Fig. 1–4).

To complete the repair, advance the lateral flap on each side inferiorly to the level of the vaginal barrel, interposing each into the space between the mucosal strip on each side and the labia minora created by the original "episiotomy," which had exteriorized the urogenital sinus.

At the conclusion of the repair, place a small Foley catheter into the bladder and a segment of a 20 or 22 French straight catheter wrapped with Vaseline gauze into the vagina as a stent to prevent hematoma formation postoperatively. A soft, bulky dressing should be taped over the perineum to minimize external swelling. The external dressing and vaginal stent should be removed in the first 24 hours and the urethral catheter in 2 or 3 days unless local tissue swelling is excessive; premature removal of the urethral catheter can cause maceration by urine of the healing suture lines. Once the catheter has been removed, start brief sitz baths and apply a topical conjugated estrogen cream to the vulva daily for 5 to 7 days for its temporary stimulating effect on the healing genital epithelium.

COMPLICATIONS

Short-term complications include hematoma formation, infection, and suture line separation. Problems from improper positioning at surgery have been described earlier. Most hematomas do not require drainage and can be monitored expectantly. Local infection is uncommon and rarely needs drainage. The most common suture line separation (1) involves the base of the perineal flap laterally, (2) is slight, and (3) readily heals secondarily with sitz baths and local hygiene. Rarely, the tip of one or both labia minora becomes detached in the early postoperative period. This not serious and should be disregarded for at least 6 months, after which it is easily reattached by making an incision in continuity along the underside of the labium through the opposing interface between the ipsilateral major labium and the mucosal strip and then suturing the adjacent medial and lateral edges. Although some surgeons perform periodic vaginal dilations in the early postoperative months, this is painful and traumatic unless done under anesthesia and is probably unnecessary; a tendency to early stricture formation in this setting suggests a technical problem at the original procedure. In any event, overdilation of the vaginal outlet should be avoided; this will tear the area of reconstruction and may result in more dense, iatrogenic stricture formation.

The major long-term complication has been vaginal stenosis, mainly at the level of the apex of the vaginal inlay flap. Between one third and two thirds of patients have required late revision, depending on the series.[12–16] Some of the patients in these earlier series had been managed by simple episiotomies or long, narrow-based perineal flap vaginoplasties. The problem of late, distal vaginal stenosis appears to be less common for patients who have had the more recent technique of repair using a relatively short, broad-based inlay flap with a rounded tip, but there is a paucity of long-term reviews to document this impression. Absent a rare catastrophe with an obliterative stricture, local vaginal stenosis should not interfere with menstruation; thus, repair of a rigid or narrow zone in the distal vagina is best handled after puberty and at a time when the patient is willing to perform subsequent self-dilatation if necessary after revision. Elevate the inlay perineal flap, and debride any underlying scar tissue beneath this flap and the dorsal aspect of the distal vagina until the pelvic outlet is soft and elastic. The dorsal vaginal wall can be dissected and separated from the surrounding tissues more proximally to provide exposure and mobility. If the vagina at this level is hypoplastic and somewhat narrow, incise it dorsally in the midline proximally until reaching the normal-caliber, elastic vagina. The debrided perineal flap should easily fit into this vaginal defect.

LONG-TERM RESULTS

The success of feminizing genitoplasty should be measured by the following outcome criteria: genital appearance, sexual responsiveness, sexual adequacy (i.e., a vagina adequate for sexual penetration without pain or discomfort), and, for those syndromes (CAH, some true hermaphrodites) compatible with fertility and pregnancy. Unfortunately, only a few long-term studies exist, none of which cover all of these matters in detail. Observations from the earlier era of clitoridectomy indicate that sexual response and orgasm are not necessarily lost in that setting, although erotic sensitivity may have been reduced.[16, 17, 18] With current, nerve-sparing clitoroplasty, glans innervation is likely to be adequate; measurement of pudendal evoked potentials intraoperatively by dorsal neurovascular bundle electrostimulation has documented preservation of electromyographic responses after phallic reduction.[19] Occasionally, late revision of the clitoroplasty is performed when there is excessive redundancy of overlying genital skin or when the glans reduction appears to be inadequate.

Postpubertal vaginal stenosis is more likely to occur in patients with the salt-losing form of CAH.[11] These patients have inherently more severe virilization and more marked lower (or distal) vaginal hypoplasia. In addition, patients with salt-losing CAH have a lower rate of satisfactory intercourse, and pregnancy is rare; in one series, 15 of 25 women with simple CAH had 25 pregnancies producing 20 normal children, whereas only 1 of 15 with the salt-losing form became pregnant.[14] A high incidence of cesarean section has been reported for CAH patients because of cephalopelvic disproportion, possibly from early epiphyseal closure or from an android pelvis.[20] In addition, cesarean section may be important to avoid disruption of a major genital reconstruction.

In conclusion, the overall management of infants and children with intersex is complex. Gender assignment and the associated family support generally require a team approach. Although early gender assignment is the goal, a hasty decision should be avoided until assessment is completed. A gender assignment that is acceptable to the family and supported by appropriate counseling should inevitably lead to appropriate family behavior and an unambiguous gender role and thus to normal gender identity by the growing child.

Contemporary techniques of feminizing genitoplasty should result in cosmetically acceptable genital reconstructions, with an acceptable complication rate and a reasonable likelihood of later satisfactory heterosexual functioning and, for CAH patients, the feasibility of later fertility.

REFERENCES

1. Federman DD, Donahoe PK. Ambiguous genitalia—Etiology, diagnosis and therapy. Adv Endocrinol Metab 6:91, 1995.
2. Mininberg DT, Levine LS, New MI. Current concepts in congenital adrenal hyperplasia. Invest Urol 17:169, 1979.
3. Feldman KW, Smith DW. Fetal phallic growth and penile standards for newborn male infants. J Pediatr 80:395, 1975.
4. Danish RK, Lee PA, Mazur T, et al. Micropenis: II. Hypogonadotropic hypogonadism. Johns Hopkins Med J 146:177, 1980.
5. Lee PA, Danish RK, Mazur T, et al. Micropenis: III. Primary hypogonadism, partial androgen insensitivity syndrome, and idiopathic disorders. Johns Hopkins Med J 147:175, 1980.
6. Ehrlich RM, Koyle MA, Shanberg AM. A technique for ureteral stump ablation. J Urol 140:1240, 1988.
7. Lewis VG, Money J. Adrenogenital syndrome: The need for early surgical feminization in girls. In Lee PA, Plotnick LP, Kowarski AB, et al (eds), Congenital Adrenal Hyperplasia. Baltimore: University Park Press, 1977, p 463.
8. Hendren WH, Crawford JD. Adrenogenital syndrome: The anatomy of the anomaly and its repair. Some new concepts. J Pediatr Surg 4:49, 1969.
9. Ansell JS, Rajfer J. A new and simplified method for concealing the hypertrophied clitoris. J Pediatr Surg 16:681, 1981.
10. Stefan H. Surgical reconstruction of the external genitalia in female pseudohermaphrodites. Br J Urol 39:347, 1967.
11. Kogan SJ, Smey P, Levitt SB. Subtunical total reduction clitoroplasty: A safe modification of existing techniques. J Urol 130:746, 1983.
12. Azziz R, Mulaikal RM, Migeon CJ, et al. Congenital adrenal hyperplasia: Long-term results following vaginal reconstruction. Fertil Steril 46:1011, 1986.
13. Jones HW, Garcia SC, Klingensmith GJ. Secondary surgical treatment of the masculinized external genitalia of patients with virilizing adrenal hyperplasia. Obstet Gynecol 48:73, 1976.
14. Mulaikal RM, Migeon CJ, Rock JA. Fertility rates in female patients with congenital adrenal hyperplasia due to 21-hydroxylase deficiency. N Engl J Med 316:178, 1987.
15. Nihoul-Fekete C, Philippe F, Thiband E, et al. Resultants a

moyen et long terme de a chirurgie reparatice des organes genitaux chez les filles aheintes d'hyperplasie congenitale viriusande des surrenales. Arch Fr Pediatr 39:13, 1982.
16. Sotiropoulos A, Morishima A, Homsy Y, et al. Long-term assessment of genital reconstruction in female pseudohermaphrodites. J Urol 115:599, 1976.
17. Money J. Intersexual problems. Clin Obstet Gynecol 16:169, 1973.
18. Money J, Schwartz M. Dating, romantic and non-romantic friendships and sexuality in 17 early treated adrenogenital females aged 16–25. In Lee PA, Plotnick LP, Kowarski AB, et al (eds), Congenital Adrenal Hyperplasia. Baltimore: University Park Press, 1977, pp 429.
19. Gearhart JP, Burnett A, Owen JH. Measurement of pudendal evoked potentials during feminizing genitoplasty: Technique and applications. J Urol 153:486, 1995.
20. Edmonds DK, Dewhurst J. Reproductive potential in adolescent girls with ambiguous genitalia. Pediatr Ann 15:530, 1986.

PART II

The Kidney

2

BARTLEY G. CILENTO, JR. AND GEORGE W. KAPLAN

Ureteropelvic Junction Obstruction

We were asked by the editor to discuss the evaluation, diagnosis, and treatment of ureteropelvic junction (UPJ) obstruction but from a practical, rather than an encyclopedic, approach. The interested reader is referred to standard urologic textbooks for details not contained herein. Nevertheless, this discussion would be incomplete without a brief discussion of the history, embryology, histology, physiology, and etiology of this disorder.

HISTORY

The term hydronephrosis was introduced by Rayer in 1841 and slowly thereafter gained acceptance. Before Rayer's description, dilatation of the renal collecting system was given many names, including expanis renum, hernia renalis, hydrops renis, hydrops renalis, hydrorenal distention, cystonephrosis, sackniere, and hydropyelosis, to name only a few! In 1641, Nicholas Tulp clinically described a patient with "ishuria lunatica" who monthly, coincident with the full moon, would experience urinary retention, severe pain, and fever. Bloodletting was the only treatment that offered relief. At the postmortem examination of this patient, a large hydronephrotic left kidney and an empty bladder were noted, convincing Tulp that this large mass compressed the great vessels and explaining to his satisfaction why phlebotomy offered symptomatic relief. Bonetus in 1679 described a child with a hydronephrotic kidney in whom the ureter was merely a fibrous cord. Rayer in 1841 described a patient with hydronephrosis caused by reduplication of the ureter with folds and contractions at the level of the ureteropelvic junction.[1] Gustave Simon in 1869 performed the first deliberate (and successful) nephrectomy and showed conclusively that a kidney could be removed without permanent impairment to the health of the individual. This event is notable because it paved the way for renal surgery.[2]

In the late 1800s, surgeons began conserving renal tissue rather than proceeding directly to nephrectomy. The first reported attempt at surgical repair of hydronephrosis is credited to Trendelenburg in 1886. He used an abdominal approach, which resulted in a colonic injury, and the patient died shortly after surgery. The case was not reported until 4 years later. Kuster is credited with the first successful procedure for the relief of hydronephrosis performed June 14, 1891. The patient was a 13-year-old boy with a solitary kidney who had previously undergone a nephrostomy, which would not close. Kuster found the upper ureter to be entirely obliterated, resected the obliterated tissue, and anastomosed the ureter into the most dependent portion of the renal pelvis. The operation was successful and stimulated great interest in the repair of hydronephrosis. Kuster reported his case to the 21st German Surgical Congress on June 8, 1892. At that time, Trendelenburg described his case and endorsed the concept of conservative surgery for hydronephrosis. Christian Fenger of Chicago, unaware of Kuster's work, simultaneously and independently surgically corrected UPJ obstruction using the Heineke-Mikulicz principle. Fenger has been given credit for introducing conservative renal surgery in the United States. By 1899, he had reported seven cases; four patients were clinically relieved and free of symptoms and three cases failed, requiring nephrectomy.

Conservative renal surgery for the relief of hydronephrosis was considered so important that it was the main topic of discussion at the 13th International Congress of Medicine in Paris in 1900. Five papers were delivered by pioneers in the field: Kuster, Fenger, Bazy, Albarran, and Legueu. As operations to correct hydronephrosis became more widely performed, comparisons of primary nephrectomy versus pyeloplasty were published. In 1903, primary nephrectomy had an 80% cure rate but a 20% mortality rate. Pyeloplasty had a 37% cure rate and a 10% mortality rate.

Some surgeons, led by Pasteau, were convinced that hydronephrosis was the result of a movable kidney resulting in obstruction of the ureter by anomalous blood vessels, adhesive bands, or torsion of the ureter. Their preferred surgical approach involved nephropexy and lysis of these bands. Others believed that hydronephrosis was caused by constriction of the upper ureter and was best corrected by pyeloplasty. In 1921, von Lichtenberg described a technique for pyeloureteroplasty in which an inverted U-shaped incision was made in the adjacent walls of the renal pelvis and ureter through the obstructed UPJ. The anterior and posterior edges of the pelvis and ureter were then sutured together. In 1923, Schwyzer described a technique for correcting UPJ obstruction, based on principles of pyloroplasty in which the ureter was first freed of adhesive bands. A Y-shaped incision was then made, extending from the renal pelvis to the ureter. The flap was pulled down into the split ureter and sutured in place, forming a "V." Resection of the redundant renal pelvis and nephrostomy drainage was introduced in the late 1920s by Papin and Walters. In 1937, Foley modified Schwyzer's Y procedure by extending the upper limbs of the Y onto the posterior and anterior walls of the renal pelvis. The lower limb of the Y extended down the lateral aspect of the ureter. In 1943, Davis described intubated ureterostomy in which a longitudinal incision is made in the narrowed portion of the ureter; a tube is left in place for 6 weeks until the ureter regenerates around the tube. In 1949, Anderson and Hynes described dismembered pyeloplasty (although it was the method used by Kuster almost 60 years earlier). Their objectives were to excise the obstructing lesion, resect the redundant pelvis if necessary, and place a dependent flap of renal pelvic tissue into the split ureter. Maintenance of ureteral continuity was considered important by many, and in 1951 and 1953 flap pyeloplasties were described by Culp and Scardino, respectively. However, as favorable results with the dismembered pyeloplasties accumulated, it became clear that maintenance of ureteral continuity was not essential to success, and the flap and intubated procedures were relegated to secondary roles for the treatment of long ureteral strictures.

EMBRYOLOGY

The collecting system of the kidney develops from the ureteric bud, which contacts and penetrates a cap of metanephric blastema. The ureteric bud dilates, forming a primitive renal pelvis. The UPJ is formed during the fifth week of embryogenesis. The primitive renal pelvis splits into a cranial and caudal portion, forming the future major calices. Each major calix continues to divide and further penetrate the metanephric blastema. There will be 12 or more such divisions, continuing until the end of the fifth month of gestation, when the second-generation tubules enlarge and absorb the tubules of the third and fourth divisions, resulting in the formation of the minor calices. The fifth and successive generations converge on the minor calices and form the renal pyramids. The ureteric bud thus gives rise to the ureter, renal pelvis, major and minor calices, and the 1 to 3 million collecting ducts.[3] By the 10th week of embryogenesis, urine is formed and can pass from the glomerulus to the bladder.[4]

HISTOLOGY

The renal pelvis is composed of three layers: mucosa, muscularis, and adventitia. The inner layer is mucosal and is lined by transitional epithelium supported by a lamina propria. The epithelium is two to three cells thick in the renal pelvis and four to five cells thick in the ureter. The epithelium sits on a thin basal lamina, which rests on the lamina propria composed of dense fibroconnective tissue with prominent elastic fibers. In transverse section, the ureteral lumen appears stellate as a result of the folds of mucosa resulting from the looseness of the lamina propria, the elastic fibers, and the muscularis. The muscularis is composed of interdigitating fibers of smooth muscle separated by strands of connective tissue. These muscle fibers are arranged into an inner longitudinal layer and an outer circular layer. This orientation is variable, is often indistinct, and changes from the papillae to the ureterovesical junction. The adventitia is external to the muscular layer and is composed of fibroelastic tissue, which is continuous with the capsule of the kidney. The ureter has a rich blood supply with extensive vascular and lymphatic plexus within the muscularis and lamina propria. Ganglion cells are present within the ureter and supply motor (autonomic) function to the muscularis. Sensory fibers within the muscularis penetrate between the cells of the epithelium.[5]

PHYSIOLOGY

The origin of the electrical activity for ureteral peristalsis begins at pacemaker sites located in the proximal portion of the collecting system. Muscular contractions occur within the calices and renal pelvis more frequently than in the upper ureter. Hence, the renal pelvis fills, producing a rise in the renal pelvic pressure. A bolus of urine is then delivered from the pelvis into the upper ureter, after which ureteral contractions move the bolus down the ureter. The UPJ remains closed during these ureteral contractions to prevent flow of urine back into the renal pelvis. Two to six ureteral peristaltic contractions occur per minute and are propelled at a rate of 2 to 6 cm/s. Efficient transport of urine is dependent on coaptation of the pelvic and ureteral walls. Resting baseline intraureteral and intrapelvic pressures range from 0 to 5 cm H_2O. Ureteral pressures during a contraction range from 20 to 60 cm H_2O. As the volume of urine increases, there is a 1:1 correlation between conduction of caliceal contractions and ureteral contractions.

ETIOLOGY

The etiology of UPJ obstruction is often divided into intrinsic and extrinsic causes. Intrinsic causes are the most common and are usually congenital.[4] Obstruction may be the result of valvelike folds or polyps[6] but most often is caused by intrinsic stenosis or aperistaltic segments. Extrinsic causes include kinks, inflammation, aberrant vessels, and tumors, so obstruction may be secondary rather than primary.

PATHOPHYSIOLOGY

Obstruction at the UPJ is assumed, by definition, to affect renal function adversely. The changes in renal function are dependent on the degree and duration of the obstruction. With impeded urine flow, there is an increase in intraluminal hydrostatic pressure, which eventually results in dilatation of the collecting system proximal to the obstruction. In addition to these anatomic changes, there are physiologic changes. Glomerular filtration rate (GFR) begins to fall because of a reduction in the pressure gradient favoring filtration (capillary hydrostatic pressure minus tubular hydrostatic pressure). If obstruction is complete, then the intratubular pressure will continue to rise until glomerular filtration virtually stops. If the obstruction is partial, glomerular filtration will not stop entirely. Experimental studies have shown that, with complete obstruction, the elevated intrapelvic pressures begin to fall after 24 hours and reach normal values at 28 weeks.[7] Because the intrapelvic pressures do not remain elevated, some other factor must be responsible for the persistent decrease in GFR. Micropuncture studies on rats have demonstrated that the proximal tubular pressure may return to normal values within 24 hours in unilateral obstruction.[8, 9] This effect is due to the constriction of the afferent arteriole, which results in reductions in the hydrostatic pressure favoring filtration. Therefore, GFR is reduced. The hemodynamic changes in bilateral obstruction are different. In bilateral obstruction the proximal tubular pressure remains elevated for longer periods as a result of renal vasodilation instead of renal vasoconstriction.[9]

Tubular function becomes progressively impaired with obstruction. The net effects are high urinary sodium concentration, reduction in urinary acidification, and decreased concentrating ability.[10] Decreased water and sodium absorption accounts for the observation that such patients have normal or increased urine output.[11] Urine flow across the obstructed UPJ has been described as being either pressure dependent or volume dependent.[12] The pressure-dependent flow pattern is seen with intrinsic obstruction in which increases in urine flow across the UPJ are produced by increased intrapelvic pressures. There is a linear relationship between intrapelvic pressure and flow across the UPJ. The volume-dependent flow pattern is seen with extrinsic obstruction where flow increases as intrapelvic pressure increases but at some point flow suddenly decreases. This decrease in flow is caused by angulation of the UPJ, with increasing pelvic volume resulting in increased resistance to flow.

The ability of the renal pelvis to dilate appears to have a nephron-sparing effect. This finding correlates with the observation that hydronephrotic kidneys can maintain their renal function over prolonged periods of time.[4] Some investigators have attempted to characterize the compliance of the renal pelvis with pelvimetry.[13, 14] Koff found that all sizes and shapes of renal pelves have similar compliance to the point of capacity. At capacity the intraluminal pressure rises sharply. It appears that this is related to the point at which the elastic fibers and smooth muscle reach their point of maximum distensibility. Progressive renal damage is seen with increasing hydronephrosis dependent on the capacity for further pelvic distention and the change in intrapelvic pressure with increasing volume. In a large and distended renal pelvis, the intrapelvic pressure rises slowly. In contrast, there can be rapid increases in pressure in a small renal pelvis. These observations explain why a kidney with a small intrarenal pelvis is more susceptible to renal damage than one with a large extrarenal pelvis.

NATURAL HISTORY OF HYDRONEPHROSIS

The nearly universal use of maternal ultrasonography has led to the early detection of fetal hydronephrosis. The fetal kidney is first detectable by ultrasonography at 15 weeks gestation, several weeks after the onset of urine production.[15] The internal renal architecture is better imaged at 20 weeks when the kidney is surrounded by fat. The medullary pyramids are sonolucent, and the renal parenchyma is slightly less echogenic than the liver. There should be a clear corticomedullary junction distinction.

Hydronephrosis is the most common abnormality detected on prenatal ultrasonogram. Fetal hydronephrosis may be the result of several factors and does not necessarily indicate obstruction. Vesicoureteral reflux, congenital nonobstructing megaureter, transient hydronephrosis, and prune-belly syndrome are some examples of nonobstructive collecting system dilatation. The majority of hydronephrosis cases detected antenatally are physiologic and resolve spontaneously. In one large series of nearly 7000 women, antenatal hydronephrosis was detected in 1.4% and confirmed in 0.65% postnatally.[16] Prenatally detected hydronephrosis of a mild nature is usually clinically insignificant. Thomas and colleagues observed 29 children (39 kidneys) with mild dilatation (anteroposterior pelvic [AP] diameter between 0.5 and 1.5 mm). Four years later, 69% of the kidneys were normal, and 31% had persistent mild dilation. Renal growth was normal in 97% of the kidneys.[17]

Hydronephrosis secondary to obstruction is most commonly the result of UPJ obstruction. However, not all cases of UPJ obstruction necessitate surgical repair. Homsy evaluated 60 renal units with pyelocaliectasis with renal sonogram, diuretic renography, and intravenous pyelogram (IVP).[18] Twenty-one renal units were partially obstructed or dilated without obstruction. Of the 17 renal units available for follow-up; 7 (41%) deteriorated, 8 (47%) improved, and 2 (12%) remained stable. Those renal units that deteriorated did so within 6 months. Homsy recommended a 6-month observation period and repeat diuretic renography in those patients in whom initial obstruction cannot be documented.[18]

In perhaps the only true study of the natural history of hydronephrosis, Koff monitored 45 neonates with unilateral hydronephrosis for 30 months regardless of the degree of hydronephrosis, results of diuretic renogram, or degree of function. Thirty patients had mild hydronephrosis with greater than 40% differential function. None of these kidneys demonstrated deterioration in function. Fifteen patients had severe hydronephrosis and parenchymal thinning; seven of the 15 (47%) exhibited decreased renal function. Follow-up ultrasonography showed no change in 8, mild to marked improvement in 5, and complete disappearance of hydronephrosis in 2. Follow-up diuretic renography showed an unobstructed pattern in 4 patients. All kidneys, including the severely hydronephrotic, showed rapid improvement in the absolute GFR and no evidence of contralateral compensatory hypertrophy. On the basis of these findings, Koff concluded that obstruction could not be proven because there was no postnatal deterioration of renal function, no progression of hydronephrosis, and no contralateral renal hypertrophy. He suggested that these patients undergo observation until a change in one of these parameters is observed.[19]

In contrast, the Society for Urology conducted a multicenter study involving 33 pediatric urologists from 21 cities registering 464 cases (582 kidneys) of hydronephrosis. A uniform method of hydronephrotic grading and performance parameters for diuretic renography were established. In this study, 275 cases (59%) were managed by observation and 189 (41%) were treated surgically. The surgically treated kidneys showed hydronephrosis grade 3 or greater and obstruction on diuretic renography. Six-month postoperative evaluation showed significant improvement in hydronephrosis (mean grade, 1.8) and no obstruction on diuretic renography. The postoperative mean grade of hydronephrosis, results of diuretic renography, and percentage of differential function were then similar to age-matched observed kidneys. They concluded that when radiographic tests are done properly, they are accurate in distinguishing which infants with hydronephrosis will do well with surgery and which with observation.[20]

Our approach to the patient with hydronephrosis is similar to the latter philosophy. Patients are evaluated with renal-bladder ultrasonography to document the degree of hydronephrosis, internal renal architecture, presence or absence of ureteral dilation, absence of bladder thickening, or dilated posterior urethra. A voiding cystourethrogram (VCUG) is performed to rule out vesicoureteral reflux, and renal scan is used to determine differential renal function and evidence of obstruction. We perform surgical correction in those patients in whom the sonogram shows grade 3 to 5 hydronephrosis and diuretic renography implies obstruction. When hydronephrosis is mild or when the renal scan shows no obstruction or is equivocal, we will re-evaluate these patients in 3 to 6 months.

CLINICAL PRESENTATION

The UPJ is the most common site of obstruction in the urinary collecting system. It occurs once in 1500 births and is more common in males than females (65% vs. 35%). There is bilateral involvement in 5% of cases. There is a slight left-sided preponderance (60%). Before the advent of prenatal ultrasonography, most infants with UPJ obstruction presented with hematuria, urinary tract infections, abdominal masses, or gastrointestinal discomfort. Most cases are now detected during prenatal ultrasonographic screening. In fact, the fetal kidney and collecting system are often detectable by ultrasonographic scanning as early as 15 weeks' gestation.[21] In those children with detectable abdominal masses on physical examination, 50% of masses are genitourinary in origin and of these 40% are secondary to hydronephrosis caused by a UPJ obstruction.[22] In 1977, Johnston reviewed 219 cases of UPJ obstruction and showed that urinary tract infection was the most common presentation.[23] Older children usually present with gastrointestinal or abdominal discomfort, hematuria following minimal trauma, nausea or vomiting, or UTIs.[24] Conditions associated with UPJ obstruction are multicystic dysplastic kidney, duplication of the collecting system, imperforate anus, congenital heart disease, VATER (vertebral defects, anal atresia, tracheoesophageal fistula with esophageal atresia, and radial and renal anomalies) association, and esophageal atresia.

DIAGNOSIS

Presently, there is no standard means by which one can diagnose obstruction. All available studies have their benefits and limitations. Current diagnostic modalities are constantly being refined in an attempt to find a simple test that has a high degree of sensitivity and specificity for the detection of obstruction.

ULTRASONOGRAM

Hydronephrosis is the most common anomaly diagnosed in utero.[24a] With the advent of maternal ultrasonography, hydronephrosis is frequently detected in utero and the diagnostic workup is completed shortly after birth. Before the widespread use of maternal sonography, infants would present with urosepsis, abdominal masses, failure to thrive, and hematuria. At Boston Children's Hospital, Brown and coworkers[25] reviewed two periods of time: presonography and postsonography. In the 6-year period from 1979 to 1985, 142 neonates with hydronephrosis were seen. Seventy-eight percent of cases were discovered by fetal screening during maternal ultrasonography. UPJ obstruction was the most common lesion detected (41%). During the 30-year presonography era (1947–1977), 146 neonates with significant hydronephrosis were seen. Most cases were discovered because of abdominal masses or urosepsis. UPJ obstruction was the most common cause of hydronephrosis (22%).[25]

Obstruction of the UPJ is the most common congenital anomaly of the urinary tract. In a large, retrospective study of 6292 pregnant women, sonography demonstrated UPJ obstruction in 12 (1.9 per 1000 live births).[26] Is UPJ obstruction being overdiagnosed with the nearly universal use of maternal ultrasonography? Weiner and others addressed this question.[27] They determined that UPJ obstruction was being detected and corrected at an earlier age but the number of pyeloplasties overall was not increased. Specifically, the number of pyeloplasties was increased in infants and decreased in older children and adults since the advent of fetal ultrasonography.

UPJ obstruction is suspected when there is dilatation of the renal pelvis and no visualization of the ureters. On ultrasonogram, the dilated pelvis should also communicate with the dilated calices (Figs. 2–1, 2–2). Lack of communication suggests a multicystic dysplastic kidney.

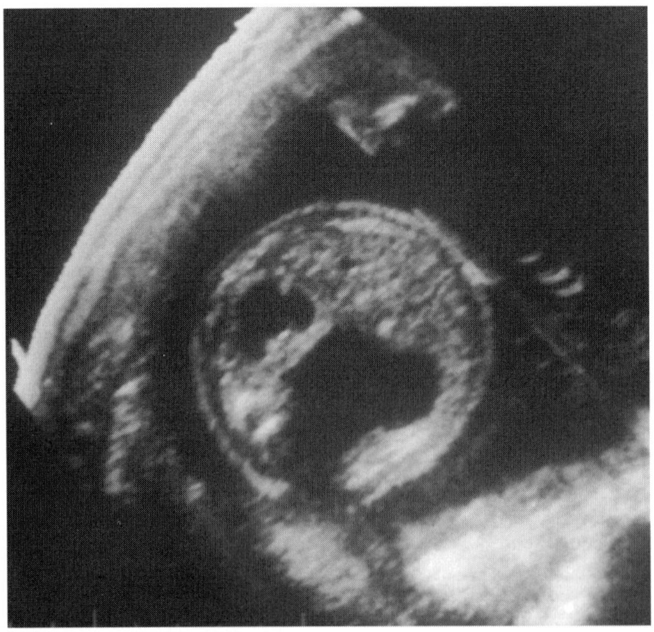

Figure 2–1 Antenatal ultrasonogram demonstrating bilateral hydronephrosis.

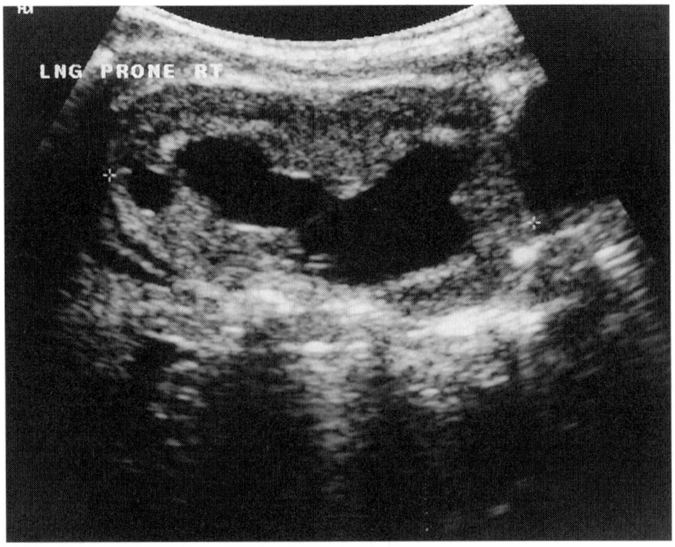

Figure 2–2 Postnatal ultrasonogram demonstrating left hydronephrosis and caliceal dilatation.

In one prenatal series, sonography had a 77% accuracy rate in diagnosing UPJ obstruction.

It has become increasingly evident that the diagnosis of UPJ obstruction is basically physiologic rather than purely anatomic; consequently, there have been multiple attempts to find a study or group of studies that will reliably determine the presence of obstruction. It is generally agreed that dilation of the urinary tract as seen in ultrasonography, intravenous urography, or retrograde pyelography is alone insufficient to diagnose obstruction of the upper urinary tract. Attempts to use physiology and ultrasonography have been made. In recognition that renal blood flow decreases with obstruction, a parameter called the *resistive index* has been studied. The resistive index is defined as the peak systolic velocity of blood flowing through the arcuate arteries divided into the lowest diastolic velocity in the same vessels. Renal resistive indexes of less than 82% correlate well with intrarenal pressures of less than 14 cm H_2O. To expand the utility of this study further, furosemide can be administered in the course of this study. An increase of 15% in the postfurosemide resistive index over the prefurosemide resistive index does correlate with the presence of obstruction with 88% specificity and 76% sensitivity. Thus far, the use of resistive indexes to define the presence of obstruction has not gained widespread acceptance in most pediatric centers, however.

Efforts have been made to use the counterbalance theory to determine the significance of unilateral functional obstruction. Koff and associates recorded the growth rate and size of the normal contralateral kidney to determine whether the occurrence or degree of compensatory growth would provide an accurate means to determine the significance of obstruction of the contralat-

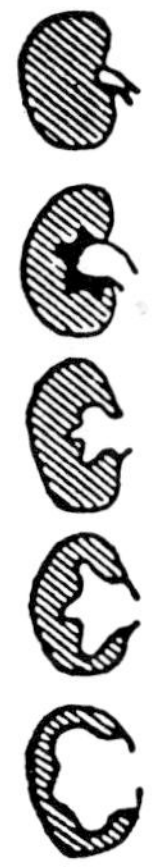

	Caliceal dilation	Size of pelvis
Grade I	Physiologic	1 cm
Grade II	Normal calyces	1 - 1.5 cm
Grade III	Slight dilation	> 1.5 cm
Grade IV	Moderate dilation	> 1.5 cm
Grade V	Severe dilation + atrophic cortex	> 1.5 cm

Figure 2–3 Classification of in utero urinary tract dilation.

eral hydronephrotic kidney. It was shown that normal kidneys opposite obstructed kidneys undergo compensatory hypertrophy. In addition, normal kidneys opposite nonobstructed but poorly functioning hydronephrotic kidneys whose function rapidly improved were smaller than normal for age.[28] To improve the diagnostic accuracy in newborns with hydronephrosis, Koff combined the sonographic measurement of renal growth with the differential renal function of the hydronephrotic kidney as determined by renal scan. Serial measurements are plotted on a renal growth–renal function chart. Four reproducible diagnostic patterns emerged: (1) obstructed, (2) corrected obstruction, (3) no obstruction with good differential function (>40%), and (4) no obstruction but poor differential growth (<40%). He concluded that this modality helped to identify and exclude obstruction as well as to provide reassurance that nonobstructive hydronephrosis was not injurious.[29]

With the universal use of maternal-fetal ultrasonography and the common finding of fetal hydronephrosis, Grignon and colleagues proposed a classification of in utero urinary tract dilatation. The classification grades dilatation on a scale ranging from 1 to 5 (Fig. 2–3). The AP diameter is measured. Grade I dilatation is pelvic dilation less than 10 mm and is considered normal. Grade II (10–15 mm) and Grade III (>15 mm with slight caliceal dilatation) represent intermediate hydronephrosis, which requires corrective postnatal surgery in 50% of cases. Grade IV dilatation has greater than 15 mm of AP separation with moderate caliceal dilatation. Grade V dilatation has greater than 15 mm of AP separation and cortical atrophy.[30]

WHITAKER TEST

In 1973 Whitaker described a study in which the pressure needed to propel fluid across a presumed area of obstruction was determined at high rates of flow (10 mL/min). A rise in pressure greater than 15 cm H_2O was believed to be indicative of obstruction. Although there was correlation between obstruction (as defined by this study) and progressive deterioration of renal function over time, the correlation was not complete. Additionally, the test is invasive, requiring a catheter in the renal pelvis and in the bladder. This study is currently used only selectively in cases in which there is a diagnostic uncertainty with less invasive modalities.

DIURETIC RENOGRAPHY

Not all dilatation of the upper urinary tract is the result of obstruction. The magnitude of hydronephrosis is not a reliable criterion by which to diagnose obstruction. The Whitaker test is invasive and may reliably diagnose obstruction, but it does not provide information concerning renal function. Renal diuretic renography provides information concerning both urinary obstruction and differential renal function. Its role can be expanded by using furosemide to produce a high urine flow noninvasively. The time required to wash the tracer from the renal pelvis is used rather than intrapelvic pressure as a measure of obstruction (Fig. 2–4). When furosemide is administered 20 minutes after the isotope, half the isotope is expected to exit the unobstructed pelvis in less than 10 minutes. When more than 20 minutes is required for half of the radioactivity to wash out of the renal pelvis, obstruction is believed to be evident. Once again, there is correlation (but not perfect correlation) with the presence of obstruc-

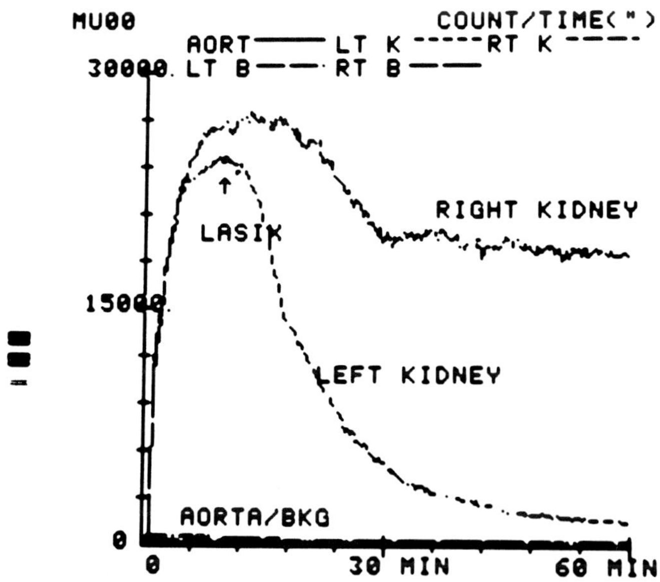

Figure 2–4 Furosemide (Lasix) renal scan demonstrating both normal radiotracer washout of the left kidney and delayed radiotracer washout of the right kidney.

tion and these parameters. Decreased renal function, state of hydration, marked hydronephrosis, and administration of furosemide before the isotope is excreted all lead to errors in interpretation. This study is usually performed on an outpatient basis without sedation, and the risk of hypersensitivity reactions is negligible.

Diuretic renography has been performed in children for more than 15 years, during which time it has undergone modification and refinement. It has become the procedure of choice in the evaluation of suspected obstruction because it is relatively noninvasive, providing information about differential function and reliably diagnosing functional obstruction. However, it should be cautioned that this test is critically dependent on technique, and adherence to technique is essential to obtain reliable information. The two agents most widely used are technetium 99m–diethylenetetraminepenta-acetic acid (^{99m}Tc–DTPA) and technetium 99m–mercaptoacetyltriglycine (MAG3). MAG3 is a newer compound that gives better anatomic detail but is much more expensive. DTPA is excreted by glomerular filtration and is not secreted or absorbed by the renal tubules. Glomerular filtration can be measured by determining the rate of its removal from the blood. The ^{99m}Tc emits a 140 keV gamma ray with no harmful beta emission. The estimated absorbed dose by the kidney is 0.04 mrad and total body absorption is 16 mrad, which is less than with an IVP. MAG3 is cleared primarily by tubular secretion and provides estimates of renal function similar to DTPA.

To reduce interinstitutional differences in technique when performing the diuretic renogram, the Society for Fetal Urology and the Society of Nuclear Medicine Council proposed a uniform methodology for performing the diuretic renogram called the "well-tempered" renogram.[31] To reduce the likelihood of immature renal function interfering with interpretation, infants should be older than 2 weeks. Oral hydration is begun 2 hours before the study. Intravenous hydration of 15 mL/kg over 30 minutes is started as a bolus 15 minutes before injection of the radionucleotide followed by maintenance fluid at a rate of 200 mL/kg/24 hours. The bladder is catheterized throughout the study.

VOIDING CYSTOURETHROGRAPHY

Approximately 10% of children with UPJ obstruction will also have vesicoureteral reflux. Additionally, hydronephrosis produced by vesicoureteral reflux can mimic UPJ obstruction on ultrasonogram. For both of these reasons, VCUG is helpful in the evaluation of children with suspected UPJ obstruction.

RETROGRADE UROGRAPHY

Retrograde pyelography is rarely needed to diagnose UPJ obstruction because the diagnosis is ascertained by ultrasonography and diuretic renal scan. The value of retrograde pyelography lies in the preoperative evaluation of the ureter to rule out missed ureterovesical obstruction and to anatomically characterize the UPJ obstruction (Fig. 2–5). Rushton and colleagues believe that retrograde pyelography is not necessary before pyeloplasty because ultrasonography and diuretic renography in their hands can reliably exclude the possibility of distal obstruction. Others (Hendren as well as ourselves) believe that retrograde pyelography is an important adjunct to pyeloplasty.[32, 33]

SURGERY

Pyeloplasty

The usual preoperative laboratory investigation before pyeloplasty in our institution includes a complete blood count, serum electrolytes, blood urea nitrogen, serum creatinine, and urine culture. Because the need for intraoperative blood transfusion is remote, blood is not routinely typed or cross-matched. Patients are admitted to the hospital the morning of surgery and are seen by the anesthesiologist immediately before surgery (assuming the patient is American Standards Association [ASA] class I or II).

After the administration of general anesthesia and the placement of a secure peripheral intravenous catheter, the patient is placed in lithotomy position for cystoscopy and retrograde pyelography. Although these studies might seem superfluous or redundant to some, the additional 15 to 20 minutes of anesthesia time seems well

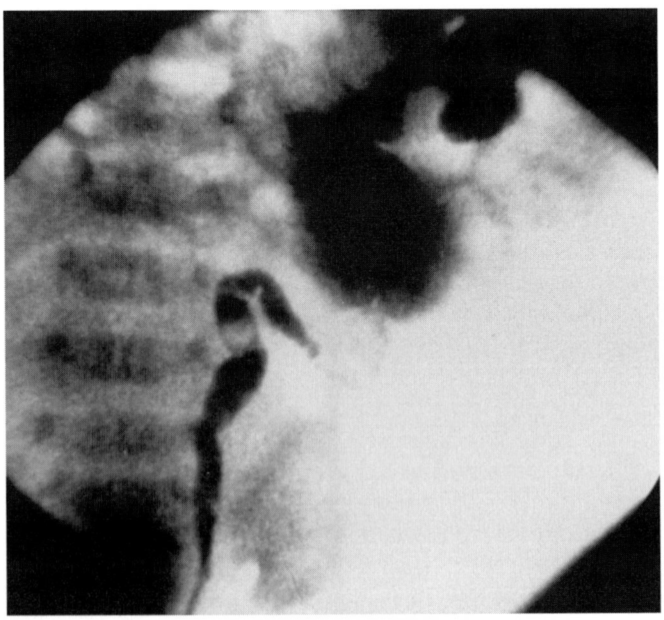

Figure 2–5 Retrograde pyelogram delineating segment of narrowing at the ureteropelvic junction.

spent to ensure that the bladder is normal and that the distal ureter on the affected side is normal and to anatomically visualize the lesion to be repaired before making an incision. The ureteral orifice on the affected side is cannulated with a 3 French ureteral catheter, and a retrograde pyelogram is obtained using portable fluoroscopy.

Surgical positioning is dictated largely by the type of repair being contemplated. For unilateral pyeloplasty, we prefer the flank position. Various combinations of table flexion, kidney rest height, and placement of a roll under the dependent flank are used to obtain a flexed torso in which the overlying flank musculature is taut, so that the space between the lower ribs and the iliac crest is maximally spread. Support and padding are provided to the axilla and to other pressure points (e.g., knees, ankles, and heels). The patient is taped to the table in this position using wide adhesive tape at the level of the hip and shoulder.

After skin preparation, older children are draped with towels and sheets. Infants are draped with Vi-Drape dressing (after an adhesive spray is applied to the patient and to the ether screen). A split sheet is applied with the tails toward the patient's head. This manner of draping helps to retain body heat and also allows the anesthesiologist a view of the operative field to estimate blood loss better. An oblique subcostal incision extending from the tip of and paralleling the 12th rib is used. The skin incision is made with a scalpel, but deeper dissection uses electrocautery down to and through the transversalis fascia and muscle. Care is taken to identify and preserve the 12th intercostal nerve.

In most infants and children, the peritoneum extends further posteriorly than in adults; hence, dissection deep to the transversalis muscle is first carried back to the psoas muscle before Gerota's fascia is opened. This usually ensures avoiding an inadvertent peritoneotomy. Once Gerota's fascia is opened, the lower pole to the kidney, the UPJ, distal renal pelvis, and proximal ureter are divested of fat in preparation for repair. In infants, hand-held Deaver retractors are used to provide exposure. In older children, a self-retaining (Balfour) retractor is often used.

There are instances in which both sides are obstructed and are best repaired. Such repairs can be performed sequentially or simultaneously. If the patient is otherwise well and there are no comorbidities that suggest the need for sequential operations, it is generally our practice to approach both sides in a single operation. In doing so, one must choose from a number of incisional approaches. Theses include two separate flank incisions, two dorsal lumbotomy incisions, two anterior extraperitoneal incisions, or a single transperitoneal incision. As a rule, the latter is our preferred approach because it is direct and expeditious. It does carry with it the postoperative risk of bowel obstruction, but this small risk seems offset by the other advantages of this approach. A transverse incision below the rib margin and above the umbilicus is used because this provides excellent exposure. Once the peritoneum is entered, the colon is reflected medially after incising the white line of Toldt. A self-retaining retractor such as an Omni or Thompson retractor is quite helpful in providing exposure.

As noted in the earlier discussion of the history of pyeloplasty, the theoretical objection to transecting the ureter and pelvis led to the development of flap (Foley, Culp, Scardino) and folding (Hamilton-Stewart) techniques for repair. Additionally, the failure to recognize that most obstructions of the UPJ in children are due to intrinsic problems in the wall of the ureter where it joins the renal pelvis led to operations in which extrinsic bands were lysed to straighten kinks and in which crossing vessels that were thought to be obstructing were transected or moved (Hellstrom). In our opinion, the flap techniques are rarely indicated, the folding techniques rarely efficacious, and extrinsic obstructions as isolated lesions quite uncommon. Consequently, the Anderson-Hynes dismembered pyeloplasty is used in almost all patients. The Foley Y-V plasty is used in some instances of high insertion of the ureter into the renal pelvis, especially in cases associated with a horseshoe kidney. The Davis intubated ureterostomy has been successfully used when there was a long area of stenosis in the ureter and insufficient pelvic size or ureteral length to bridge the gap. Ureterocalicostomy has been used in some redo cases in which the renal pelvis is encased in scar and the renal parenchyma is thin.

Our technique for dismembered pyeloplasty is similar to that generally described, but it has some nuances that we believe are helpful. After the ureter has been identified and isolated with a silicone tape (vessel loop), the distal renal pelvis, UPJ, and proximal ureter are dissected free of overlying tissue. Holding (stay) sutures are placed through the medial aspect of the ureter below the UPJ but also below the area of the ureter felt to be abnormal (i.e., at the transition from abnormal to normal proximal ureter). A holding (stay) suture is also placed at the inferior lateral aspect of the renal pelvis (presumably the most dependent point of the renal pelvis). Lastly, a holding (stay) suture is placed on the medial aspect of the renal pelvis superior to the UPJ such that the distance between the two pelvic stay sutures equals the length of the proposed ureteral spatulation. The ureteral holding suture is then pulled cephalad to confirm that the ureter, once transected, will reach the renal pelvis without tension. If this is not confirmed, the entire kidney should be mobilized so that it can be displaced inferiorly, and, if necessary, more of the proximal ureter should be mobilized. The ureter should not be transected until it is confirmed that there will be a tension-free anastomosis. If this cannot be confirmed, other techniques of repair should be used.

Once it is determined that a tension-free anastomosis can be performed, the ureter is transected just cephalad to the ureteral stay suture. In most instances, the renal pelvis will remain distended with urine, confirming an obstruction at the UPJ. The renal pelvis is transected below the two pelvic stay sutures, at which point the obstructed renal pelvis empties. The ureter is spatulated along its lateral aspect so that the length of the spatulation conforms to the length of the pelvic transection (1–2 cm). The ureter is then anastomosed to the renal pelvis using fine (5-0 or 6-0) chromic catgut suture. The lateral (dependent) tongue of the renal pelvis is brought down into the apex of the ureteral spatulation. The anastomosis is usually performed using interrupted sutures rather than a continuous closure (Figs. 2–6 and 2–7). Many authors believe that a continuous closure is preferable to produce a watertight anastomosis. It is our prejudice that these anastomoses are never completely watertight and that a continuous closure risks narrowing the newly created UPJ, especially in small infants.

In most instances, it is neither necessary nor desirable to reduce the size of the renal pelvis. It is our prejudice that once the obstruction is eliminated the renal pelvis will spontaneously reduce in size if the pelvis is not fibrotic. If the renal pelvis musculature has been sufficiently replaced by fibrosis, reduction of the renal pelvic size may reduce the size of the reservoir but will do nothing to promote emptying of the pelvis. The dissection necessary to reduce the pelvis often is considerably in excess of that needed to repair the obstruction alone. If renal pelvis reduction is deemed necessary or desirable, there will be a discrepancy in the length of the pyelotomy and the ureteral spatulation, such that a "tennis racket" closure will be necessary. The long limb of the racket is usually closed with a continuous suture.

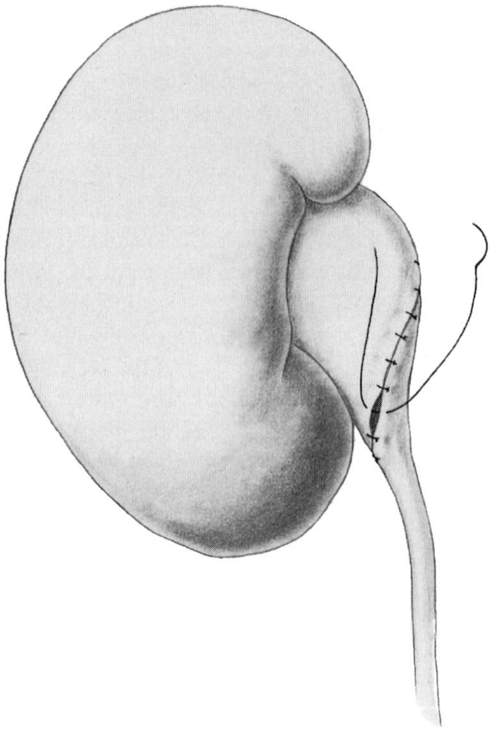

Figure 2–7 Completed dismembered pyeloplasty.

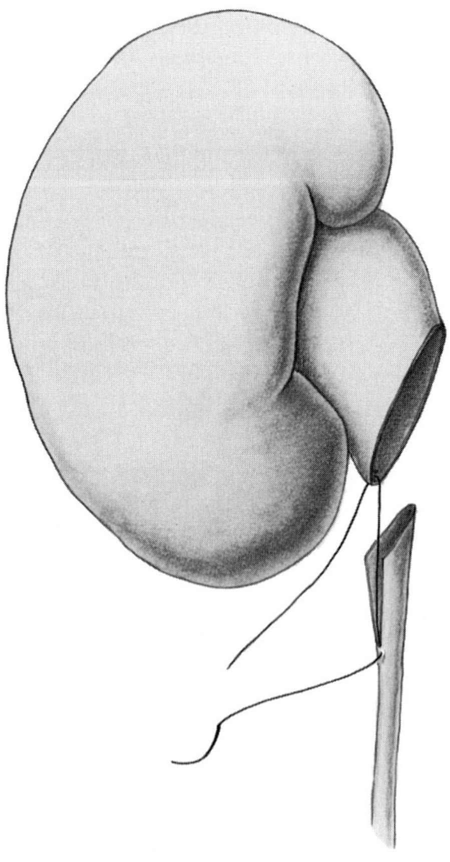

Figure 2–6 Dismembered pyeloplasty showing renal pelvic tongue and lateral spatulation of the ureter.

When there is a long area of stenosis or when, despite downward displacement of the kidney and mobilization of the ureter, there will not be a tension-free anastomosis, the Davis intubated ureterotomy is a useful procedure. It is based on the premise that a buried strip of urothelium will form itself into a tube as it heals. After the stenotic area is identified, stay sutures are placed in the ureter roughly 1 cm above and 1 cm below the stenotic area (Fig. 2–8). A longitudinal ureterotomy is created between the stay sutures. A nephrostomy is placed in the kidney, and a ureteral stent is placed through the ureterotomy, extending from the kidney into the bladder (Fig. 2–9). The stent is left indwelling for approximately 6 weeks. It is preferable to have the stent exit the renal parenchyma and the skin of the flank rather than to internalize it, because the stent can then be removed without another anesthetic. Once the stent has been removed, a nephrostogram is performed to ascertain that there is no extravasation and that there is transport of contrast down the ureter. At that point, the nephrostomy is clamped for a trial for a day or two and, if successful, removed at that time.

There are some instances in reoperation cases in which there is so much fibrosis around the renal pelvis that a dismembered pyeloplasty would be quite difficult to accomplish. In these instances, a ureterocalycostomy becomes the procedure of choice (Figs. 2–10 and 2–11). The lower pole of the kidney is amputated sufficiently to expose the lower calices. The ureter is transected where it enters the cicatrix surrounding the renal pelvis, is spatulated, and is anastomosed to the lower pole calix with fine, interrupted chromic catgut sutures using magnification and gentle tissue handling. If, as is usually true, the overlying renal parenchyma is thin, this is relatively easily accomplished. It is important that the parenchyma be resected to a point above the calicoureteral suture line to prevent the parenchyma from contracting about the anastomosis and thereby obstructing it. It is our practice to use both a stent and a nephrostomy when this type of procedure is performed. Placing omentum or fat over the repair may reduce scarring and facilitate success.[34]

The Foley Y-V pyeloplasty can be used if there is a high insertion of the ureter into the renal pelvis and if there is an extrarenal pelvis (Figs. 2–12 and 2–13). These criteria are most often fulfilled when there is a UPJ obstruction associated with a horseshoe kidney. After the renal pelvis and proximal ureter have been sufficiently exposed, stay sutures are placed in the renal pelvis at the UPJ, in the ureter through the wall adjacent to but well below the UPJ, and in the renal pelvis anteriorly and posteriorly at a distance equivalent to the distance from

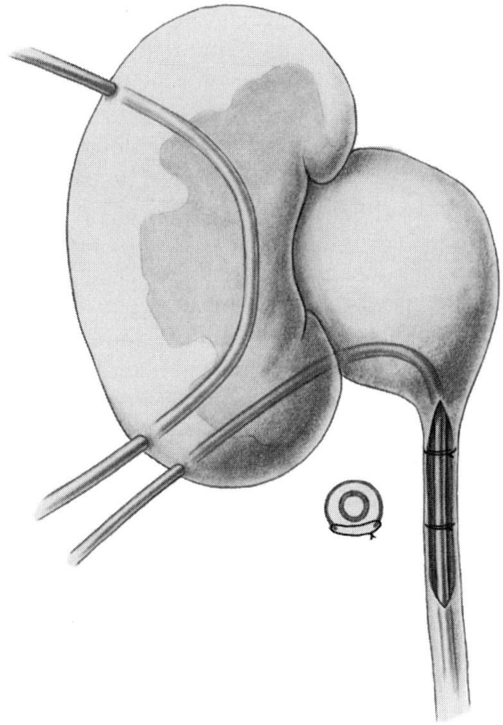

Figure 2–9 Davis intubated ureterotomy with stent and circle nephrostomy in place.

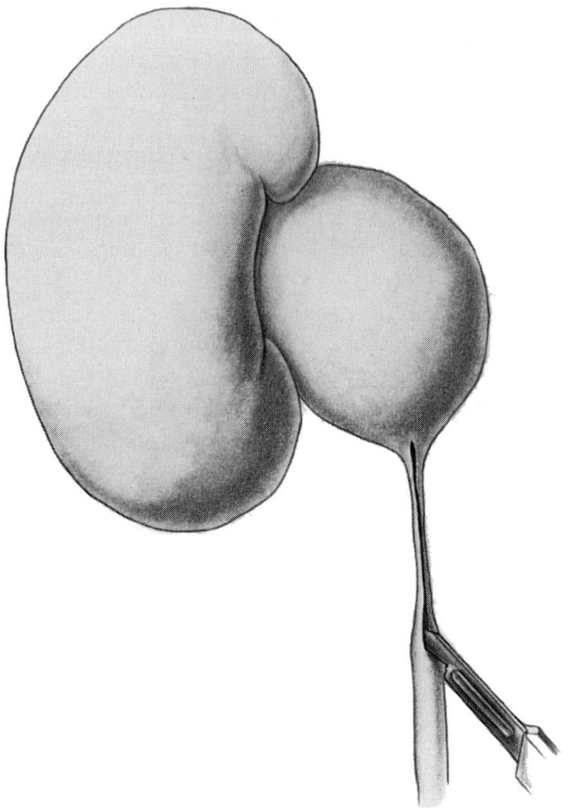

Figure 2–8 Long ureteropelvic junction obstruction.

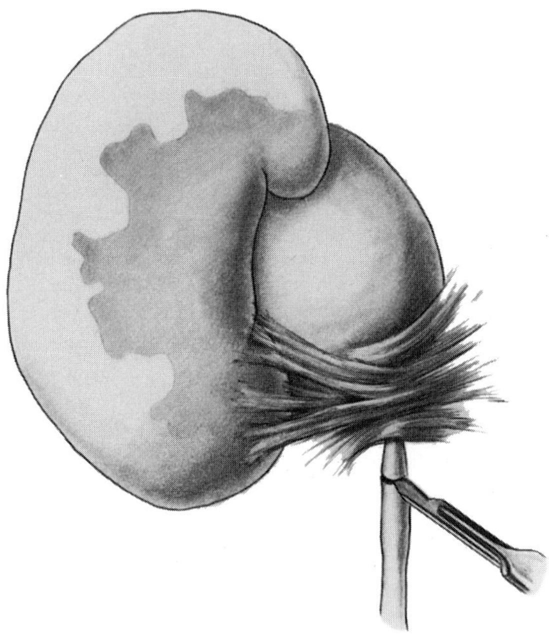

Figure 2–10 Intense ureteropelvic junction fibrosis.

the UPJ to the ureteral stay suture. The renal pelvis is then incised from each stay suture to the UPJ and the ureter is incised from the ureteropelvic junction to the distal stay suture. The dependent tongue of renal pelvis is then advanced to the apex of the ureterotomy and the resulting V-shaped incision is closed with interrupted chromic catgut sutures.

In general, ureteral stents, splints, or nephrostomies are not routinely used, but situations do arise in which stenting may be valuable (recent infection or inflammation with friable tissue or technically difficult dissection and repair). It is believed that nephrostomy drainage should also be used when a stent is necessary, but the converse is not necessarily true. Azotemia or recent infection would mandate nephrostomy drainage, but a stent would not be necessary.

In all cases, Penrose drains are placed after the completion of the anastomosis. Our preference is to place two separate Penrose drains through two separate stab incisions. It has been George W. Kaplan's experience that a single Penrose drain has not always adequately drained the retroperitoneum, resulting in a urinoma. Placement of drains in this manner has appeared to alleviate this uncommon but significant complication. The drains are arbitrarily left in place for at least 1 week. The patient is discharged home with the Penrose drains in place and returns to the office for removal. Care of the Penrose drains by the parent is rarely a point of concern because there is usually little drainage. The presence of the drains provides an added measure of safety, however, as the repair heals. A Foley catheter is placed at the conclusion of the cystoscopic examination and is usually removed on the first or second postoperative day. A nasogastric tube is placed when an anterior transperitoneal approach is used. It too is removed on the first or second postoperative day when active bowel sounds return or when the patient is passing flatus.

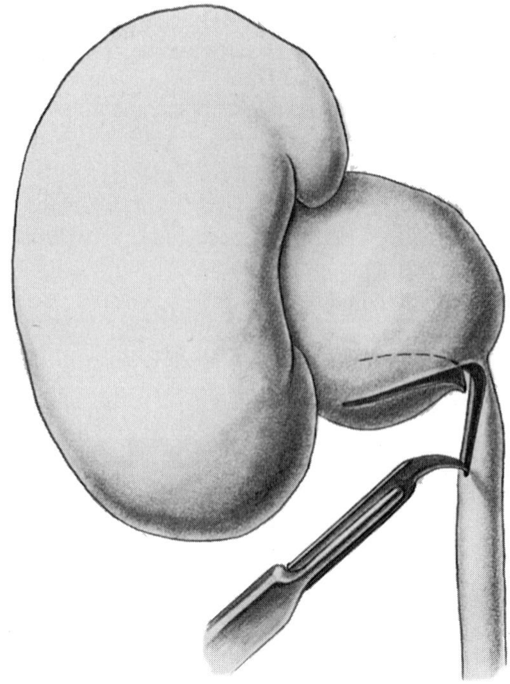

Figure 2–12 Initial incision for creation of a Y-V pyeloplasty.

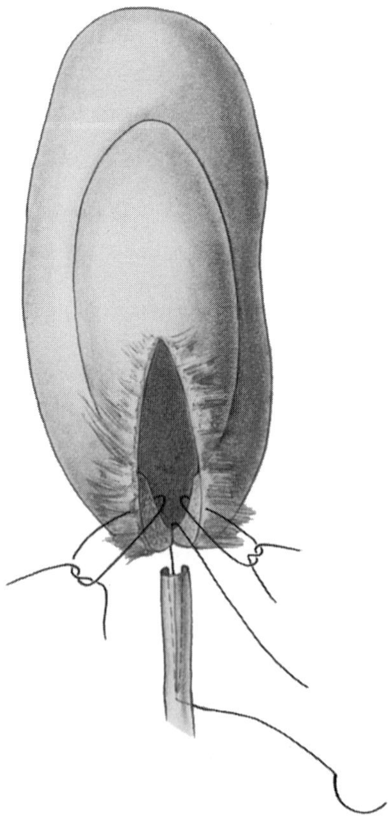

Figure 2–11 Ureterocalicostomy.

It has been our practice to obtain a renal biopsy at the time of UPJ obstruction repair. An elliptical wedged-shaped piece of renal cortex measuring 6 to 7 mm in length is obtained from the lower pole of the kidney. The biopsy site is closed with a horizontal mattress suture of 3-0 chromic. The specimen is sent to the pathology department for standard hematoxylin and eosin staining. We have found microscopy results helpful in reconciling the results of the postoperative differential renal function. Stock and others[34] studied 17 patients undergoing unilateral pyeloplasty and renal biopsy. Six patients had an abnormal renal biopsy, five of whom demonstrated preoperative differential renal function on radionuclide renal scanning of less than 35%. None of these kidneys showed postoperative improvement in renal function despite a technically successful result, and some lost function relative to the other kidney. All remaining 11 kidneys had normal biopsies and preoperative differential renal function of greater than 44%. It was concluded that patients with a differential renal function of less than 35% have an increased probability of adverse histologic changes

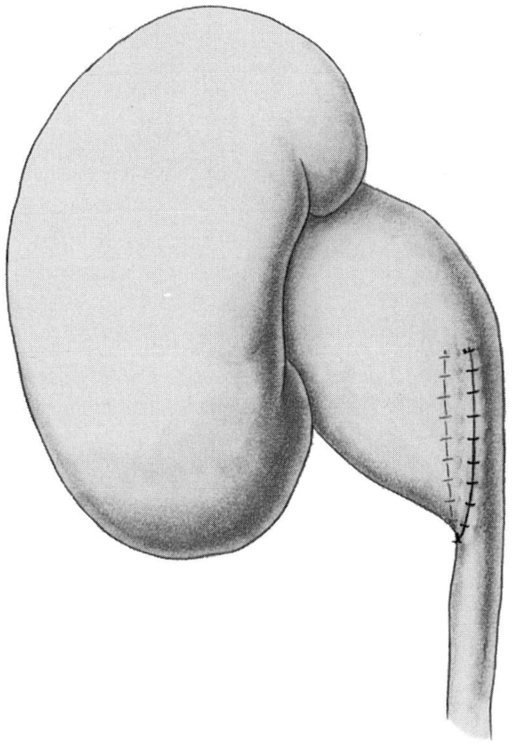

Figure 2–13 Completed Y-V pyeloplasty.

and a lower chance of postoperative improvement in differential function.[34]

Gerota's fascia is not routinely closed. The muscles of the flank incision are closed in layers using suture of the surgeon's preference. The authors have used Dexon, Vicryl, Maxon, and chromic catgut with equally satisfactory results. The anterior transperitoneal incision is closed in two layers. The first layer incorporates the peritoneum, transversalis fascia, and posterior rectus sheath. The second layer incorporates the anterior rectus sheath. Again, the suture type and size are the surgeon's choice, although chromic catgut is generally advised. Scarpa's fascia is reapproximated with a running 4-0 chromic suture, and the skin is closed with a running subcuticular 5-0 PDS suture.

Postoperatively, the diet is advanced as tolerated once bowel activity is present. Several doses of perioperative intravenous antibiotics are given followed by oral prophylactic doses (usually trimethoprim-sulfamethoxazole [Septra]) in those children older than 2 months. Children younger than 2 months are given amoxicillin or ampicillin. The gauze dressings overlying the Penrose drains are changed regularly and weighed, and output is recorded at the bedside chart. Immediate postoperative pain management currently varies between standard intravenous narcotics, single-injection caudal anesthetic followed by intravenous narcotics, or an epidural catheter administering a mixture of bupivacaine (Marcaine) and fentanyl, depending on the preferences of the parents and anesthesiologist. The epidural catheter, if used, is generally in place for 24 to 48 hours, after which it is removed and the child is started on oral analgesics. Patients are generally discharged on the third or fourth postoperative day.

The patients are seen in the office 7 to 10 days after surgery for removal of the Penrose drain. A MAG3 furosemide (Lasix) renal scan is obtained at 3 months to document the postoperative result. A renal ultrasonogram is repeated yearly. If the sonogram shows poor interval growth, a furosemide renal scan is then repeated. The renal biopsy is especially helpful in this situation, because when the renal scan shows poor differential function postoperatively without evidence of obstruction, the intraoperative renal biopsy has invariably been abnormal, predicting poor renal function postoperatively. If follow-up renal ultrasonogram demonstrates increased hydronephrosis, a diuretic renal scan is repeated. If there is not prompt washout of isotope, a Whitaker test may be needed to ascertain whether there is recurrence of obstruction.

Endopyelotomy

Open pyeloplasty is the current standard by which all other modalities are gauged. The success of open surgical correction of UPJ obstruction is greater than 95%.[35, 36] Endopyelotomy in children, although seemingly less invasive, is reserved for secondary UPJ obstruction after failure of primary open pyeloplasty. In general, there is no good instrumentation for this procedure, especially in small children. Experience with endopyelotomy is much greater in adults, and the instrumentation is better. King and colleagues reported the first series of endoscopic incision of ureteral strictures in two children.[37] Other investigators have reported small series involving endopyelotomy in children for secondary UPJ obstruction, with success rates ranging from 67 to 100%.[38–41] Presently, there is no standard established method for the performance of this procedure in children. We have on occasion used balloon dilation of a narrowed anastomosis through a percutaneous nephrostomy. We have also incised the UPJ using a cold knife through a 20 French sheath in two older boys with less than stellar results. Further experience is needed to establish the indications and efficacy of this procedure. Endopyelotomy is not recommended as a primary method of repair for UPJ obstruction given the high success rate and low morbidity of open surgical repair. Because of its decreased morbidity compared with open repair, it may be appropriate to use endopyelotomy in failed cases of open repair in an attempt to avoid a repeat open operation.

SUMMARY

The UPJ is the most common site of urinary tract obstruction, occurring in 1 in 1500 births. Most cases are now detected during prenatal screening. Symptomatic patients have UTIs, abdominal masses, gastrointestinal discomfort, or hematuria. Hydronephrosis does not equate with obstruction. Further evaluation of hydronephrosis with serial ultrasonography, diuretic renography, and the Whitaker test help to identify obstructing lesions. A VCUG is necessary to exclude vesicoureteral reflux. Open surgical repair with a dismembered pyeloplasty is well tolerated in the neonate and has a high rate of success (95%). Endopyelotomy is reserved for failed pyeloplasties.

REFERENCES

1. Murphy L. The history of urology. In The Kidney. Springfield, IL: Charles C Thomas, 1972, p 197.
2. Mathe CP. Kidney surgery. In Bellenger EG, Frontz WA, Homer HG, Lewis B (eds), History of Urology. Baltimore, MD: Williams & Wilkins, 1933, p 281.
3. Langman J. Urogenital system. In Medical Embryology, 4th ed. Baltimore, MD: Williams & Wilkins, 1981, p 234.
4. Flashner SC, King LR. UPJ. In Kelalis PP, King LR, Belman AB (eds), Clinical Pediatric Urology. Philadelphia: WB Saunders, 1992, p 693.
5. Leeson TS, Leeson CR. The urinary system. In Histology. Philadelphia: WB Saunders, 1981, p 451.
6. Maizels M, Stephens FD. Valves of the ureter as cause of primary obstruction of the ureter: Anatomic, embryologic and clinical aspects. J Urol 123:742, 1980.
7. Gillenwater JY. Hydronephrosis-induced change in renal hemodynamics and function. Cardiovasc Med 4:701, 1979.
8. Arendhorst WJ, Finn WF, Gottschalk CW. Nephron stop flow pressure response to obstruction for 24 hours in the rat kidney. J Clin Invest 53:1497, 1975.
9. Yarger WE, Aynedijian HS, Bank N. A micropuncture study of postobstructive diuresis in the rat. J Clin Invest 51:625, 1972.
10. Gillenwater JY, Westervelt FB Jr, Vaughan E Jr, Howards SS. Renal function after release of chronic unilateral hydronephrosis in man. Kidney Int 7:179, 1975.
11. Rose BD: Pathophysiology of Renal Disease. New York: McGraw-Hill, 1981, p 350.
12. Koff SA, Hayden LJ, Cirulli C, et al. Pathophysiology of ureteropelvic junction obstruction: Experimental and clinical observations. J Urol 136:336, 1986.
13. Koff SA. The diagnosis of obstruction in experimental hydronephrosis. Invest Urol 19:85, 1981.
14. Olsen PR. The renal pelvis and ureteral peristalsis. T pelvometry. Scand J Urol Nephrol 13:269, 1979.
15. Mandell J, Peters CA, Retik AB. Current concepts in the perinatal diagnosis and management of hydronephrosis. Urol Clin North Am 17:247, 1990.
16. Blyth B, Snyder HM, Duckett JW. Antenatal diagnosis and subsequent management of hydronephrosis. J Urol 149:693, 1993.
17. Thomas DFM, Madden NP, Irving HC, et al. Mild dilatation of the fetal kidney: A follow up study. Br J Urol 74:236, 1994.
18. Homsy YL, Willot P, Danais S. Transitional neonatal hydronephrosis: Fact or fantasy? J Urol 136:339, 1986.
19. Koff SA, Campbell K. Nonoperative management of unilateral neonatal hydronephrosis. J Urol 148:525, 1992.
20. Maizels M, Mitchell B, Kass E, et al. Outcome of nonspecific hydronephrosis in the infant: A report from the registry of the Society for Fetal Urology. J Urol 152:2324, 1994.
21. Mandell J, Peters CA. Antenatal diagnosis and intervention in urologic disease. In Kelalis PP, King LR, Belman AB (eds), Clinical Pediatric Urology. Philadelphia: WB Saunders, 1992, pp 1–12.
22. Bryan PJ, Azimi F. Ultrasound in diagnosis of congenital hydronephrosis due to obstruction of pelviureteric junction. Urology 5:17, 1975.
23. Johnston JH, Evans JP, Glassberg KI, Shapiro SR. Pelvic hydronephrosis in children: A review of 219 personal cases. J Urol 117:97, 1977.
24. Valayer J, Adda G. Hydronephrosis due to pelviureteric junction obstruction in infancy. Br J Urol 54:451, 1982.

24a. Flashner SC, King LR: UPJ. In Kelalis PP, King LR, Belman AB (eds), Clinical Pediatric Urology. Philadephia: WB Saunders, 1992, p 699.

25. Brown T, Mandell J, Lebowitz RL. Neonatal hydronephrosis in the era of sonography. AJR 148:959, 1987.
26. Livera LN, Broolfield DSK, Egginton JA, Hawnaur JM. Antenatal ultrasonography to detect fetal renal abnormalities: A prospective screening program. Brit Med J 298:1421, 1989.
27. Wiener JS, Emmert GK, Mesrobian HG, et al. Are modern imaging techniques over diagnosing ureteropelvic junction obstruction. J Urol 154:659, 1995.
28. Koff SA, Peller PA, Young DC, Pollifrone DL. The assessment of obstruction in the newborn with unilateral hydronephrosis by measuring the size of the opposite kidney. J Urol 152:596, 1994.
29. Koff SA, Peller PA. Diagnostic criteria for assessing obstruction in the newborn with unilateral hydronephrosis using the renal growth-renal function chart. J Urol 154:662, 1995.
30. Grignon A, Filion R, Filiatrault D, et al. Urinary tract dilatation in utero: Classification and clinical applications. Radiology 160:645, 1986.
31. Conway JJ. The "well tempered" diuretic renogram: A standard method to examine the asymptomatic neonate with hydronephrosis or hydroureteronephrosis. J Nucl Med 33:2047, 1992.
32. Cockrell SA, Hendren WH. The importance of visualizing the ureter before performing a pyeloplasty. J Urol 144:588, 1990.
33. Heffernan JP, Stock JA, Packer MG, Kaplan GW. In support of routine visualization of the ureter prior to pyeloplasty in children. Presented at AUA Western Section. Seattle, WA, August 1994.
34. Stock JA, Krous HF, Heffernan J, et al. Correlation of renal biopsy and radionuclide renal scan differential function in patients with unilateral ureteroplevic junction obstruction. J Urol 154:716, 1995.
35. Scardino PT, Scardino PL. Obstruction at the ureteropelvic junction. In Bergman H (ed), The Ureter, 2nd ed. New York: Springer-Verlag, 1981, p 617.
36. Hendren WH, Radhakrishman J, Middleton AW Jr. Pediatric pyeloplasty. J Pediatr Surg 15:133, 1980.
37. King LR, Coughlin PWF, Ford KK, et al. Initial experience with percutaneous and transurethral ablation of postoperative urethral strictures in children. J Urol 145:345, 1991.
38. Kovoussi LR, Meretyk S, Dierks SM, et al. Endopyelotomy for secondary ureteropelvic junction obstruction in children. J Urol 145:345, 1991.
39. Tan HL, Najmaldin A, Webb DR. Endopyelotomy for pelvi-ureteric junction obstruction in children. Eur Urol 24:84, 1993.
40. Towbin RB, Wacksman J, Ball WS. Percutaneous pyeloplasty in children: Experience in three patients. Radiology 163:381, 1987.
41. Faerber GJ, Ritchey ML, Bloom DA. Percutaneous endopyelotomy in children and young children after failed open pyeloplasty. J Urol 154:1495, 1995.

3

GREGOR K. EMMERT, JR.

Multicystic Kidney

Before the advent of fetal ultrasonography, multicystic dysplastic kidney (MCDK), defined as a unilateral grossly dysplastic organ with little or no function in which cystic elements predominate, was the most common abdominal, usually flank, mass detected in the neonate by physical examination. The incidence was approximately 1 in 4300 live births.[1, 2] When the cysts are larger, there usually is very little stroma between them, giving the kidney an appearance suggestive of a "bunch of grapes" (Fig. 3–1). The kidneys vary in size from massive, crossing the midline and filling most of the abdomen, to those somewhat smaller than a normal kidney. MCDKs diagnosed at autopsy usually are smaller than those found at nephrectomy.[3, 4] Also included in the category are kidneys that have small or microscopic cysts. Potter referred to the large cystic variety as type IIA cystic disease and the smaller variety as type IIB cystic disease. Others have used the term *solid cystic dysplasia* to describe the smaller but still cystic variety (Fig. 3–2). Both types exemplify severe renal dysplasia and differ mainly in the relative amount of stroma and the size of the cysts. In general, those kidneys with small cysts tend to be smaller and have relatively more stroma. What is common to all kidneys within this group is the finding of cysts, whether large or small, and primitive ducts.[5]

Schwartz, in 1936, was the first to propose the term *unilateral multicystic kidney*. However, subsequently, it was shown that the condition may occasionally be bilateral.[6–8] Bilateral disease, of course, is incompatible with life because of the lack of functional tissue. Neonates affected bilaterally have the classic features of Potter's syndrome (abnormal compressed facies from oligohydramnios).[7] Historically, the term *multicystic kidney* had been used interchangeably with polycystic kidney until Spence emphasized the need to separate these entities completely. He argued that the term multicystic kidney should mean a situation in which all the cysts are confined to one nonvisualizing kidney. The other kidney is always noncystic but is associated with a high risk of another abnormality. This contralateral disease may consist of ureteropelvic junction (UPJ) obstruction, reflux, ureterovesical junction (UVJ) obstruction or bladder outlet obstruction. It is now clear that the pathologic lesion that is multicystic kidney may be bilateral, but the convention of using "multicystic kidney" to describe the common unilateral lesion is useful and conveys the idea that the contralateral kidney must be carefully evaluated. In any case, bilateral multicystic kidney disease is incompatible with life, although one infant was reported to have survived 69 days.[5, 9]

CLINICAL FEATURES

Multicystic dysplasia is the most common form of renal cystic disease in infants, and in the majority of studies it has been reported as the most common or second most common entity responsible for an abdominal mass in

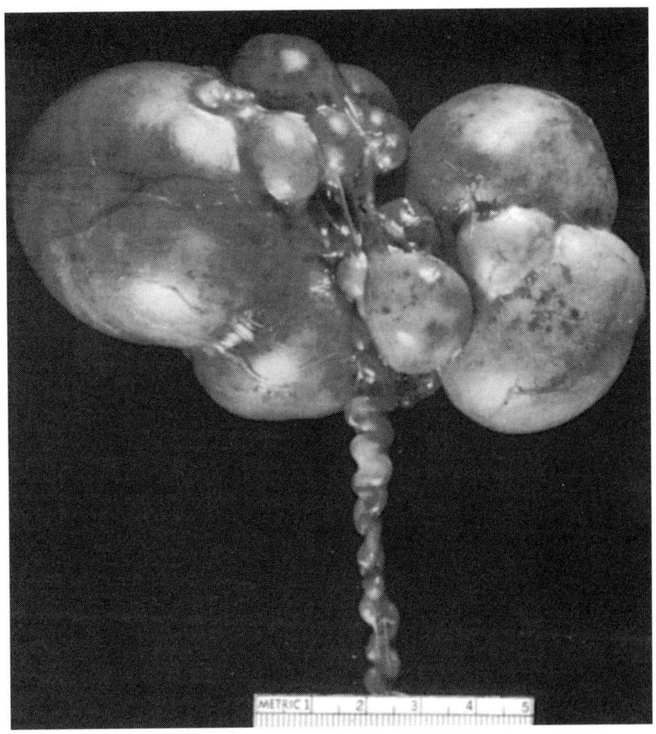

Figure 3–1 This type IIA multicystic kidney has a tortuous, atretic ureter and cysts that vary in size. From Glassberg KI, Filmer RB. Renal dysplasia, renal hypoplasia, and cystic disease of the kidney. In Kelalis PP, King LR, Belman AB (eds), Clinical Pediatric Urology. Philadelphia: WB Saunders, 1992, p 1155. Used with permission.

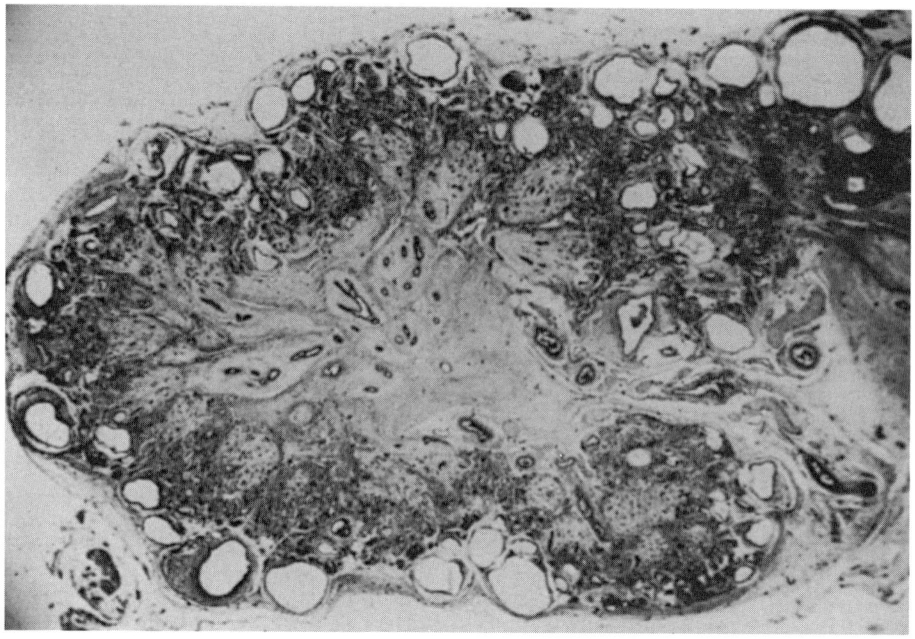

Figure 3–2 Less obvious cysts and a smaller kidney are seen in this Potter's type IIB cystic kidney. From Potter EL. Normal and Abnormal Development of the Kidney. Chicago: Year Book Medical Publishers, 1972. Used with permission.

infants.[10–12] Because of the widespread use of in utero ultrasonographic scanning, there are now a large number of cases being identified prenatally. In the adult, the diagnosis is usually made as an incidental finding during a workup for unrelated symptoms or for abdominal pain, hypertension, or hematuria.[5]

The natural history of the multicystic kidney both antenatally and postnatally, is unfolding because of the increased use of sonography. One finding is a high incidence in some series of bilaterality of the disease or the association of a multicystic kidney with contralateral renal agenesis, neither condition being compatible with life.[5] A 19% incidence of bilateral multicystic kidneys was detected in a series of 27 MCK patients evaluated antenatally.[13] Another feature of the multicystic kidney is the involution that can occur either before or after birth.[14, 15] At times, the involution can be so extreme that the cystic kidney cannot be detected on follow-up ultrasonographic examination. Although the pathogenic process causing a multicystic kidney probably takes place by the eighth week in utero, the mean age at diagnosis of the multicystic kidney in utero is about 28 weeks, with a range of 21 to 35 weeks in most series.[14] The cause for this is not clearly understood. It is important to remember that cystic disease of the kidney cannot be definitively excluded by a midtrimester sonogram alone.[5]

The sex incidence has varied among reports, but overall it is probably equal or slightly more common in males. Blacks are probably less affected than whites, as evidenced by one series of 49 patients, of whom only 4 were black (in an institution in which a third of the patients admitted are black).[4] Multicystic kidney is almost always a unilateral condition, encountered most often on the left side.[10, 16–19] Cases of horseshoe kidney have been reported in which only one side was affected.[5, 6, 20]

In most cases, the multicystic kidney does not in itself cause any further problems. However, the opposite urinary tract is often diseased. Contralateral UPJ or primary obstructive megaloureter is common.[6, 19] The presence of associated urologic abnormalities in patients with MCDK is as high as 51%, with most patients having contralateral vesicoureteral reflux or a UPJ obstruction, and others having UVJ obstruction, contralateral renal hypodysplasia, and fetal ureteral folds.[5, 10, 21–24] Although fetal ureteral folds may be a normal transient finding in infants, the high incidence of this finding suggests a possible ureteral anomaly as the cause of multicystic kidney.

PATHOLOGY

Multicystic kidneys vary in size. The kidneys with large cysts tend to be large with little stroma between the cysts; those with small cysts are larger and more solid in appearance. The blood supply to the multicystic kidney is also variable, ranging from a definite pedicle with small vessels to no pedicle at all.[5, 18]

Microscopically, primitive dysplastic elements are located centrally and between the cysts.[25] Mature glomeruli, although sparse, may be present. Most often, the cysts are lined by low cuboidal epithelium and are separated by thin septa of fibrous tissue in primitive elements. Most multicystic kidneys are associated with atresia of part or all of the accompanying ureter. The renal pelvis may or may not be present. The MCDK without histologic evidence of communication between cysts and without a pelvis has been referred to as pyeloinfundibular atresia.[10] Yet contrast has been shown radiographically in other patients to pass from one cyst to another via tubules located in the cysts.[26] A variety of multicystic kidney with a renal pelvis and with communication between the cysts and pelvis has also been reported and has been referred to as the hydronephrotic type of multicystic kidney.[5, 27]

ETIOLOGY

Because of the high association of ureteral atresia, various investigators have tried to produce multicystic kidneys in animals by ligating the ureter at different times during gestation. Multicystic dysplasia could not be induced in animal studies when the ureter was tied off during mid or late gestation.[28–30] However, ligation of the fetal ureter in the lamb during early gestation did produce dysplasia.[29] This suggested that urinary obstruction may be a cause of dysplasia, but only when the obstruction is present during early gestation. However, dysplasia could not be induced in the chick embryo even with ligation of the ureter at a very early stage.[5, 31]

MCDK may represent an extreme form of hydronephrosis that develops secondary to atresia of the ureter, pelvis, or both.[27] Also suggesting the possibility of obstruction as the cause is the fact that the left kidney—the one more often affected with multicystic dysplasia—is also the kidney more often found to have primary obstructive megaloureter and UPJ obstruction.[5, 32, 33]

Other theories have been offered on the cause of MCDK, including a failure of union between the ureteric bud and the metanephric blastema, resulting in cystic dilatation of the blastema, a theory that is supported clinically by the high incidence of associated ureteral atresia.[34] It has also been suggested that type IIA kidneys (those with large cysts) result from an ampullary abnormality in which the ampullae stop dividing before they normally would and, therefore, produce fewer generations of tubules. The last generation of tubules is cystic, and they fail to induce normal metanephric differentiation. The occasional normal or near-normal nephron that is sometimes found in these kidneys occurs only in rare instances when the ampullae and collecting tubules are normal enough to induce them.[5, 8, 35]

INVESTIGATION

Ultrasonography is particularly useful in differentiating fluid-filled structures from solid tissue in evaluating abdominal masses of renal origin in infants, and therefore sonography has become a prime tool for diagnosing multicystic kidneys (Fig. 3–3). However, in some cases, it may be difficult to differentiate multicystic kidney disease from severe hydronephrosis, because the cysts may be arranged to mimic a dilated pelvis with peripheral dilated calices.[5, 36, 37] An interface between cysts, a nonmedial location of the larger cysts, and an absence of an identifiable renal sinus are typical ultrasonographic features diagnostic of MCDK.[38] However, when a large cyst appears medial on ultrasonogram, it mimics the renal pelvis in appearance. When lateral cysts seem to communicate and radiate from a larger medial cyst, the diagnosis of hydronephrosis becomes more likely. This may be important clinically to some surgeons who may choose not to remove the multicystic kidney, but who may prefer to remove a nonfunctioning hydronephrotic kidney or repair a UPJ obstruction when function is detected only on renal scan.[5]

The unusual so-called hydronephrotic form of

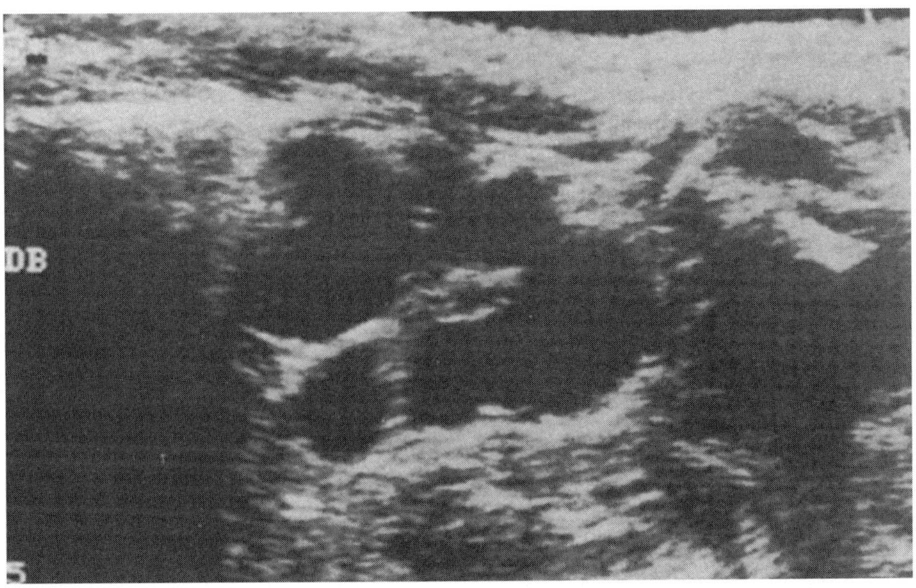

Figure 3–3 An irregular arrangement of cysts is present on this renal ultrasonogram of a multicystic dysplastic kidney. From Glassberg KI, Filmer RB. Renal dysplasia, renal hypoplasia, and cystic disease of the kidney. In Kelalis PP, King LR, Belman AB (eds), Clinical Pediatric Urology. Philadelphia: WB Saunders, 1992, p 1161. Used with permission.

MCDK, in which a renal pelvis may be present, can cause a diagnostic dilemma. Nuclear studies are helpful in differentiating a poorly functioning hydronephrotic kidney from a multicystic kidney. In most cases of hydronephrotic kidney that do not visualize on excretory urogram, some evidence of renal function is found on dimercaptosuccinic acid scan, whereas renal visualization is rare in an MCK. Because of immature renal function, the intravenous pyelogram (IVP) is of limited use in neonates. The diagnosis can also be confirmed with a technetium 99m–mercaptoacetyltriglycine scan. Angiography, although rarely indicated for the evaluation of the mass, may not demonstrate a renal artery in multicystic kidney. When one is seen, it is likely to be very small. Cystoscopy is also usually unwarranted, but if performed may reveal a hemitrigone with absent ipsilateral ureteric orifice. More commonly, an orifice is present, but retrograde catheterization is likely to demonstrate an atretic ureter.[5, 39]

MANAGEMENT

Historically, before the era of sonography, MCDK was recognized as a common cause of abdominal mass in the newborn and was frequently removed surgically because of difficulty in determining the precise diagnosis, as well as concern about potential complications such as malignancy, hypertension, urinary tract infection or abscess, and pain.[21, 40] Successful cyst aspiration for the rare case of respiratory embarrassment has also been reported.[40, 41] The security with which the diagnosis can be established today and the relatively few late complications of MCDK have led to the suggestion that patients may be managed with surveillance instead of by nephrectomy, and the treatment of this entity thus remains controversial. The National Multicystic Kidney Registry was established in 1968 through the American Academy of Pediatrics, Section of Urology, to help track the natural history of patients with this disorder.[21, 40]

Clear indications for surgical management have presented in numerous patients. One report reviewed 27 adults who required surgery for pain or infection.[42] Furthermore, nine cases of malignancy in association with MCDK have been reported since 1957, including six cases in children: four Wilms' tumors, one adenosarcoma, and one renal cell carcinoma.[1] Two additional malignancies were reported in 1997, both in 4-month-old infants with multicystic kidneys. Of the first 508 patients registered in the National Multicystic Kidney Registry, misdiagnosis occurred in 6 of the first 181 operated cases, but the hydronephrosis was so severe that the kidneys were not salvageable (J. Wacksman and L. Phipps, personal communication, 1994).[2] Thirteen patients in the registry had urinary tract infections, and two had hematuria. One of the patients had pain, but no tumors were reported.[40]

Four patients in the registry were also noted to be hypertensive, although it can be argued that the hypertension is not always related to the MCDK. However, a number of other reports implicate the MCDK in development of hypertension. Susskind and colleagues reported two patients with hypertension cured by removal of an MCDK.[1] Gordon and others previously reported nine cases with associated hypertension, of which three became normotensive after nephrectomy.[43] That a single physician (L. R. King) observed three of those reported cases indicates that the incidence of hypertension associated with MCDK may be under-reported. There is personal knowledge of an additional three patients with hypertension cured by removal of an MCDK (J. Elder, personal communication, 1994). Indeed, 15 of 136 (11%) pediatric urologists in reply to a survey stated that they had seen or treated patients with MCDK and hypertension.[40, 44]

Furthermore, many MCDKs have been discovered in older children and adults during evaluation for hypertension. Nephrectomy has rarely cured hypertension of long or unknown duration. This does not mean that the hypertension was not caused initially by the MCDK, because arteriolar thickening in the contralateral, usually originally normal, kidney would occur if such hypertension were sustained; the contralateral arteriolar thickening would tend to produce continued hypertension after removal of the MCDK, even if the cystic kidney was the original cause of the elevated blood pressure.[1, 40]

If patients with MCDK are to be managed by surveillance, following for hypertension must be rigorous. Unfortunately, it is relatively difficult to obtain blood pressure measurements in infants, and the fact that such infants do not appear ill discourages regular and costly return visits at regular but lengthy intervals. In fact, of the first 508 patients enrolled in the National Multicystic Kidney Registry, 42 (8.3%) were lost to follow-up even by physicians who made a special effort to keep track of these patients.[2] If such patients are to be managed nonoperatively, it remains to be determined how much follow-up is required as well as whether or not such follow-up is practical in terms of out-of-pocket cost and actually achieving the degree of follow-up that was initially planned.[40]

NEPHRECTOMY

Nephrectomy can be performed by either open or laparoscopic techniques.[45] With an open technique, the patient is placed in the extended flank position, and a regional block is often performed, usually with an intracostal block between the 10th, 11th, and 12th ribs with 0.25% bupivacaine with epinephrine (1 per 300,000 parts) with 0.25 to 0.5 mL injected per level through a 25-gauge butterfly needle. A small incision is made off the tip of the 12th rib, and the incision is extended through the muscle layers until the retroperitoneum is identified. Gerota's fascia is incised posteriorally, and Deaver retractors are inserted into the wound. The kidney is mobilized with the help of a traction suture. If necessary, a distended renal pelvis or fluid-filled cysts may be aspirated, facilitating separation of the kidney from adjacent structures. After the kidney is mobilized completely, the vascular pedicle is suture ligated with two sutures of 2-0 or 3-0 polyglycolic acid. Typically, the artery and vein cannot be easily distinguished and are usually ligated as a single entity. The ureter is also suture ligated with 4-0 polyglycolic acid.

Children are fed on awakening and are discharged home after they have eaten. Mean operating time is approximately 45 minutes. Some difficulties with exposure can be expected with this technique, because the appendix, the pancreas, and the aorta have all been partially removed with the specimen at one time or another. These misadventures are prevented by staying on the cysts and being certain that no other tissues are removed. If the multicystic kidney has a solid component and tumor is suspected, transperitoneal or thoracoabdominal exploration is recommended to facilitate radical nephrectomy.

Laparoscopic nephrectomies have been performed in the management of renal tumors, renal vascular hypertension, multicystic or otherwise dysplastic kidneys, chronic pain, or infection in a nonfunctioning kidney and in infected kidneys containing a calculus.[46, 47] The usual technique for the more commonly performed transperitoneal laparoscopic nephrectomy includes the use of four or five trocar sites (at the umbilicus, midclavicular, and anterior axillary lines), full mechanical and antimicrobial bowel preparation, and cystoscopy with placement of a ureteral catheter.[48] A nasogastric tube and Foley catheter are inserted. These are removed in the recovery room or later.[44, 48] Four trocar sites have also been used to perform retroperitoneal laparoscopic nephrectomy.[49] However, surgical exposure has been found to be excellent for left transperitoneal laparoscopic nephrectomy without mechanical bowel cleansing. Placement of a ureteral catheter cystoscopically to guide the dissection is unnecessary, and surgical dissection may be accomplished successfully using only three trocar sites.[47]

After administration of general anesthesia, a nasogastric tube and Foley catheter are placed. The patient is placed in approximately 40-degree right lateral decubitus position to remove the left kidney (Fig. 3–4). Approximately 40-degree left lateral rotation is then applied to the table to make the abdomen horizontal with the floor. The patient is prepared from just above the nipples to the midthighs and is sterile draped.[47]

An 11-mm curved skin incision is made at the base of the umbilicus, and electrocautery is used to extend the incision through the rectus fascia. The peritoneum is opened sharply, taking care to avoid injury to the under-

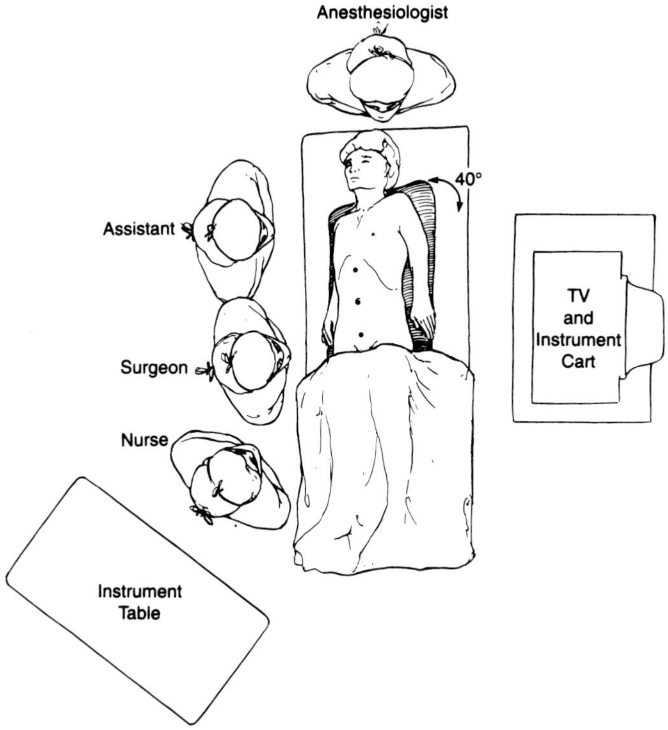

Figure 3–4 Illustration showing the patient's 40-degree lateral decubitus position; the position of the surgeons, scrub nurse, and camera; and the three sites for trocar placement. From Emmert G Jr, Eubanks S, King L. Improved technique of laparoscopic nephrectomy for multicystic dysplastic kidney. Urology 44:423, 1994. Used with permission.

lying viscera. Vicryl sutures are placed in the opposing edges of rectus fascia. A 10-mm Hassen trocar is passed intraperitoneally, and carbon dioxide is insufflated to a pressure of 12 mm Hg. At this time, both surgeons and the scrub nurse are positioned on the side of the table opposite the multicystic kidney, a 0-degree lens is inserted, and the entire abdomen is inspected for possible injury. It should be noted that the complication of major vascular or bowel injuries encountered with use of the Veress needle is reduced or eliminated using this open technique. Regardless, blood type and screen are necessary, and a full set of laparotomy instruments must be immediately available in the operating room at all times.[47]

Next, under direct vision, a 10-mm trocar is placed in the midepigastrium, a 5-mm trocar is placed in the suprapubic midline, and the table is rotated to place the patient in a right lateral decubitus position to provide gravity retraction of the colon and facilitate exposure of the left kidney. Grasping forceps and electrocautery scissors are introduced, and the posterior parietal peritoneum lateral to the descending colon is grasped and incised along the line of Toldt from the aortic bifurcation to the splenic flexure. Blunt dissection is used to further mobilize the colon medially. After the left ureter is identified, the overlying peritoneum is incised. Sharp and blunt

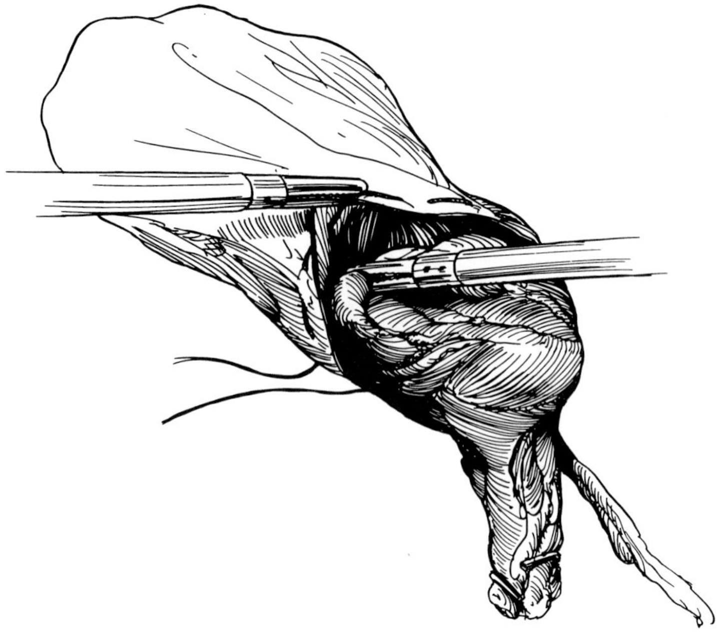

Figure 3–5 The multicystic dysplastic kidney is placed in the Cook-Lapsac bag. From Emmert GJ Jr, Eubanks S, King L. Improved technique of laparoscopic nephrectomy for multicystic dysplastic kidney. Urology 44:424, 1994. Used with permission.

dissection is used to free the ureter up to the level of the renal pelvis, and traction on the ureter with the grasping forceps permits easy identification of the kidney. Gerota's fascia is incised laterally, and the perinephric fat is dissected off the kidney laterally, superiorly, inferiorly, and finally medially toward the pedicle. At this point, the ureter is grasped with Babcock forceps and held up toward the anterior abdominal wall to provide traction and exposure for dissection of the renal pedicle. After sharp and blunt dissection expose the renal pedicle, the entire vascular pedicle is ligated with a 2-0 silk suture passed around the vessels with a laparoscopic right-angle clamp. Ten-millimeter endoclips passed through the epigastric trocar are applied twice on the vessel side and once on the specimen side of the pedicle to ensure hemostasis, and the pedicle is then divided sharply. The ureter is grasped and divided with electrocautery. Suction and irrigation of the surgical site affirm good hemostasis. A Cook-Lapsac bag is inserted through the epigastric trocar and opened with the grasping forceps. The entire specimen is placed in the bag, and the drawstrings are tightened around the bag (Fig. 3–5). With the lens and camera placed through the epigastric trocar, forceps advanced through the umbilical trocar are used to grasp the drawstrings and remove the bag with specimen through the umbilical site. The umbilical trocar is removed from the wound at the same time.[47]

Inspection of the surgical site with reduced insufflation pressure avoids the complication of undetected venous hemorrhage. The umbilical trocar site is inspected for bleeding, as is the suprapubic site on removal of its trocar. Finally, the lens and epigastric trocar are removed. Care is taken to ensure complete desufflation of the abdomen, and figure-eight and interrupted 2-0 Vicryl sutures are used to close the fascia at all wound sites. The nasogastric tube and Foley catheter are usually removed in the operating room.[47]

Alternatively, after the umbilical trocar is placed, the two additional trocars may be placed in the upper and lower abdominal quadrants, between the anterior axillary and midclavicular lines. Operating times as short as 60 to 90 minutes have been reported. Most children have been kept routinely overnight for observation with discharge home the following day.[47, 50] Attempting a retroperitoneal laparoscopic approach in children would require placement of multiple trocars in a very small area, likely resulting in poor instrument maneuverability.[47] Immediate complications, including difficulty with insufflation, hemorrhage, and injury of intraperitoneal structures, can be largely avoided, as noted previously, by using open technique for placement of the initial trocar. Provisions should, of course, be made for a full laparotomy if that becomes a necessity. Viewing the abdominal contents at reduced insufflation pressure will detect troublesome venous bleeding. The incidence of late complications such as bowel obstruction is extremely low, averaging about 0.2%.[47, 51]

Although laparoscopic procedures are expensive, if a child is old enough to be concerned by the cosmetic effects of a scar and too large to permit removal of a kidney through a small open incision, laparoscopy may be quite worthwhile psychologically in preserving or enhancing body image.[51]

REFERENCES

1. Susskind MR, Kim KS, King LR. Hypertension and multicystic kidney. Urology 34:362, 1989.

2. Wacksman J, Phipps L. Report of the multicystic kidney registry: Preliminary findings. J Urol 150:1870, 1993.
3. Bloom DA, Brosman S. The multicystic kidney. J Urol 120:211, 1978.
4. Filmer RB, Taxy JB. A nephrectomy and autopsy review of multicystic kidney dysplasia. unpublished data, 1994.
5. Glassberg KI, Filmer RB. Renal dysplasia, renal hypoplasia, and cystic disease of the kidney. In Kelalis PP, King LR, Belman AB (eds), Clinical Pediatric Urology. Philadelphia: WB Saunders, 1992, p 1121.
6. Greene LF, Feinzaig W, Dahlin DC. Multicystic dysplasia of the kidney: With special reference to the contralateral kidney. J Urol 105:482, 1971.
7. Johannessen JV, Haneberg B, Moe PJ. Bilateral multicystic dysplasia of the kidneys. Beitr Pathol 148:290, 1973.
8. Potter EL. Normal and Abnormal Development of the Kidney. Chicago: Year Book, 1972.
9. Kishikawa T, Toda T, Ito H, et al. Bilateral congenital multicystic dysplasia of the kidney. Jpn J Surg 11:198, 1981.
10. Griscom NT, Vawter FG, Fellers FX. Pelvoinfundibular atresia: The usual form of multicystic kidney; 44 unilateral and two bilateral cases. Semin Roentgenol 10:125, 1975.
11. Longino LA, Martin LW. Abdominal masses in newborn infant. Pediatrics 21:596, 1958.
12. Melicow MM, Uson AC. Palpable abdominal masses in infants and children: A report based on a review of 653 cases. J Urol 81:705, 1959.
13. Kleiner B, Filly R, Mack L, et al. Multicystic dysplastic kidney: Observations of contralateral disease in the fetal population. Radiology 161:27, 1986.
14. Avni E, Thoua Y, Lalmand B, et al. Multicystic dysplastic kidney: Natural history from in utero diagnosis and postnatal follow-up. J Urol 138:1420, 1987.
15. Hashimoto B, Filly R, Cullen P. Multicystic dysplastic kidney in utero: Changing appearance on US. Radiology 159:107, 1986.
16. Fine MG, Burns E. Unilateral multicystic kidney: Report of six cases and discussion of the literature. J Urol 81:42, 1959.
17. Friedman H, Abeshouse BS. Congenital unilateral multicystic kidney: A review of the literature and a report of three cases. Sinai Hosp J (Baltimore) 6:51, 1957.
18. Parkkulamen KV, Hjelt L, Sirola K. Congenital multicystic dysplasia of kidney: Report of nineteen cases with discussion on the etiology: Nomenclature and classification of cystic dysplasia of the kidney. Acta Chir Scand (Suppl) 244:5, 1959.
19. Pathak IG, Williams DI. Multicystic and cystic dysplastic kidneys. Br J Urol 36:318, 1964.
20. Walker RD, Fennell R, Garin E, et al. Spectrum of multicystic renal dysplasia: Diagnosis and management. Urology 11:433, 1978.
21. Mentser M, Mahan J, Koff S. Multicystic dysplastic kidney. Pediatr Nephrol 8:113, 1994.
22. Atiyeh B, Husmann D, Baum M. Contralateral renal abnormalities in multicystic-dysplastic kidney disease. J Pediatr 121:65, 1992.
23. Johnston JH. The pathogenesis of hydronephrosis in children. Br J Urol 41:724, 1969.
24. Ostling K. The genes of hydronephrosis. Acta Chir Scand 86:1, 1942.
25. Bernstein J. Developmental abnormalities of the renal parenchyma — Renal hypoplasia and dysplasia. Pathol Annu 3:213, 1968.
26. Saxton HM, Golding SJ, Chantler C, et al. Diagnostic puncture in renal cystic dysplasia (multicystic kidney): Evidence on the aetiology of the cysts. Br J Urol 54:555, 1981.
27. Felson B, Cussen LJ. The hydronephrotic type of congenital multicystic disease of the kidney. Semin Roentgenol 10:113, 1975.
28. Beck AD. The effect of intra-uterine urinary obstruction upon development of the fetal kidney. J Urol 105:784, 1971.
29. Fetterman GH, Ravitch MM, Sherman FE. Cystic changes in fetal kidneys following ureteral ligation: Studies of microdissection. Kidney Int 5:111, 1974.
30. Tanagho EA. Surgically induced partial urinary obstruction in the fetal lamb: III. Ureteral obstruction. Invest Urol 10:35, 1972.
31. Berman DJ, Maizels M. Role of urinary obstruction in embryo. J Urol 128:1091, 1982.
32. Glassberg KI. The dilated ureter: Classification and approach. Urology 9:1, 1977.
33. Johnston JH, Evans JP, Glassberg KI, et al. Pelvic hydronephrosis in children: A review of 219 personal cases. J Urol 117:97, 1977.
34. Hildebrandt O. Weiterer beitrag zur patologischen Anatomie der Nierengeschwulste. Arch Klin Chir 48:343, 1894.
35. Osathanondh V, Potter EL. Pathogenesis of polycystic kidneys: Historical survey. Arch Pathol 77:459, 1964.
36. Gates GF. Ultrasonography of the urinary tract in children. Urol Clin North Am 7:215, 1980.
37. Hadlock FP, Deter RL, Carpenter P, et al. Sonography of fetal urinary tract anomalies. Am J Radiol 137:261, 1981.
38. Stuck KJ, Koff SA, Silver TM. Ultrasonic features of multicystic dysplastic kidney: Expanded diagnostic criteria. Radiology 143.217, 1982.
39. Tyrrell PN, Boivin CM, Burrell DN, et al. Multicystic dysplastic kidney: Another application of 99mTcMAG3. Clin Radiol 49:400, 1994.
40. Emmert G Jr, King L. The risk of hypertension is underestimated in the multicystic dysplastic kidney: A personal perspective. Urology 44:404, 1994.
41. Peterson NE. Percutaneous decompression: Treatment for respiratory distress secondary to multicystic dysplastic kidney. J Urol 147:171, 1992.
42. Ambrose SS. Unilateral multicystic renal disease in adults. Birth Defects 13:349, 1976.
43. Gordon AC, Thomas DF, Arthur RJ, Irving HC. Multicystic dysplastic kidney: Is nephrectomy still appropriate? J Urol 140:1231, 1988.
44. Bloom DA, Brosman S. The Multicystic Kidney. J Urol 120:211, 1978.
45. Elder JS, Hladky D, Selzman AA. Outpatient nephrectomy for nonfunctioning kidneys. J Urol 154:712, 1995.
46. Albala DM, Kavoussi LR, Clayman RV. Laparoscopic nephrectomy. Semin Urol 10:146, 1992.
47. Emmert G Jr, Eubanks S, King L. Improved technique of laparoscopic nephrectomy for multicystic dysplastic kidney. Urology 44:422, 1994.
48. Clayman RV, Kavoussi LR, Soper NJ, et al. Laparoscopic nephrectomy: Initial case report. J Urol 146:278, 1991.
49. Gaur DD, Agarwal DK, Purohit KC. Retroperitoneal laparoscopic nephrectomy: Initial case report. J Urol 149:103, 1993.
50. Koyle MA, Woo HH, Kavoussi LR. Laparoscopic nephrectomy in the first year of life. J Pediatr Surg 28:693, 1993.
51. Emmert G Jr, Eubanks S, King L. Response to comment. Urology 45:1085, 1995.

MICHAEL L. RITCHEY

4

The Management of Wilms' Tumor

The management of children with solid neoplasms has advanced tremendously over the past few decades. These advances are attributable to improved methods of diagnosis, better anesthetic and surgical techniques, and availability of effective adjuvant chemotherapy or radiotherapy or both. Patients with Wilms' tumor have benefited greatly from these advances in terms of improved survival and decreased morbidity of treatment. This chapter provides an overview of the current management of nephroblastoma.

DIAGNOSIS

The typical presentation of a child with Wilms' tumor is an abdominal mass found incidentally by a family member or physician. The findings on physical examination will not clearly differentiate Wilms' tumor from other abdominal neoplasms or benign masses. Hematuria occurs in one fourth of children at diagnosis, but gross hematuria is uncommon and warrants evaluation to exclude tumor extension into the collecting system. Atypical presentations, such as abdominal pain, can result in inappropriate exploration for appendicitis.[1] Rupture of the tumor with hemorrhage into the free peritoneal cavity can also result in presentation as an acute abdomen. Extension of Wilms' tumor into the renal vein and inferior vena cava can produce varicocele, hepatomegaly from hepatic vein obstruction, ascites, and even congestive heart failure.[2]

Assessment of Local Tumor Extension

Tremendous advances have occurred in the field of imaging over the past two decades. At the outset of the National Wilms' Tumor Study Group (NWTSG) in 1969, the gold standard for assessing renal involvement was the intravenous pyelogram (IVP). Although this study is now infrequently performed in the evaluation of an abdominal mass, it did generally establish that the patient had a functioning contralateral kidney before performing a nephrectomy. The classic findings of nephroblastoma on IVP are distortion of the renal contour with splaying of the collecting system. Nonopacification of the kidney is not uncommon and may result from tumor obstruction of the collecting system,[3] complete replacement of the renal parenchyma with neoplasm, or intravascular tumor extension.[2]

Today the child is subjected to numerous imaging studies, often before the surgeon is consulted. These studies are ordered with the intent of obtaining the correct diagnosis, but there are few distinguishing radiographic features that will allow a precise preoperative diagnosis of the histology of a renal mass. In today's cost-conscious environment, it is important to be sure that important additional information is obtained from the various body imaging techniques.

Ultrasonography is probably the first study ordered in most children with abdominal masses. One important feature of ultrasonography is the ability to distinguish between solid and cystic lesions. In most cases, an experienced radiologist can determine whether the mass is of renal origin. Establishing that there is a solid renal tumor present is probably the most important finding that will help the surgeon plan a major cancer operation, which will minimize surgical morbidity.[1] Another important role for ultrasonography is to exclude intracaval tumor extension, which occurs in 4% of Wilms' tumor patients.[2] Real-time ultrasonography can document the presence of tumor thrombi in the inferior vena cava (IVC).

The important issue is whether more expensive body imaging studies (e.g., computed tomography [CT] or magnetic resonance imaging [MRI]) provide information that will alter management. Some authors have suggested that these studies can provide important staging information.[4] However, the current staging system used by the NWTS group relies on surgical findings and pathologic examination. Clearly, defining tumor extent before treatment is fundamental for Wilms' tumor patients when outcome is highly correlated with stage.[5] Staging involves detection of distant metastases and defining the local extent of the tumor. The local tumor burden determines whether the child receives abdominal irradiation and also the intensity of the chemotherapy regimen. As is discussed more extensively later, it is the group of patients with stage III tumors (positive regional lymph nodes, residual disease, diffuse tumor spillage) that need to be identified.

Preoperative CT can suggest extrarenal tumor extension into the perirenal fat and evidence of regional adenopathy. However, prospective correlation with pathologic findings has not been done. Enlarged benign retroperitoneal lymph nodes are common in children. Correlation between lymph node evaluation at surgical exploration and pathologic findings in Wilms' tumor patients have found false-positive and false-negative error rates of 18% and 31%, respectively.[6] It should not be expected that CT or MRI will have greater accuracy. As noted, ultrasonography is particularly helpful in the assessing the patency of the IVC. If this study is inconclusive, MRI has been shown to be superior to CT in confirming intravascular tumor extension.[7]

Many years ago, it was noted that a number of children with presumed unilateral Wilms' tumor were found to have bilateral lesions at surgical exploration.[8] This led to the recommendation that all patients with suspected Wilms' tumor be explored through a generous transperitoneal approach. Gerota's fascia is opened over the contralateral kidney to allow both inspection and palpation of all surfaces to exclude synchronous bilateral Wilms' tumor (BWT).

When this recommendation was made, IVP was the predominant preoperative imaging study available. It later became obvious that the introduction of CT scanning resulted in considerable improvement in the detection of bilateral disease. One report noted that IVP was accurate in 42% of children with synchronous BWT, whereas CT scanning was able to detect disease in 83% of such patients.[9] As experience with ultrasonography, CT, and MRI increased, several authors questioned whether a negative preoperative imaging evaluation of the contralateral kidney might preclude the need for formal surgical exploration.[10, 11] However, a review of 122 patients with synchronous BWT enrolled in NWTS-4 demonstrated that, despite the availability of improved imaging modalities, 7% of bilateral lesions were still missed by preoperative imaging.[12] Most of the missed lesions were 1 cm or smaller, but early identification of synchronous BWT is important because the therapeutic approach of such patients is different from that of children with unilateral Wilms' tumors: they should not undergo nephrectomy at diagnosis.[9, 13] The authors concluded that formal exploration of the contralateral kidney with opening of Gerota's fascia to allow both palpation and inspection of all surfaces should continue to be performed.

Obviously, the indication for adequate exploration of the contralateral kidney needs to be balanced against possible increased morbidity from the added procedure.[10] However, for most children with Wilms' tumor, a large, transverse transperitoneal incision is required for tumor removal alone because of the relatively large size of the tumor. Therefore, modification of the incision is not routinely necessary to afford adequate exposure of the opposite kidney in the young child. Significant vasospasm with subsequent ischemic damage can occur after operative manipulation of the kidney in young infants, but a review of nearly 2000 NWTS-3 patients found no instance of renal injury from examination of the contralateral kidney.[1]

Assessment of Metastatic Disease

The most common site of distant metastases is within the lungs, present at diagnosis in 8% of Wilms' tumor patients. The majority of these lesions can be identified on routine chest x-ray films. If the patient is documented to have metastases on chest radiographs, chest CT scan will provide little additional information. Other smaller metastases may be discovered, but the CT findings will not alter the adjuvant treatment required (whole lung irradiation and addition of doxorubicin to the chemotherapy regimen). There is debate on the need for a chest CT scan in children with negative chest x-ray films and whether those patients discovered to have lesions on CT scan alone need additional treatment.[14–16]

Clearly, some stage IV patients will be identified only by chest CT scan. Some may be children with benign lesions, necessitating lung biopsy to confirm malignancy. The other question regarding chest x-ray–negative, CT scan–positive patients is whether pulmonary irradiation is needed. Green and colleagues reviewed 32 children enrolled in NWTS-3 who had metastatic lesions on a chest CT scan and a negative chest roentgenogram.[14] The survival in patients treated according to the local extent of the abdominal disease alone was equivalent to that in patients receiving pulmonary irradiation. However, others have reported that when pulmonary radiation was omitted in patients whose histologic examination results were favorable with pulmonary densities detected on CT scan alone, 40% experienced recurrent disease.[15]

The next most common site of distant metastasis is the liver. Most are evident during surgical exploration. Isolated deep-seated lesions are uncommon. Direct invasion of the liver is particularly difficult to assess by CT scan. Dynamic scanning of the liver after bolus injection is recommended to obtain the most reliable imaging.

Additional studies are recommended to detect the presence of metastases in selected renal tumors with unfavorable histology.[17] Clear cell sarcoma of the kidney (CCSK) and renal cell carcinoma have a propensity to metastasize to the skeleton. Rhabdoid tumor of the kidney (RTK) and CCSK are also associated with brain metastases. Skeletal surveys, bone scans, and MRI of the brain are recommended after the histologic diagnosis is confirmed.

Screening for Nephroblastoma

Patients with aniridia, hemihypertrophy, and the Beckwith-Wiedemann syndrome are at increased risk for nephroblastoma. Periodic screening ultrasonogram is recommended for the detection of new renal tumors. A review from the NWTS group did find more stage I tumors in patients whose tumor was detected radiographically,[18] but could not determine whether early detection had an impact on patient survival. The current recommendation for screening of high-risk patients is listed in Table 4–1.

SURGICAL MANAGEMENT

The preoperative evaluation of a child discovered to have an abdominal mass can generally be completed in 48 hours. Emergent operation is not necessary unless there is evidence of active bleeding. Laboratory evaluation should include kidney function tests, evaluation of both kidneys, a complete peripheral blood count, platelet count, liver function tests, serum calcium, and urinalysis. Elevation of the serum calcium can occur in children with congenital mesoblastic nephroma and RTK.

Surgery was once the only means of cure in a child with nephroblastoma and remains today an important cornerstone of therapy for Wilms' tumor patients. The surgeon has an important role in assessing the extent of local tumor spread. As noted, this information cannot be accurately assessed by any other modality. Accurate staging is essential for determining the need for radiation therapy and the appropriate chemotherapy regimen. It is also the surgeon's responsibility to perform safe and complete removal of the tumor. Intraoperative events that can have an adverse impact on patient survival include tumor spill, incomplete removal, and surgical complications. These are discussed more extensively later.

The transperitoneal approach has become the standard procedure in patients with Wilms' tumor. Once the peritoneal cavity is entered, thorough exploration of the abdominal cavity is carried out. One should assess the liver and regional lymph nodes in the periaortic area and look for other evidence of tumor spread. Exploration of the contralateral kidney should be performed before nephrectomy. The colon is reflected and Gerota's fascia opened so that the kidney can be palpated and inspected on all surfaces. Any abnormalities of the opposite kidney should undergo biopsy to exclude occult Wilms' tumor or the presence of nephrogenic rests.

Radical nephrectomy is performed with sampling of regional lymph nodes, but formal lymph node dissection is not required.[6] The colon is mobilized off the tumor and reflected medially, preserving the colonic blood supply. Gentle handling of the tumor throughout the procedure is mandatory to avoid tumor spillage, because these patients have a sixfold increase in local abdominal relapse.[5] Although early ligation of the renal vein does not appear to have an appreciable effect on survival, separate ligation is performed before mobilization of the tumor but only if exposure is adequate. More importantly, the surgeon

Table 4–1
Recommended Follow-Up Imaging Studies for Children With Renal Neoplasms of Proven Histology and Free of Metastases at Diagnosis

Tumor Type	Study	Schedule After Therapy
Favorable histology Wilms' tumor; stage I anaplastic Wilms' tumor	Chest films	6 wk and 3 mo postop; then every 3 mo × 5, every 6 mo × 3, yearly × 2
Irradiated patients only	Irradiated bony structures*	Yearly to full growth, then every 5 yr indefinitely†
Without NRs, stages I and II	Abdominal ultrasonogram	Yearly × 3
Without NRs, stage III	Abdominal ultrasonogram	As for chest films
With NRs, any stage‡	Abdominal ultrasonogram	Every 3 mo × 10, every 6 mo × 5, yearly × 5
Stage II and stage III anaplastic	Chest films	As for favorable histology
	Abdominal ultrasonogram	Every 3 mo × 4; every 6 mo × 4
Renal cell carcinoma	Chest films	Like favorable histology
	Skeletal survey and bone scan	Like CCSK
CCSK	Brain MRI and/or opacified CT	When CCSK is established; then every 6 mo × 10
	Skeletal survey and bone scan	As for favorable histology
	Chest films	
Rhabdoid tumor	Brain MRI and/or opacified CT	As for CCSK
	Chest films	As for favorable histology
Mesoblastic nephroma§	Abdominal ultrasonogram	Every 3 mo × 6

* To include any irradiated osseous structures.
† To detect second neoplasms, benign (osteochondromas) or malignant.
‡ The panelists at the first International Conference on Molecular and Clinical Genetics of Childhood Renal Tumors, Albuquerque, New Mexico, May 1992, recommended a variation: every 3 month for 5 years or until age 7, whichever comes first.
§ Data from the files of Dr. J. B. Beckwith reveal that 20 of 293 mesoblastic nephroma patients (7%) relapsed or had metastases at diagnosis; 4 of the 20 in the lungs, 1 of the 4 at diagnosis. All but 1 of the 19 relapses occurred within 1 year. Chest films for mesoblastic nephroma patients may be elected on a schedule such as every 3 months × 4, every 6 months × 2.
NR, nephrogenic rest; CCSK, clear cell sarcoma of the kidney; MRI, magnetic resonance imaging; CT, computed tomography.
Modified, with permission, from D'Angio GJ, Rosenberg H, Sharples K, et al. Position paper: Imaging methods for primary renal tumors of childhood: Cost versus benefits. Med Pediatr Oncol 21:205, 1993. Used with permission.

should be certain that the contralateral renal vessels, aorta, iliac, or superior mesenteric arteries have not been mistakenly ligated.[19]

The renal vein and IVC should be palpated to exclude intravascular tumor extension before vessel ligation. Identification of intracaval extension on the preoperative imaging studies will allow the surgical team to prepare for the operative procedure adequately. For vena caval involvement below the level of the hepatic veins, the caval thrombus can be removed via cavotomy after proximal and distal vascular control is obtained. Generally, the thrombus will be free floating, but if there is adherence of the thrombus to the caval wall, the thrombus can often be delivered with the passage of a Fogarty or Foley balloon catheter.

Patients with extension of intracaval tumor thrombus above the level of the hepatic veins should receive preoperative chemotherapy to shrink the tumor and thrombus.[20, 21] This will facilitate complete removal of the tumor with decreased morbidity. There has been one report of tumor embolus during chemotherapy,[22] but this complication can also occur before or during surgical removal of the tumor.[23]

Although radical nephrectomy is advocated to ensure complete tumor removal, heroic efforts to excise en bloc all or parts of adjacent organs to which the tumor appears to be adherent are generally not warranted. Wilms' tumors are generally very large, and the gross appearance of the tumor at the time of surgery can be misleading in interpreting tumor extent. These tumors often compress and adhere to adjacent structures without frank invasion, and in the majority of cases tumor invasion is not confirmed after the adjacent visceral organs are removed.[1] If the tumor is found to be unresectable, biopsy of the tumor is followed by chemotherapy or radiation therapy or both. This will generally produce tumor shrinkage, allowing resection.[24, 25] Radical en bloc resection of the tumor is probably not justified in most children because of the increased surgical morbidity.

Surgery should not be overlooked as a cause of morbidity in children with Wilms' tumor. A review of NWTS-3 patients undergoing primary nephrectomy found a 19% incidence of surgical complications.[1] The most common complications were hemorrhage and small bowel obstruction.[26] Several risk factors for increased surgical complications were identified, including higher local tumor stage, intravascular extension, en bloc resection of other visceral organs, and incorrect preoperative diagnosis. Increased bleeding can be secondary to acquired von Willebrand's disease found in 8% of newly diagnosed Wilms' tumor patients.[27]

PATHOLOGY AND STAGING

Analysis of early NWTS patients identified a group of tumors with "unfavorable" histologic features that were associated with increased rates of relapse and death.[28] These characteristics included tumors of extreme nuclear atypia (anaplasia) and monomorphic sarcomatous-appearing tumors. These latter tumors have been reclassified as rhabdoid tumors and clear cell sarcomas of the kidney and are now considered to be entities distinct from Wilms' tumors. These unfavorable features occurred in approximately 10% of patients but accounted for almost half of the tumor deaths in early NWTS reports.[29] Identification of these high-risk patients allows stratification of patients, with greater treatment intensity reserved for patients with a poor prognosis.

Anaplasia. The cytopathologic features of anaplasia are threefold: nuclear enlargement, hyperchromatism of enlarged nuclei, and increased mitotic figures. Anaplasia is rare in the first 2 years of life, but the incidence increases to 13% in children age 5 years or older.[30] Anaplastic features can occur focally, requiring thorough sampling of the primary tumor to avoid missing this poor prognostic feature. The new definition of focal anaplasia requires that the anaplastic nuclear changes be confined to a specified region of the primary tumor and not be present in any site outside the kidney parenchyma.[31] Diffuse anaplasia is diagnosed when anaplasia is present in more than one portion of the tumor, present in a random biopsy specimen, or found in any extrarenal or metastatic site.

Clear Cell Sarcoma of the Kidney. CCSK accounts for 3% of renal tumors reported to the NWTS. Although not currently considered a variant of Wilms' tumor, the age at diagnosis and location are the same as for nephroblastoma. CCSK is associated with a much higher rate of relapse and death than favorable histology Wilms' tumor. These patients have a strikingly increased number of bone as well as brain metastases. Unlike tumors with anaplasia, even stage I CCSK lesions are associated with increased rates of relapse. Studies have demonstrated that doxorubicin is associated with a significant improvement in outcome for these children.[5]

Rhabdoid Tumor of the Kidney. This is a highly malignant tumor of the kidney that accounts for 2% of renal tumors registered to the NWTS. This tumor is typically seen in infants and very young children (mean age, 13 months). RTK metastasizes to the brain, which is exceedingly uncommon for Wilms' tumor. The prognosis of RTK remains dismal with conventional chemotherapeutic regimens, and new treatment strategies are being developed for management of these children.

Precursor Lesions of Wilms' Tumor

Renal lesions apparently representing Wilms' tumor precursors have been recognized for many years. These lesions are present in 1% of kidneys in infants on postmortem examination[32] and in 30 to 40% of kidneys removed for Wilms' tumor. The current preferred term for this precursor lesion is *nephrogenic rest,* which is defined as foci of abnormally persistent nephrogenic cells that can form a Wilms' tumor.[33] Two types of nephrogenic rests have been identified—perilobar nephrogenic rest (PLNR) and intralobar nephrogenic rest (ILNR)—based on the location of these lesions within the kidney. PLNRs are located peripherally, whereas ILNRs can be found anywhere within the renal lobe (Fig. 4–1). It is inferred that ILNRs situated deep in the renal lobe reflect an earlier developmental event. The presence of multiple or diffuse nephrogenic rests leads to the diagnosis of nephroblastomatosis.

Nephrogenic rests display a spectrum of appearances. Given that the incidence of nephrogenic rests is much greater than that of Wilms' tumor, it is not surprising that regression of the rests is common. Hyperplasia of the rest can occur and be easily mistaken for a small Wilms' tumor.[33]

Nephrogenic rests are of theoretical interest in the pathogenesis of Wilms' tumor, but they are also of clinical importance. When multifocal rests are found in a kidney removed for Wilms' tumor, this implies that nephrogenic rests are present in the contralateral kidney. Such a patient is at risk for a metachronous tumor, and they need careful imaging follow-up to detect contralateral recurrence (see Table 4–1). Because metachronous Wilms' tumors occur in patients previously treated with conventional chemotherapeutic regimens, one infers that nephrogenic rests cannot always be eradicated.

Biologic Parameters

Because of the excellent survival of most patients with favorable histology Wilms' tumor, it becomes increasingly difficult to find histologic features of a given tumor that will predict the risk of relapse. Therefore, the search is on for biologic features that can further stratify favorable histology Wilms' tumor patients into low- and high-risk groups. Such a test might allow a further reduction in treatment intensity for a large number of patients.

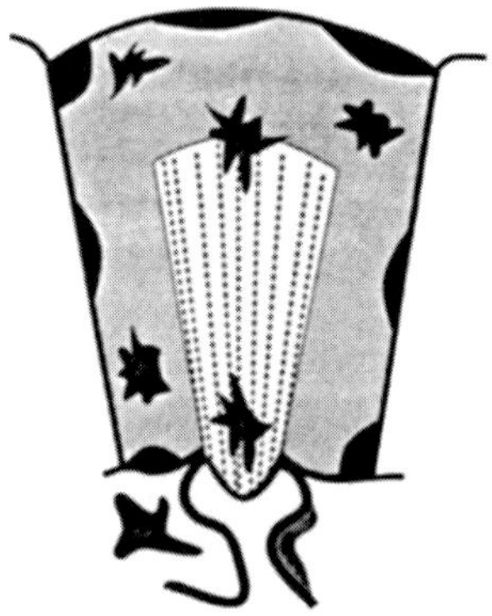

Figure 4–1 Renal lobe showing characteristic locations of intralobar nephrogenic rest (dark gray) and perilobar nephrogenic rest (black). Used with permission from Beckwith JB. Precursor lesions of Wilms tumor: Clinical and biological implications. Med Pediatr Oncol 21:158, 1993.

Tumor Markers. Several biologic markers for Wilms' tumor are under investigation, including serum renin, neuron-specific enolase, hyaluronic acid, hyaluronidase, and hyaluronic acid–stimulating activity.[34] At present, studies of these markers have been limited to assessing the response of the tumor to treatment or detecting tumor recurrence.

Deoxyribonucleic Acid Content

Flow cytometry is used to measure deoxyribonucleic acid (DNA) content and to estimate the proliferative rate of populations of cells comprising solid malignancies. An analysis of 47 Wilms' tumors found that patients with a diploid or aneuploid DNA histogram had a 100% survival at 5 years.[35] Stage III and IV patients with tetraploid patterns fared significantly worse, with a 25% 5-year survival. However, others have found that DNA ploidy was not a more accurate predictor of survival than histology and stage.[36]

Nuclear morphometric techniques have been evaluated in patients with Wilms' tumors to predict clinical outcome.[37] A report of 108 Wilms' tumor patients with favorable histology identified two shape factors that could be used to distinguish patients with an unfavorable outcome.[37] Further studies are ongoing to determine whether this technique will prove to be a reliable and reproducible method of predicting response to therapy.

Chromosomal Abnormalities. Wilms' tumor specimens have been noted to have numerous karyotypic abnormalities on cytogenetic examination. This led to the discovery of genes on chromosome 11 believed to be responsible for the induction of Wilms' tumor. Investigation for other sites of DNA gain or loss have found loss of heterozygosity (LOH) for a portion of chromosome 16q in 20% of Wilms' tumor patients.[38] This is not a germline mutation, suggesting that this region may play a role in tumor progression rather than tumor initiation. A prospective study of 232 patients registered on the NWTS found LOH for 16q in 17% of the tumors.[39] Patients with tumor-specific LOH for chromosome 16q had a statistically significantly poorer 2-year relapse-free survival than patients without LOH for chromosome 16q. This difference in outcome persisted after adjustment for histology and stage. If this information is confirmed in NWTS-5, molecular markers may one day serve to further stratify Wilms' tumor patients for treatment.

TREATMENT

Patterns of Spread

The most important determinants of outcome in children with Wilms' tumor are histopathology and tumor stage. Assignment of local tumor stage is a responsibility of both the surgeon and pathologist. Examination for extension through the capsule, residual disease, and lymph node involvement is essential to assess the extent of the tumor properly. Stage I tumors are limited to the kidney and completely resected. The first signs of spread outside the kidney are in the renal sinus and lymphatic vessels. Penetration through the renal capsule is the next most common site of extrarenal spread. Tumors that penetrate the renal capsule are considered stage II lesions. Clear demonstration of tumor cells in the perirenal fat is required to document capsular penetration. Tumor extension into the soft tissues of the sinus and the presence of tumor cells in blood or lymphatic vessels of the renal sinus are now considered stage II.

The presence of lymph node metastases has an adverse outcome on survival; therefore, it is important that adequate lymph node sampling be performed during the course of nephroblastoma removal. Local tumor extension is another important factor in identifying risk of tumor relapse. Patients with diffuse tumor spill are at increased risk for abdominal relapse; therefore, their disease is considered to be stage III, and patients are given whole abdominal irradiation. The current staging system used by the NWTS group is summarized in Table 4–2. For NWTS-3, the distribution by stage of favorable histology tumors was as follows: stage I, 47%; stage II, 22%; stage III, 22%; stage IV, 9%.[5]

Table 4–2
Staging System of the National Wilms' Tumor Study

Stage	Description
I	Tumor is limited to the kidney and is completely excised. The renal capsule is intact and the tumor was not ruptured before removal. There is no residual tumor. The vessels of the renal sinus are not involved.
II	Tumor extends beyond the kidney but is completely excised. There is regional extension of tumor (i.e., penetration of the renal capsule, extensive invasion of the renal sinus). A biopsy of the tumor may have been performed, or there may be local spillage of tumor confined to the flank. Extrarenal vessels may contain tumor thrombus or may be infiltrated by tumor.
III	Residual nonhematogenous tumor confined to the abdomen: lymph node involvement, diffuse peritoneal spillage either before or during surgery, peritoneal implants, tumor beyond surgical margin either grossly or microscopically, or tumor not completely removed.
IV	Hematogenous metastases (e.g., lung, liver, bone, brain) or lymph node metastases outside the abdominopelvic region are present.
V	Bilateral renal involvement at diagnosis.

Identification of unfavorable histology tumors is more important than even stage assignment because these tumors are responsible for 50% of tumor deaths.[29] Patients with anaplastic tumors are twice as likely to present with stage IV disease than those with favorable histology tumors.[40] Anaplastic Wilms' tumors are stratified into focal and diffuse anaplasia.[31] In NWTS-4, children with stage I anaplastic tumors were treated in a similar fashion to those with favorable histology. Patients with stage II–IV focal anaplasia were treated with AMD, dactinomycin, vincristine, and doxorubicin (Adriamycin) and received irradiation to the tumor bed. If there was evidence of diffuse anaplasia, stage II–IV patients received more aggressive therapy.

Results of Intergroup Studies

The current staging system for Wilms' tumor has allowed stratification of patients into high- and low-risk treatment groups. This permits a reduction in the intensity of therapy for the majority of children, decreasing the morbidity of treatment. The last intergroup study, NWTS-4, recently closed for patient entry. Final results have not been published, but some preliminary results are available. This study used a pulse-intensive chemotherapy regimen to decrease the number of days of hospitalization required for administration of chemotherapy. These regimens produce less hematologic toxicity than the standard regimens[41] and achieve equivalent survival compared with the standard chemotherapy regimen.

The 4-year survival of patients with favorable histology Wilms' tumor now approaches 90%. Current recommendations for treatment to be used in the recently opened intergroup study NWTS-5 are outlined in Table 4–3. Patients with a stage I or II favorable histology Wilms' tumor are treated with a regimen of vincristine and dactinomycin for 18 weeks. Radiation therapy is now omitted for all stage I and stage II tumors.[5] Stage III favorable histology patients continue to receive abdominal irradiation external radiation therapy, but the dosage has been reduced to 1080 cGy. Patients with stage IV favorable histology tumors receive abdominal irradiation based on the local tumor stage and also receive 1200 cGy to both lungs. Less than one fourth of children with favorable histology tumors entered on NWTS-4 received postoperative abdominal irradiation.[42]

One new approach to be tested during NWTS-5 will be the treatment of a small group of stage I patients with surgery alone. Omission of postoperative adjuvant therapy has been proposed for small stage I tumors of favorable histology that occur in children younger than 2 years (Cassady tumor).[43] The NWTS pathologists have identified several variables predictive of tumor relapse that could be used to stratify stage I tumors[44]: invasion of

Table 4–3
Protocol for National Wilms' Tumor Study-5

Variable	Radiotherapy	Chemotherapy
Stages I and II FH and anaplasia	None	EE-4A: pulse-intensive AMD plus VCR (18 wk)
Stages III and IV FH and focal anaplasia stage II–IV	1080 cGy	DD-4A: pulse-intensive AMD, VCR, and DOX (24 wk)
Stages II–IV diffuse anaplasia and CCSK	Yes*	Regimen I†
Stages I–IV RTK	Yes*	Regimen RTK‡

* Radiation therapy is given to all clear cell sarcoma patients. Stage IV FH patients are given radiation based on the local tumor stage. Consult protocol for specific treatment.
† Regimen I: AMD, VCR, DOX, cyclophosphamide, and etoposide.
‡ Regimen RTK: carboplatin, etoposide, and cyclophosphamide.
AMD, dactinomycin; VCR, vincristine; DOX, doxorubicin; FH, favorable histology; UH, unfavorable histology; CCSK, clear cell sarcoma of the kidney; RTK, rhabdoid tumor of the kidney.

the tumor capsule, presence of an inflammatory pseudocapsule, renal sinus invasion, and tumor in the intrarenal vessels. A study of NWTS-4 favorable histology stage I patients found that the 2-year relapse-free survival rate was 96.5% if all microsubstaging variables were negative.[45] There was good correlation among age less than 2 years, tumor weight less than 550 g, and negative microsubstaging variables. Therefore, it was concluded that the variables of age and weight could be more easily applied in clinical practice to stratify patients for treatment, because they are easily determined.

Preoperative Chemotherapy

Unilateral Tumors

The majority of North American children with Wilms' tumor are treated according to clinical trials conducted by the NWTS. The NWTS recommends initial surgical resection for children with unilateral tumors. In Europe, most patients are treated according to protocols conducted by the International Society of Pediatric Oncology (SIOP). Their protocols have included preoperative chemotherapy since the early 1970s.[46, 47] They reported significant "downstaging" of the tumor with a greater number of patients having "postchemotherapy stage I" tumors. The SIOP investigators use the post-treatment stage to determine therapy. Therefore, fewer patients needed adjuvant radiation because of the greater percentage of "stage I" tumors. Over the course of time, however, it also became apparent to NWTS investigators that radiation therapy was unnecessary for patients with stage I and II tumors.[5] As a result, the number of children receiving abdominal irradiation is now quite comparable between the two groups.[8]

One major concern regarding the routine use of preoperative chemotherapy is whether the postchemotherapy stage adequately defines the risk of relapse or recurrence. An important variable is the presence of lymph node involvement. For NWTS patients, positive lymph nodes mandate postoperative irradiation as well as the addition of doxorubicin to the chemotherapy regimen. In SIOP-6, postchemotherapy stage II node-negative patients were randomized to receive or not receive abdominal irradiation. Investigators noted an excessive number of intra-abdominal recurrences in nonirradiated patients.[48] Although the overall outcome between the two treatment arms was reported as showing no significant difference, subsequent SIOP trials added anthracyclines to the chemotherapy regimen for postchemotherapy stage II node-negative patients. This experience suggests that staging the patient after chemotherapy may inadequately define the risk of relapse. Although preoperative therapy may destroy the evidence of extrarenal spread of disease (e.g., lymph node involvement or extracapsular extension), these patients are still at an increased risk for relapse.

The most recently completed and published studies by both NWTS and SIOP report very similar survival for patients with nonmetastatic, favorable histology Wilms' tumor.[5, 48] There are differences in staging systems, but both groups have achieved excellent results.

There has been concern about the late occurrence of renal dysfunction in children who have undergone unilateral nephrectomy. There is both clinical and experimental evidence of hyperfiltration damage of remnant nephrons after a loss of renal mass.[49] This concern over renal dysfunction has led some surgeons to recommend parenchyma-sparing procedures for unilateral tumors.[50, 51] The majority of Wilms' tumors are too large for a partial nephrectomy at initial presentation. After preoperative chemotherapy, 10% of patients may become amenable to partial nephrectomy. The use of partial nephrectomy is probably a sound idea for those with solitary kidneys or renal insufficiency. However, for the majority of patients with unilateral Wilms' tumor, the indication for partial nephrectomy is less clear. The incidence of renal failure in unilateral Wilms' tumor patients reported to the NWTS is less than 0.2%, and the majority of these had Drash syndrome, which itself is associated with end-stage renal disease.[52]

Bilateral Tumors

Synchronous BWTs account for 4 to 6% of all Wilms' tumors.[13, 53] For most of this century, ablative surgery was considered to be essential for cure, and these patients were thought to have a poor survival. Consequently, many patients with synchronous BWT ended with significant renal insufficiency, some to the extent of requiring dialysis and renal transplantation.[54] Multidisciplinary treatment combining chemotherapy, radiation therapy, and surgery has resulted in a markedly improved outcome.

In 1987, Blute and colleagues reported a large series of 145 BWT patients enrolled in NWTS-2 and NWTS-3.[9] They noted that patients undergoing initial biopsy followed by postoperative chemotherapy had a survival—83% at 2 years—equivalent to that of patients undergoing initial surgical resection. Other investigators have reported similar results.[13, 53] With improved survival comparable to other Wilms' tumor patients, attention has now turned to the preservation of renal units in these patients. One advantage of preoperative chemotherapy for patients with bilateral tumors is that more renal units will be spared if surgery is deferred until after the tumor burden is reduced.[13, 55, 56] Blute and coworkers noted that nephrectomy could be avoided entirely in almost 50% of the kidneys in patients undergoing initial biopsy. This is important because renal failure is a significant risk in patients with bilateral tumors.[52]

A child with BWT should undergo the appropriate clinical workup, including imaging studies, and subsequently be explored surgically. Grossly abnormal lymph nodes or other lesions suggestive of extrarenal spread should undergo biopsy and a surgical stage assigned to both kidneys. Bilateral biopsies should be obtained to confirm the presence of Wilms' tumor in both kidneys and establish the histologic type of each tumor, although sampling errors may still occur. Primary excision of the tumor masses should not be attempted; rather, patients should be given preoperative chemotherapy appropriate to the stage and histology of the tumor. After 8 weeks of chemotherapy, the patient is reassessed with an abdominal CT scan to determine the feasibility of resection.

Some patients may not have a measurable response to preoperative chemotherapy. Failure of the mass to shrink is not always due to persistent viable tumor. Second-look surgery is recommended, and partial nephrectomy or wedge excision of the tumor can still be considered. If the tumors are not amenable to partial resections, biopsies should again be performed. Patients with persistent viable tumor are then treated with a different chemotherapeutic regimen or radiotherapy or both. Patients who have been on dactinomycin and vincristine should then be given doxorubicin. Those who have received all three of these drugs should receive radiotherapy (150 cGy/day for 10 days). The patient should be reassessed after an additional 12 weeks of chemotherapy or 4 weeks after radiotherapy to determine the feasibility of resection of residual tumors. If it appears that either or both of the kidneys can be salvaged, partial nephrectomies or wedge excisions of the tumors are performed. Radical nephrectomy is accomplished to remove the kidney with extensive tumor involvement when only one of two can be preserved.

Bilateral nephrectomies and dialysis may rarely be required when the tumors fail to respond to chemotherapy and radiation therapy. The recommended interval between successful completion of treatment of the Wilms' tumor and renal transplantation varies. Some advocate a waiting period of 2 years to ensure that metastatic disease does not develop: others have found that a 1-year interval is sufficient.[54]

Inoperable Tumors

There are occasional patients with massive tumors judged by the surgeons to pose too great a risk for surgical removal. Past experience[24, 25] has shown that pretreatment with chemotherapy generally reduces the bulk of the tumor, allowing subsequent removal. However, this method does not result in improved survival rates and does result in the loss of important staging information. Unresectable tumors treated by preoperative therapy should be considered stage III, and these patients should be treated accordingly.[25] In general, the operative procedure can be performed within 6 weeks of initiating treatment. Patients who fail to respond can be considered for preoperative irradiation because this may produce enough shrinkage to facilitate nephrectomy. Patients with progressive disease in spite of therapy have a very poor prognosis, and these patients require treatment with a different chemotherapeutic regimen.[25]

REFERENCES

1. Ritchey ML, Kelalis PP, Breslow N, et al. Surgical complications following nephrectomy for Wilms' tumor: A report of National Wilms' Tumor Study—3. Surg Gynecol Obstet 175:507, 1992.
2. Ritchey ML, Kelalis PP, Breslow N, et al. Intracaval and atrial involvement with nephrobalastoma: Review of National Wilms' Tumor Study—3. J Urol 140:1113, 1988.
3. Nakayama DK, Ortega W, D'Angio GJ, O'Neill JA. The nonopacified kidney with Wilms' tumor. J Pediatr Surg 23:152, 1988.
4. Cohen MD. Staging of Wilms' tumor. Clin Radiol 47:77, 1993.
5. D'Angio GJ, Breslow N, Beckwith JB, et al. Treatment of Wilms' tumor: Results of the Third National Wilms' Tumor Study. Cancer 64:349, 1989.
6. Othersen HB Jr, DeLorimer A, Hrabovsky E, et al. Surgical evaluation of lymph node metastases in Wilms' tumor. J Pediatr Surg 25:3:1, 1990.
7. Weese DL, Applebaum H, Taber P. Mapping intravascular extension of Wilms' tumor with magnetic resonance imaging. J Pediatr Surg 26:64, 1991.

8. Martin LW, Kloecker RJ. Bilateral nephroblastoma (Wilms' tumor). Pediatrics 28:101, 1961.
9. Blute ML, Kelalis PP, Offord KP, et al. Bilateral Wilms' tumor. J Urol 138:968, 1987.
10. Koo AS, Koyle MA, Hurwitz RS, et al. The necessity of contralateral surgical exploration in Wilms' tumor with modern noninvasive imaging technique: A reassessment. J Urol 144:416, 1990.
11. Goleta-Dy A, Shaw PJ, Stevens MM. Re: The necessity of contralateral surgical exploration in Wilms' tumor with modern noninvasive imaging technique: A reassessment (letter). J Urol 147:171, 1992.
12. Ritchey ML, Green DM, Breslow NE, Norkool P. Accuracy of current imaging modalities in the diagnosis of synchronous bilateral Wilms tumor. Cancer 75:600, 1995.
13. Montgomery BT, Kelalis PP, Blute ML, et al. Extended follow-up of bilateral Wilms' tumor: Results of the National Wilms Tumor Study. J Urol 146:514, 1991.
14. Green DM, Fernbach DJ, Norkool P, et al. The treatment of Wilms' tumor patients with pulmonary metastases detected only with computed tomography: A report from the National Wilms' Tumor Study. J Clin Oncol 9:1776, 1991.
15. Wilimas J, Douglass EC, Magill HL, et al. Significance of pulmonary computed tomography at diagnosis in Wilms' tumor. J Clin Oncol 6:1144, 1988.
16. Cohen MD. Current controversy: Is CT scan of the chest needed in patients with Wilms tumor? J Pediatr Hematol Oncol 16:191, 1994.
17. D'Angio GJ, Rosenberg H, Sharples K, et al. Position paper: Imaging methods for primary renal tumors of childhood: Cost versus benefits. Med Pediatr Oncol 21:205, 1993.
18. Green DM, Breslow NE, Beckwith JB, Norkool P. Screening of children with hemihypertrophy, aniridia, and Beckwith-Wiedemann syndrome in patients with Wilms' tumor: A report from the National Wilms Tumor Study. Med Pediatr Oncol 21:188, 1993.
19. Ritchey ML, Lally KP, Haase GM, et al. Superior mesenteric artery injury during nephrectomy for Wilms' tumor. J Pediatr Surg 27:612, 1992.
20. Dykes EH, Marwaha RK, Dicks-Mireaux C, et al. Risks and benefits of percutaneous biopsy and primary chemotherapy in advanced Wilms' tumour. J Pediatr Surg 26:610, 1991.
21. Ritchey ML, Kelalis PP, Haase GM, et al. Preoperative therapy for intracaval and atrial extension of Wilms' tumor. Cancer 71:4104, 1993.
22. Borden TA. Wilms tumor and pulmonary embolism. Soc Pediatr Urol Newsletter, August, 1992, p 27.
23. Zakowski MF, Edwards RH, McDonough ET. Wilms' tumor presenting as sudden death due to tumor embolism. Arch Pathol Lab Med 114:605, 1990.
24. Bracken RB, Sutow WW, Jaffe N, et al. Preoperative chemotherapy for Wilms' tumor. Urology 19:55, 1982.
25. Ritchey ML, Pringle K, Breslow N, et al. Management and outcome of inoperable Wilms tumor: A report of National Wilms' Tumor Study. Ann Surg 220:683, 1994.
26. Ritchey ML, Kelalis P, Breslow N, et al. Small bowel obstruction following nephrectomy for Wilms' tumor. Ann Surg 218:654, 1993.
27. Coppes MJ, Zandvoort SWH, Sparling CR, et al. Acquired von Willebrand disease in Wilms tumor patients. J Clin Oncol 10:1, 1993.
28. Beckwith JB, Palmer NP. Histopathology and prognosis of Wilms tumor: Results from the National Wilms Tumor Study. Cancer 41:1937, 1978.
29. Breslow NB, Churchill G, Beckwith JB, et al. Prognosis for Wilms' tumor patients with nonmetatastic disease at diagnosis—Results of the Second National Wilms' Tumor Study. J Clin Oncol 3:521, 1985.
30. Bonadio JF, Storer B, Norkool P, et al. Anaplastic Wilms' tumor: Clinical and pathological studies. J Clin Oncol 3:513, 1985.
31. Faria P, Beckwith JB. A new definition of focal anaplasia (FA) in Wilms tumor identifies cases with good outcome. A report from the National Wilms Tumor Study (abstract). Mod Pathol 6:3, 1993.
32. Bennington JL, Beckwith JB. Tumors of the kidney, renal pelvis, and ureter. In Firmingen HI (ed), Atlas of Tumor Pathology, Second Series, Fasicle 12. Bethesda, MD: Armed Forces Institute of Pathology, 1975.
33. Beckwith JB. Precursor lesions of Wilms tumor: Clinical and biological implications. Med Pediatr Oncol 21:158, 1993.
34. Coppes MJ. Serum biological markers and paraneoplastic syndromes in Wilms tumor. Med Pediatr Oncol 21:213, 1993.
35. Rainwater LM, Hosaka Y, Farrow GM, et al. Wilms tumors: Relationship of nuclear deoxyribonucleic acid ploidy to patient survival. J Urol 138:974, 1987.
36. Layfield LJ, Ritchie AWS, Ehrlich R. The relationship of deoxyribonucleic acid content to conventional prognostic factors in Wilms' tumor. J Urol 142:1040, 1989.
37. Partin AW, Gearhart JP, Leonard MP, et al. The use of nuclear morphometry to predict prognosis in pediatric urologic malignancies: A review. Med Pediatr Oncol 21:222, 1993.
38. Maw MA, Grundy PE, Millow LJ, et al. A third Wilms' tumor locus on chromosome 16q. Cancer Res 52:3094, 1992.
39. Grundy PE, Telzerow PE, Breslow N, et al. Loss of heterozygosity for chromosomes 16q and 1p in Wilms tumor predicts an adverse outcome. Cancer Res 54:2331, 1994.
40. Green DM, Breslow NE, Evans I, et al. Treatment of children with stage IV favorable histology Wilms tumor: A report from the National Wilms Tumor Study Group. Med Pediatr Oncol 26:147, 1996.
41. Green DM, Breslow NE, Evan I, et al. Effect of dose intensity of chemotherapy on the hematological toxicity of the treatment of Wilms tumor. A report from the National Wilms Tumor Study. Am J Pediatr Hematol Oncol 16:207, 1994.
42. Green DM, D'Angio GJ, Kelalis PP, et al. The risks associated with prenephrectomy chemotherapy for unilateral Wilms' tumor patients. Dial Ped Urol 15:7, 1992.
43. Larsen E, Perez-Atayde A, Green DM, et al. Surgery only for the treatment of patients with stage I (Cassady Wilms' tumor). Cancer 66:264, 1990.
44. Weeks DA, Beckwith JB. Relapse-associated variables in stage I, favorable histology Wilms' tumor. Cancer 60:1204, 1987.
45. Green DM, Beckwith JB, Weeks DA, et al. The relationship between microsubstaging variables, tumor weight and age at diagnosis of children with stage I/favorable histology Wilms tumor. A report from the National Wilms Tumor Study. Cancer 74:1817, 1994.
46. Lemerle J, Voute PA, Tournade MF, et al. Preoperative versus postoperative radiotherapy, single versus multiple courses of actinomycin D, in the treatment of Wilms' tumor: Preliminary results of a controlled clinical trial conducted by the International Society of Paediatric Oncology (SIOP). Cancer 38:647, 1976.
47. Lemerle J, Voute PA, Tournade MF, et al. Effectiveness of preoperative chemotherapy in Wilms' tumor: Results of an International Society of Paediatric Oncology (SIOP) clinical trial. J Clin Oncol 1:604, 1983.
48. Tournade MF, Com-Nougue C, Voute PA, et al. Results of the sixth International Society of Pediatric Oncology Wilms' tumor trial and study: A risk-adapted therapeutic approach in Wilms' tumor. J Clin Oncol 11:1014, 1993.
49. Anderson S, Meyer TW, Brenner BM. The role of hemodynamic

factors in the initiation and progression of renal disease. J Urol 133:363, 1985.
50. McLorie GA, McKenna PH, Greenburg M, et al. Reduction in tumor burden allowing partial nephrectomy following preoperative chemotherapy in biopsy proved Wilms' tumor. J Urol 146:509, 1991.
51. Cozzi F, Schiavetti A, Clerico A, et al. Tumor enucleation in unilateral Wilms' tumor: A pilot study. Med Pediatr Oncol 25:313, 1995.
52. Ritchey ML, Green DM, Thomas P, et al. Renal failure in Wilms tumor. Med Pediatr Oncol 23:264, 1994.
53. Coppes MJ, deKraker J, vanKijken PJ, et al. Bilateral Wilms' tumor: Long-term survival and some epidemiological features. J Clin Oncol 7:310, 1989.
54. Penn I. Renal transplantation for Wilms' tumor: Report of 20 cases. J Urol 122:793, 1979.
55. Shaul DB, Srikanth MM, Ortega JA, Mahour GH. Treatment of bilateral Wilms' tumor: Comparison of initial biopsy and chemotherapy to initial surgical resection in the preservation of renal mass and function. J Pediatr Surg 27:1009, 1992.
56. Horwitz J, Ritchey ML, Moksness J, et al. Renal salvage procedures in patients with synchronous bilateral Wilms tumors: A report of the NWTSG. J Pediatr Surg (in press).

PART III

The Ureter

R. DIXON WALKER

5

Vesicoureteral Reflux

The surgical management of vesicoureteral reflux is based on principles that were developed by pioneers who played an integral part in pediatric urologic history. The most basic principle is that vesicoureteral reflux occurs because of an incompetent flap valve. It is corrected by creating a competent flap valve with a sufficient tunnel length to ureteral diameter ratio to prevent reflux. Sampson and Young in 1903 simultaneously recognized that the obliquity of the ureter, as it coursed through the bladder wall, prevented reflux.[1, 2] Coffey, in an eloquent presentation to the Surgical Section of the American Medical Association in 1910, declared that, in dealing with a severed ureter, tunneling the ureter through the bowel wall would prevent regurgitation of bowel contents to the kidney.[3] He provided proof by citing an experiment involving two groups of dogs, one with a tunneled ureterointestinal anastomosis and the other with an end-to-side anastomosis. The latter group experienced sepsis and pyelonephritis. This same principle was supported by Gilchrist and colleagues in their attempt to create a continent diversion, which failed only because there was no knowledge of clean intermittent catheterization.[4] Leadbetter and Clarke,[5] in 1955, applied this principle to ureterosigmoidostomy, and in 1958 Politano took Leadbetter's application and applied it first in animal experimentations and then to children with reflux.[6] Paquin provided a more accurate assessment of the ureterovesical junction and found that the ratio of tunnel length to ureteral diameter necessary to prevent reflux was approximately 5:1.[7] All of these early pioneers applied this principle to the new techniques they developed, and their success with these new procedures set the stage for the development of pediatric urology as a specialty.

The purpose of this chapter is to elaborate on how this historic information is still so vitally important in our present-day decision making about the management of reflux. The reflux described previously is *primary* vesicoureteral reflux and occurs because there is an inadequate flap valve in the bladder. This inadequate flap valve is a result of a deficient tunnel length to ureteral diameter ratio. Secondary reflux may also occur because of an inadequate flap valve but is in part related to an underlying problem that alters bladder function. Conditions that cause secondary reflux include sphincter dyssynergia, posterior urethral valves, prune-belly syndrome, and neurogenic bladder. Initial management decisions must be based on how the patient presents to the physician.

PRESENTATION OF VESICOURETERAL REFLUX

Prenatal Hydronephrosis

The most common presentation of reflux in the neonate is hydronephrosis on prenatal ultrasonogram. It has been estimated that as much as 17% of prenatal hydronephrosis cases may be related to reflux.[8] Many more cases without pyelocaliectasis may involve mild reflux. One of the important characteristics of prenatal reflux is that it often appears worse because of the elasticity of the newborn collecting system. Thus, even high-grade reflux may improve or resolve quickly in neonates. Reflux that is prenatal may be associated with dysmorphic kidneys, often a result of dysplasia.

Febrile Urinary Tract Infection

Infants and young children with reflux are most likely to present with a history of febrile urinary tract infection (UTI) with or without failure to thrive. Body temperature greater than 38.5°C is considered significant. Febrile UTI is much more often associated with acute pyelonephritis, whereas nonfebrile UTI is more often associated with cystitis. The most basic concept of the relationship of reflux to renal scarring is that the combination of UTI and significant reflux results in acute pyelonephritis, characterized by fever, which, if left untreated, causes renal scarring.[9] That relationship is depicted in Figure 5–1. Although there are exceptions to this algorithm, it is the model that most of us accept. Confirmation of this relationship is documented by several studies. Woodard and Holden evaluated a large number of children with febrile UTI. They found that 90% of the children with reflux presented with fever, whereas only 40% of children without reflux presented with fever.[10] Govan and Palmer found clinical evidence of acute pyelonephritis, including

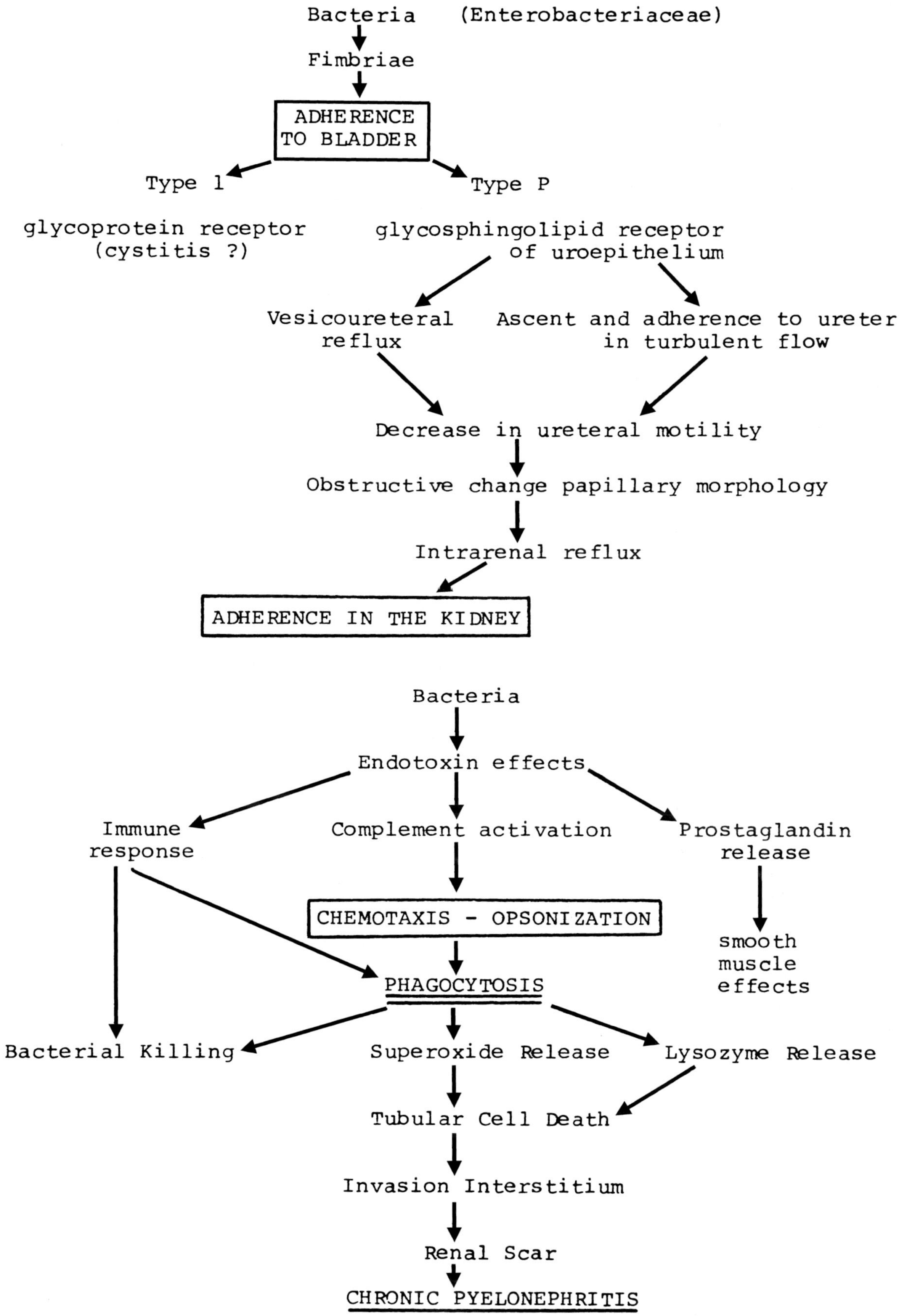

Figure 5–1 Algorithm of pathophysiology of pyelonephritis. From Roberts JA. Pathogenesis of pyelonephritis. J Urol 129:1102, 1983. Used with permission.

fever, in 79% of children with reflux but only 39% of children without reflux.[11]

Abdominal Pain

Abdominal pain is common in children and is difficult to relate to reflux. Some children appear to have colicky pain with voiding and another subset have pain when the bladder is full. Improvement of this pain after reflux resolves is not predictable.

Incontinence

Dysfunctional voiding is common in children with reflux, and the presentation of a wet child with or without UTI may prompt the cystographic evaluation of the bladder with the discovery of reflux. Taylor and coworkers have indicated that as many as 75% of girls with reflux have evidence of bladder instability,[12] and the results of the International Reflux Study clearly showed that a large number of children with reflux were dysfunctional voiders when evaluated by parent questionnaire.[13] The spectrum of dysfunctional voiding can range from nocturnal enuresis to the Hinman syndrome, but intermittent daytime wetting in an uninfected child is the most common sign.

Inherited Reflux

For some patients the reflux is discovered as part of family screening. Jerkins and Noe found that 33% of siblings of patients with reflux will have reflux and 66% of children of patients with reflux will have reflux.[14, 15]

Secondary Reflux

Secondary reflux is discovered when a cystogram is done in patients with posterior urethral valves, prune-belly syndrome, imperforate anus, or neurogenic bladder.

EVALUATION

The basis for judging the severity of reflux is the grading system developed as part of the International Reflux Study,[16] depicted in Figure 5–2. The key to interpretation is assessing the calices and papillary impression; the grade is determined by the effect on the majority of calices in the kidney. Grade I is reflux into the ureter, Grade II is reflux to the kidney with maintenance of the sharp angles of the fornix, Grade III is reflux into the kidney with mild loss of the forniceal angle, Grade IV is reflux involving mild papillary blunting and more severe loss of the forniceal angle, and Grade V is reflux with loss of papillary impression and loss of the forniceal angle. These demarcations among grades are not rigid, and one must use some flexibility in interpretation to adapt to the variations actually seen in clinical practice.

The initial radiologic evaluation of the patient with suspected reflux depends, in part, on how the patient presents. For the initial assessment of suspected reflux, a contrast voiding cystourethrogram (VCUG) is preferred because this allows one to grade the reflux accurately and to assess the bladder for evidence of a duplex system, diverticula, or other disease. This approach also allows one to assess the urethra in males. For those patients evaluated because of prenatal hydronephrosis, the diagnosis is established on a postnatal VCUG, which is recommended as a part of postnatal evaluation in

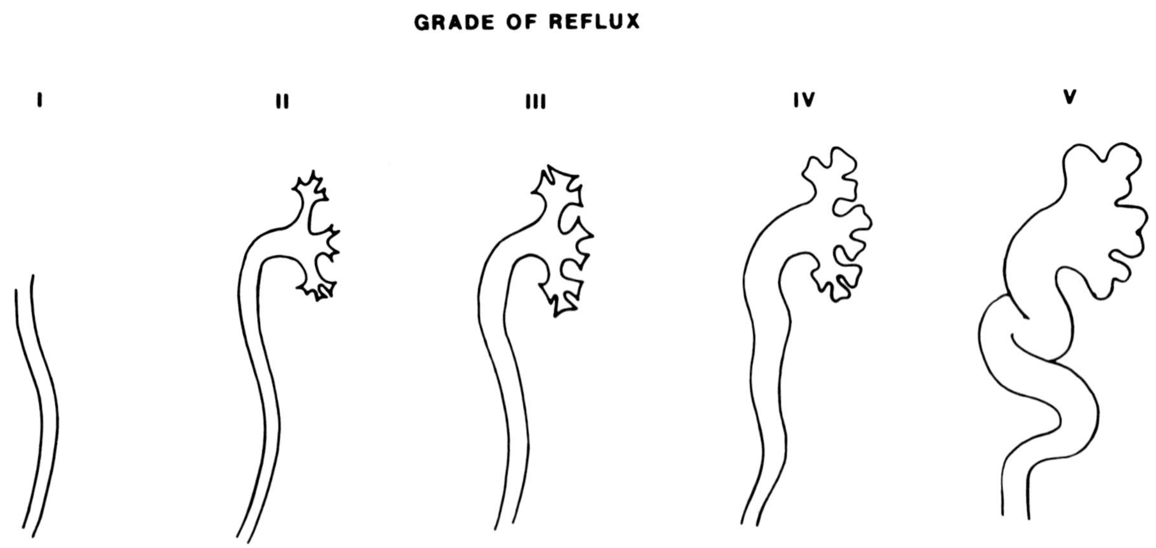

Figure 5–2 International Reflux Study Grading System.

conjunction with an ultrasonogram and a diethylenetriamine-pentaacetic acid renal scan. These studies then delineate whether the hydronephrosis is a result of the reflux or whether reflux is simply an associated finding (Fig. 5–3). This determination is most often made on the basis of the grade of reflux because low-grade reflux (Grades I and II) would be unlikely to be associated with hydronephrosis, and if present, most likely coincidental. Grade III and especially Grades IV and V are more likely to cause hydronephrosis.

Reflux is most frequently discovered as part of the evaluation of UTI. The appropriate radiologic evaluation after UTI depends on whether the child presents with fever. For children who present with a febrile UTI, an ultrasonogram should be obtained while treating the initial infection with intravenous therapy. This will rule out hydronephrosis and often suggest acute pyelonephritis. In selected cases (such as children with augmented bladders) a technetium 99m–dimercaptosuccinic acid (DMSA) renal scan will confirm acute pyelonephritis. Children who are afebrile at presentation are treated with appropriate antibiotics or antibacterials, and the ultrasonogram is obtained at the time of the VCUG. In both groups of children, the VCUG can be done approximately 2 to 4 weeks after initiating therapy for the UTI. This time frame is arbitrary but does allow some of the inflammatory process in the bladder to subside.

Nuclear cystography has its advocates. It has the advantage of decreased radiation dosage and perhaps increased sensitivity. The indications for its use are primarily in screening female patients and in follow-up studies in either sex. The disadvantage of the nuclear cystogram is that the grading system does not allow a strict comparison to the International Reflux Study (IRS) grading system and does not allow visualization of the urethra or other bladder disease. Abdominal ultrasonography is not satisfactory for diagnosing reflux. Blane and coworkers found that ultrasonography was completely normal in 74% of reflux patients evaluated.[17] This also indicates that ultrasonography is a poor method of screening siblings of children with reflux.

Intravenous urography (IVU) is not required for patients with reflux. The disadvantage of IVU is the radiation dosage, the possibility of contrast reaction, and the inadequacy of adequate visualization in many children. Ultrasonography will adequately assess renal length and growth and is less invasive when used repeatedly in follow-up. DMSA renal scans are the most sensitive test for assessment of renal scarring. Because DMSA scintigraphy is not widely available, IVU may be used in its place to assess scarring. The relative sensitivity of these three studies in assessing scarring is 60% for ultrasonography, 90% for IVU, and 98% for DMSA renal scan.[18, 19] IVU is also useful in instances in which it is suspected

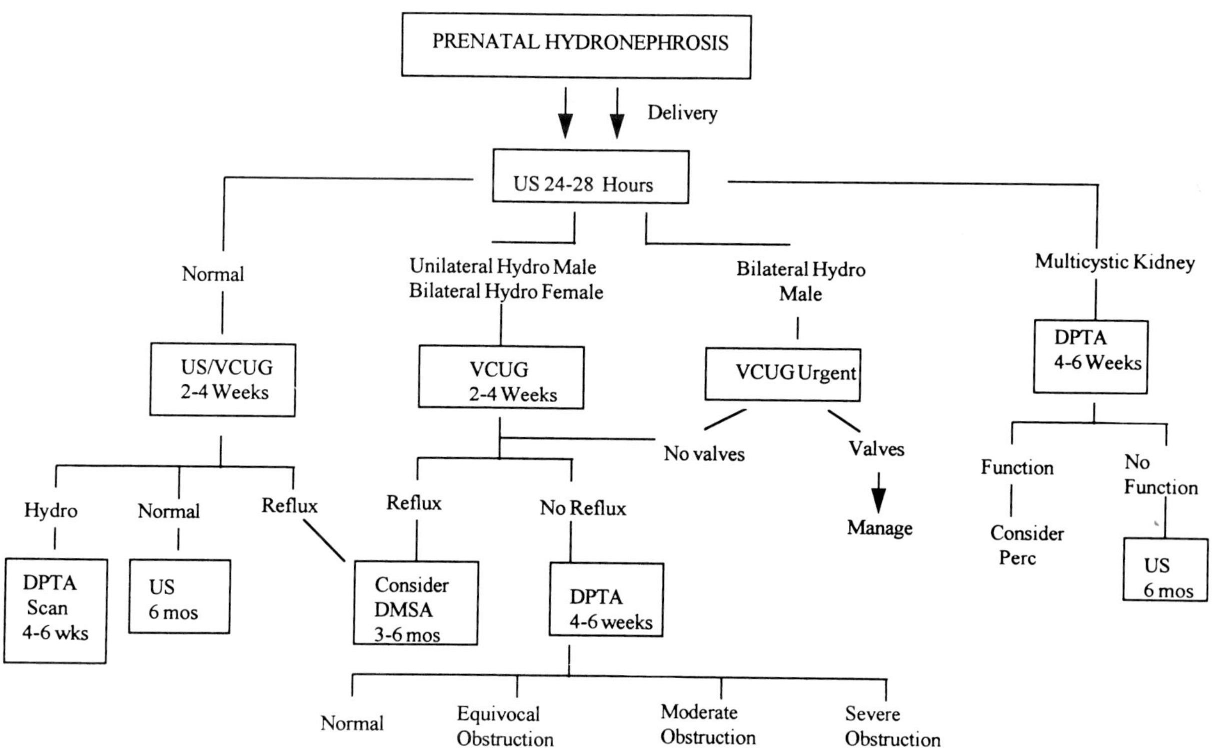

Figure 5–3 The relationship of reflux to prenatal hydronephrosis. (US, ultrasonogram; VCUG, voiding cystourethrogram; DTPA, diethylenetriamine-pentaacetic acid; DMSA, 99m-technetium-dimercaptosuccinic acid; Perc, percutaneous nephrostomy.)

that the vesicoureteral reflux is into the lower pole of a duplex system.

MANAGEMENT

The initial management of reflux when first detected depends on a variety of factors. Probably the two most important are the age of the child at diagnosis and the grade of reflux. The basis for medical management is that reflux will resolve spontaneously, with growth of the intravesical ureter, in a majority of patients. Edwards and coworkers[20] did the pioneering work with medical management and found that reflux resolved in 41% of dilated ureters and 85% of nondilated ureters. This study was done before the IRS classification system, and it is likely that those ureters that were dilated were those with high-grade reflux. The prospective study on low-grade reflux by the Southwest Pediatric Nephrology Group indicated excellent resolution in Grades I and II; 82% and 80%, respectively, within 5 years.[21] Contrasting this is the retrospective study of high-grade reflux from Toronto that showed that 70% of patients with Grade IV persisted at 5 years.[22] The results of the IRS also showed that resolution was heavily dependent on grade.[23] These data confirmed the findings of others that children with low-grade reflux (Grades I and II) had an excellent chance of spontaneous resolution, whereas those with high-grade reflux (Grade IV and V) had much less chance of resolution. Grade III reflux has an intermediate resolution. Resolution rates of reflux for different grades are depicted in Table 5–1. The IRS data also showed that resolution depends on whether the reflux is unilateral or bilateral; the latter has less chance of resolution. The data from other prospective studies do not refute the data from the IRS. Resolution of Grade IV reflux was higher in studies by Scholtmeijer, but the number of patients studied was small.[24] The prospective study by Goldraich and Goldraich showed poor resolution of Grade IV reflux, and it appeared that resolution in males was less likely.[25]

Table 5–1
Five-Year Resolution or Improvement Rates for Vesicoureteral Reflux

Grade	No. Ureters	Resolution (%)	Improvement (%)
I	23*	86*	NA
II	71*	78*	8*
III	111†	59*	26*
IV	229‡	16‡	33‡

* Data from International Reflux Study, European arm[23] and Scholtmeijer.[24]
† Data from International Reflux Study, European arm,[23] Southwest Pediatric Nephrology Group,[21] and Scholtmeijer.[24]
‡ Data from Southwest Pediatric Nephrology Group[21] and Scholtmeijer.[24]
NA, not applicable.

Resolution may also be altered by the presence of other anomalies such as a duplex collecting system, the presence of a diverticulum, or dysfunctional voiding. The actual resolution of reflux with complete duplication is not known but is almost certainly related to grade and is probably slightly worse than would be expected with single systems. Peppas and colleagues reviewed 56 children with duplex systems and reflux and found that reflux did resolve in some patients (18%) and another 23% who were monitored medically did not have deterioration of their kidneys.[26] Ben-Ami and associates found resolution of reflux in most of their children with low-grade reflux but no resolution in patients with Grade IV reflux into a duplex system.[27] Resolution of reflux in a ureter that enters a diverticulum is unlikely to occur and is probably decreased when associated with a paraureteral diverticulum. Aladjem and coworkers noted failure of even low-grade reflux to resolve when associated with a paraureteral diverticulum, but their length of follow-up was short.[28] Resolution of reflux associated with a paraureteral diverticulum probably relates to the size of the diverticulum and the degree of its damage to the muscular hiatus. Resolution may also be delayed in patients who are dysfunctional voiders. Dysfunctional voiding is common in refluxing patients. Taylor and others found that 75% of girls with reflux and clinical symptoms of urgency or incontinence had evidence of unstable bladder activity on urodynamic studies.[12] Koff and Murtagh identified 62 children with uninhibited bladder and reflux and found that they could significantly improve resolution rates with anticholinergic treatment.[29] Seruca found, in a similar group of patients, not only increased resolution of reflux with anticholinergic treatment but also conversion of the bladder from an unstable to stable pattern.[30] Sill'en and others showed that this was not age dependent and the voiding dysfunction occurred not only in young children but in infants with high-grade reflux.[31] The data from the IRS examined the incidence of dysfunctional voiding in the cohort of patients selected for the study and found it to be 18%. A strong negative correlation was found between the presence of dysfunctional voiding and the resolution of reflux.[13]

Another important factor in the initial management is the status of the kidneys. A solitary kidney may call for more aggressive management of reflux, although data to support this are largely biased. Hypertension, renal insufficiency, and extensive renal scarring may also be relative factors favoring surgical management. The basis for this latter decision would be to protect all remaining renal parenchyma from further damage. Finally, the objective findings in the patient need to be coordinated with the patient's family and their expectations, because some families are interested in medical management and will likely be compliant, whereas others want a more direct solution to the problem.

Thus, the initial recommendation for management in a child with reflux will be heavily weighted toward medical management. Children with unilateral or bilateral Grade V reflux should often be managed surgically. The exception would be an infant with Grade V reflux who would be given at least a short period of close medical management to determine whether there was improvement in grade. The reason for this is the concept that the neonatal ureter may be more elastic and compliant and even very dilated ureters might improve quickly. Another alternative for infants with persistent Grade V reflux would be temporary cystostomy, which has the advantage of allowing the reflux to decrease in grade. The disadvantage of cystostomy is that the thin-walled bladder is more prone to prolapse and other complications.[32] Early surgical management should also be considered in an older child or adolescent with Grade IV reflux, particularly if bilateral. The selection of an age is arbitrary, but after 7 to 8 years of age resolution of Grade IV reflux is unlikely. This initial decision would also be based on the status of the kidneys at initial evaluation and an assessment of the willingness of the parents to comply with medical management. The presence of single kidneys or extensive scarring would weigh in favor of initial management by surgery. All other patients than those who fit these criteria would initially be medically managed.

Medical Management

Treatment and Prevention of Infection. Febrile UTI will require specific intravenous antibiotic therapy, with an attempt to deliver the first dose within 12 hours of the initiation of fever. Ransley and Risdon, in their elegant work in swine, showed that early treatment of pyelonephritis can prevent renal scarring.[33] In many of the children who require intravenous antibiotic therapy, hospitalization can be avoided and the medication administered by a home health care team. The most common antibiotics are ceftazidime or ceftriaxone until the results of the culture are available. Nonfebrile UTI can be treated with oral antibacterials or antibiotics in a full therapeutic dose for 7 to 10 days. Prevention is best accomplished by giving antibacterials such as nitrofurantoin or trimethoprim-sulfamethoxazole in a dose that is one half the therapeutic dose. These drugs can have side effects for infants up to 3 months of age, and the best choice is amoxicillin, ampicillin, or cephalexin. Prophylactic therapy with antibacterials is the cornerstone of medical management. Breakthrough UTI while on antibacterial medication, particularly if associated with fever, represents an indication for conversion to surgical management. Thus, compliance by the parents in giving the medication is important. Compliance may be difficult to measure, and pharmacologic compliance testing, although available, is not always practical. A good measure of compliance is the presence of a breakthrough UTI with a bacterium sensitive to the antibacterial that the child is currently on. Side effects of low-dose antibacterial therapy are uncommon. Other than obtaining periodic history and physical examination, the only other study necessary is a yearly blood count for patients taking trimethoprim. Parents often have questions about the development of resistance to antibacterials or long-term side effects. Antibacterials are less likely than antibiotics to develop a resistant strain, and both nitrofurantoin and trimethoprim-sulfamethoxazole can be tolerated for extended periods of time with infrequent side effects. When breakthrough UTI does occur, it should be treated as with the initial infection: intravenous therapy for febrile infections and oral therapy for nonfebrile infections for 7 to 10 days and then resumption of the prophylactic antibacterials.

Treatment of Associated Dysfunctional Voiding. This is an integral part of the management of reflux. The diagnosis of dysfunctional voiding is suggested by a history of incontinence and can be confirmed by urodynamic study. Dysfunctional voiding associated with reflux in small children before toilet training should be treated with oxybutynin. Older children with incontinence and reflux can be treated with oxybutynin, propantheline, or hyoscyamine or by bladder retraining.

Frequency of Urine Cultures

Urine cultures should be done at no greater than 3-month intervals. Any febrile episode between office visits requires a urine culture to rule out breakthrough UTI. Many parents are interested in more frequent surveillance. Home culture can be performed by parents who are taught an office methodology by dedicated clinic nursing personal. The home culture is done after obtaining a voided specimen in a clean container. An advantage to a home culture program is that siblings can be screened. An alternative to home cultures is to teach parents to use a dipstick to test for nitrites and leukocytes. Positive home cultures or dipsticks then require a laboratory culture and sensitivity to confirm infection.

Frequency of Radiological Studies

The initial radiological study most often is a contrast VCUG and abdominal ultrasonogram. In children younger than 2 years, a VCUG or nuclear cystogram is repeated at 1-year intervals. After 2 years of age, alternating contrast and nuclear cystograms are done every 18 months. Indications for a cystogram more often include breakthrough UTI or new renal scarring on IVU or DMSA scan. After resolution of the reflux has been confirmed on cystogram, the study does not have to be repeated unless the child has febrile UTI. It has been suggested that reflux can be absent on one study and present on another in as many as 30% of children. Thus, some recommend two negative studies to declare reflux resolved.[34] Although this is scientifically more accurate, it is not cost effective and many parents will not accept it.

Renal growth can be adequately assessed with follow-up abdominal ultrasonogram, which is not satisfactory to assess renal scarring. Renal growth is assessed by obtaining an ultrasonogram at yearly intervals. More frequent ultrasonograms are done if the kidney is not growing or the child has febrile UTI. After reflux has resolved, an ultrasonogram should be done annually for at least 2 years to monitor renal growth and longer if there is extensive renal scarring. Ideally, all children with vesicoureteral reflux should have an early renal assessment with IVU or DMSA renal scan. DMSA renal scan provides the best measure of function and scarring but is not available in all areas. Because it may not be cost effective to perform DMSA scanning in all children with reflux, strict criteria should at least include those who have Grade IV or V reflux and all children with febrile UTI. The timing of these studies in relation to UTI is important. A reasonable time is 2 to 4 months after evidence of a febrile infection to allow the acute effects of the UTI to resolve. As shown by Friedland, renal scarring may take up to 2 years to develop.[35] For this reason DMSA renal scan is also recommended 2 years after reflux is medically or surgically resolved; a normal scan portends a prognosis without future renal scarring.

Criteria for Switching to Surgical Management

Criteria for switching to surgical management include breakthrough UTI, evidence of new renal scarring, failure of the kidney to grow, noncompliance by the parents in giving antibacterial therapy, and failure of the reflux to resolve with medical management. All of these indications for surgical management are subject to interpretation and are dependent on a joint decision with the family.

Breakthrough UTI is a relative indication for converting to surgical management depending on the type of breakthrough infection and the grade of reflux. The need for individualized management is nowhere more evident than in this important group of patients. The presence of asymptomatic bacteriuria in a patient being monitored for low-grade reflux is not often a reason to convert to surgical management. Alternatively, the clearest indication for immediate conversion to surgical therapy would be a severe febrile breakthrough UTI with confirmed pyelonephritis followed by a demonstrated renal scar on DMSA scan. Most of the patents with breakthrough UTI fall between these extremes. Factors that favor continued medical management are low-grade reflux and asymptomatic or afebrile breakthrough infection occurring infrequently and associated with no new renal scars. Frequent infection, particularly when associated with fever, is a factor that favors conversion to surgical management. Parents who are noncompliant in giving antibacterials present a particular dilemma because some of those children will maintain a sterile urine and be at low risk. Parents who are noncompliant on medication are also likely to be noncompliant on follow-up visits; thus, most often their children should be surgically managed. A different group of parents are those whose children did not present with or have UTI and who request not to have antibacterials as part of a joint decision-making process with the surgeon. These children are ideal candidates for a home culture program and may often be successfully managed without medication.

Changes in the kidney structure, either new renal scars or failure of the kidney to grow, direct one to consider surgical management even if there are no breakthrough UTIs. Most often, renal growth is assessed over several years before making a decision to convert. Bauer and coworkers have shown improvement in renal growth, even in very small kidneys, after reflux resolves.[36]

The age at which complete resolution of reflux is no longer to be expected is not known. The management of reflux persisting into late childhood has been a subject for debate. Despite the lack of specific data about the natural history of reflux in adolescents, four pediatric urologists and one pediatric nephrologist concluded that reflux in the adolescent girl should be repaired.[37] The basis for this is the opinion that women entering childbearing age who have reflux are more likely to experience pyelonephritis and renal scarring. The infection is also more difficult to treat because of a decreased choice of antibacterial therapy. Low-grade reflux in males is unlikely to cause long-term damage to the kidney, but this has to be balanced by the data on sterile reflux, which are largely short term. Last, most patients will not be compliant for the remainder of their life with long-term antibacterials, frequent office visits, and repeat radiological studies. Thus, the reality is that many adolescent and adult patients who are medically managed will subsequently be lost to follow-up.

SURGICAL MANAGEMENT

The options for surgical management should be discussed with the family. These options include periureteral injection of collagen or an open surgical procedure. Injection of collagen is advantageous in that it can be done as an outpatient procedure with little discomfort to the patient. Other substances for subureteric injection have been described but are not approved in the United States for use in children. The major disadvantage of collagen injection is that the short-term success rates are poorer than with an open procedure, and there are no data on long-term success. Additionally, the substance is quite expensive and may not be covered by insurance. The clearest advantage of an open surgical repair of reflux is that there is a long track record of success. The chances of correcting reflux, without simultaneously causing obstruction, are better than 95% in most current series. The success rate in the American arm of the IRS was 99% when the procedure was done by an experienced surgeon.[38] Similar success rates have been enjoyed with all open techniques. Operative success is less when the patient has an abnormal thick-walled bladder or a dilated ureter that will require tapering. The success rate with collagen injection is much less. Frey and others injected 97 ureters in 66 children and had a short-term success rate of 59% after one injection and 77% after two.[39] Short term, in the context of reflux correction, is not well defined, but data are available for 2 to 3 years of follow-up. Long term is intended to mean correction of reflux for the life of the patient. Our current knowledge of collagen biology is that the substance will degrade and be absorbed over a period of time and then reflux may recur.

The choice of an open operative procedure is a decision to be made by the surgeon. The Cohen,[40] or transtrigonal, procedure is widely done and has the advantage of having a very low rate of postoperative obstruction with high resolution of reflux. It is also the procedure of choice for patients with a small bladder. The disadvantage of the Cohen procedure is that reflux or obstruction, if either develops, may be more difficult to manage because of the inability to view the ureteral orifice directly through the cystoscope. The Glenn-Anderson procedure[41] is another excellent advancement procedure that has most of the advantages of the Cohen procedure: it is easily viewed cystoscopically if there is a complication but is not always applicable because it requires a very laterally placed refluxing orifice. The Politano-Leadbetter[6] procedure is one of the most popular procedures worldwide. It is a more technically demanding procedure than the others and can result in an unacceptably high complication rate in inexperienced hands. Complications that are associated with this procedure only are placing the ureter through peritoneum or bowel. The disadvantage of the Paquin[42] procedure is the extensive amount of extravesical dissection required, but this dissection is advantageous when one has to perform extensive tapering of a ureter, particularly when used with a psoas hitch. It is also an excellent procedure for use with renal transplantation. The Lich-Gregoire procedure is undergoing a resurgence of popularity in the United States.[43, 44] The advantage of this procedure is that the patient has fewer postoperative complaints such as hematuria or bladder spasms. Additionally, catheter drainage may be shortened as might hospital stays. The disadvantage is that one is not able to view the interior of the bladder and the opposite orifice and thus may be unaware of intravesical disease such as a diverticulum, small ureterocele, or trabeculation. This problem can be avoided by examining the patient cystoscopically before beginning the procedure.

Surgical Technique of Collagen Injection

Before using collagen clinically, the patient should be given a skin test to ensure that he or she is not reactive to the collagen. This is done by injecting the collagen into the volar surface of the forearm and observing for a reaction over the next month. A reaction will usually be erythematous.

Children receiving collagen injection require an outpatient general anesthetic. Ideally, a urine culture should be done 48 hours before the injection to ensure its sterility, but this is not always practical. Indeed, some patients who are chronically bacteriuric will still require injection. An alternative to a urine culture is a dipstick urinalysis of a catheterized specimen obtained at the beginning of the procedure. If the urine is infected, consideration should be given to canceling the procedure, particularly in a patient in whom the infection is unexpected. All infected patients should be treated with appropriate antibiotic therapy.

The patient is placed in the lithotomy position and the perineum draped as for cystoscopy. In female children, the urethra may be dilated with urethral sounds so as to accommodate a 17 French cystourethroscope through which can be inserted the 22-gauge Bard needle. The alternative is to use a 10 French cystoscope through which one can pass a 21-gauge, 20-cm Yale endourology needle. At cystoscopy the bladder should be initially inspected and both orifices identified. With the bladder approximately one-third full, the needle is advanced into view and, upon visualization of the appropriate orifice, is placed at the 6 o'clock position at the lowest edge of the orifice.[45] The needle is then advanced underneath the ureteral mucosa for a distance of 2 to 4 mm and held steadily in place. The collagen is then slowly injected submucosally so that the floor of the ureter is elevated, creating a crescentic orifice. Once the lumen is obliterated, the needle is held in place for 30 to 60 seconds to allow the collagen to "sit" and then slowly withdrawn. The amount injected depends on the size of the orifice and may vary from 0.5 to 1.5 mL. The cystoscope is then withdrawn, and the patient is allowed to void normally (Fig. 5–4).

It is not unusual for two injections, and sometimes three, to be required. If the collagen has not worked with three injections, then it is unlikely to do so, and an open surgical procedure should be considered. Open surgical procedures to correct reflux done after collagen injection do not appear to be made more difficult because of the collagen.

Technique of Advancement Ureterocystoplasty

The techniques for ureteral reimplantation that are described in detail are those that I prefer, predominately

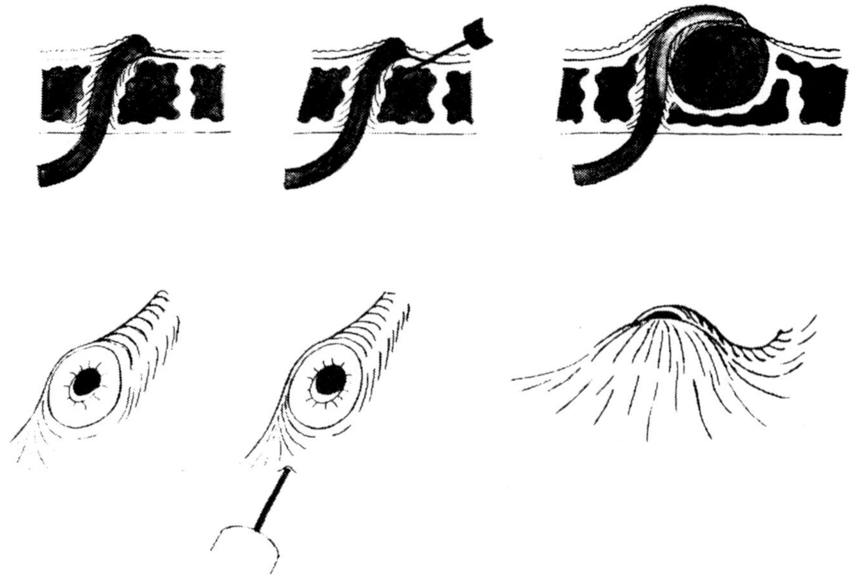

Figure 5–4 Technique of collagen injection. From Lipsky H. Endoscopic treatment of vesicoureteral reflux with bovine collagen. Eur Urol 18:52, 1990. Used with permission.

advancement-type procedures. (The urologist should, however, be familiar with all techniques because conditions that are present intraoperatively may alter one's plans.) The two advancement operations that meet this criterion are the Cohen[40] and the Glenn-Anderson[41] operations. The advantages of these operations have been discussed. The decision as to which to use is based on the laterality of the refluxing orifice. For those orifices that are far lateral, in which a tunnel can be directed toward the bladder neck, the Glenn-Anderson procedure is appropriate. In the patient with the smaller bladder base, the Cohen procedure is more appropriate.

The positioning of the patient for the procedure is important. A pad of one to two folded towels placed underneath the sacrum will elevate the pelvis and allow improved access to the bladder. Having the legs spread slightly allows preparation of the genital area for placement of a Foley catheter during the procedure (Fig. 5–5). General anesthesia with sufficient muscle relaxation is required for adequate intravesical exposure. Once the retractor is placed, it should not be continually adjusted because this will increase bladder edema.

The incision is a standard suprapubic incision that is one fingerbreadth above the pubis and runs to the lateral border of the rectus muscle. The rectus fascia is freed up extensively from the underlying muscle, allowing adequate retraction. Once the rectus muscle has been split in the midline, the anterior bladder wall is gently dissected and two holding sutures are placed through the bladder wall. No attempt is made to dissect lateral to the bladder. The bladder is opened in the midline only sufficiently to accommodate the Denis-Browne retractor. Although more modern retractors are available, the Denis-Browne type is still optimal in the majority of cases.

Once the retractor is placed, the decision is made, based on the anatomy, to perform a Cohen or a Glenn-Anderson procedure. They are both started in the same manner (Fig. 5–6). The refluxing orifice is catheterized with a 5 French feeding tube, and a figure-eight suture is placed through the orifice and held for traction. Frequent suction should be avoided because it can cause bladder edema, and moist saline sponges allow cleaning of the area. The bladder wall should also be frequently irrigated with saline. The mucosa around the orifice is scored with the electrocautery. The scored mucosa is incised, and,

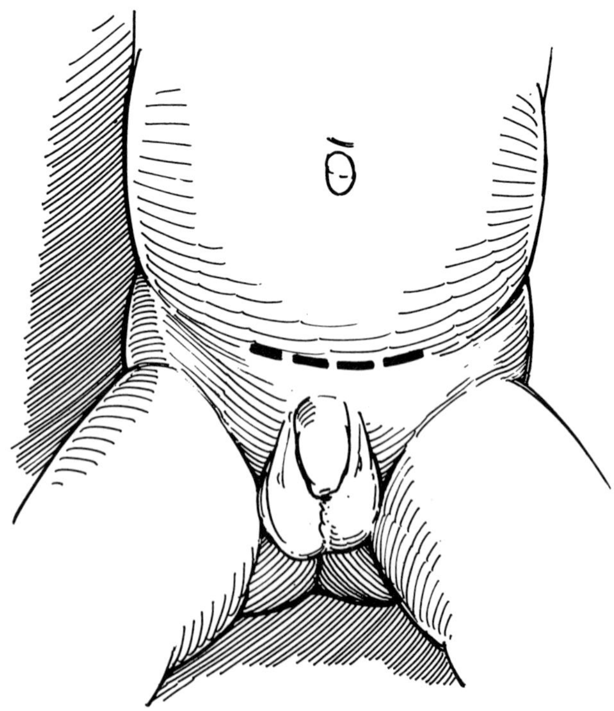

Figure 5–5 Position of patient.

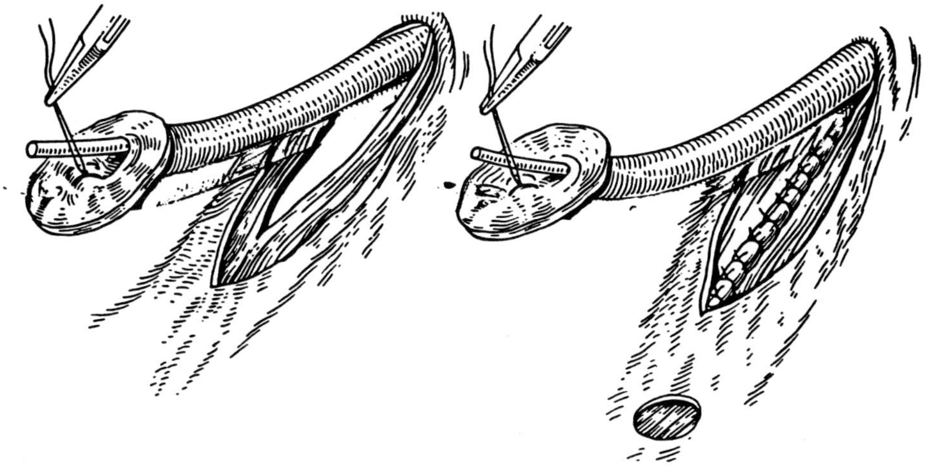

Figure 5–6 Ureter catheterized, tagged with holding suture, and mobilized. Hiatus closed with interrupted absorbable suture.

using the tenotomy or DeMartel scissors, dissection is carried through the bladder wall at the inferior aspect of the orifice. The muscle bundles of Waldeyer's sheath are elevated with a sharp right-angle clamp and cauterized well away from the ureter. As one dissects the retrovesical space, the retrovesical fat and peritoneum come into view and are dissected from the ureter with a Kitner dissector. This last maneuver usually frees the ureter adequately for sufficient tunnel length. The mucosa at the hiatus is then dissected free from the underlying muscle, and the muscle is closed with interrupted absorbable suture of sufficient strength and without unduly tightening the hiatus, which should admit a clamp alongside the ureter. If tight, the hiatus should be reopened because a narrow passage in the bladder wall will produce obstruction. The diameter of the ureter is measured with an ophthalmic caliper, and a submucosal tunnel, five times this diameter in length is designed. A tunnel length that is too long or too narrow may lead to obstruction, and one that is too short will predispose to persistent reflux. Dissection is then made with DeMartel scissors across the bladder for the Cohen procedure (Fig. 5–7) or toward the bladder neck for the Glenn-Anderson procedure (Fig. 5–8). When there is not quite enough tunnel length to perform a Glenn-Anderson repair, the hiatus can be enlarged as described by Mathisen[46] (Fig. 5–9).

The ureter is brought through the tunnel and the end trimmed and spatulated if necessary. Most refluxing orifices are large and usually do not require spatulation. Spatulation or cutting at a bias to create a larger orifice should be done on the top of the ureter. The new orifice is then sewn in place with interrupted, fine, absorbable suture. Sutures at the distal portion of the ureter should incorporate muscle (Fig. 5–10). All mucosal openings are then closed with fine, absorbable suture. Each orifice is then catheterized with a feeding tube to ensure patency of the ureter. Any difficulty passing this catheter must be resolved, even if it means redoing the reimplant. This is the most opportune time to prevent obstruction. If obstruction is encountered, it may be necessary to explore lateral to the bladder to determine whether the ureter has been obstructed outside the bladder. Obstruction is a rare complication with either of the advancement procedures. A decision will also be made as to whether to stent the ureters during the postoperative period. Stents are most often required when the operation has been difficult or the ureter is quite small. Adequate stenting can be done with two small feeding tubes (3–5 French) passed alongside a 12 to 14 French urethral Foley catheter. After the Foley balloon is inflated, a sterile adhesive Band-Aid is wrapped around the catheter, and the catheters are sewn to the Band-Aid with silk suture. The bladder is then closed in three layers, with a watertight closure ensured by irrigation. No drains are used. The remainder of the closure is in standard fashion. A caudal anesthetic is initiated at the end of the operation and before the patient wakes from anesthesia.

The patient is given intraoperative antibiotics, which are continued postoperatively. Pain is managed with intravenous morphine and acetaminophen with codeine once fluids are tolerated. Bladder spasms are managed with chips of belladonna and opium suppositories for 24 hours and then oral oxybutynin. The catheter and stents are removed on day 3; after voiding, the patient is discharged home.

The Paquin Reimplantation

The Paquin reimplant is ideal for renal transplant ureteroneocystotomy as well as for cases in which extensive tapering and remodeling of the lower ureter is required.[42] The procedure lends itself to an associated psoas hitch when tapering and remodeling are done.

The preoperative preparation and positioning of the patient are the same as for the Cohen or Glenn-Anderson repairs. An incision is made in the same location, extended slightly cephalad if tapering of the ureter is expected. As the prevesical space is entered, the bladder is identified and tagged with two holding sutures. The bladder is emptied by either a catheter or a small cystotomy incision. Attention is then directed toward mobilizing each lateral aspect of the bladder by blunt dissection, with particular attention to sweeping off the peritoneum. The Denis-Browne retractor is placed so as to retract the rectus muscles laterally. The obliterated umbilical artery is identified, clamped, divided, and ligated. Following the obliterated artery retroperitoneally by placing slight traction on it, the ureter is identified just medial to the vessel. Although placing a ureteral catheter before this maneuver may aid in identification, it is not necessary and it is preferable to leave the bladder undisturbed. A vessel loop is placed around the refluxing ureter, and blunt dissection is continued distally, dividing and ligating small bleeders as encountered. Where the ureter enters the bladder, the bladder wall is tented up, the ureter is clamped with a right-angle clamp and divided, and the ureteral stump and surrounding detrusor muscle are closed with a heavy absorbable ligature. If there is concern about weakness at the hiatus, one can close a second layer inverting the ureteral stump. Gentle blunt dissection of the ureter is then performed proximally; one must be especially careful to dissect free the peritoneum. Any ureteral tapering or remodeling is done as described in Chapter 6. The tunnel is then created by dissecting, with Metzenbaum scissors or a tonsil clamp, from the outside in, beginning at the lateral edge of the bladder base until the clamp or scissors are visualized submucosally. Using a combination of blunt and sharp dissection, the submucosal dissection is carried caudally toward the bladder neck until a tunnel has been created that is five times as long as the diameter of the ureter (Fig. 5–10*A*). A small transverse incision is then made at the distal tunnel and, with a clamp, a 12 French red Robinson catheter is grasped and brought through the tunnel. The distal ureter is then sewn to the tip of the catheter, and the catheter and ureter are brought distally through the tunnel (Fig.

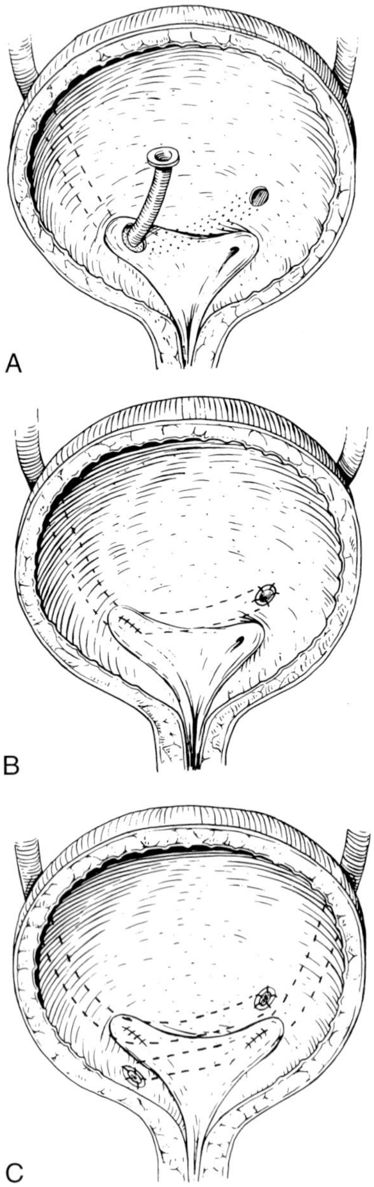

Figure 5–7 Cohen or cross-trigonal repair. *A*, Mobilization of ureter. *B*, Reimplantation of single ureter. *C*, Reimplantation of two ureters.

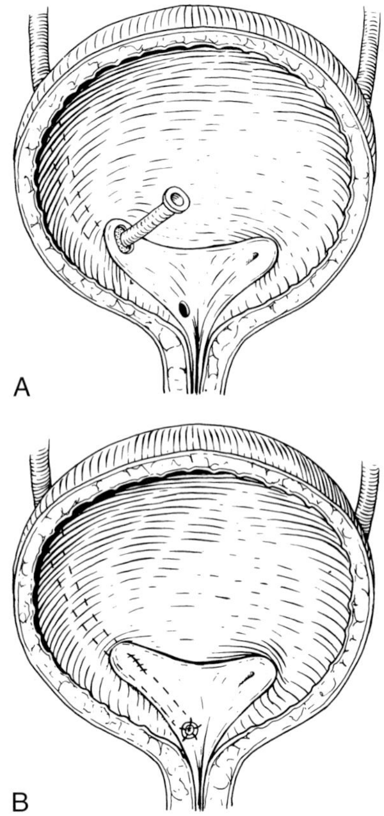

Figure 5–8 Glenn-Anderson repair. *A*, Mobilization of ureter. *B*, Advancement toward bladder neck.

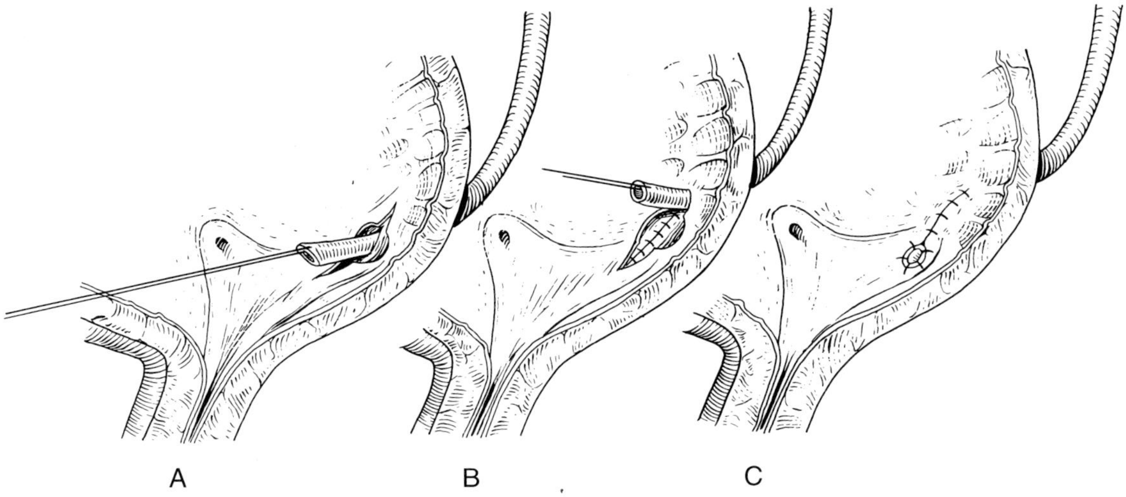

Figure 5–9 Mathisen repair. Modification can be used with Glenn-Anderson repair to increase tunnel length. The ureteral hiatus is recessed.

5–10*B*). The ureter is then trimmed and anchored with 4-6 interrupted, fine, absorbable sutures (Fig. 5–10 *inset*). The ureter is also secured with a fine absorbable suture on the outside of the bladder at the muscular hiatus that is placed from detrusor to ureteral adventitia. The bladder is drained with a Foley catheter, a ureteral stent is used if desired, and the bladder is closed in standard fashion.

There are several areas where one can have difficulty with this procedure. The ureter can be devascularized by extensive and careless dissection. Forceps for fine vascular work should be used. Electrocautery should be used judiciously on the ureter. Great care must be taken in dissecting free the peritoneum; if it is entered, caution must be used in closing it because a suture may incorporate the ureter and lead to obstruction. The tunnel needs to be made with precision and a wide enough dissection made so that the tunnel accommodates the ureteral width. A narrow tunnel may compromise vascularity. Last, the tunnel should be made on the bladder base rather than the side wall of the bladder because the latter can lead to J hooking and obstruction. The bladder base can be enlarged with a psoas hitch[47] (Fig. 5–11).

Duplex Reimplant

Reimplantation of duplex ureters can be accomplished satisfactorily with a Cohen or Glenn-Anderson–type repair (Fig. 5–12). Care must be taken not to twist the ureters and to make sufficient tunnel length.

Extravesical Reimplant

Extravesical reimplantation has gained in popularity, although is still done as the preferred procedure by a minority of pediatric urologists. The procedure may have some advantages over an intravesical procedure that will increase its usage.[48, 49] These advantages include a decrease in hospital stay and less postoperative symptomatology, particularly bladder spasms and hematuria. The disadvantages of the extravesical procedure are the inability to assess the bladder for associated disease (diverticula, stones, unsuspected duplex ureters, abnormal contralateral ureteral orifices) and the occurrence of postoperative urinary retention in some patients who have bilateral extravesical repair. Because the procedure is gaining in popularity and because it has a legitimate role in the armamentarium of the pediatric urologist, the procedure is described with the recent modifications that have improved surgical success of intravesical procedures[50] (Fig. 5–13).

Patient positioning, skin incision, and exposure of the bladder are the same as with the intravesical procedure. After separation of the rectus muscles and exposure of the bladder, the bladder is emptied with a Foley catheter. The perivesical space is bluntly dissected on each side of the bladder; special care is taken to sweep the peritoneum cephalad to avoid entry. The Denis-Browne retractor is placed in the perivesical space, and the bladder is retracted medially with a Deaver retractor. The obliterated umbilical vessel (often patent) is identified, divided, and suture ligated. Medial to the proximal portion of the obliterated umbilical vessel, the retrovesical space is entered, and the ureter is located, bluntly dissected, and retracted with a vessel loop. Extreme care must be taken not to enter the peritoneal cavity or to damage the blood supply to the ureter. The ureter is then followed and freed from the umbilical artery distally to its junction with the bladder. The vascular and muscular attachments of the lower ureter are divided, with vessels either electrocoagulated or ligated.

Once the ureter is mobilized, a detrusor incision is made in a cephalad direction in the axis of the ureter for

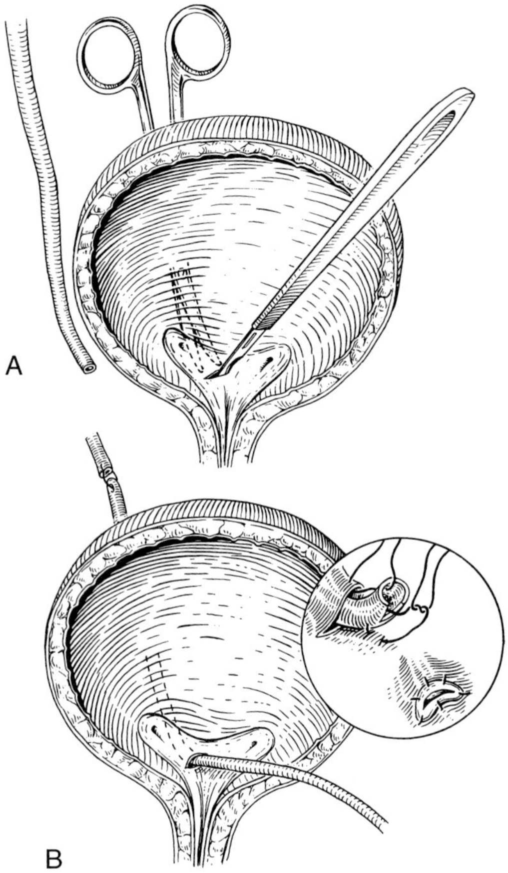

Figure 5–10 Paquin repair. *A*, Creating the tunnel with scissors or clamp. *B*, Ureter sewn to red Robinson catheter and brought through tunnel.

a distance of 2 to 3 cm, with care taken not to enter the bladder. This incision can be made with needle point electrocautery to maintain hemostasis. Once the mucosa is exposed, it is bluntly dissected to make a wide trough and also dissected distally and circumferentially around the attachment of the ureter to the bladder mucosa. This is one of the most important aspects of the procedure because it allows advancement of the ureter. This concept was first proposed by Daines and Hodgson[51] and is the prime factor that has allowed for the improved results over the classic Lich procedure. The ureter is advanced with the placement of two parallel sutures from the more distal bladder wall to the lateral aspect of the ureter. Once the sutures are tied, the ureter is advanced and fixed distally. The ureter is then laid in the wide detrusor trough, and the muscle is closed loosely over the ureter with interrupted, absorbable suture. No stents are used, and the Foley catheter is left in place for 2 to 3 days.

MANAGEMENT OF COMPLICATIONS OF URETERAL REIMPLANTATION

Prevention of complications of reimplantation surgery is the first priority of the surgeon. Prevention can be divided into those aspects that pertain to proper patient selection and those that are related to proper surgical technique.[52]

Bladder dysfunction represents the most common reason for improper patient selection. For that reason, it is important to elicit the findings on history or physical examination that might indicate dysfunctional voiding. Historically, one should be concerned about day- or night-time wetting, urgency, squatting, or encopresis. Physical examination should include examination of the buttocks and lower spine. Older children with these symptoms should have urodynamic studies and radiological evaluation of the lower spine. The latter may simply require a plain pelvic film, but, if indicated, a magnetic resonance imaging (MRI) of the lower spine should be performed. The finding of dysfunctional voiding does not preclude proceeding with ureteral reimplantation, but one must expect an increase in the complication rate. For that reason, it is better to stabilize the bladder, first using anticholinergic therapy and clean intermittent catheterization if necessary. Noe reviewed his experience with ureteral reimplantation and found that 66% of patients with failures had dysfunctional voiding.[53]

In addition to dysfunctional voiding, one must recognize that any pathologic process that leads to a thickened bladder wall will result in a decreased success rate. In almost all such situations, the reflux is secondary rather than primary, and management of the underlying primary disease is the first priority. Such conditions may include

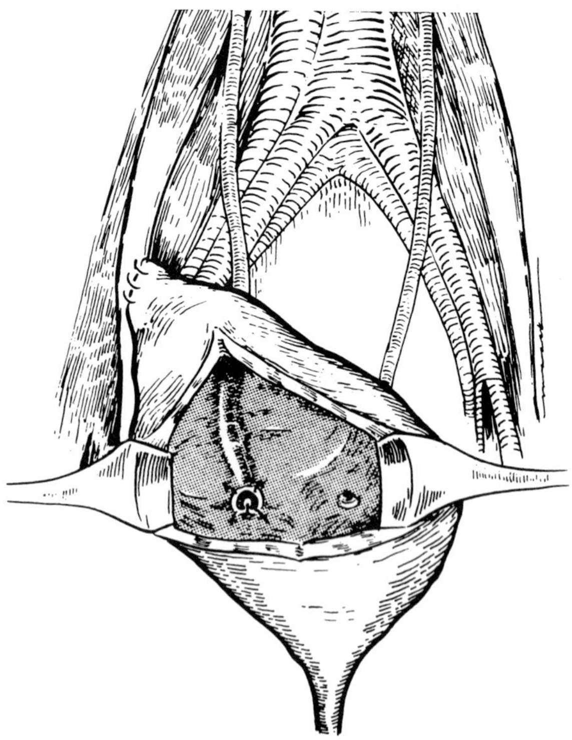

Figure 5–11 Psoas hitch. From Middleton RG. Routine use of the psoas hitch in ureteral reimplantation. J Urol 123:352, 1980. Used with permission.

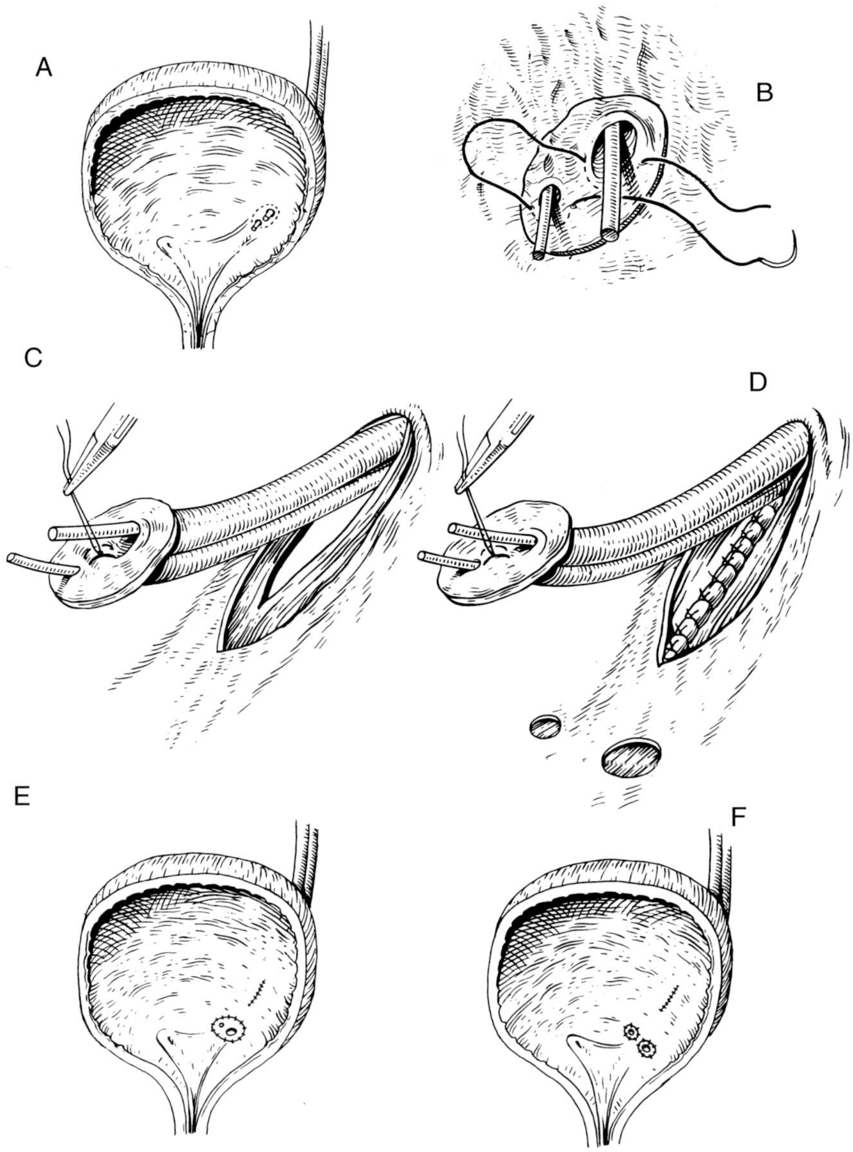

Figure 5–12 *A–F,* Reimplantation of duplex ureters with Glenn-Anderson procedure.

posterior urethral valves, neurogenic bladder, and prune-belly syndrome.

The technical problems that one can experience have been alluded to in previous discussion, but, to summarize, the tunnel should be approximately five times the diameter of the ureter in length, and it should be wide enough to accommodate the ureter without compressing it. The tunnel should be located on the posterior bladder wall, and extravesical dissection should not damage the peritoneum, müllerian structures, or rectum.

Complications will still occur despite best efforts to prevent them. Obstruction that occurs within the first 3 to 6 months can often be managed with balloon dilation and a short period of ureteral stenting. Obstruction that persists after 6 months should be approached endoscopically first. Most often, that can be done through the cystoscope, but a percutaneous nephrostomy may be required. The standard technique involves using a guidewire over which an endoureterectomy is performed. The incised area is then stented with an appropriate stent for 4 to 6 weeks. For those patients who fail an endourologic procedure, a repeat reimplant is the next step. Hendren outlined the basic principles for repeat reimplantation surgery.[54] These include minimal handling of the ureter, a combined intravesical-extravesical approach often with ureteral tailoring, and psoas hitch. Other alternatives would be transureteroureterostomy or even nephroureterectomy if the kidney has very poor function.

Patients with persistent reflux should initially be managed conservatively because it is quite possible that, on subsequent cystograms, the reflux will resolve. Those patients in whom the reflux does not resolve should undergo cystoscopy; if there is reasonable tunnel length, an attempt should be made to bolster the floor of the ureteral orifice with collagen injection. Two or even three injections may be required; one must realize that there is

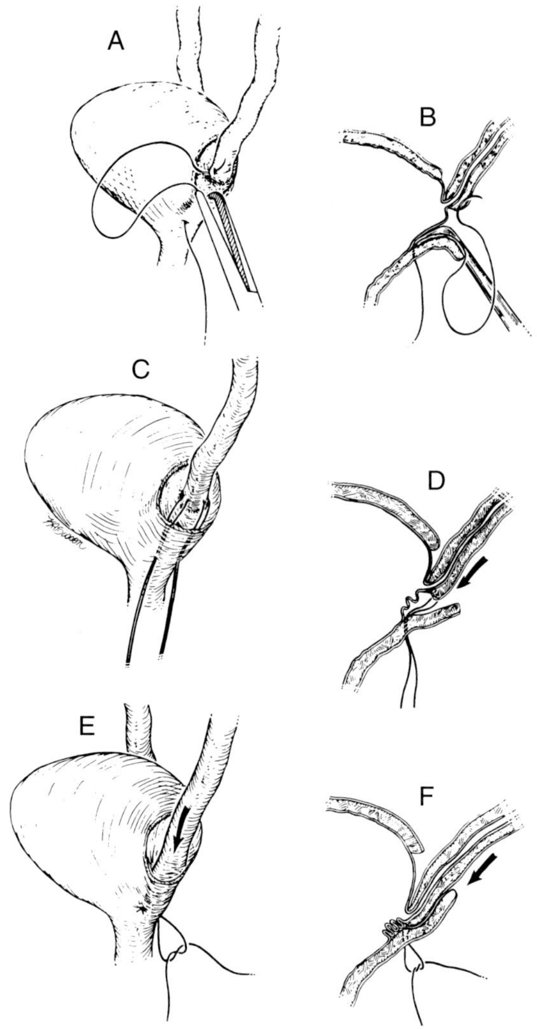

Figure 5–13 Extravesical reimplant. *A*, Dissection of trough and mucosa. *B* and *C*, Placement of advancement suture. *D–F*, Suture tied advancing ureter.

only a 50% success rate for the failed reimplant. In those situations in which the reflux persists despite collagen injection, a repeat open reimplantation of the ureter must be performed.

REFERENCES

1. Sampson JA. Ascending renal infection: With special reference to the reflux of urine from the bladder into the ureters as an etiological factor in its causation and maintenance. Johns Hopkins Hosp Bull 14:334, 1903.
2. Young HH. Comment on "ascending renal infection with special reference to the reflux of urine from the bladder into the ureters as an etiological factor in its causation and maintenance. Johns Hopkins Hosp Bull 14:340, 1903.
3. Coffey RC. Physiologic implantation of the severed ureter or common bile duct into the intestine. JAMA 56:397, 1911.
4. Gilchrist RK, Merricks JW, Hamlin HW, et al. Construction of a substitute bladder and urethra. Surg Gynecol Obstet 90:752, 1950.
5. Leadbetter WF, Clarke BG. Five years experience with ureteroenterostomy by the combined technique. J Urol 72:67, 1955.
6. Politano VA, Leadbetter WF. An operative technique for the correction of vesicoureteral reflux. J Urol 79:932, 1958.
7. Paquin AJ. Ureterovesical anastomosis: The description and evaluation of a technique. J Urol 82:573, 1959.
8. Nitzsche EU, Zimmerhackl LB, Hawkins A, et al. Correlation of ultrasound and renal scintigraphy in children with unilateral hydronephrosis in primary workup. Pediatr Nephrol 7:138, 1993.
9. Roberts JA. Pathogenesis of pyelonephritis. J Urol 129:1102, 1983.
10. Woodard JR, Holden S. The prognostic significance of fever in childhood urinary infections. Clin Pediatr 15:1051, 1976.
11. Govan DE, Palmer JM. Urinary tract infection in children: The influence of successful antireflux operations on morbidity from infection. Pediatrics 44:677, 1969.
12. Taylor CM, Corkery JJ, White RHR. Micturition symptoms and unstable bladder activity in girls with primary vesicoureteral reflux. Br J Urol 54:494, 1982.
13. Van Gool JD, Hjalmas K, Tamminen-Mobius T, et al. Historical clues to complex of dysfunctional voiding urinary tract infection and vesicoureteral reflux. J Urol 148:1699, 1992.
14. Noe HN. The long term results of prospective sibling reflux screening. J Urol 148:1739, 1992.
15. Noe HN, Wyatt RJ, Peeden JN, et al. The transmission of vesicoureteral reflux from parent to child. J Urol 148:1869, 1992.
16. International Reflux Study Committee. Medical versus surgical treatment of primary vesicoureteral reflux. Pediatrics 67:392, 1981.
17. Blane CE, DiPietro MA, Zerin JM, et al. Renal sonography is not a reliable screening examination for vesicoureteral reflux. J Urol 150:752, 1993.
18. Smellie JM. The intravenous urogram in the detection and evaluation of renal damage following urinary tract infection. Pediatr Nephrol 9:213, 1995.
19. Goldraich NP, Goldraich IH. Update on dimercaptosuccinic acid renal scanning in children with urinary tract infection. Pediatr Nephrol 9:221, 1995.
20. Edwards D, Normand ICS, Prescod N, et al. Disappearance of vesicoureteral reflux during long-term prophylaxis of urinary tract infection in children. Br Med J 2:286, 1977.
21. Arant BS. Medical management of mild and moderate vesicoureteral reflux: Follow-up studies of infants and young children. Preliminary report of Southwest Pediatric Nephrology Study Group. J Urol 148:1683, 1992.
22. McLorie GA, McKenna PH, Jumper BM, et al. High grade vesicoureteral reflux: Analysis of observational therapy. J Urol 144:537, 1990.
23. Tamminen-Mobius T, Brunier E, Ebel KD, et al. Cessation of vesicoureteral reflux for 5 years in infants and children allocated to medical treatment. J Urol 148:1662, 1992.
24. Scholtmeijer RJ. Treatment of vesicoureteral reflux: Results of a prospective study. Br J Urol 71:346, 1993.
25. Goldraich NP, Goldraich IH. Follow-up of conservatively treated children with high and low grade vesicoureteral reflux: Prospective study. J Urol 148:1688, 1992.
26. Peppas DS, Scoog SJ, Canning DA, et al. Nonsurgical management of primary vesicoureteral reflux in complete ureteral duplication: Is it justified? J Urol 146:1594, 1991.
27. Ben-Ami T, Gayer G, Hertz M, et al. The natural history of reflux in the lower pole of duplicated collecting systems: A controlled study. Pediatr Radiol 19:308, 1989.
28. Aladjem MA, Bolchis H, Hertz M, et al. The conservative management of vesicoureteral reflux: A review of 121 children. Pediatrics 65:78, 1980.
29. Koff SA, Murtagh DS. The uninhibited bladder in children: Effect

of treatment on recurrence of urinary infection and on vesicoureteral reflux resolution. J Urol 130:1138, 1983.
30. Seruca H. Vesicoureteral reflux and voiding dysfunction. J Urol 142:494, 1989.
31. Sill'en U, Hjalmas K, Aili M, et al. Pronounced detrusor hypercontractility in infants with gross bilateral reflux. J Urol 148:598, 1992.
32. Duckett JW, Ziylan O. Uses and abuses of vesicostomy. AUA Update Series 16:130, 1995.
33. Ransley PG, Risdon RA. Reflux nephropathy: Effects of antimicrobial therapy on the evaluation of the early pyelonephritic scar. Kidney Int 20:733, 1981.
34. Amar AD. Delayed recurrence of reflux after initial success of antireflux operation. J Urol 119:131, 1978.
35. Friedland GW. Post-reimplantation renal scarring. In Hodson J, Kincaid-Smith P (eds), Reflux Nephropathy. New York: Masson, 1979, p 323.
36. Bauer SB, Willscher MK, Zammuto PJ, et al. Dilemma of small pyelonephritic kidney associated with vesicoureteral reflux. Urology 15:466, 1980.
37. Galansky SH, Walker RD, Elder JS, et al. Management of unresolved vesicoureteral reflux in school age children. Dial Pediatr Urol 18:1, 1995.
38. Duckett JW, Walker RD, Weiss R. Surgical results: International Reflux Study in children—United States Branch. J Urol 148:1674, 1992.
39. Frey P, Lutz N, Jenny P, et al. Endoscopic subureteral collagen injection for the treatment of vesicoureteral reflux in infants and children. J Urol 154:804, 1995.
40. Cohen SJ. Ureterozystoneostomic, eine neue antirefluxtechnik. Aktuel Urol 6:1, 1975.
41. Glenn JF, Anderson EE. Distal tunnel ureteral reimplantation. J Urol 97:623, 1967.
42. Woodard JR, Keats G. Ureteral reimplantation: Paquin's procedure after 12 years. J Urol 109:891, 1973.
43. Lich R, Howerton LW, Goode LS, et al. The ureterovesical junction of the newborn. J Urol 92:436, 1964.
44. Gregoire W, van Regemorter GU. Le reflux vesicoureteral congenital. Urol Int 18:122, 1964.
45. Lipsky H. Endoscopic treatment of vesicoureteral reflux with bovine collagen. Eur Urol 18:52, 1990.
46. Mathisen W. Vesicoureteral reflux and its surgical correction. Surg Gynecol Obstet 118:965, 1964.
47. Middleton RG. Routine use of the psoas hitch in ureteral reimplantation. J Urol 123:352, 1980.
48. Burbidge KA, Miller M, Connor JP. Extravesical ureteral reimplantation: Results in 128 patients. J Urol 155:1721, 1996.
49. Wacksman J, Gilbert A, Sheldon CA. Results of the renewed extravesical reimplant for surgical correction of vesicoureteral reflux. J Urol 148:359, 1992.
50. Zaontz MR, Maizels M, Sugar E, et al. Detrusorrhaphy: Extravesical ureteral advancement to correction of vesicoureteral reflux in children. J Urol 138:947, 1987.
51. Daines SL, Hodgson NB. Management of reflux in total duplication anomalies. J Urol 105:720, 1971.
52. Flack CE, Walker RD, Kelalis PP. Prevention and management of the failed ureteral reimplant. AUA Update Series 14:70, 1995.
53. Noe HN. The role of dysfunctional voiding in failure or complication of ureteral reimplantation for primary reflux. J Urol 134:1172, 1985.
54. Hendren WH. Reoperation for the failed ureteral reimplantation. J Urol 111:403, 1974.

JOHN R. WOODARD

6

Megaloureter

Although the term megaloureter is purely descriptive, it has, through common usage, come to have a certain connotation. It has also been the basis of a rather detailed classification of disorders in which a dilated ureter is a feature. For the basis of this discussion, however, we confine our comments to "obstructive megaloureter." In using this term, most of us refer to a specific, albeit incompletely understood, entity (Fig. 6–1), and it is safe to assume that this disorder occurs in a spectrum of severity. Its milder forms are probably not obstructive at all, simply dilated; the opposite side of the spectrum represents severe degrees of obstruction. It is those in the middle in which the degree and significance of obstruction can be very difficult to delineate, especially at a single point in time.

The typical configuration of obstructive megaloureter includes a fusiform dilation of the lower, lower and central, or entire ureter, with a narrow distal segment approximately 1 cm in length above the ureterovesical junction. This narrow distal segment seldom resists the retrograde passage of a ureteral catheter. Therefore, it is not thought of as a true stricture or stenosis. Although there is some variation in the morphologic characteristics of the narrow distal segment,[1–3] there is general consensus that it does not transmit a peristaltic wave. The retrograde peristaltic wave thus produced may lead to progressive dilation in some instances, whereas others improve with time for reasons that are less evident.

Successful surgical repair of megaloureter was once considered to be challenging enough to warrant a preliminary indwelling nephrostomy[4]; however, it is now an operation that most reconstructive surgeons approach with confidence.[5] As surgeons have become more confident in repair, the indications for surgical intervention have become somewhat more restrained if not more precise.[6] This has been most obvious since the advent and extensive use of diagnostic fetal sonography. The widespread incidental discovery of dilated ureters has challenged the pediatric urologist to delineate the natural history of megaloureter better and to define the indications for surgical correction.

CLINICAL PRESENTATION

In the past, it was not uncommon for a child with obstructive megaloureter to present with a symptomatic urinary infection, flank pain, or hematuria (secondary to minor trauma or stones in the distal ureter). Although this type of clinical presentation is still encountered, the vast majority now present before birth after a prenatal ultrasound study.[5,6] Some argue that early diagnosis allows the surgeon to repair all cases before complications occur. However, we have known for many years that some cases of apparent obstructive megaloureter improve or even resolve spontaneously (Fig. 6–2). In recent years we have seen that this occurs more often than previously suspected and that in other instances a dilated ureter may persist with no apparent detrimental effects on the kidney itself.[6] The long-term outcome in these infants after fetal discovery is yet to be documented.

For completeness it should be mentioned that this

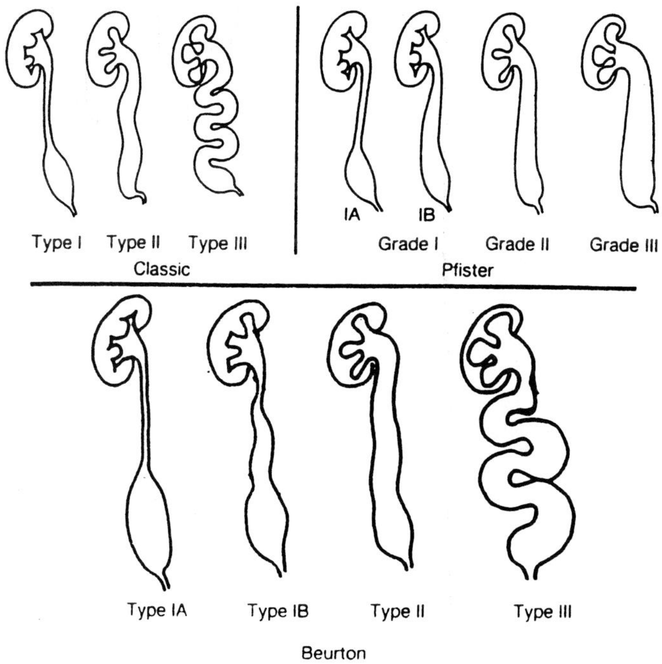

Figure 6–1 Primary obstructive megaloureter has been classified according to ureteral morphology (classic), degree of renal distortion (Pfister), and a combination of both (Beurton). From Beurton D. Primary megaureter, retrocaval ureter, and ureteral valves. In Retik AB, Cukier J (eds), Pediatric Urology. Baltimore: Williams & Wilkins, 1986, p 429. Used with permission.

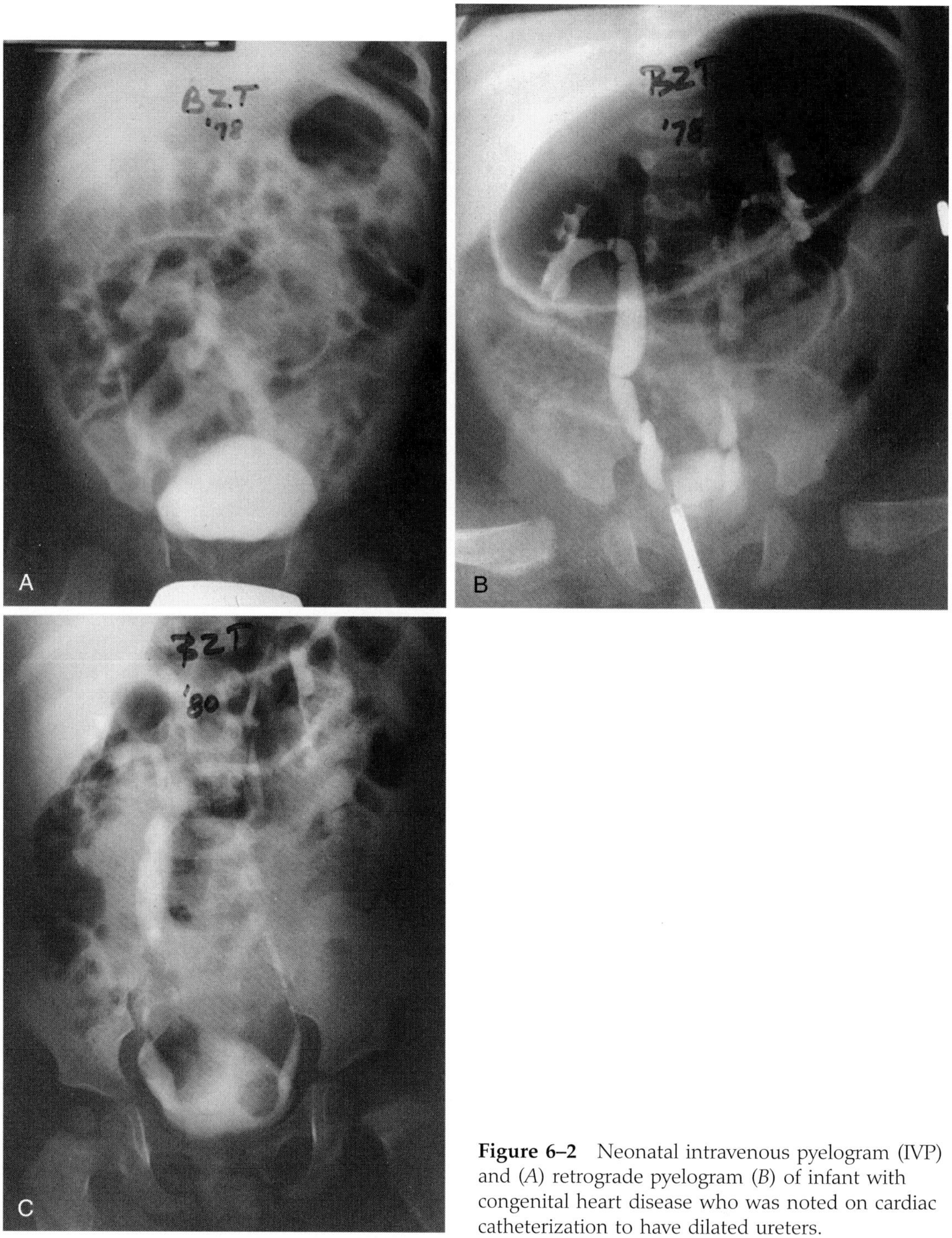

Figure 6–2 Neonatal intravenous pyelogram (IVP) and (*A*) retrograde pyelogram (*B*) of infant with congenital heart disease who was noted on cardiac catheterization to have dilated ureters.

disorder occurs much more often in males, in whom, in unilateral cases, the left side is much more likely to be affected.

DIAGNOSTIC EVALUATION

The diagnostic windfall offered by fetal ultrasonography has been an impetus to refine and standardize the diagnostic regimen and to learn more of the natural history of this disorder. It logically follows that a prenatal fetal ultrasonogram showing a dilated ureter with an apparent normal bladder should be confirmed by a neonatal ultrasonogram shortly after birth (Fig. 6–3). Once the megaloureter is confirmed, reflux must be ruled out as a cause. In addition, it is necessary to have some evidence that the bladder itself is normal to rule out a secondary megaloureter. Therefore, a voiding cystourethrogram is neces-

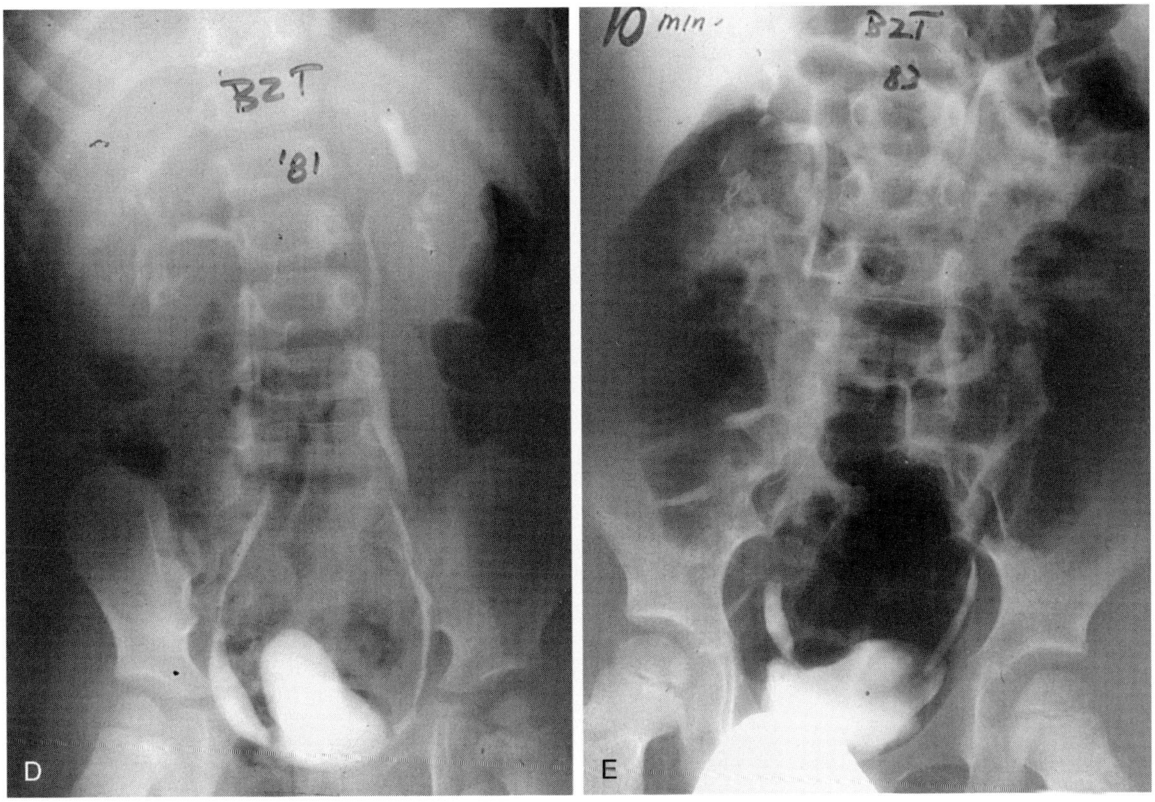

Figure 6–2 *Continued* IVPs 2(*C*), 3(*D*), and 5(*E*) years later show complete resolution on the left and almost complete resolution on the right without surgical intervention.

sary and is usually next in order. If there is no reflux and the bladder does appear to be normal with no outflow obstruction or neuropathic stigmata, a renal excretory function study should be obtained next. In the past this would have routinely been an intravenous pyelogram. However, the current standard functional study is either a diethylenetetramine-pentaacetic acid (DTPA) or mercaptoacetyltriglycine (MAG3) radionuclide scan with a furosemide (Lasix) renogram (Fig. 6–3*D, E*). In unilateral cases and in those with obviously good renal function, it may be wise to wait 2 to 4 weeks through the "transitional nephrology" stage for more unequivocal results. From the radionuclide renal scan, we can obtain several potentially useful types of information, including the differential renal function, extraction fraction, and tracer transit time (i.e, half-life, or T½).

These three studies—renal ultrasonogram, voiding cystogram, and DTPA or MAG3 renal scan—have become the standard basic imaging modalities used in patients suspected of having obstructive megaloureter. Surgeons differ in their conclusions using these parameters, but each can be helpful in deciding whether to operate on a patient with uncomplicated megaloureter. The most agreement centers around differential function in unilateral cases in which surgical intervention is usual when the kidney on the side of the megaloureter has 35% or less of the total renal function with an apparently normal contralateral kidney.

The use of retrograde pyelography varies with individual surgeons. Although many still find it useful, retrograde pyelograms rarely add essential information. Whitaker pressure-flow[7] studies are also not necessary in most patients but can be helpful in those in whom doubt remains concerning the necessity of surgical intervention after the standard studies have been completed. It should also be emphasized, especially in bilateral cases, that abnormal bladder function (secondary megaloureter) must be ruled out.

INDICATIONS FOR SURGERY

Given a significantly dilated ureter with a narrow distal segment typical of obstructive megaloureter, the indications for surgery include (1) differential function by radionuclide scan of less than 35% in the involved kidney, (2) persistent accumulation of tracer material on a DTPA or MAG3 scan, after furosemide, despite normal drainage on the contralateral side, (3) severe hydroureteronephrosis with marked thinning of the renal parenchyma, (4) hypertension, hematuria, infection, or pain assumed to be secondary to the megaloureter, (5) calculi, or (6)

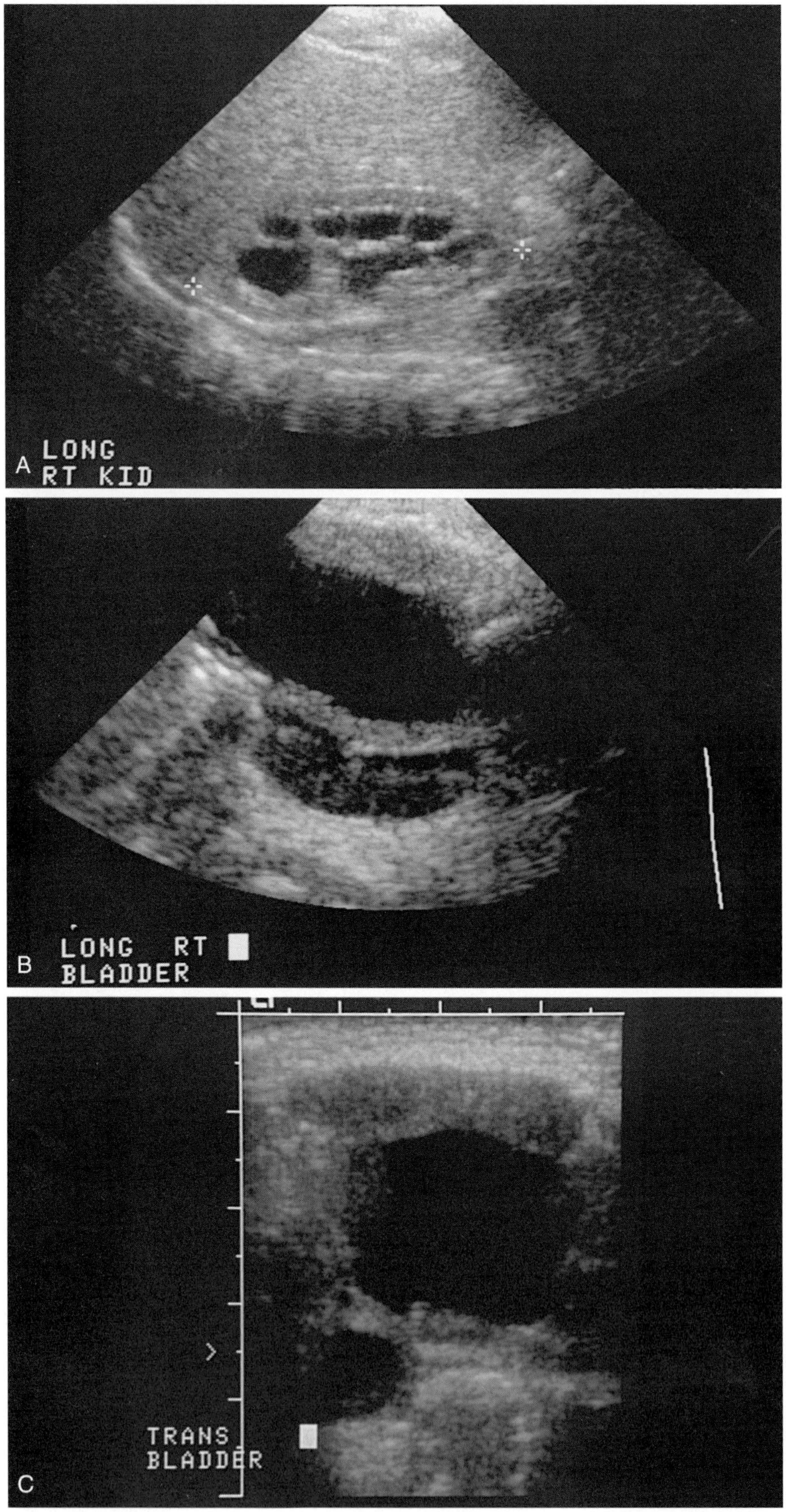

Figure 6–3 Sonograms in 4-month-old boy show right hydronephrosis with thin renal pelvis (*A*) and longitudinal (*B*) and transverse (*C*) veins of bladder showing markedly dilated right ureter. The DTPA acid scan in the same patient shows differential function and renogram curves

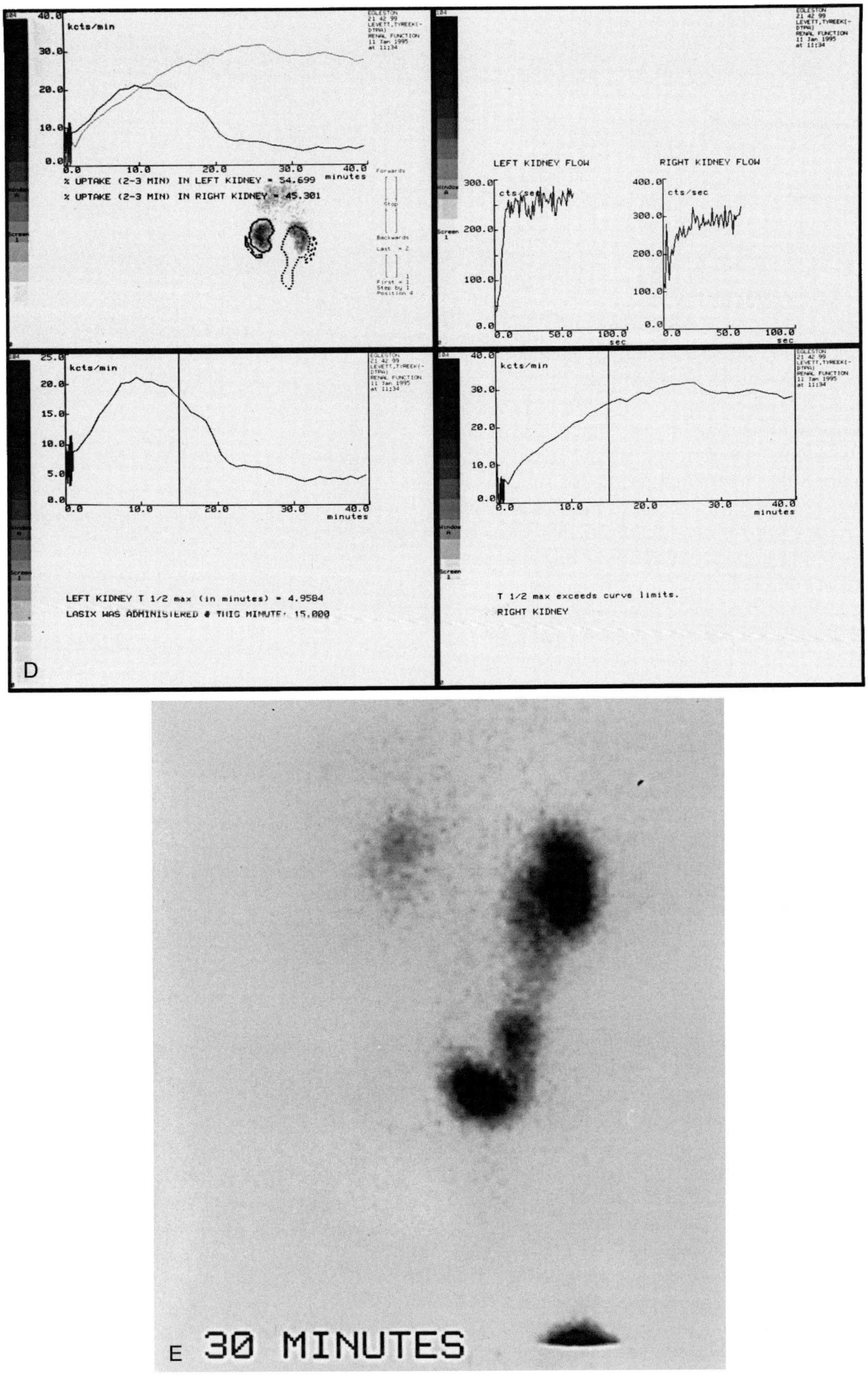

Figure 6–3 *Continued* (*D*) and delayed image (*E*) of the dilated ureter.

definite progression of the disease during a period of surveillance.

If one is to use the slope of the renogram curve or the T½ in deciding when surgical intervention is necessary, it is important to standardize the study itself. This at least means having the bladder on constant catheter drainage and keeping it empty during the study. Even with highly standardized nuclear studies, most surgeons are hesitant to base a surgical decision on a prolonged T½ alone.

SURGICAL TECHNIQUES

The techniques for the surgical repair of megaloureter have evolved over several decades. Initially, this was almost in a trial and error endeavor. Now the techniques for tapering and reimplanting megaloureters are fairly standard and based on established anatomic and surgical principles. Credit is due many individuals for the development of the principles and techniques that have led to the excellent results we now expect from these procedures.[8–11] The surgical principles governing management of megaureter include (1) reduction of the caliber of the distal ureter to facilitate improved effectiveness of ureteral peristalsis and a favorable ratio of ureteral diameter to submucosal tunnel length (1:5) to prevent postoperative reflux; (2) careful preservation of the distal ureteral blood supply to prevent postoperative ureteral obstruction secondary to fibrosis and stricture; and (3) a comfortable passage of the ureter into the muscular hiatus of the bladder to avoid angulation or J hooking of the ureter as the bladder fills. In the past, it was not unusual to see J hooking of the ureter (Fig. 6–4) in cases in which the tapered ureter entered the new muscular hiatus of the bladder too far lateral or too high on the posterior bladder wall. This is largely avoidable by transvesical procedures in which the same muscular hiatus is used or by the judicious use of psoas hitch.

Ureteral tailoring may be done either by excision of a wedge of ureteral wall and reconstruction of the distal ureter or by ureteral folding as described by Kalicinski and others.[12] The latter technique excludes the lateral portion of the distal megaloureter, folding the excluded segment under the ureter, and results in better preservation of ureteral blood supply than might occur with excisional tailoring, thus decreasing the possibility of postoperative fibrosis and stricture. It also decreases the time necessary for postoperative ureteral stenting and may thereby reduce hospital stay. There are other techniques for nonexcisional ureteral tapering. The Kalicinski technique is used because the results have been good and reproducible. Although our experience with ureteral folding has been very successful, excisional tailoring may be better than folding for those extremely dilated or thick-walled ureters.[11]

A sterile urine is desirable before any urologic recon-

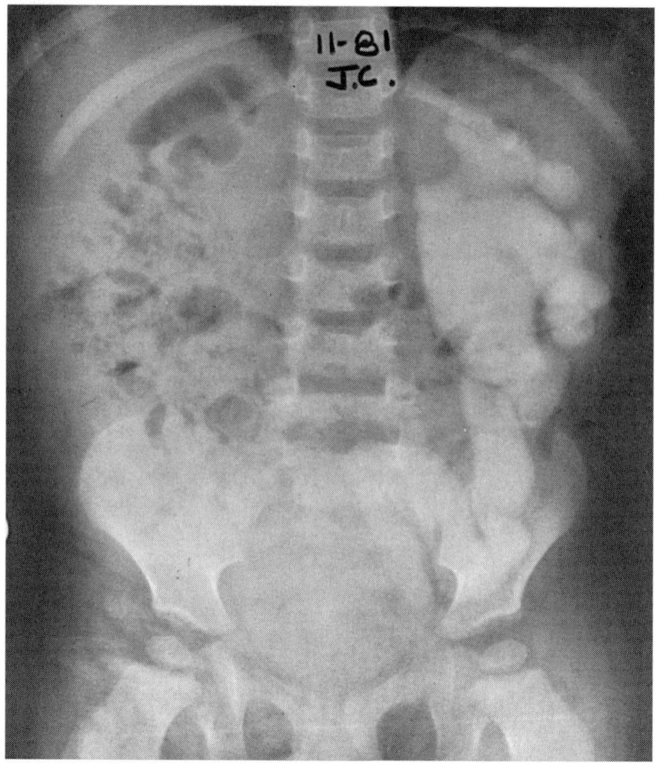

Figure 6–4 Intravenous pyelogram in 3-year-old boy after reimplantation of solitary left ureter into bladder. Note the persistent hydroureteronephrosis, full bladder, and J hooking of ureter.

structive procedure. Antibiotics are given intraoperatively and during the early postoperative convalescence. For the uncomplicated megaloureter with a moderate degree of dilatation, a transvesical approach is preferred. For the more complicated cases with massive dilatation or reoperations, a combined intravesical-extravesical approach may facilitate exposure and allow for a psoas hitch.

Transvesical Approach

In the transvesical approach (Fig. 6–5), cystoscopy always precedes the operation. A retrograde pyelogram, if deemed necessary, is performed at this time. The bladder is then exposed through a Pfannenstiel incision and entered through a longitudinal cystotomy. A self-retaining ring retractor is placed and a 5 or 8 French plastic feeding tube is passed up the involved ureter and sutured in place. The bladder mucosa around the ureteral orifice is incised and the ureter mobilized within Waldeyer's sheath in the same manner as would be done with a routine ureteral reimplantation. In the male patient, care must be exercised to avoid injury to the vas deferens during this type of ureteral mobilization. It is also important to avoid unnecessary disruption of ureteral vasculature. In the usual case of megaloureter, it is easy to obtain considerable intravesical ureteral length with this type of intraves-

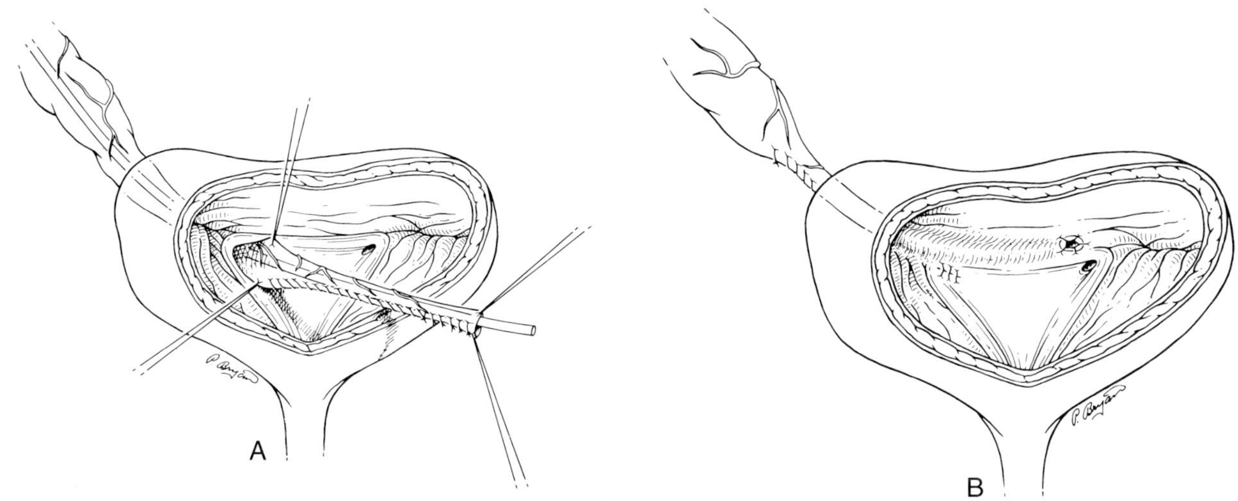

Figure 6–5 *A*, Ureter after transvesical mobilization and excisional tapering over 8 or 10 French catheter. *B*, The ureter has been reimplanted across the base of the trigone.

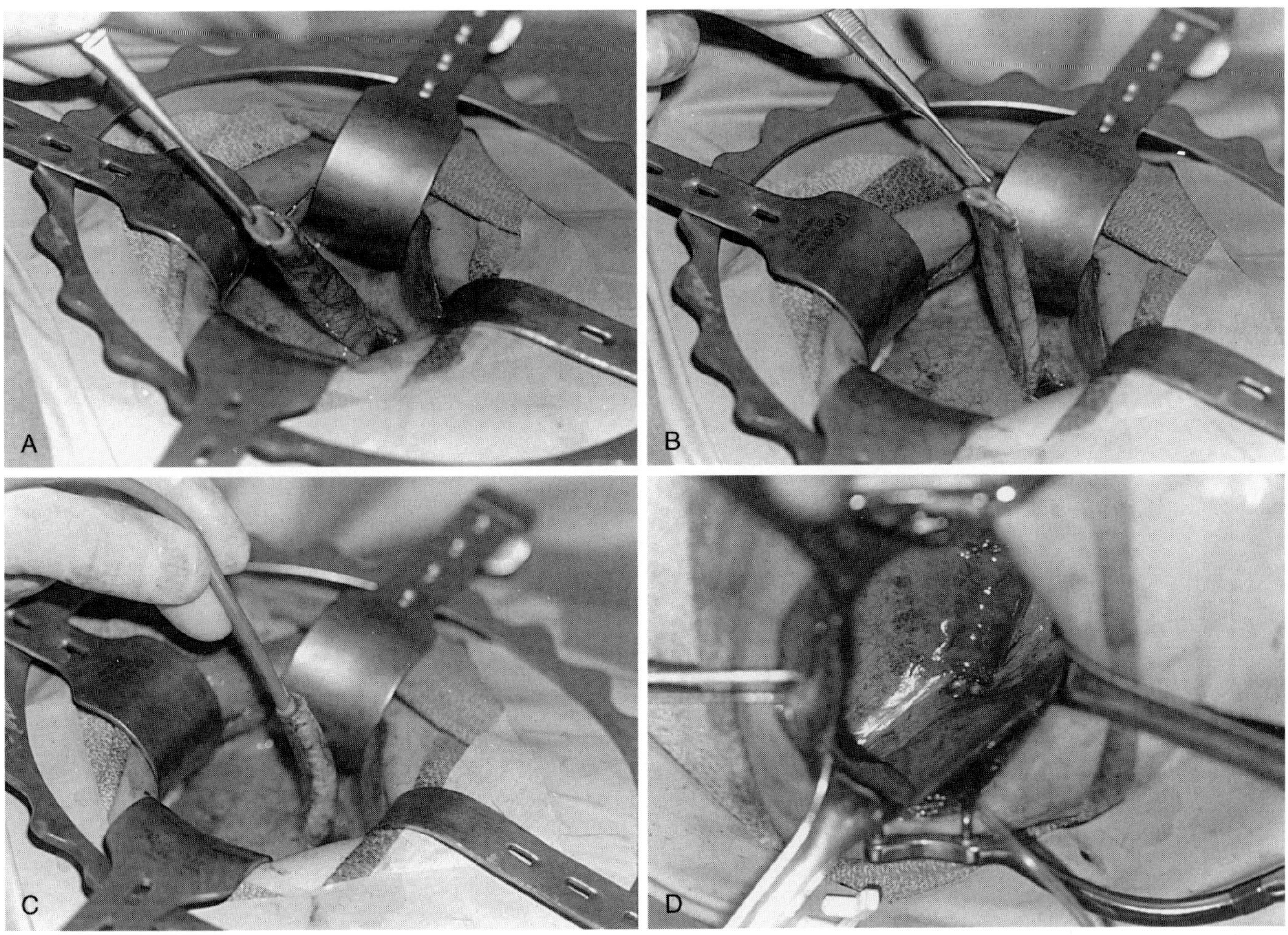

Figure 6–6 Photographs of megaloureter repair in 3-month-old boy showing transvesical mobilization of ureter (*A*), placement of initial suture line for Kalicinski folding (*B*), completion of folding (*C*), and completion of submucosal reimplantation (*D*).

ical mobilization (Fig. 6–6). Additional cephalad incision of the muscular hiatus may be used to facilitate exposure and visualization and may also make it possible to obtain a longer submucosal tunnel across the base of the bladder. The peritoneum can usually be identified as it is dissected off of the ureter as the mobilization extends proximally. Care should be taken to avoid injury to the peritoneum.

When advancement of the ureter is completed, the "narrow distal segment" is completely excised. It is necessary at this time to decide whether the ureter is to be folded or an excisional tailoring is to be carried out (see Fig. 6–6). Unless the ureter is massively dilated or very thick walled, we would select a Kalicinski or folding procedure. The folding is performed over an 8, 10, or 12 French catheter by placing a continuous horizontal mattress suture of 5-0 polyglycolic acid (PGA) along the lateral aspect of the ureter, excluding a portion of the lumen of the distal ureter. This segment is then folded under the patent distal ureter and is attached to the medial edge with a continuous suture of the same material. A wide submucosal tunnel is then fashioned across the base of the bladder in a manner that would ensure a tunnel length–ureteral tapered diameter ratio of at least 5:1. As the ureter is passed through this tunnel to its new position on the opposite side of the bladder, it is important to avoid angulation or twisting. After the ureter has passed through the submucosal tunnel, a ureterovesical anastomosis is performed, with 4-0 or 5-0 PGA sutures firmly anchoring the ureteral orifice to the detrusor. Bladder mucosa is then reapproximated over the ureteral hiatus with continuous 5-0 chromic catgut. The ureter is stented with a 5 or 8 French feeding tube for 3 to 4 days. The bladder is closed in two layers and is drained with a ureteral catheter for approximately 4 days.

Combined Intravesical-Extravesical Approach

For the most severely dilated ureter or the ureter requiring reoperation, we often prefer a combined intravesical-extravesical surgical approach (Fig. 6–7). The bladder is exposed and opened in the usual manner. Once the ureter has been freed transvesically, the ipsilateral paravesical space is exposed by bluntly dissecting the peritoneum from the bladder wall to the iliac vessels and dividing the obliterated hypergastric artery as it crosses the ureter. This allows the previously mobilized ureter to be extracted from the muscular hiatus of the bladder and mobilized to the level of the iliac bifurcation, taking care to preserve small vascular collaterals from the internal iliac artery.

For the larger, more tortuous, or reoperated ureters, a classic wedge excision ureteral tapering is generally the more appropriate technique. First, the narrow distal ureteral segment and redundant distal ureter are excised, taking care to estimate the amount of ureteral length that

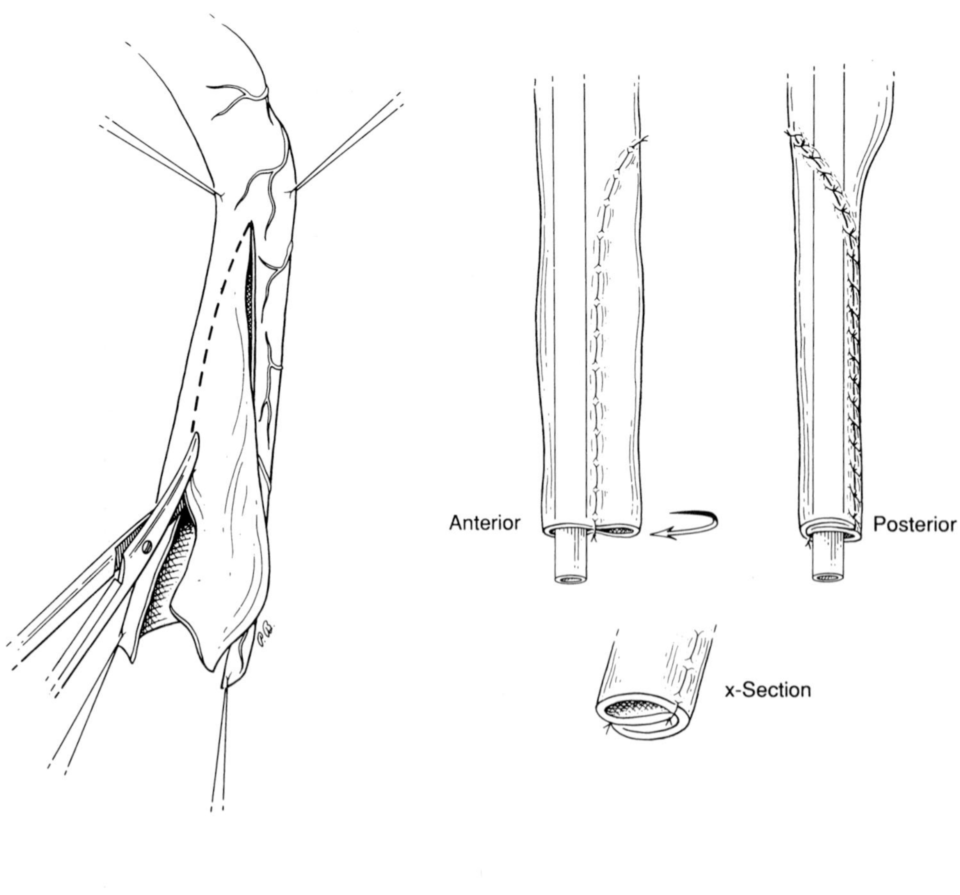

Figure 6–7 Two methods of ureteral tapering. *A*, classic excisional tapering with an attempt to avoid cutting major vessels. *B*, The Kalicinski folding technique.

will be necessary to carry out a suitable reimplantation. A 10 or 12 French catheter is placed in the ureter. It is often possible to identify one or two arterial branches entering the posterolateral ureteral wall. In such instances, we prefer to excise a wedge of the anterolateral aspect of the ureter. This wedge is first outlined with a marking pen. The wedge excision is performed with straight Potts scissors, taking care to avoid excessive ureteral resection. The ureter is symmetrically reconstructed over a 10 or 12 French catheter. To define proper alignment of the suture line, the ureteral walls are reapproximated with several 5-0 PGA sutures placed at 1-cm intervals from the apex of the wedge to the distal end of the ureter. A second continuous running suture of 5-0 PGA completes a watertight repair. If there is any likelihood of the need for further resection of the terminal end of the ureter, the continuous suture should be stopped short of the end and the layer completed with interrupted sutures to allow for further resection. In some cases the ureter may now be brought back inside the bladder through the original musculature hiatus and reimplanted across the base of the bladder as described in the transvesical technique. This may reduce the chance of angulation or J hooking at the ureterovesical junction. In other instances, a new muscular hiatus is required and is placed cephalad and medial to the old hiatus, although care must be taken not to place the new hiatus too cephalad or too lateral if one is to avoid ureteral obstruction during bladder filling. Once the site of the new hiatus has been selected, the detrusor is incised transversely and a submucosal tunnel developed from the new hiatus down to a selected spot on the base of the bladder toward the trigone. The mucosa is incised and the ureter brought through the hiatus, down the tunnel, and into the bladder.

In cases in which the ureteral hiatus has been repositioned, a psoas hitch lateral to the iliac vessels provides stabilization of the ureterovesical junction, maintains the length of submucosal tunnel, and prevents ureteral angulation (J hooking) (Fig. 6–8). Redundant tapered ureter is excised and the ureter sutured to the bladder as previously described. We routinely stent an excisionally tapered ureter for 10 days and leave a Penrose drain in the paravesical area until after the stent has been removed.

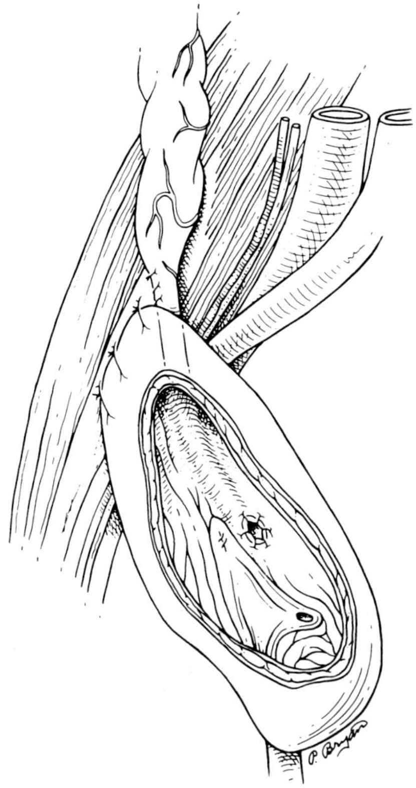

Figure 6–8 Diagram of combined intravesical-extravesical operation with a psoas hitch to stabilize the base of the bladder and prevent J hooking.

RESULTS AND COMPLICATIONS

A success rate of approximately 95% should be attainable with either excisional tailoring or folding techniques. The degree of anatomic improvement is often impressive (Fig. 6–9). However, the most common complications following megaureter repair are reflux and obstruction.[13] The two most important factors contributing to postoperative reflux are an inadequate ratio of submucosal tunnel length to ureteral diameter and abnormal bladder function. It is well established that a 5:1 ratio of submucosal tunnel length to ureteral diameter is usually sufficient to prevent reflux. Vesicoureteric fistulas are an uncommon cause of reflux in ureters tapered by excision. This can usually be prevented by positioning the ureteral suture line posteriorly toward the detrusor rather than toward the bladder lumen. Abnormal bladder function is a cause of failed ureteral reimplantation that has received relatively little attention in the literature. In 1979, Retik and colleagues[15] reported a 97% success rate after tapered reimplantation of megaloureters in patients with normal bladders compared with a 55% success rate in those with abnormal bladder urodynamics. Thus, it is important to rule out abnormal bladder function in these patients.

Postoperative ureteral obstruction is a serious complication that may lead to loss of renal function. The most common cause of obstruction—distal ureteral ischemia and angulation at the ureterovesical junction—can usually be prevented by meticulous surgical technique and attention to detail. Excessive ureteral dissection and tapering predisposes to devascularization of the distal ureter and is unnecessary in most cases. Total ureteral remodeling has been abandoned in favor of a more limited distal ureteral tapering starting 2 to 3 cm proximal to the ureteral entrance into the muscular hiatus. The use of the original muscular hiatus or the judicious use of a psoas

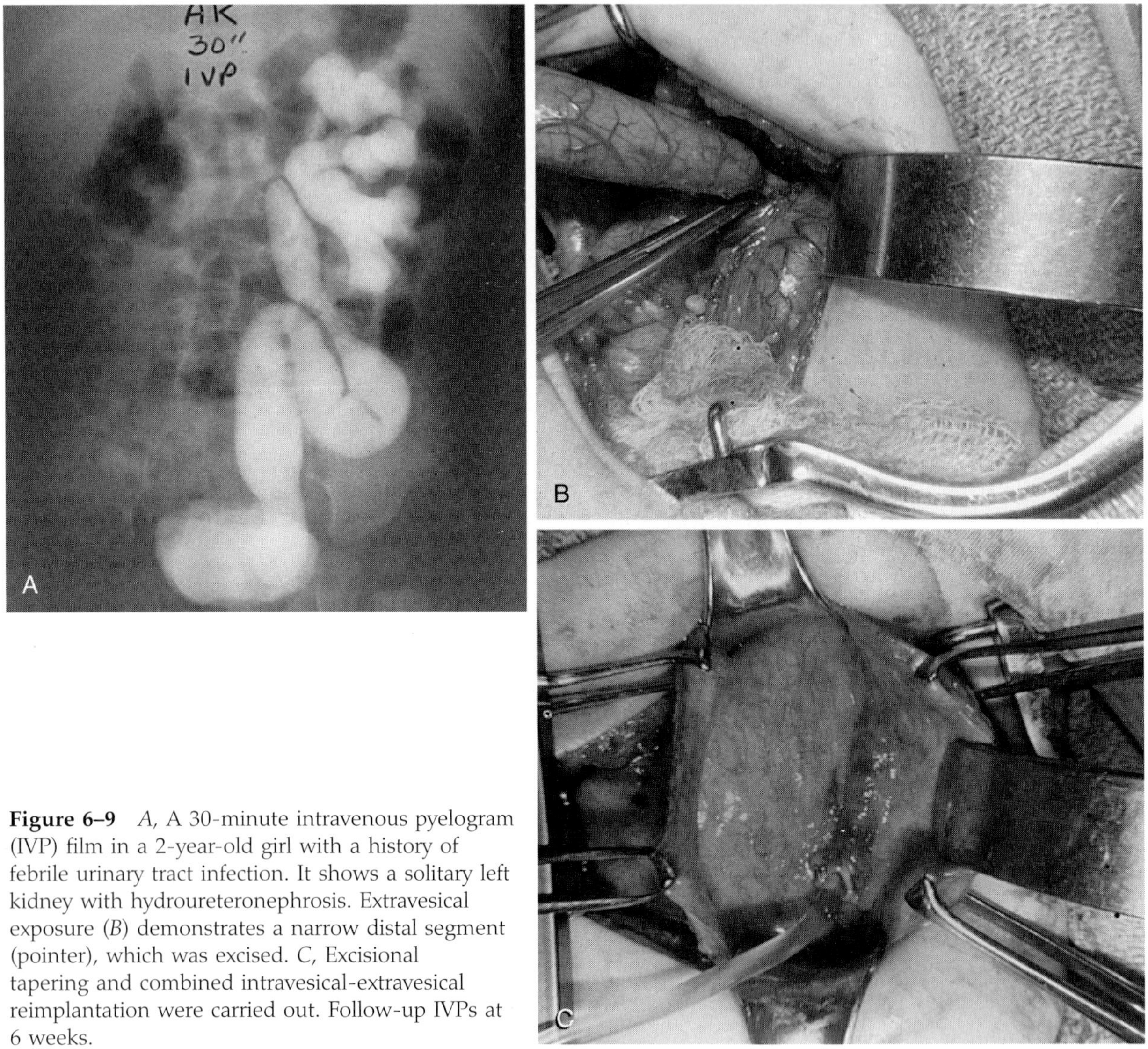

Figure 6–9 *A*, A 30-minute intravenous pyelogram (IVP) film in a 2-year-old girl with a history of febrile urinary tract infection. It shows a solitary left kidney with hydroureteronephrosis. Extravesical exposure (*B*) demonstrates a narrow distal segment (pointer), which was excised. *C*, Excisional tapering and combined intravesical-extravesical reimplantation were carried out. Follow-up IVPs at 6 weeks.

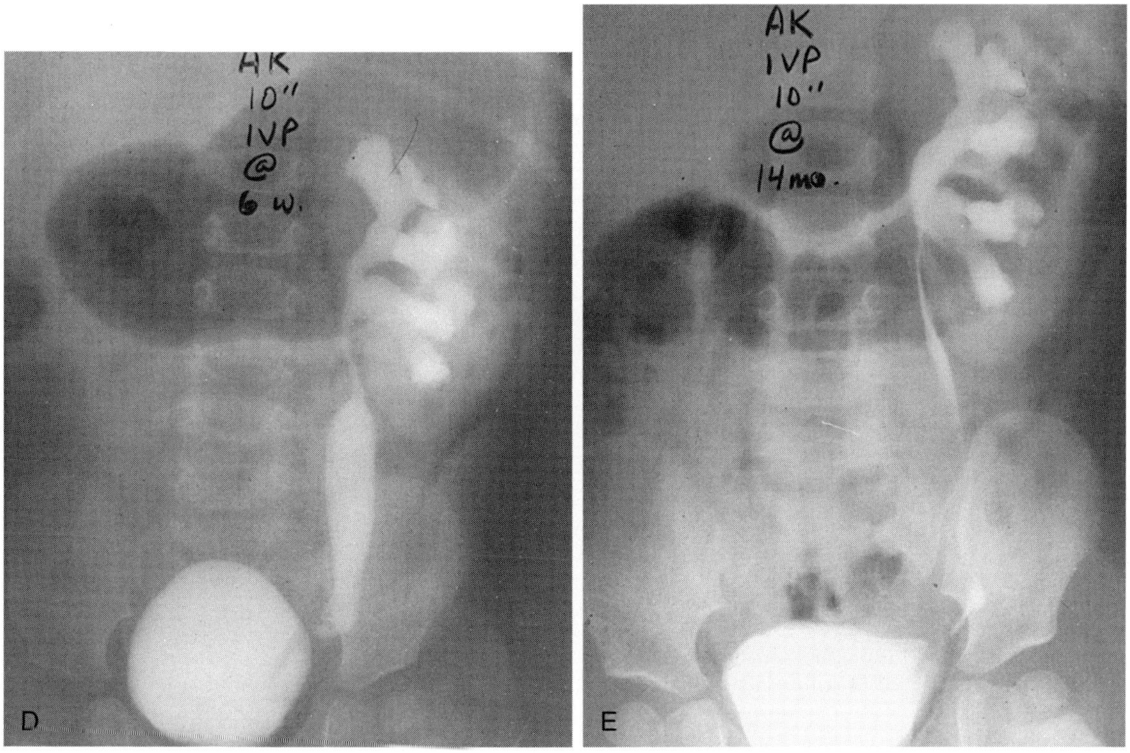

Figure 6–9 *Continued* (*D*) and 14 months (*E*) show impressive progressive improvement.

hitch has been very helpful in eliminating intermittent ureteral obstruction during bladder filling or so-called J hooking.

SUMMARY

Primary megaloureter is being discovered more often than in the past because of the widespread use of maternal-fetal diagnostic sonography. This has led to refinements in diagnostic evaluation and more precise indications for surgical intervention in this condition. It has also helped to increase our understanding of the natural history of primary megaloureter. There has also been a progressive improvement in the results of surgical repair of megaloureter and the introduction of useful modifications of ureteral tapering techniques.

REFERENCES

1. Paguin AJ Jr. Ureterovesical anastomosis: The description and evaluation of a technique. J Urol 82:573, 1959.
2. Tanagho EA, Smith DR, Guthrie TH. Pathophysiology of functional ureteral obstruction. J Urol 104:73, 1970.
3. McLaughlin AP III, Pfister RC, Leadbetter WF, et al. The pathophysiology of primary megaureter. J Urol 109:805, 1973.
4. Paguin AJ Jr. Considerations for the management of some complex problems for ureterovesical anastomosis. Surg Gynecol Obstet 118:75, 1964.
5. Peters GA, Mandell J, Lebowitz RL, et al. Congenital obstructive megaureter in early infancy: Diagnosis and treatment. J Urol 142:641, 1989.
6. Keating MA, Escala J, Snyder HM III, et al. Changing concepts in management of primary obstructive megaureter. J Urol 142:636, 1989.
7. Whitaker RH. Methods of assessing obstruction in dilated ureters. Br J Urol 45:15, 1973.
8. Hendren WH. Technical aspects of megaureter repair. Birth Defects 13:21, 1977.
9. Paguin AJ Jr. Ureterovesical anastomosis: The description and evaluation of a technique. J Urol 82:573, 1959.
10. Johnston JH. Reconstructive surgery of megaureter in children. Br J Urol 39:17, 1967.
11. Parrott TS, Woodard JR, Wolpert JJ. Ureteral tailoring: A comparison of wedge resection and infolding. J Urol 144:328, 1990.
12. Kalicinski ZH, Kansy J, Kotarbinska B, et al. Surgery of megaureters—Modification of Hendren's operation. J Pediatr Surg 12:183, 1977.
13. Kelalis PP, Kramer SA. Complications of megaureter surgery. Urol Clin North Am 10:417, 1983.
14. Beurton D. Primary megaureter, retrocaval ureter, and ureteral valves. In Retik AB, Cukier J (eds), Pediatric Urology. Baltimore: Williams & Wilkins, 1986, p 429.
15. Retik AB, McEvoy JP, Bauer SB: Megaureters in children. Urology 11:231, 1978.

EDMOND T. GONZALES, JR.

7

Ureteroceles

A ureterocele is a cystic enlargement of the intravesical segment of the ureter. Ureteroceles are multifaceted, complex anomalies that present clinically in many different ways. Ureteroceles can be tiny or may be so large as to fill the entire space within the bladder (Fig. 7–1). Ureteroceles can be single, or there can be one involving each side of the trigone. They may subtend a single ureter or one of the ureters in a complete ureteral duplication (almost always the ureter draining the upper segment). A ureterocele may be positioned wholly within the bladder (an intravesical ureterocele) or in a position at or beyond the bladder neck (an extravesical ureterocele). Although the ureter draining into the ureterocele usually is dilated and presumed obstructed, the location and size of the ureterocele can also distort the other ureteral orifices or obstruct the bladder neck. Varying degrees of effacement of the detrusor muscle behind the ureterocele can result in the eversion of the ureterocele into a pseudodiverticulum during micturition. In other cases, the ureterocele might prolapse through the urethra, presenting at the external urethral meatus as a congested, indurated introital mass (Fig. 7–2). Ureteroceles often distort the trigone, causing vesicoureteral reflux to occur into the other ureters.

In addition to these anatomic variations at the level of the ureteral orifice, trigone, and bladder neck, varying degrees of abnormality of the involved renal parenchyma are also present. In the face of obstruction and infection, there is, of course, the likelihood of progressive renal damage. However, many children with a ureterocele have

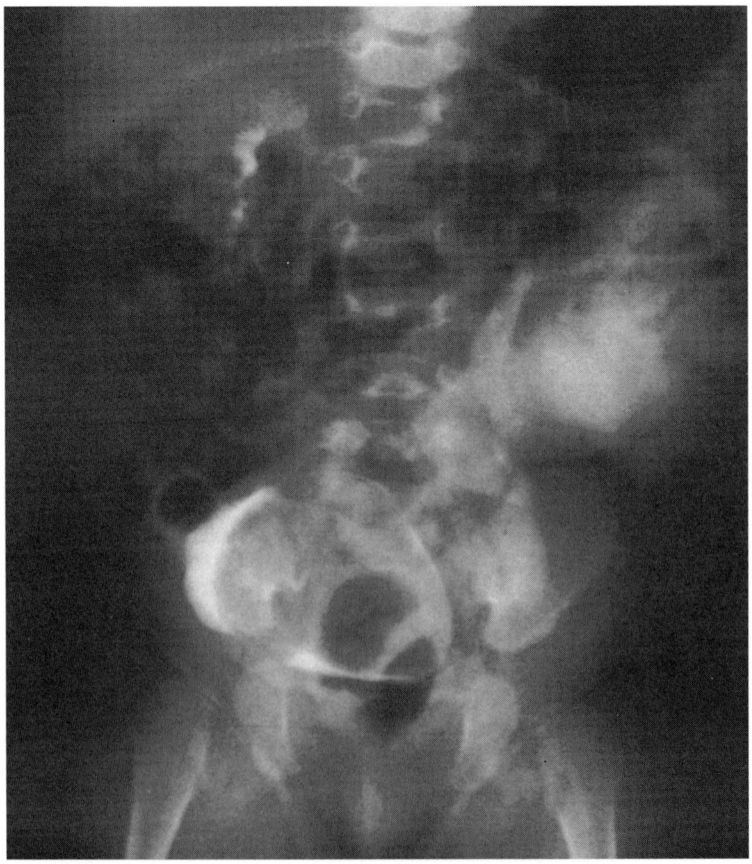

Figure 7–1 Intravenous pyelogram in a 3-month-old girl who presented with a palpable left flank mass. This study demonstrates a large, extravesical, duplex ureter ureterocele on the left side with nonvisualization of the left upper pole and massive hydronephrosis and hydroureter of the lower segment. From Gonzales ET, Decter RM. Management of ureteroceles in the newborn. In King LR (ed), Urologic Surgery in Neonates and Young Infants. Philadelphia: WB Saunders, 1989. Used with permission.

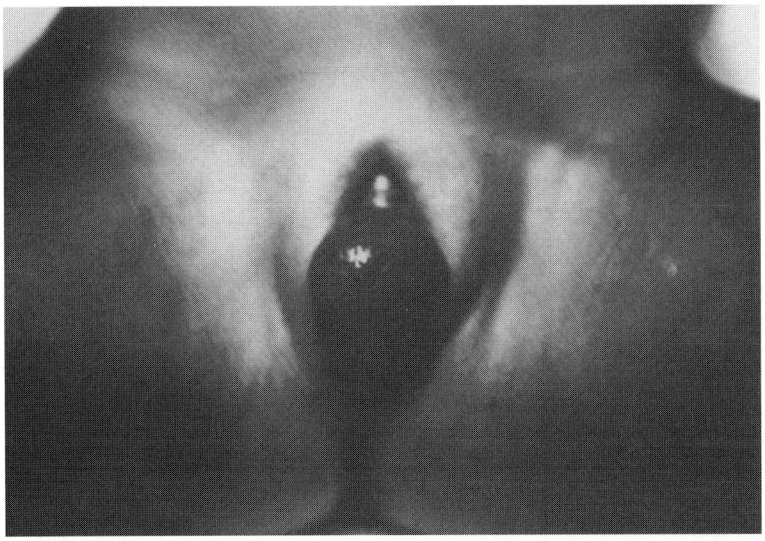

Figure 7–2 The congested, tense, and somewhat ecchymotic prolapsed ureterocele presenting as an interlabial mass. From Gonzales ET, Decter RM. Management of ureteroceles in the newborn. In King LR (ed), Urologic Surgery in Neonates and Young Infants. Philadelphia: WB Saunders, 1989. Used with permission.

some element of renal parenchymal dysplasia that affects the involved segment. In several series of duplex system ureteroceles, approximately 40% of resected segments have histologic evidence of severe dysplasia.[1] The extent of dysplasia often seems to correlate with the position of the ureteral orifice, such that ureteroceles terminating distally in the urethra are associated with more severe parenchymal dysplasia than are those that are completely intravesical (Fig. 7–3).[2] Therefore, in planning management for a child with a ureterocele, some estimate of the degree of renal function, especially from the segment draining into the ureterocele, is essential. This information most often is obtained with a radionuclide renal scan (Fig. 7–4).

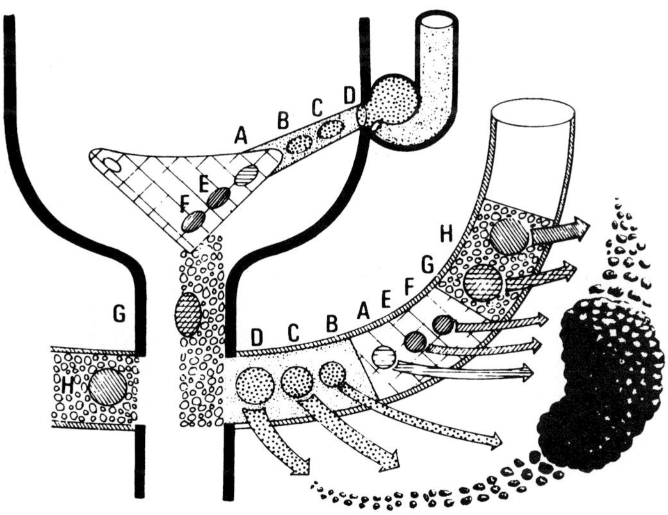

Figure 7–3 Diagram depicting how the position of the ureteral bud on the wolffian duct (mesonephric duct) will correspond to the final position of the ureteral orifice in the bladder. Ureteral buds that originate at the E position and more proximally on the wolffian duct will tend to hit less normal metanephric blastema and therefore induce dysplastic tissue. From Mackey GG, Stephens FD. Duplex kidneys: A correlation of renal dysplasia with position of ureteral orifice. J Urol 114:274, 1975. Used with permission.

The concept of dysplasia in association with ureteroceles can be extended to include the ureter also. Studies have shown that some ureteroceles have an incomplete, patchy muscular coat, and the muscularization of the lower ureter tends to be more abnormal than a similar segment of ureter in children who have an ectopic ureter without a ureterocele.[1, 3] This observation may also be important in planning the amount of abnormal ureter to resect (or leave) during surgical reconstruction.

EMBRYOLOGY

The cause of ureteroceles remains somewhat controversial and may be multifactorial. Truly intravesical ureteroceles often appear to have a pinhole ureteral meatus, and, to some extent, these lesions may result from true ureteral meatal stenosis. It has been proposed that intravesical ureteroceles result from incomplete dissolution of a thin embryonic membrane that temporarily occludes the ureteral orifice (Chawalla's membrane).[4] This is in distinction from the ureterocele that drains extravesically, in which cases the orifice often appears to be large, gaping, and poorly supported within the urethra.

Ureteroceles that are located extravesically are thought to be the result of a primary anomaly of the distal segment of the mesonephric duct and the primitive ureter as it buds from the mesonephric duct. In normal embryogenesis of the ureter, the distal segment of the mesonephric duct widens as it is incorporated into the differentiation of the trigone, the bladder neck, and the proximal urethra. In a child with a ureterocele, it is proposed that this widening is excessive and extends up to

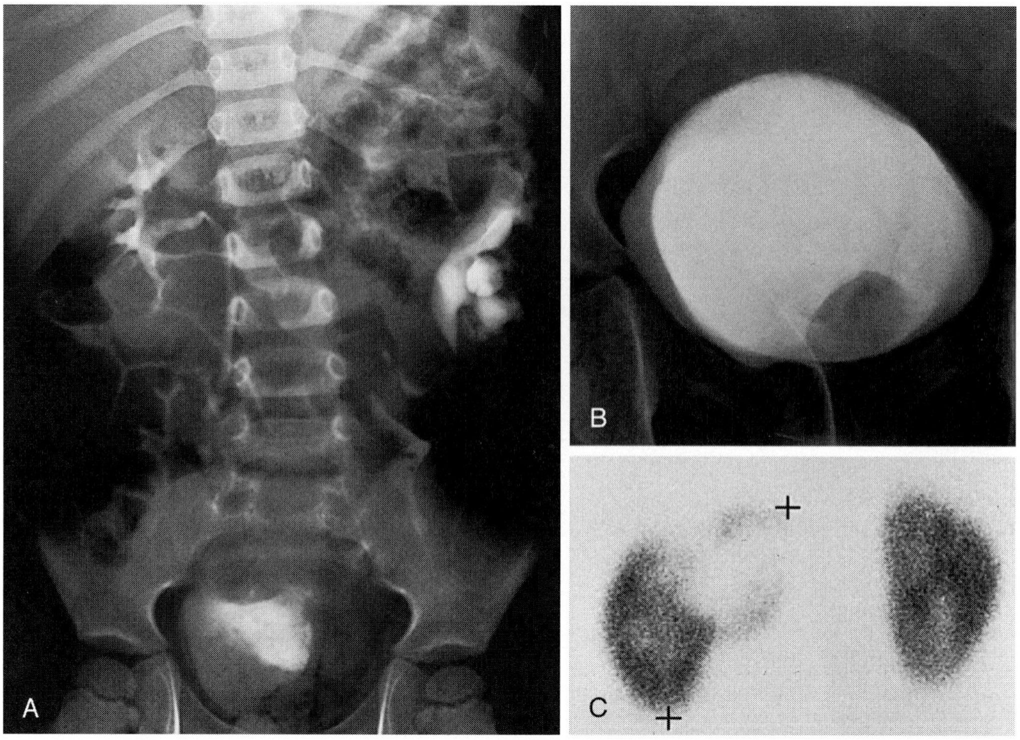

Figure 7–4 Use of radionuclide renal scan to assess the level of renal function in segments of the kidney in a patient with an extravesical, duplex ureter ureterocele. *A,* An intravenous urogram demonstrates inferior and lateral displacement of the visualized collecting system of the left kidney, suggesting an upper pole mass. *B,* A cystogram shows a small cystic lesion on the left side of the bladder neck. *C,* Radionuclide renal scan demonstrating very poor function of the left upper pole.

and includes the distal portion of the ureter.[5] Because of this, the more normal-caliber ureter is unable to reach the trigone and a ureterocele results (Fig. 7–5). Obstruction at the ureterovesical junction is thought to result as the ureter passes through the bladder sphincter on its way to a distal, ectopically located ureteral orifice.

These extravesical ureteroceles are located anatomically between the detrusor and the transitional epithelium of the bladder and urethra. Although the detrusor muscle may be effaced and thin behind the ureterocele, the ureteral hiatus at the trigone is generally much smaller than the ureterocele. At the bladder neck and into the urethra, the ureterocele is totally enclosed by the detrusor and the sphincter mechanism.

In the great majority of cases, the orifice of the ureterocele drains at the most distal edge of the ureterocele. In a small minority, an anatomic variant of ureteroceles termed a *cecoureterocele* is present. In this situation, the orifice of the ureterocele opens more proximally and a distal, blind mucosal extension of the ureterocele continues into the bladder neck and proximal urethra. These types of ureteroceles are especially prone to obstruction of the bladder neck which may worsen if the more proximal ureterocele is incised (Fig. 7–6).

PRESENTATION

Children with ureteroceles will eventually experience urinary infection and risk sustaining renal parenchymal damage from pyelonephritis. Because there is a high incidence of reflux into the other ureters, urinary infection may put the patient's entire complement of renal parenchyma at risk. A few children present because of introital abnormalities: prolapse of the ureterocele or presentation of the orifice on the perineum. At times purulent drainage may be seen at the introitus or in the diaper if the orifice drains onto the perineum directly. In a few cases, the hydronephrotic segments may be palpable. Today, however, most ureteroceles are being recognized on prenatal ultrasonogram, and appropriate intervention can eliminate the risk of infection and allow for more organized and planned reconstruction (Fig. 7–7).

GOALS OF THERAPY

Because ureteroceles present such a complex, multifaceted problem, the approach to and timing of therapy varies considerably. As in all congenital anomalies, the spectrum of disease is wide, and no single approach will address all the permutations one encounters in dealing with ureteroceles. In general, though, planning a management algorithm for a patient with a ureterocele involves consideration of four separate factors: prevention of urinary tract infection; assessment and management of the renal segment draining into the ureterocele; assessment and management of the bladder, trigone, and bladder neck defect; and preservation of the remaining renal parenchyma.

In the past, nearly all patients with a ureterocele presented because of urinary infection or recognition of

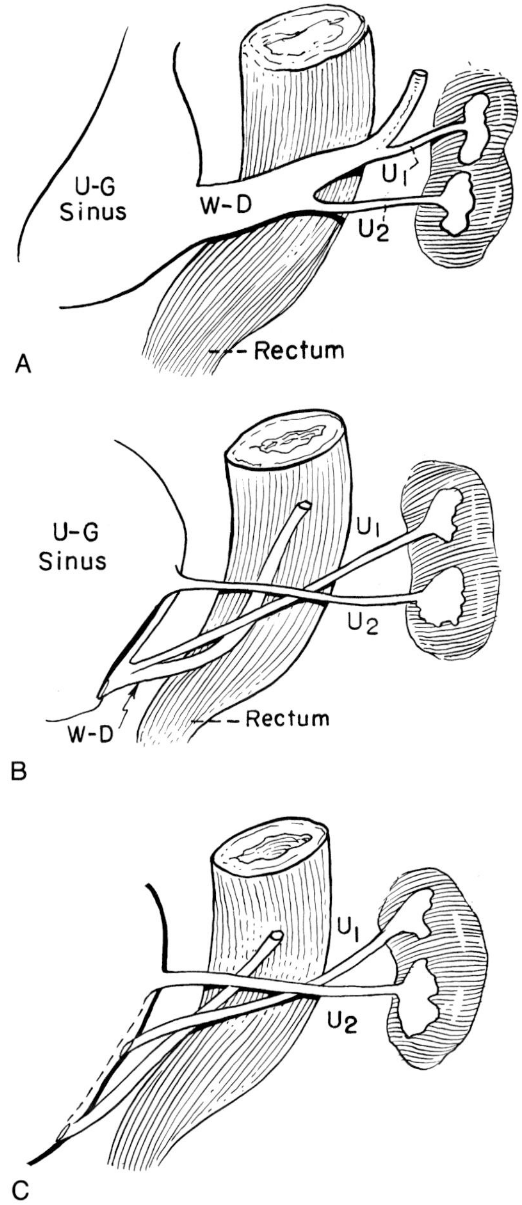

Figure 7–5 Embryology of the duplex ureter. Because the lower segment ureter (U_2) reaches the developing bladder first and, therefore, migrates more lateral and proximal along the trigone, it is the upper pole ureter (U_1) that is at risk of opening in an ectopic position. A ureterocele might then develop if the expanded portion of the wolffian duct (W-D) is incompletely incorporated into the bladder base. (U-G, urogenital; U, ureter.) From Gonzales ET. Anomalies of the renal pelvis and ureter. In Kelalis PP, King LR, Belman AB (eds), Clinical Pediatric Urology, 3rd ed. Philadelphia: WB Saunders, 1992. Used with permission.

purulent drainage at the introitus. When the dilated, atonic, obstructed segment becomes infected, it often functions much like an abscess in that adequate antibiotic levels may not be achievable in the abnormal parenchyma or dilated system. The acute period of sepsis may be able to be controlled by adequate treatment of the perinephric inflammation, but recurrence of the symptoms is common when antibiotics are discontinued. Therefore, some form of direct intervention is often necessary to control this sepsis completely after the acute febrile episode has resolved. This may include placing a percutaneous nephrostomy into the hydronephrotic system, endoscopic ureterocele incision and decompression, cutaneous ureterostomy, ureterocele excision and reimplantation, or open (in some centers laparoscopic) partial nephrectomy (or nephrectomy for a single system) or upper ureter to lower ureter ureteroureterostomy. Because current chemotherapeutic drugs will almost always control the symptoms of acute sepsis, urgent percutaneous or open temporizing drainage (nephrostomy or ureterostomy) is rarely needed. Surgical management after presentation with urinary infection is nearly always urgent but unlikely to require emergent decompression of the obstructed system.

Today, most patients with ureteroceles are identified on prenatal ultrasonogram, and immediate initiation of appropriate antibiotics (usually ampicillin in the neonate) will protect the infant from infection while a plan of management is being devised.

The renal segment draining into the ureterocele will be abnormal because of dysplasia or hydronephrotic atrophy. It is not possible to be absolutely certain how much dysplasia is present, and several studies have shown that the histologic appearance of a majority of excised upper pole segments is more often compatible with hydronephrotic atrophy rather than dysplasia. Infection, of course, should it occur, will result in varying degrees of additional damage. Nevertheless, it is essential that an accurate assessment of the function of the involved renal segment be obtained. Currently, this is best done using the information obtained with a renal ultrasonogram and a radionuclide renal scan.

The renal ultrasonogram provides information on parenchymal thickness, corticomedullary differentiation, the presence of cysts within the parenchyma, and the echogenicity of the parenchyma. Because dysplasia is often associated with many microcysts, dysplastic parenchyma often appears very echodense compared with normal renal tissue or surrounding tissues. The radionuclide renal scan is the standard for assessing function. Either an agent that measures flow and filtration—diethylenetetramine-pentaacetic acid (DTPA) or mercaptoacetyltriglycine—or a tissue-staining agent (dimercaptosuccinic acid [DMSA]) will allow for quantification of function and differentiation of functional differences between the upper and lower segments of the involved kidney as well as comparison to the contralateral kidney. My preference is for DMSA. An intravenous pyelogram is not a satisfactory technique to estimate function in the various renal segments.

Because of the location of the ureterocele on the trigone and at the bladder neck, there are often abnor-

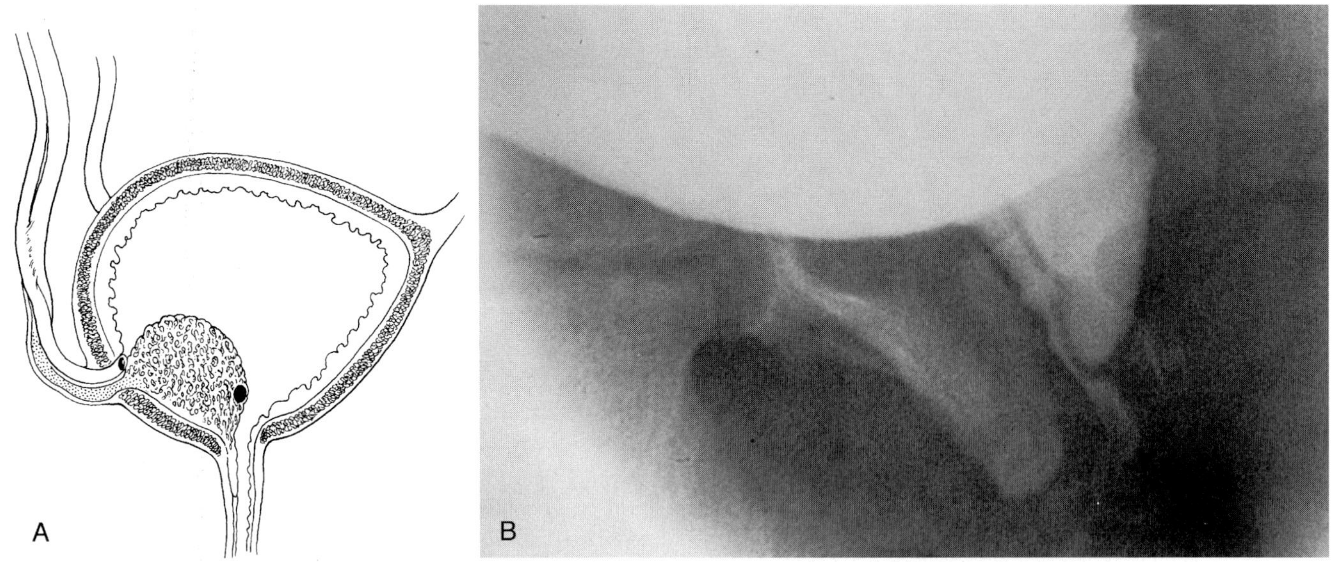

Figure 7–6 Cecoureterocele. *A,* The anatomy of a cecoureterocele. If the intravesical portion of the ureterocele is opened widely (i.e., endoscopic incision or incomplete resection), the blind mucosal extension will fill with urine during voiding. This results in a flap valve that can cause severe outlet obstruction. *B,* A voiding cystourethrogram of a child who had endoscopic "unroofing" of a ureterocele and could not void postoperatively. The blind urethral extension is clearly outlined. From Gonzales ET. Lower tract surgery for ureterocele and duplication anomalies. In Marshall FF (ed), Textbook of Operative Urology. Philadelphia: WB Saunders, 1996. Used with permission.

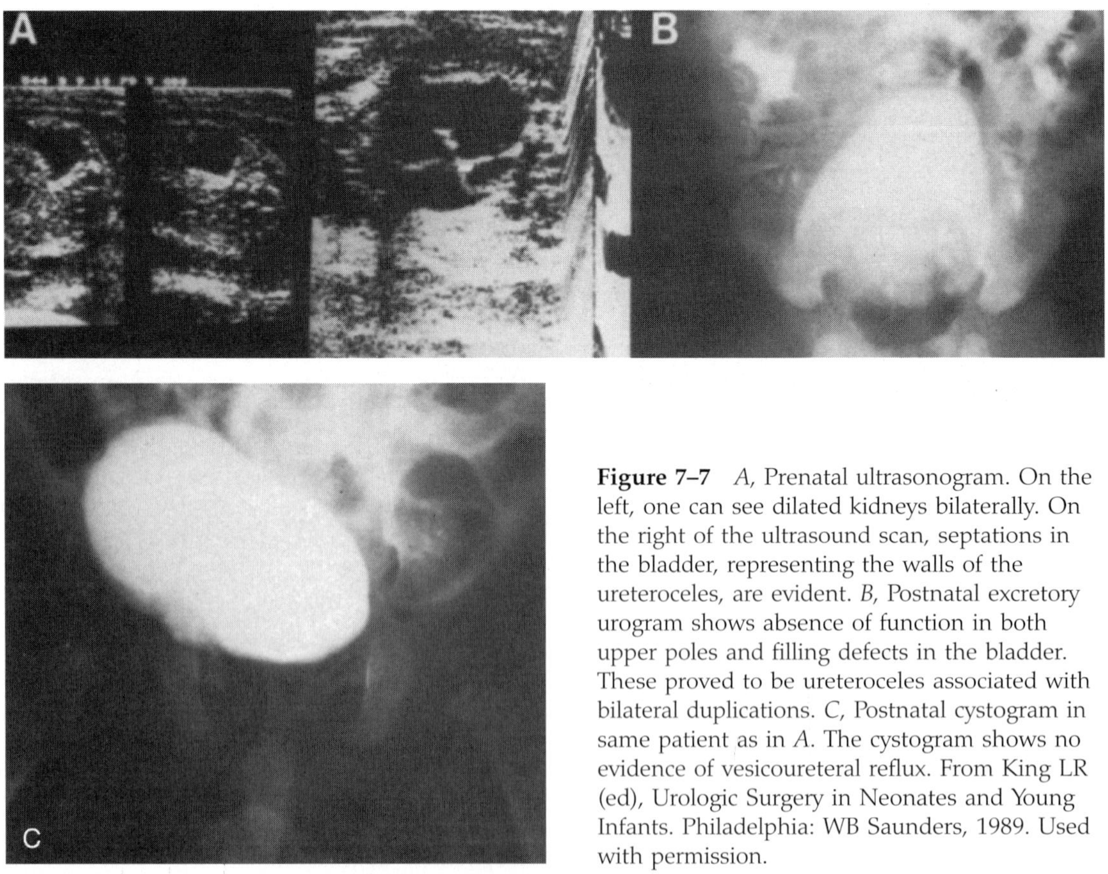

Figure 7–7 *A,* Prenatal ultrasonogram. On the left, one can see dilated kidneys bilaterally. On the right of the ultrasound scan, septations in the bladder, representing the walls of the ureteroceles, are evident. *B,* Postnatal excretory urogram shows absence of function in both upper poles and filling defects in the bladder. These proved to be ureteroceles associated with bilateral duplications. *C,* Postnatal cystogram in same patient as in *A.* The cystogram shows no evidence of vesicoureteral reflux. From King LR (ed), Urologic Surgery in Neonates and Young Infants. Philadelphia: WB Saunders, 1989. Used with permission.

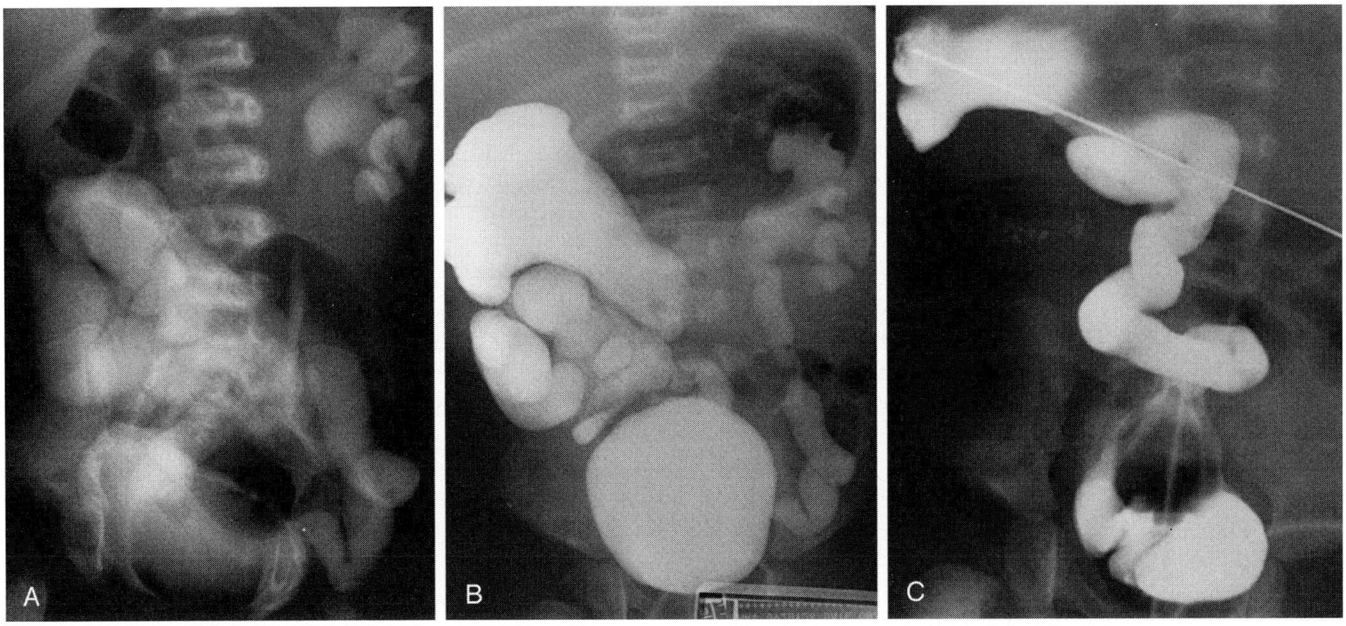

Figure 7–8 Intravenous urogram *(A)* and voiding cystourethrogram *(B)* demonstrating a right extravesical duplex ureter ureterocele with massive reflux into the other ureters. On the cystogram, the right upper pole is visualized because a percutaneous nephrostomy had been placed *(C)*.

malities that disturb bladder emptying and place the remaining renal parenchyma in jeopardy. Reflux into the other ureters may be present, making it likely that urinary infection will most likely involve all the renal parenchyma; or there may be obstruction to ureteral efflux, causing hydronephrosis and additional parenchymal loss. At times, the source of obstruction is at the bladder neck, resulting in high intravesical pressures and global effects on the upper urinary tract. A properly done voiding cystourethrogram is essential to evaluate completely the full extent of the anomaly (Fig. 7–8).

Management of the ureterocele also must correct these other problems. This can all be taken care of in a single surgical session, or the approach may be staged, relieving obstruction and reducing infection risk with the first procedure and addressing the reflux and bladder abnormality later if necessary.

MANAGEMENT

Because ureteroceles can present in so many ways, several options have been developed to effectively treat these anomalies. When discussing treatment, it is customary to separate ureteroceles into those affecting single systems and those associated with the upper pole of a complete ureteral duplication. However, this distinction, in my view, is artificial. As discussed, the surgeon should focus on the concept of whether the ureterocele is intravesical or extravesical. Although it is true that a greater proportion of single-system ureteroceles will be classified as intravesical than those associated with duplex ureters, the pathophysiology is more dependent on ureterocele location than on ureteral number. Considerations in planning therapy must consider the quality of the affected renal parenchyma (how much function, how much dysplasia) and the effect of the ureterocele on bladder function (obstruction, reflux; how will simple decompression of the ureterocele alter these effects). Treatment options include the following:

1. Observation
2. Endoscopic incision and decompression of the ureterocele
3. Either a renal procedure that might include a nephrectomy (total for a single system or partial for a duplex system) if there is significant dysplasia or severe atrophy from hydronephrosis or infection, or improved drainage for the upper segment by performing upper to lower ureteropyelostomy if the upper pole is salvageable; a subtotal ureterectomy would also be performed in the case of a duplex ureter
4. A bladder procedure (this might include excision of the ureterocele, reinforcement of any attenuated detrusor muscle, and reimplantation to correct reflux)
5. A combination of options 3 and 4, performed as a staged procedure
6. A total reconstruction, including upper renal surgery and bladder repair at one operative session.

Observation

Symptomatic ureteroceles, those associated with significant hydronephrosis or reflux or presenting with urinary infection, are not candidates for observation. However, recognition of a small ureterocele incidentally (either prenatally or when a renal ultrasonogram is done for other symptoms, such as urinary incontinence) does not always demand urgent attention. Careful surveillance or initiation of maintenance chemoprophylaxis will allow for a period of time to assess whether this small lesion is likely to be a problem or not. The sophistication of modern endoscopic instruments and the development of effective endoscopic management (discussed next) make it tempting to consider incision of these small lesions. However, the associated complications of acquired vesicoureteral reflux or ureteral obstruction will then demand an open repair. It behooves the responsible surgeon to recognize that current diagnostic techniques can identify some ureteroceles that do not require immediate or perhaps any intervention.

Endoscopic Incision and Decompression

Endoscopic management of ureteroceles is an old, once-discarded technique that has been reactivated with the introduction of better endoscopic instruments as well as improved understanding of the pathophysiology associated with ureteroceles. Initially, endoscopic management consisted of "unroofing" of the ureterocele, which was seen as a convenient and expedient means to drain a dilated, atonic, infected system. Although this was very effective at controlling sepsis, these infants nearly always experienced massive vesicoureteral reflux into the ureterocele unit (as well as recurring episodes of pyelonephritis), and clinicians subsequently moved to a more open reconstructive surgical approach.

About a decade ago, Tank rekindled interest in endoscopic management of ureteroceles.[6] He reasoned that decompression of the ureterocele would delay an open surgical reconstruction in the tiny infant and would allow for possible recovery of function in some of the affected renal parenchyma. He demonstrated that current nonoperative management for vesicoureteral reflux could forestall the need for urgent surgical treatment. In a series of 40 consecutive children with duplex-system ureteroceles managed by endoscopic drainage, all with postdecompression reflux, only 6 (15%) required surgery for breakthrough urinary infection. In half of the cases, improvement was believed to occur in upper pole function, but the extent of improvement was not quantitated. In addition, hydronephrosis generally improved significantly in all ureters so treated.

The success of this initial series encouraged other investigators to re-evaluate endoscopic management. Monfort and colleagues reported on a small series of single-system intravesical ureteroceles in male infants.[7] In this series they purposely attempted to incise the ureterocele such that reflux would not occur, as opposed to the technique used by Tank. In each instance, they were successful at relieving obstruction and preventing reflux. At the time of the report, the procedure appeared definitive. Rich and coworkers reported similar success in a somewhat larger series.[8]

However, as surgeons became more familiar with endoscopic techniques and extended these procedures to more complex, extravesical, and duplex ureteroceles, long-term results were not nearly as successful (Table 7–1).[9, 10] It was not as easy to prevent reflux and, because of the more serious defect at the bladder neck, many children ultimately did experience problems with urinary infection. However, as noted by Tank, endoscopic decompression of the large complex lesions generally can buy sufficient time to allow the newborn or infant to grow and plan an elective reconstruction, when needed, in an older, healthy infant. Endoscopic decompression is an option for almost any child with a ureterocele and is the procedure of choice, I believe, for those children with intravesical lesions (especially with single systems) and no vesicoureteral reflux into other ureters.

Surgical Reconstruction

The disappointing short-term results of endoscopic unroofing several decades ago prompted a closer look at primary surgical reconstruction for ureteroceles. When planning this reconstruction, one must consider that the effects of a ureterocele are felt at the level of both the kidney and the bladder. These effects may be a result of simple obstruction but often are primary developmental abnormalities and include renal parenchymal dysplasia, abnormal ureteral function, and anatomic maldevelop-

Table 7–1
Experience With Endoscopic Incision of Duplicate Ureter Ureteroceles[9]

Location of Ureterocele	Satisfactory Decompression (%)	Preservation of Upper Pole (%)	Postdecompression Reflux (%)	Needed Second Surgery (%)
Intravesical	93	96	18	7
Extravesical	75	50	47	50

ment of the bladder neck and proximal urethra. Each of these factors impacts on the timing and extent of reconstruction.

The primary decision in any reconstructive effort is to evaluate the degree of function in the renal unit drained by the ureterocele. Because renal dysplasia is commonly present, very poor or nonfunction of that segment would prompt a nephrectomy as opposed to any reconstructive effort to salvage the kidney. For a single-system ureterocele, this would, of course, be a total nephrectomy; for a duplex ureterocele, an upper pole ("partial") nephrectomy is all that would be required. If renal function is good and the upper segment is worth saving, the most frequently used procedure involves an upper segment ureter to lower segment pelvis or upper ureter (a ureteropyelostomy) with excision of the abnormal, dilated ureter (Fig. 7–9). Alternatively, renal salvage can be achieved by lower ureteral reconstruction, which might include primary ureteral reimplantation (tailoring where necessary) for a single-system anomaly or a common sheath reimplantation or lower segment reimplant with a lower ureteroureterostomy in the case of a duplication anomaly. Although a low ureteroureterostomy can be successful and has been advocated as the procedure of choice by some authors,[11] a high ureteropyelostomy is preferred by most pediatric urologic surgeons. A low ureteroureterostomy deep in the pelvis leaves a long segment of dilated, atonic ureter that can result in stasis and is at presumed increased risk for urinary infection. With a high ureteropyelostomy, a significant portion of the abnormal ureter can be discarded, even through a flank incision alone.

The second portion of the reconstruction for a ureterocele involving a duplex ureter includes excision of the ureterocele and reimplantation of any associated refluxing ureters. However, the timing and extent of vesical reconstruction remain somewhat controversial. King and coworkers suggested that a total reconstruction for a ureterocele was best staged in most instances, but especially in infants, with the upper procedure being accomplished first and the lower bladder reconstruction delayed for several months.[12] The justification for this approach was based on the observation that, in most cases, simple decompression of the ureterocele after the upper procedure relieved obstruction at the bladder neck and the other ureteral orifices and resulted in improvement of the hydronephrosis, better emptying of the bladder, and a decrease in detrusor hypertrophy (Fig. 7–10). Subsequent bladder reconstruction was believed to be easier and, in the hands of those authors, was more successful than when they performed total one-stage reconstruction.

Several publications have subsequently established the efficacy and safety of this staged approach when managing an infant with a large, duplex ureterocele with marked reflux or hydronephrosis in all ureteral units.[13–15] However, other surgeons take issue with this premise. Hendren and colleagues advocated a total one-stage repair, arguing that leaving the ureterocele and significant vesicoureteral reflux increases the risk of additional urinary infections and further damage to the healthier segments of renal parenchyma.[16, 17] In their series, a total one-stage upper and lower reconstruction was as efficacious as that reported for the staged repairs.

DEVISING A TREATMENT ALGORITHM

Considering the many facets of ureteroceles and the multitude of surgical options available to manage them, any treatment plan will require a thorough knowledge of all these parameters; but certain basic principles seem to hold:

1. Endoscopic decompression of a ureterocele effectively relieves obstruction to the involved renal unit and will improve urethral drainage and bladder emptying in almost all cases (single and duplex ureteroceles). Beware of the cecoureterocele, the one anatomic variant in which making a large intravesical opening into the ureterocele will increase bladder outlet obstruction. In these cases, the distal urethral extension must be marsupialized into the urethra.
2. Endoscopic decompression can be definitive management for an intravesical ureterocele when the incision into the ureterocele is made medial and inferior so as to prevent vesicoureteral reflux. However, this form of therapy is more often only temporizing when used for an extravesical ureterocele.
3. Decompression of a ureterocele by excision of the associated renal parenchyma and most of the ureter is also effective in relieving obstruction. It may also be definitive therapy if the ureterocele is not too large and there is no reflux into the other ureters. If one hopes that an upper pole procedure only will be definitive, it is important to leave as short a segment of the distal portion of the ureter as possible. The experience in the literature, however, is that 50 to 70% of children managed in this way will ultimately need bladder reconstruction also.
4. If marked vesicoureteral reflux is present on the preoperative cystogram, it is almost certain that a bladder reconstruction will be necessary, although endoscopic decompression of the ureterocele and antibiotic chemoprophylaxis are generally effective in preventing urinary infection in neonates and young infants, thereby allowing ureterectasis to decrease before the necessary reconstruction is done electively in an older, healthy infant.
5. Definitive one-stage reconstruction is safe and effective when done by one skilled in the

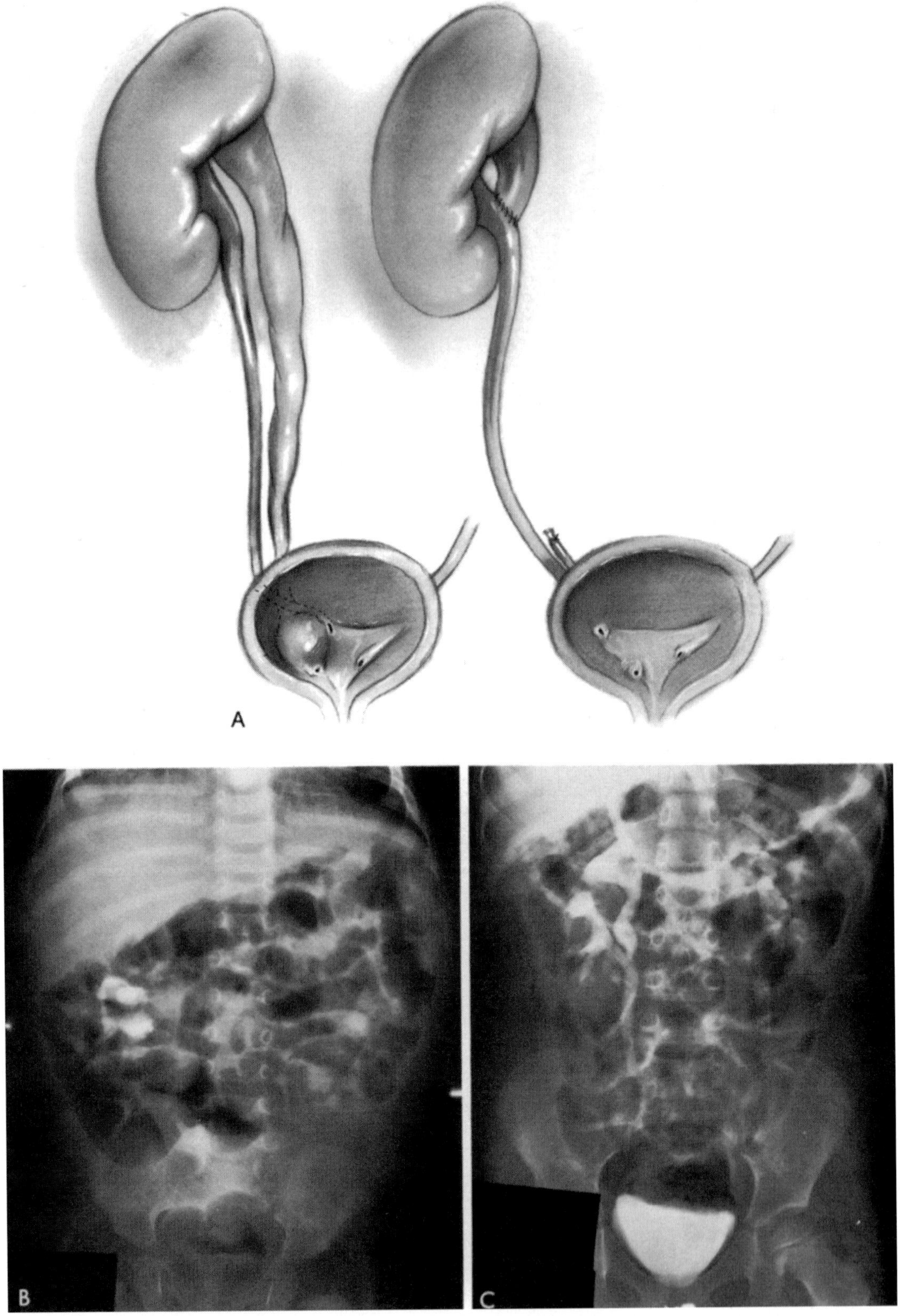

Figure 7–9 *A*, Ureteropyelostomy for treatment of ectopic ureterocele. *B*, Excretory urogram. Bilateral duplication and ectopic ureteroceles. Poorly functioning hydronephrosis, upper segment on right, salvageable according to dimercaptosuccinic acid scan. *C*, Excretory urogram after right ureteropyelostomy, left upper heminephrectomy, and bilateral subtotal ureterectomy. Note return of function in upper segment on right and collapse of both ureteroceles. From Gonzales ET. Anomalies of the renal pelvis and ureter. In Kelalis PP, King LR, Belman AB (eds), Clinical Pediatric Urology, 3rd ed. Philadelphia: WB Saunders, 1992. Used with permission.

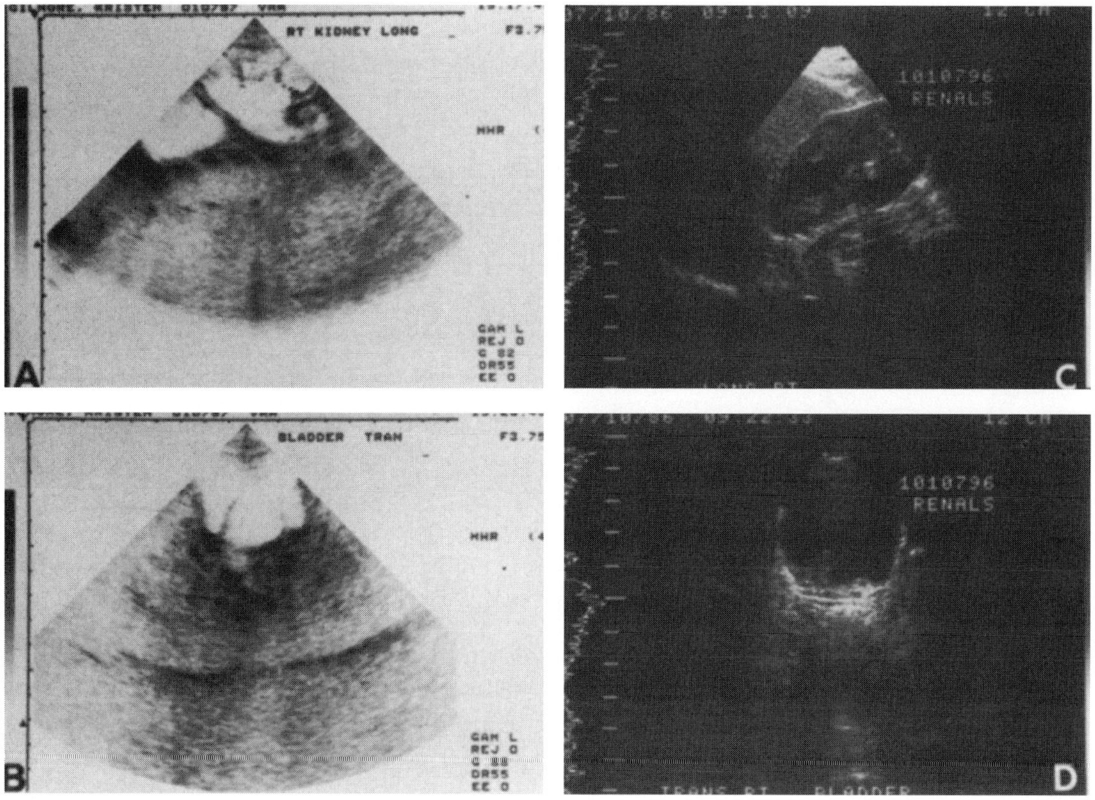

Figure 7–10 The preoperative ultrasonogram of the right kidney *(A)* shows hydronephrosis of both segments of the kidney. The bladder view of this ultrasound examination *(B)* shows the wall of the ureterocele clearly. Postoperatively, after right upper pole heminephrectomy, the hydronephrosis of the lower pole moiety has considerably improved *(C)*, and the ureterocele has collapsed down to be only a small remnant that one can visualize in the bladder view *(D)*. From Gonzales ET, Decter RM. Management of ureteroceles in the newborn. In King LR (ed), Urologic Surgery in Neonates and Young Infants. Philadelphia: WB Saunders, 1989. Used with permission.

techniques of renal, ureteral, and bladder neck reconstruction.

On the basis of these principles, I have developed the following algorithm for managing ureteroceles:

1. Endoscopic decompression would be considered
   a. As definitive therapy for a small, single-system intravesical ureterocele.
   b. As a temporizing procedure in a large extravesical ureterocele in a neonate, especially if there is significant reflux into the other ureters. In my experience, these infants always need a bladder reconstruction, and I would opt to perform a total one-stage open repair at about 1 year of age when I can prevent infection by excising the ureterocele.
   c. To drain a pyoureter either in a child unresponsive to antibiotics or after an upper (renal) procedure in which the ureteral stump becomes infected.
2. In neonates with a small duplex-system ureterocele and no vesicoureteral reflux, I primarily perform an upper tract procedure and subtotal ureterectomy, with the thought that this can be definitive therapy. A secondary bladder repair can be done later as needed.
3. It is not common to see a significant ureterocele in an older child, but there are occasional delays in presentation. In these unusual situations, I would generally opt for a total, one-stage reconstruction if the ureterocele is large and extravesical and if there is associated vesicoureteral reflux. Similarly, endoscopic decompression of the extravesical, upper pole ureterocele in a neonate is done with the expectation that a total one-stage reconstruction will be done in an older infant.

TECHNICAL CONSIDERATIONS

Endoscopic Decompression

The technique of endoscopic decompression involves opening the ureterocele inferiorly and medially. In most

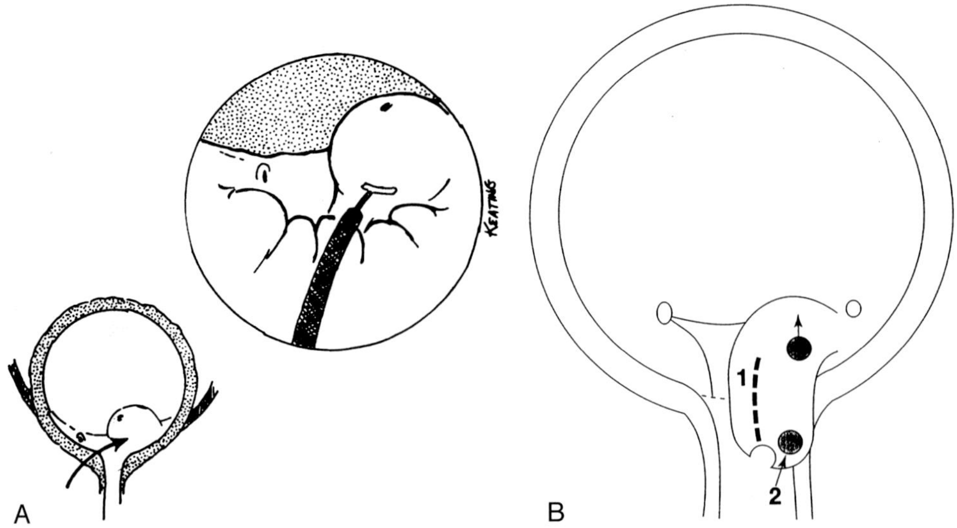

Figure 7–11 Endoscopic puncture *(A)* and incision *(B)* of a ureterocele. A large flap of the wall of the ureterocele is preserved in an attempt to prevent vesicoureteral reflux into the ureterocele segment. Figure 7–11*A* from Rich MA, Keating MA, Snyder HM, Duckett JW. Low transurethral incision of single-system intravesical ureteroceles in children. J Urol 144:120, 1990. Used with permission. Figure 7–11*B* from Blyth B, Passerini-Glazel G, Camuffo C, et al. Endoscopic incision of ureteroceles: Intravesical versus ectopic. J Urol 149:556, 1993. Used with permission.

cases, a small Bugbee electrode used to "puncture" the ureterocele is sufficient. If the orifice of the ureterocele is seen in the urethra, an incision from the orifice along the luminal wall proximally into the bladder will also drain the ureterocele effectively (Fig. 7–11). These maneuvers will often avoid the development of vesicoureteral reflux because a large surface of ureterocele persists to act as an antireflux flap. A hot loop to unroof the ureterocele is specifically avoided.[18]

If one suspects a cecoureterocele is present, then endoscopic incision is best avoided. Opening into the ureterocele may allow reflux to occur into the lumen of the ureterocele, overdistending the urethral extension and causing severe bladder outlet obstruction.

Partial (Upper Pole) Nephrectomy

The kidney is approached through an anterior subcostal incision in neonates or traditional flank incision in older children. The ureters are then identified at the level of the lower pole, and the upper and lower segment ureters are differentiated and separated. If there is a marked discrepancy in ureteral caliber, this differentiation is easy. If such is not the case, careful dissection along the two ureters proceeds proximally until separation into upper and lower ureters can be made. As the ureters are separated, the adventitial blood supply is compulsively swept away with the lower pole ureter. At this point, the upper pole ureter is transected.

The anatomic relationships at the hilum are the vessels anteriorly, the upper pole ureter medially, and the lower pole pelvis posteriorly. Careful dissection along the upper pole ureter will free this structure from the pedicle and lower pole system, allowing the ureter to be passed superior to the renal vessels.

Mobilization of the ureter in this fashion now allows the upper pole to be mobilized into the operative field. Care must be taken to identify small, accessory upper pole renal vessels at this time and to secure them with hemostatic clips. If divided, these vessels retract superiorly and can cause troublesome bleeding. Dissection then continues along the ureter and upper pole pelvis deep within the hilum of the upper pole of the kidney. The primary blood supply to the upper pole tends to run along the pelvis and is most easily identified at this time. As these vascular bundles are isolated and ligated, the upper pole tissue is clearly demarcated.

Transection of the upper pole is begun medially on either side of the renal pelvis at the line of the tissue demarcation. Because the upper pole is often "cupped" by the lower pole, dissection follows the course of the pelvis and infundibular structures so as to remove all of the upper pole parenchyma and collecting system (Fig. 7–12). Major vessels are ligated with carefully placed, atraumatic chromic sutures. The edges of the cut parenchyma can often be run with a chromic suture. Large, oozing surfaces are fulgurated with the argon beam coagulator, and Gelfoam is used as needed for hemostasis. A small Penrose drain is left overlying the upper margin of the lower pole.

The remaining distal segment of upper pole ureter is then dissected toward the bladder as far as can be safely

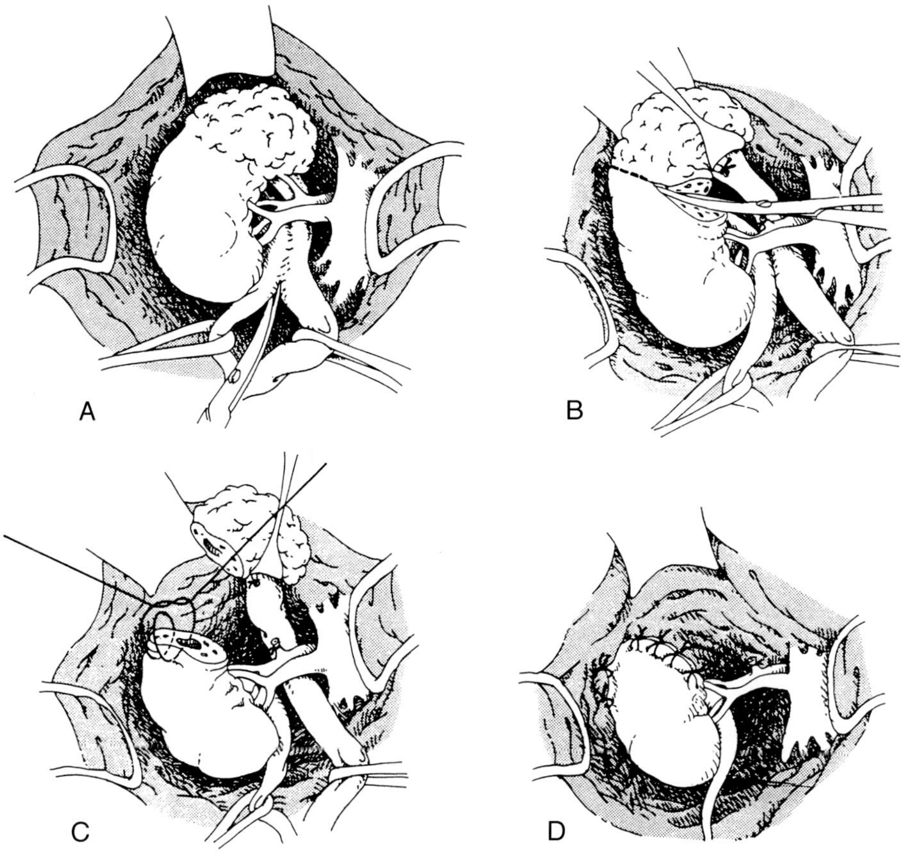

Figure 7–12 Technique of upper pole nephrectomy. The child can be either in a classic flank position or placed for a subcostal, extraperitoneal approach (neonate or young infant). *A*, The upper and lower segment ureters are separated, and the blood supply to the lower segment ureter is compulsively maintained. *B*, The upper pole vasculature is ligated, demarcating the upper pole. The dissection is generally begun medially, as portrayed. If the upper pole is significantly hydronephrotic, the lower pole will encase the upper pole collecting system, much like an "egg in a cup." *C*, Major parenchymal arteries are individually ligated with atraumatic chromic sutures. *D*, Through and through mattress sutures can approximate margins of the "excavated" lower pole, further enhancing hemostasis. The kidney can be fixed to the psoas muscle if the surgeon desires.

reached. Care is taken to preserve the blood supply to the lower pole ureter. The ureter is then transected with the coagulating current but is left open. A second Penrose drain is left in the location of the cut ureter. The lower pole is then carefully examined for bleeding and for evidence of adequate vascular flow.

Some have argued for complete excision of the ureter via a second suprapubic incision.[16] Although this may be justified in an older child in whom a long stump often remains, in the very young child a substantial portion of the upper pole ureter can be resected from the single upper incision.

Ureteropyelostomy (Ureteroureterostomy)

The approach to the kidneys and ureters is identical to that for a partial nephrectomy. The ureters are separated, and the distal portion of the upper pole ureter is discarded, as described previously.

If a large lower pole pelvis is present, I prefer to perform a ureteropyelostomy. More often, however, the pelvis is small and tapered and may be almost intrarenal. In that situation, a ureteroureterostomy is performed. The upper pole ureter is transected on a bias to lay without tension along the lower pole ureter.

The adventitia of the lower pole ureter is then incised. Major longitudinal blood supply is pushed to the side but not injured. The lower pole system is mobilized only minimally in its bed. The ureter is then supported with a proximal and distal traction suture of 6-0 chromic. A longitudinal ureterotomy sufficient in length to accommodate the caliber of the upper pole ureter is then made.

The ureteroureterostomy is generally completed using 7-0 chromic or Vicryl suture, depending on the surgeon's preference. A single apical stitch is placed proximally and distally; the side walls are closed with a running, locking suture. A stent is not left indwelling, although a feeding tube is in position at the time of placement of the apical sutures. The operative field is drained (Fig. 7–13).

Ureterocelectomy

Ureterocelectomy is generally begun intravesically. Kroovand[15] described an extravesical approach for removal of the ureterocele, but I have found this technically difficult.

With a feeding tube in the lower pole ureteral orifice and a traction suture in the ureterocele, the bladder mucosa is opened along the lateral and medial edges of the ureterocele and around the proximal margin of the lower pole orifice. By careful dissection, the lower pole ureter and the proximal portion of the ureterocele can be dissected free of the detrusor muscle. Further proximal dissection will identify the upper pole ureter, and the mobili-

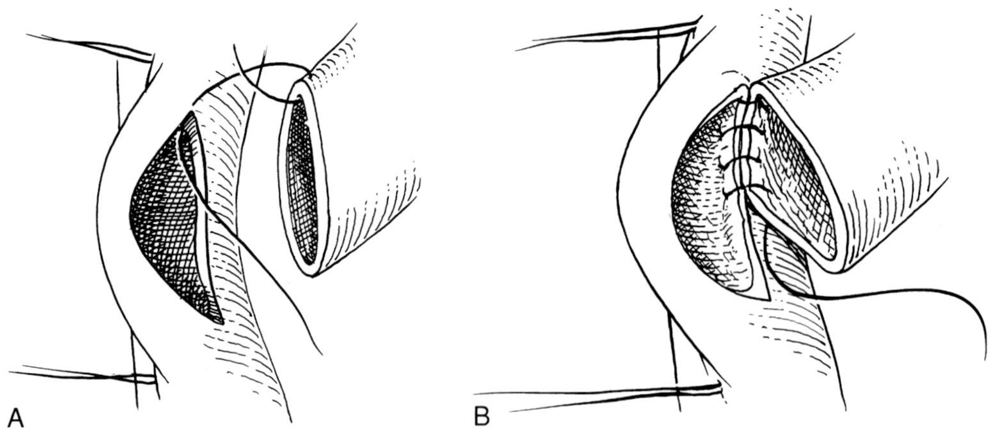

Figure 7–13 Diagram of end-to-side ureteroureterostomy. The incision in the lower pole ureter is made sufficient to accommodate the lumen of the upper pole ureter *(A)*. A carefully placed running suture improves the likelihood of a watertight anastomosis *(B)*. From Hensle TW, Kennedy WA III. Reconstruction of the lower ureter: psoas hitch, Boari flap, and transureteroureterostomy. In Marshall FF (ed), Textbook of Operative Urology. Philadelphia: WB Saunders, 1996. Used with permission.

zation then proceeds as one would for a common sheath reimplant. When the ureters can be separated, the lower pole ureter is transected and placed aside for later reimplantation. Further proximal mobilization of the upper segment ureter will finally reach the cut portion, and the entire remaining portion of the upper pole ureter can be delivered into the bladder. Most often, this dissection is done entirely intravesically, although I do not hesitate to go outside the bladder when I believe it will help the dissection.

At this point, dissection of the ureterocele proceeds distally toward the bladder neck. Care is taken to stay right on the mucosa of the ureterocele to prevent damage to the detrusor. Inferiorly (along the detrusor) and laterally, this is generally an easy dissection. Medially, the mucosa of the ureterocele and the bladder are thin and fused, and separation may be impossible. The ureterocele is transected at the bladder neck. Any extension into the urethra is incised sharply with delicate tenotomy scissors to marsupialize the ureterocele extension into the bladder or urethra. The mucosa at the bladder neck is then reapproximated to resurface the denuded detrusor.

The hiatus is narrowed, a cross-trigonal reimplant of the lower segment ureter is performed, and the remaining detrusor is resurfaced with transitional epithelium (Fig. 7–14).

COMPLICATIONS

Each treatment modality has its own list of potential risks and complications, and each is discussed individually.

Endoscopic Incision of Ureterocele

If the intention of endoscopic decompression is definitive therapy, one can assume that vesicoureteral reflux was not identified on the preoperative cystogram. The most common complication, then, would be the development of reflux into the ureterocele system. When dealing with a salvageable single-system ureterocele, options in reconstruction would be either endoscopic incision or ureteral reimplantation. The development of vesicoureteral reflux after endoscopic incision is disappointing but does not deter too much from more conventional therapy. When dealing with a duplex system, another alternative is an upper renal procedure only with subtotal ureterectomy and extravesical ureterocele decompression. If there is no associated reflux, this might be definitive. The development of reflux after endoscopic incision likely means that, ultimately, excision of the ureterocele and, at least, reimplantation of the ipsilateral lower pole ureter will be necessary.

Upper Pole Nephrectomy

The primary complication associated with an upper pole nephrectomy is atrophy of the lower pole (Fig. 7–15). Although not common, this complication is thought to result from development of an intimal tear from stretching of the lower pole vessels. The upper pole segment in a complete duplication almost always has a discrete blood supply. However, these vessels are often very short as they separate from the lower pole vessels. They are most easily identified when dissecting the upper pole collecting system well into the hilum, thereby avoiding direct dissection along the primary renal pedicle.

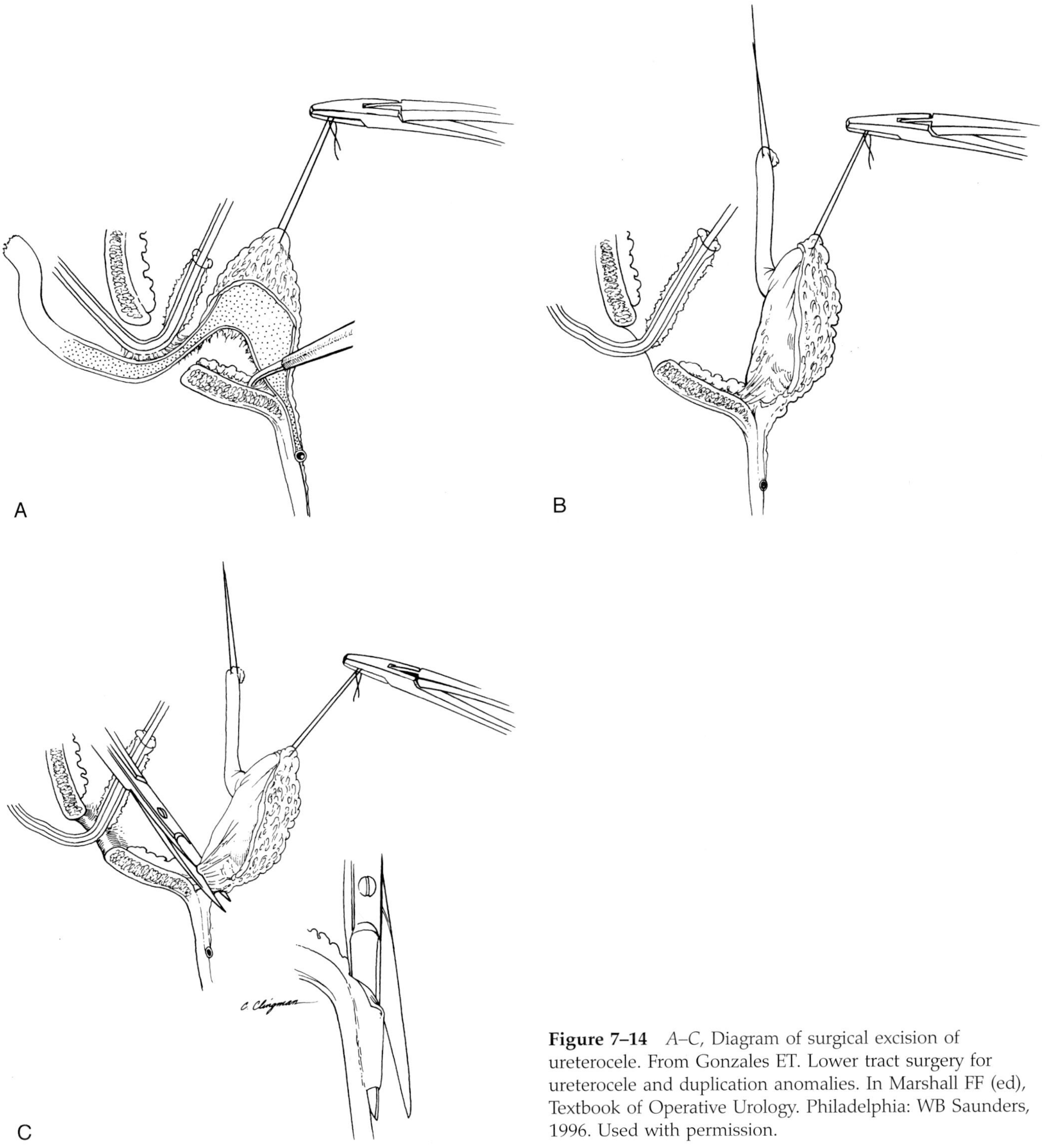

Figure 7–14 *A–C,* Diagram of surgical excision of ureterocele. From Gonzales ET. Lower tract surgery for ureterocele and duplication anomalies. In Marshall FF (ed), Textbook of Operative Urology. Philadelphia: WB Saunders, 1996. Used with permission.

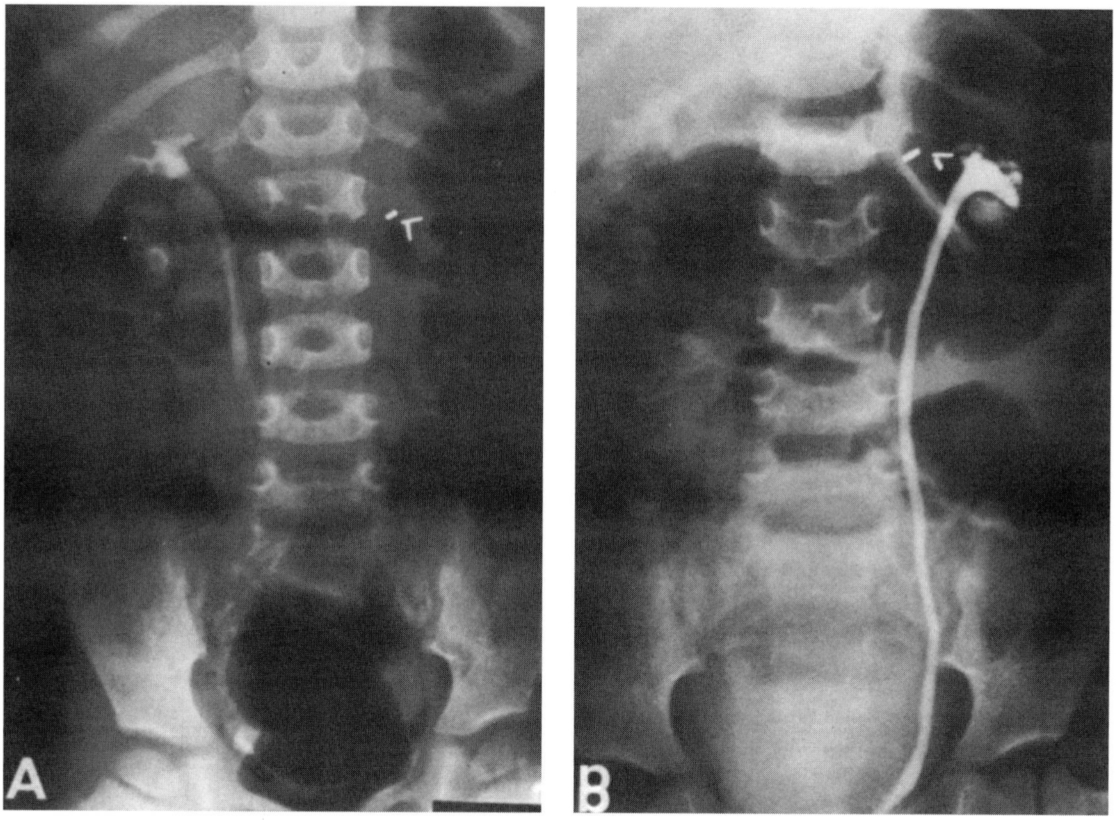

Figure 7–15 Postoperative studies after left upper segment nephrectomy and partial ureterectomy. The intravenous pyelogram *(A)* does not show any contrast excretion by the remaining lower pole of the kidney, which had visualized well before surgery. A retrograde pyelogram *(B)* demonstrates a shrunken unobstructed lower pole moiety. This is an example of a vascular injury to a lower pole moiety at the time of upper pole heminephrectomy. From Gonzales ET, Decter RM. Management of ureteroceles in the newborn. In King LR (ed), Urologic Surgery in Neonates and Young Infants. Philadelphia: WB Saunders, 1989. Used with permission.

Occasionally, a leak can develop if the lower pole collecting system is entered. However, this is usually easily recognized and should be no problem if repaired and properly drained.

Ureteroureterostomy

The primary complication of this procedure is development of a stricture of the lower pole ureter and possible loss of the better lower pole or the need for additional open procedures. Ureteroureterostomy has been a safe and effective procedure with success rates comparable to primary pyeloureterostomy for ureteropelvic junction obstruction. Significant size discrepancy between the ureters is not recognized as a cause for complications. The main consideration here preoperatively is that the responsible surgeon is confident that the upper pole is worth saving.

Ureterocelectomy

Excision of the ureterocele may result in injury to the bladder neck, which can result in urinary incontinence, or an injury to the vagina with subsequent vesicovaginal fistula. The key points, I believe, in avoiding these problems are to remember that the ureterocele itself is an intravesical structure. The detrusor may be effaced, but careful dissection on the ureterocele mucosa to, but not through, the bladder neck is generally sufficient. In fact, marsupialization of the ureterocele rather than excision has been advocated by some authors.[19] If a submucosal extension continues into the urethra, then I simply incise the extension of the ureterocele along the urethral lumen and leave the ureterocele mucosa to surface the posterolateral aspect of the urethra.

REFERENCES

1. Caldemone AA, Snyder HM, Duckett JW. Ureteroceles in children: Follow-up of management with upper tract approach. J Urol 131:1130, 1984.
2. Mackey GG, Stephens FD. Duplex kidneys: A correlation of renal dysplasia with position of ureteral orifice. J Urol 114:274, 1975.
3. Tokunaka S, Gotoh T, Koyanagi T, Tsuji I. The morphological

study of ureterocele: A possible clue to its embryogenesis as evidenced by a locally arrested myogenesis. J Urol 126:726, 1981.
4. Chawalla R. The process of formation of cystic dilation of the vesical end of the ureter and of diverticulae at the ureteral ostium. Urol Cutan Rev 31:499, 1927.
5. Tanagho EA. Embryogenic basis for lower ureteral anomalies: A hypothesis. Urology 7:451, 1976.
6. Tank ES. Experience with endoscopic incision and open unroofing of ureteroceles. J Urol 136:241, 1986.
7. Monfort G, Morrisson-Lacombe G, Coguet M. Endoscopic treatment of ureteroceles revisited. J Urol 133:1031, 1985.
8. Rich MA, Keating MA, Snyder HM, Duckett JW. Low transurethral incision of single system intravesical ureteroceles in children. J Urol 144:120, 1990.
9. Blyth B, Passerini-Glazel G, Camuffo C, et al. Endoscopic incision of ureteroceles: Intravesical versus ectopic. J Urol 149:556, 1993.
10. Smith C, Gosalbez R, Parrott TS, et al. Transurethral puncture of ectopic ureteroceles in neonates and infants. J Urol 152:2110, 1994.
11. Sen S, Akmed S. Management of double system ureterocele. Aust N Z J Surg 57:655, 1987.
12. King LR, Koslowski JM, Schacht MJ. Ureteroceles in children: A simplified and successful approach to management. JAMA 249:1461, 1983.
13. Hanson E, Enger EA, Hjalmar K. Heminephrectomy—Ureterectomy as the sole procedure in ectopic ureterocele in children. Z Kinderchir 39:355, 1984.
14. Decter RM, Roth DR, Gonzales ET. Individualized treatment of ureterocele. J Urol 142:535, 1989.
15. Kroovand RL: Ureterocele. Urol Clin North Am 10:445, 1983.
16. Hendren WH, Monfort FJ. Surgical correlation of ureteroceles in childhood. J Pediatr Surg 6:235, 1971.
17. Hendren WH, Mitchell ME. Surgical correction of ureteroceles. J Urol 121:590, 1979.
18. Coplen DE, Duckett JW. Modern approach to ureteroceles. J Urol 153:166, 1995.
19. Scherz HC, Kaplan GW, Packer MG, Brock WA. Ectopic ureteroceles: Surgical management with preservation of continence—Review of 60 cases. J Urol 142:538, 1989.

CHI K. LEE, ISRAEL FRANCO, & SELWYN LEVITT

8

Ectopic Ureter and Incontinence

The ectopic ureter is a congenital anomaly that reflects an abnormal ureteral bud site. Ureteral orifices occur in many abnormal locations, ranging from several sites within the bladder on the ectopic pathway to extravesicular sites such as the bladder neck, urethra, vestibule, and genital tract. Depending on the location of the ectopia, patients with ectopic ureters present in a myriad of ways, ranging from no symptoms to urinary tract infections, urinary incontinence, vesicoureteral reflux, and urethral obstruction. Because the ectopic ureter is a treatable entity, it is important to establish the diagnosis and implement definitive surgical intervention early to avert the development of potential consequences and complications of ectopic ureters.

EMBRYOLOGY

The cause of ureteral ectopia lies in the anomalous formation of the ureteral bud. Therefore, an understanding of the normal embryology of the ureteral bud is essential to establishing a fundamental knowledge of this ureteral abnormality.

In normal ureteral development, the ureteral bud grows from the dorsal surface of the mesonephric duct (later to become the wolffian duct) at a gestational age of about 4 weeks (Fig. 8–1). The origin of the ureteral bud is at an area of the mesonephric duct that is commonly termed the "elbow" or "knee"; this is the point at which the mesonephric duct turns sharply in an anterior direction. The growing ureteral bud quickly penetrates the metanephric blastema, a process that induces renal morphogenesis (Fig. 8–2). The renal pelvis is evident by the fifth week of gestation. By the eighth week of gestation, the portion of the mesonephric duct between the urogenital sinus and the ureteral bud, which is known as the common excretory duct, is completely absorbed and incorporated into the urogenital sinus (Fig. 8–3). The common excretory duct eventually forms the trigone and bladder neck.

Once the common excretory duct has been incorporated into the urogenital sinus, the ureter and mesonephric duct enter the urogenital sinus independently as two separate orifices. Initially, the position of the ureteral bud is caudal and medial relative to the mesonephric duct. Over the next 4 weeks, the two orifices undergo a rotational migration within the urogenital sinus, which brings the ureteral orifice to a craniolateral position and the mesonephric duct to a caudomedial position at the verumontanum. By the 12th week of gestation, each of the two orifices is approximately equidistant from the bladder neck (Fig. 8–4). The mesonephric duct ultimately forms the ejaculatory duct, vas deferens, seminal vesicles, and epididymis. A consequence of the rotational migration is the crossing of the vas deferens over the ureter ventrally.

Deviations from this embryologic process interfere

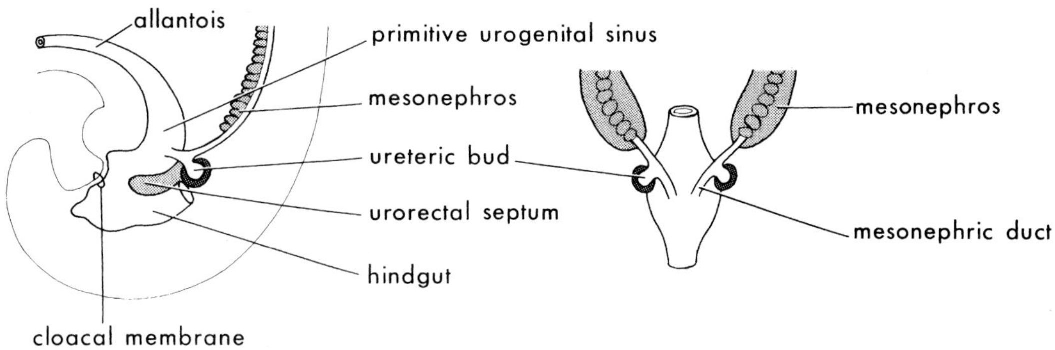

Figure 8–1 At 4 weeks' gestation, the ureteral bud emanates from the dorsal surface of the mesonephric (wolffian) duct. From Moore KL. The Developing Human, 3rd ed. Philadelphia: WB Saunders, 1992. Used with permission.

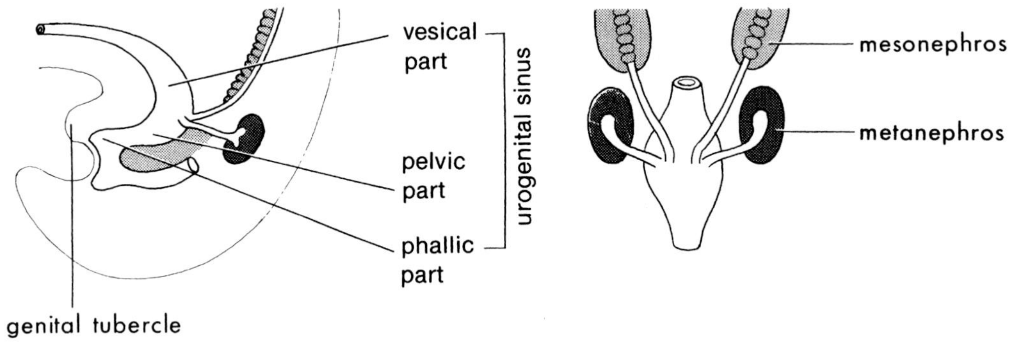

Figure 8–2 The ureteral bud penetrates the metanephric blastema to induce renal morphogenesis. From Moore KL. The Developing Human, 3rd ed. Philadelphia: WB Saunders, 1992. Used with permission.

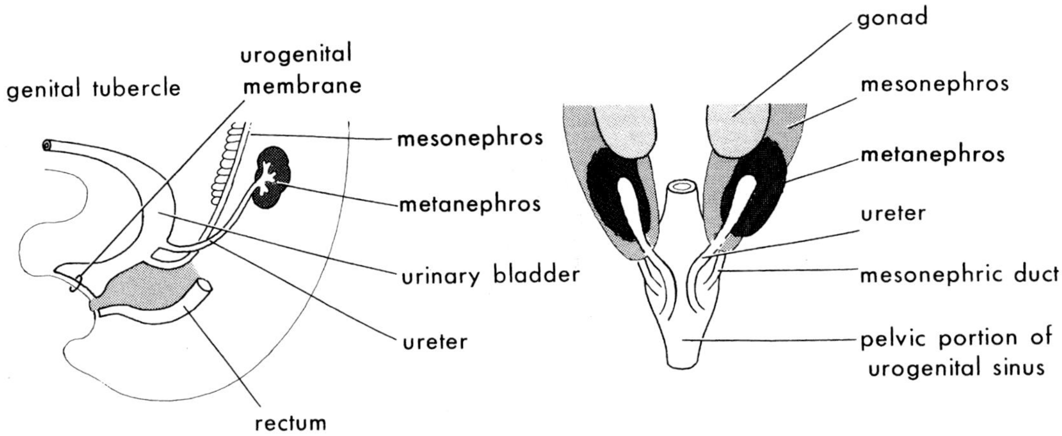

Figure 8–3 At 8 weeks' gestation, the common excretory duct is completely absorbed into the urogenital sinus and will eventually form the trigone and the bladder neck. From Moore KL. The Developing Human, 3rd ed. Philadelphia: WB Saunders, 1992. Used with permission.

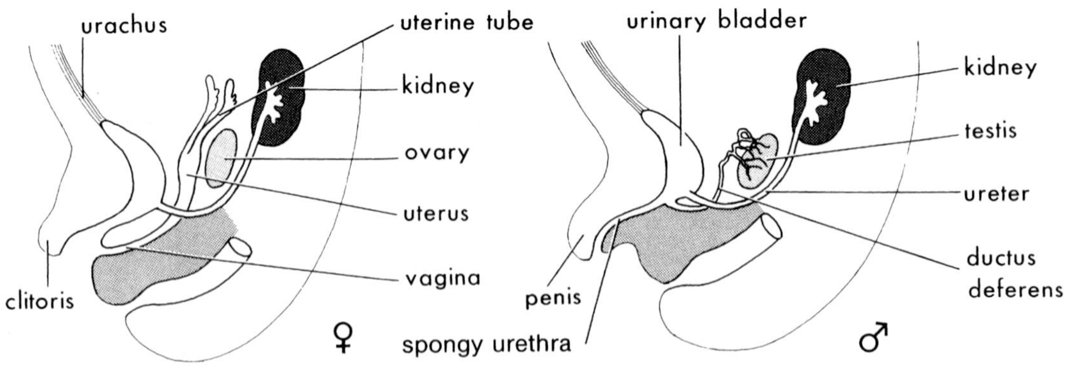

Figure 8–4 By 12 weeks' gestation, the ureteral orifice and the orifice to the mesonephric duct complete a rotational migration, bringing the ureter to a craniolateral position and the mesonephric duct to a caudomedial position. From Moore KL. The Developing Human, 3rd ed. Philadelphia: WB Saunders, 1992. Used with permission.

with normal ureteral development. Anomalies occur as a result of an abnormal site of origin of the ureteral bud as well as because of an abnormal number of ureteral buds that may arise from the mesonephric duct.

The formation of the ureteral bud at a location that is inferior to the normal "elbow" or "knee" of the mesonephric duct allows the ureteral bud to be absorbed into the urogenital sinus earlier. Hence, the ureteral orifice migrates a longer distance within the bladder and achieves a final position that is more cranial and lateral than normal. This type of ureteral ectopia is associated with a shortened submucosal ureteral tunnel, which often results in an incompetent ureterovesical junction and subsequent primary vesicoureteral reflux.[1–3]

If the ureteral bud originates at a site that is superior to the "elbow" or "knee," the complete incorporation of the ureteral bud into the urogenital sinus is delayed. The result is a shorter migration of the orifice within the bladder to a more caudal and medial final position. The severity of the ureteral ectopia depends on how far the origin of the ureteral bud was removed from the normal location on the "elbow" or "knee." A ureteral bud that grows on the mesonephric duct at a site that is only slightly more superior than normal leads to a nonpathologic condition in which the ureteral orifice is situated closer to the bladder neck than usual but remains within the bladder. However, a very distant origin of the ureteral bud superiorly results in significant caudal displacement of the ureter and, in some cases, the ureteral orifice fails to enter the bladder (Fig. 8–5). These "ectopic" ureters end in the urethra or upon mesonephric duct remnants. In the male, the mesonephric derivatives include the epididymis, vas deferens, and seminal vesicles. In the female, the ectopic ureter may drain into Gartner's duct, which is the distal remnant of the mesonephric duct. Because this duct runs from the broad ligament along the lateral wall of the vagina and ends at the hymen, ectopic ureters may open onto the vestibule, vagina, cervix, or uterus.

Ureteral ectopia has been best studied in cases in which two ureteral buds form separately from two distinct sites on the mesonephric duct. Each ureteral bud pene-

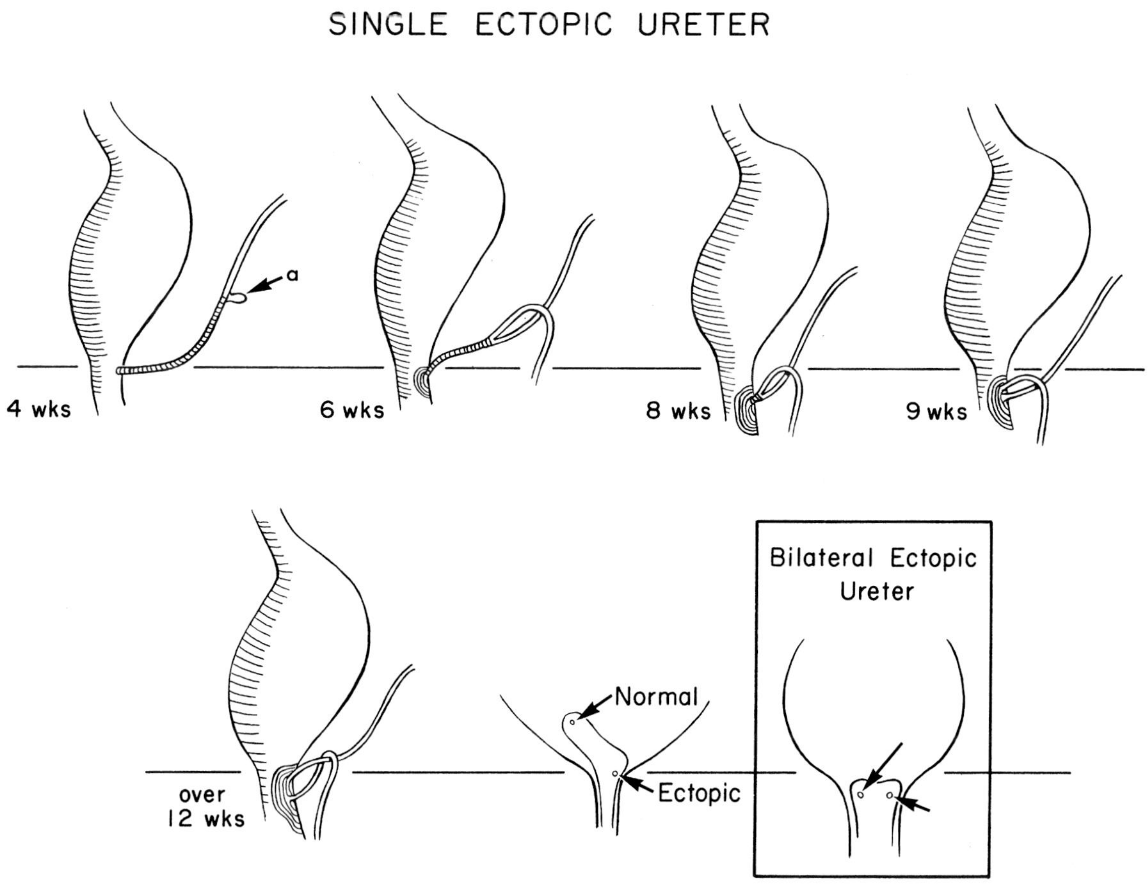

Figure 8–5 The formation of a very high ureteral bud results in the failure of the ureteral orifice to enter the bladder proper leading to the formation of an ectopic ureter. From Walsh PC, Perlmutter AD, Gittes RF, et al. Campbell's Urology, 5th ed. Philadelphia: WB Saunders 1986; as modified from Tanagho EA. Embryologic basis for lower ureteral anomolies: A hypothesis. Urology 7:451, 1976. Used with permission.

trates the metanephric blastema independently, which results in complete renal duplication. Once absorbed into the bladder, the ureteral orifices undergo rotational migration, which causes the two ureters to cross each other. As a result, the medial and inferior ureteral orifice is associated with the ureter that drains the upper pole kidney; this relationship is known as the Meyer-Weigert law.[4, 5] However, rare exceptions have been reported.[6] In completely duplicated systems, if any of the ureteral buds originate at an anomalous site on the mesonephric duct, craniolateral or caudomedial ureteral ectopia occurs as in single renal systems. The ectopic (caudal) ureter in duplicated systems drains the upper pole kidney (Fig. 8–6).

Ureteral ectopia is often associated with dysplasia or hypoplasia of the corresponding renal unit. The more ectopic the ureteral orifice, the more dysplastic the parenchyma of the kidney tends to be. To account for this observation, Mackie and Stephens[7] theorized that normal ureteral bud formation occurs at the "elbow" or "knee" of the mesonephric duct because this site of ureteral origin allows the ureter to penetrate the metanephric blastema at a position that results in optimal renal morphogenesis. Penetration of the blastema away from this optimal location, the central zone of the metanephric ridge, results in less optimal renal development; the further away from the central zone, the less likely is the formation of normal renal tissue (Fig. 8–7). This theory serves to explain the abnormal renal tissue or dysplastic renal segments induced by upper pole ureters in complete duplications that involve ectopic ureters. Nevertheless, exceptions to this theory exist in which normal renal tissue is associated with ectopic ureteral orifices.[8]

THE ECTOPIC URETER

Technically, the term *ectopic ureter* refers to a ureter that drains into a site other than the normal location at the corner of the bladder trigone. More commonly, the term has been used to describe ureters that end at the bladder neck or outside the bladder proper. When the ureteral ectopia involves structures that are outside the urinary system, the associated renal unit is commonly nonfunctional.[9, 10]

The incidence of ectopic ureters, according to data from autopsies, is estimated to be 1 in 1900 children.[11] Eighty-five percent of ectopic ureters occur in females and 15% occur in males.[12] Ten percent are bilateral.[13]

Approximately 80% of ectopic ureters drain the upper pole segment of a duplicated system.[12, 14, 15] When ectopic ureters occur in a duplex system, 80% are associated with

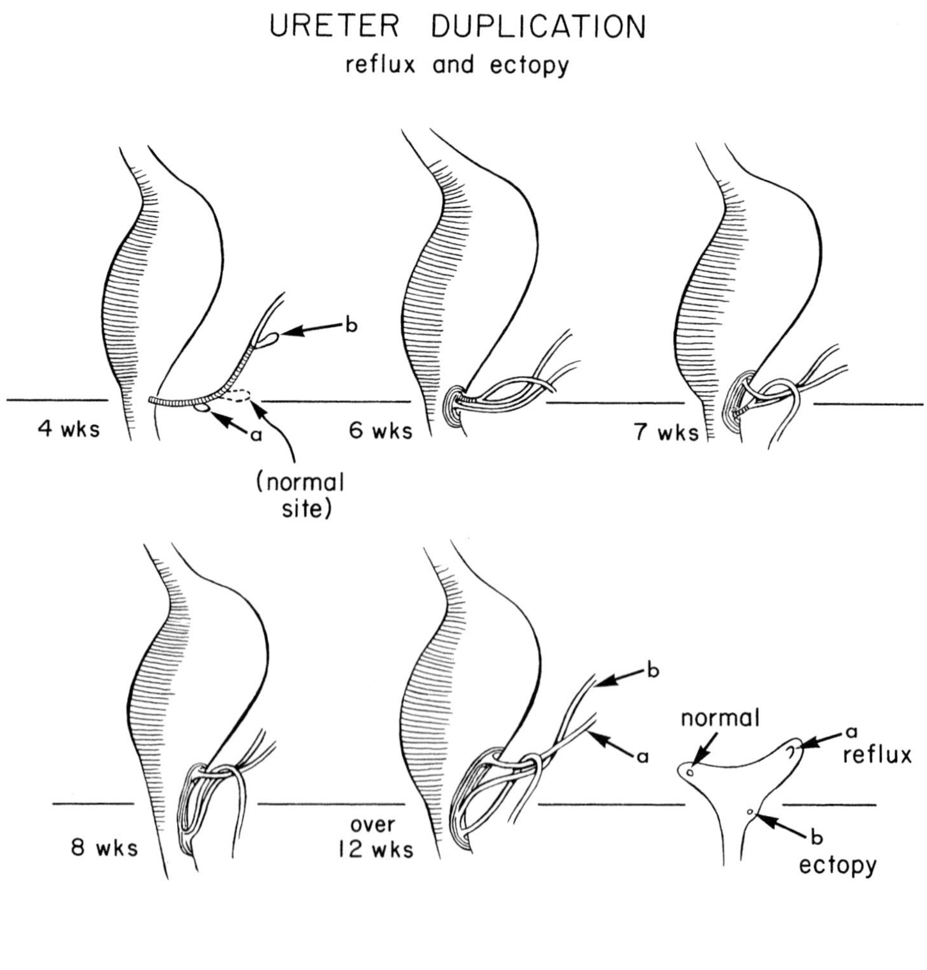

Figure 8–6 In completely duplicated systems, a very high takeoff of the ureteral bud to the upper pole kidney will result in the formation of an ectopic upper pole ureter. From Walsh PC, Perlmutter AD, Gittes RF, et al. Campbell's Urology, 5th ed. Philadelphia: WB Saunders, 1986; as modified from Tanagho EA. Embryologic basis for lower ureteral anomalies: A hypothesis. Urology 7:451, 1976. Used with permission.

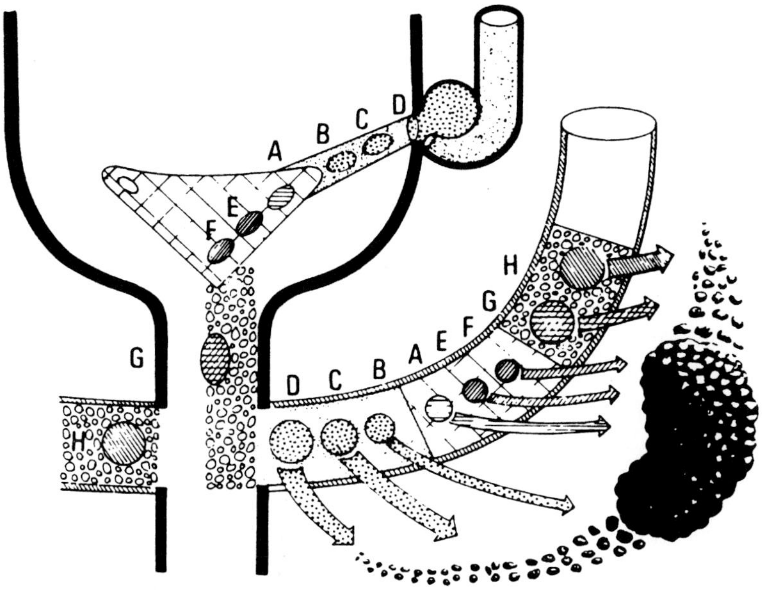

Figure 8–7 Mackie and Stephens' theory that an abnormal ureteral bud leads the ureter to penetrate the renal blastema at suboptimal locations resulting in abnormal renal development. The more abnormal the ureteral bud, the more dysplastic is the kidney. Reprinted with permission from Mackie GG, Stephens FD. Duplex kidneys. A correlation of renal dysplasia with position of the ureteral orifice. J Urol 114:274, 1975; © by Williams & Wilkins, 1975.

a contralateral renal duplication. Of note, ectopic ureters subtending single renal systems occur more frequently in males than in females.[16, 17]

Ectopic ureters are associated with renal, genital, and anal anomalies. The most common is hypoplasia or dysplasia of the renal unit, the severity of which usually correlates with the degree of ureteral ectopia. This correlation has been observed more frequently in duplex-system than in single-system ectopic ureters. In contrast, most genital and anal anomalies that occur in conjunction with ectopic ureters are more likely with single drainage systems than with duplex systems.[18] Genital and anal anomalies comprise about 33% of the congenital abnormalities associated with ureteral ectopia.[8] The most common of these is imperforate anus.

Females

In the female patient, an ectopic ureter may drain into a site that is either proximal or distal to the external urethral sphincter. The possible ectopic locations include the bladder neck, urethra, vestibule, vagina, cervix, uterus, and even the rectum.[19, 20]

When the ectopic site is distal to the external urethral sphincter, urinary incontinence usually results from the continuous drainage of urine that bypasses the sphincter mechanism. However, exceptions have been reported of ureters opening ectopically at the vaginal vestibule or distal urethra that are not associated with urinary incontinence.[21] The reason that incontinence does not occur is usually obstruction of the ureter as it traverses the continence mechanism within the bladder neck. In such cases, urine leaks from the ectopic ureter only occasionally or only during voiding.

In about one third of ureteral ectopia cases in females, the ectopic site is the bladder neck or upper urethra; both locations are proximal to the external urethral sphincter.[22] These ectopic ureters tend to be obstructed when the bladder outlet is closed during periods of continence and drain urine only when the urethral sphincter relaxes during voiding. Therefore, urinary incontinence is not likely. Paradoxically, vesicoureteral reflux (VUR) is present in more than 75% of these cases. Cyclic voiding cystourethrogram (VCUG), which evaluates two or more consecutive cycles of bladder filling and voiding, is superior to conventional single-cycle VCUG in documenting VUR in these patients. Wyly and Lebowitz reported that cyclic VCUG demonstrated reflux in 11 of 12 females (92%) with ectopic ureters. In contrast, the success rate for single-cycle VCUG in diagnosing VUR in patients with ectopic ureters has historically been about 30%.[23]

In another third of cases, the ectopic ureter drains into the vaginal vestibule, which surrounds the urethral meatus. The ureter ends at the vagina in 25% and at the cervix or uterus in less than 5%. Ureteral ectopia that involves the vagina, cervix, or uterus results from the rupture of Gartner's duct into the urovaginal canal along their common wall. Occasionally, an ectopic ureter that opens into a Gartner's duct cyst has been reported.[24]

The rectum, a rare site of ureteral ectopia, is usually noted incidentally at the autopsies of children with other severe congenital anomalies.[25] The involvement of the rectum in this type of ectopia is thought to result from an abnormal division of the cloaca by the urorectal septum or from an abnormally placed mesonephric duct that empties into the posterior half of the cloaca.

The classic presentation for the female child with an ectopic ureter is the continuous dribbling of urine despite a normal voiding pattern. However, this presentation is noted in only 50% of patients.[9, 26] More than half of the female children with ectopic ureters remain undiagnosed until adulthood because of the lack of symptoms initially.

Patients with ectopic ureters that end at the bladder neck or urethra experience ureteral obstruction by the closed urethral sphincter, and although they tend to be continent, they are prone to urinary tract infections and may present with flank pain.[27] These children may later experience incontinence after puberty, childbirth, or pelvic surgery, when the urethral sphincter tone may decrease.[28, 29]

If the ectopic ureter is very dilated, continence is maintained in the supine position, and daytime incontinence occurs only in the standing or sitting positions. This pattern has been mistaken for stress urinary incontinence, a rare condition in children. Therefore, a female child with a presentation consistent with stress urinary incontinence should be evaluated for ureteral ectopia.

Urinary tract infection is the most common presentation for small children with ectopic ureters. In these female patients, VUR and obstruction are the predisposing causes for the urinary tract infections. Less common presenting signs and symptoms include a malodorous vaginal discharge, a mass on the anterior vaginal wall,[30] and an abdominal mass that represents either an obstructed renal unit or a massively dilated ectopic ureter.[31, 32]

Males

In contrast to ureteral ectopia in females, ectopic ureters in males always open proximally to the external urethral sphincter. The most common site is the posterior urethra, seen in 50% of ureteral ectopia cases in males.[13] The next most common site, the seminal vesicles, is observed in 33% of cases.[33, 34] In the remainder, the ectopic sites are located within the genital ducts.[35]

Surprisingly, ectopic ureters that end in the genital ducts occur more frequently in single renal systems than in duplicated systems. The renal unit that is associated with the ectopic ureter is usually nonfunctional. Occasionally, such ectopic ureters have predisposed to epididymitis. Thus, a prepubertal boy with epididymitis should be evaluated for the possibility of an ectopic ureter that enters the vas deferens.[36] Other ectopic ureters that end within the genital tract do not cause symptoms until the onset of sexual activity, at which time epididymitis, prostatitis, seminal vesiculitis, or an infected seminal vesicle cyst may develop.[37]

Other presentations of ectopic ureters include flank pain and urinary tract infections. Urgency and frequency may also be manifestations of a ureter that ends at the posterior urethra; the reflex to void is triggered by the constant drip of urine into the posterior urethra. Urinary incontinence in the male with a unilateral ectopic ureter is rare but may occur in circumstances in which voided urine refluxes into a dilated ectopic ureter and subsequently leaks out the urethra through a relaxed external sphincter.[38]

Diagnostic Studies

An array of studies is available to aid in the diagnosis of an ectopic ureter. Sonography can detect hydronephrosis, hydroureter, or evidence of a duplex system. VCUG that demonstrates reflux into the ectopic ureter is diagnostic. The detection of the reflux is enhanced by the use of cyclic VCUG rather than conventional single-cycle studies.[24]

An intravenous pyelogram (IVP) offers good anatomic detail of ectopic ureters that are associated with nonobstructed, functioning renal units as well as obstructed, nonfunctioning renal units in duplicated systems. Radiological evidence of an obstructed, nonfunctioning upper pole kidney on an IVP includes a "drooping lily" sign, which characterizes a downward and lateral displacement of the functioning lower pole kidney by the obstructed upper pole kidney; lateral displacement of the lower pole ureter by the dilated upper pole ureter; an increase in the distance between the upper most calix and the upper border of the renal shadow; and a decrease in the number of calices as a result of a missing upper pole caliceal segment. Computed tomography and magnetic resonance imaging are sometimes helpful in gaining further anatomic information.

The more invasive modalities that are used to locate ectopic ureters include cystoscopy, vaginoscopy, and retrograde studies. It is important to note that the cystoscopic finding of a hemitrigone may be misinterpreted as evidence of renal agenesis. Occasionally, cystoscopy reveals a pseudoureterocele on the floor of the bladder; this finding represents the distal portion of a dilated, obstructed ectopic ureter that is bulging into the bladder.

Dyes such as methylene blue or indigo carmine can be used to suggest the presence of an ectopic ureter. The dye is administered intravesically, and the perineum is then inspected for a constant slow drip of clear urine.

In females, a flush vaginogram is useful in identifying a ureter that ends in the vagina. This study is implemented either with contrast and fluoroscopic imaging or with aerosolized saline and sonography. After injecting aerosolized saline into the vagina, the detection of air bubbles in the upper urinary tract indicates the presence of an ectopic ureter. The diagnosis of a vaginal ectopic ureter can also be established by the orange staining of cotton swabs that are placed in the vagina after the oral administration of phenazopyridine hydrochloride (Pyridium). This test is valid for renal segments with poor function as well as normal function because Pyridium is excreted by even poorly functioning kidneys.[39]

In males, a vasogram may be performed to identify ureters that drain into the genital tract.[17] This is an invasive procedure that may result in ipsilateral sterility, so it is rarely performed in practice.

Treatment

The treatment of the ectopic ureter depends on whether the ureter is associated with a functioning or nonfunctioning renal unit and whether the ureter is part of a single or duplicated collecting system. When the ectopic ureter occurs in a single collecting system and is associated with poor or nonfunctioning renal tissue, nephroureterectomy is the treatment of choice. The ectopic ureter in a single system that drains a kidney with significant function should receive a ureteral reimplantation.

In duplex collecting systems, the ectopic ureter is usually associated with the upper pole renal moiety. If the upper pole kidney has poor or no function, an upper pole partial nephroureterectomy should be performed. It is important to note that the lower portion of the upper and lower pole ureters are usually adherent along their common wall. Therefore, distal circumferential dissection of the upper pole ureter increases the risk of injury to the lower pole ureter along the common wall. This complication can be avoided by performing a partial excision of the upper pole ureter, leaving the common wall undisturbed.

If the upper pole kidney in a duplicated system has good renal function, a ureteral reimplantation is the recommended intervention. If the lower pole kidney possesses an extrarenal pelvis, an alternative treatment option is a ureteropyelostomy, anastomosing the upper pole ureter to the lower pole renal pelvis.[40] In cases in which the caliber of the lower pole ureter is large enough to accommodate the upper pole ureter, the formation of a high ureteroureterostomy between the upper and lower pole ureters is yet another option.[40] The disadvantage of the latter two options is that these surgical procedures place the lower pole collecting system at some risk of iatrogenic injury.

After a nephroureterectomy has been performed to remove a nonfunctional renal unit, proper management of any remaining ureteral stump is essential. In females, non-obstructed ectopic ureters that drain into the introitus or vagina need not be removed completely because these short ureteral stumps rarely cause postoperative complications.[41] Nevertheless, one potential complication is infection, the treatment of which is the marsupialization of the infected ureteral stump into the vaginal wall. In males, the stump of an ectopic ureter ending in the seminal vesicle or vas deferens does not require routine excision. However, ligation of the vas deferens to prevent recurrent epididymitis is beneficial in those patients who are prone to such infections.

In contrast to the benign nature of the ectopic ureteral stumps that end in the genital tract, even short segments of ectopic ureters that end at the bladder neck or urethra may give rise to problems requiring surgical intervention. A common complication is the reflux of voided urine into the ureteral stump, which results in postmicturition urinary incontinence and predisposes the patient to recurrent urinary tract infections. Therefore, such ureters require more complete excision. It is important to exercise care during the operation to avoid injury to the bladder neck, external sphincter, and vagina. Injury to any of these structures may cause postoperative urinary incontinence as a result of a compromised urinary sphincter mechanism or from the formation of a vesicovaginal fistula. In instances in which the ureteral stump is not too large, endoscopic fulguration of the ureteral lumen is a reasonable alternative to excision.

When a patient with an obstructed ectopic ureter presents with florid sepsis in association with a hydronephrotic renal unit, the initial management is usually intravenous antibiotics and drainage of the infected system by a percutaneous nephrostomy. The definitive treatment of the obstructed ectopic ureter is instituted after complete resolution of sepsis.

Bilateral Single Ectopic Ureter

Bilateral single ectopic ureters are rare anomalies. To date, just more than 50 cases have been reported in the English literature.[42–44] Patients with such single-system ectopic ureters have absent trigones, poorly developed bladder necks, and small, thin bladders. In addition, genital and anal anomalies are common.[8] Rare cases of bladder agenesis have also been reported.[45]

Three permutations of ureteral ectopia exist in both males and females with bilateral single ectopic ureters. In the first scenario, both ureteral orifices are located at the bladder neck. The bladder neck tends to be well formed and urinary continence is maintained, although the kidneys are dilated. In the second case, one ureteral orifice is located at the bladder neck, and the other orifice is situated more distally. The bladder neck is less developed, but continence usually prevails. In the third scenario, both ureteral orifices are located distal to the bladder neck. These patients have poorly formed bladders and total urinary incontinence.

The ureteral orifices of females with bilateral single ectopic ureters are most commonly situated in the distal urethra. As a result, these patients are usually incontinent of urine. In addition, the bladder necks are more poorly formed, the bladder capacities are smaller, and the associated renal anomalies are more severe than those noted in male counterparts.[42, 43]

The diagnosis of bilateral single ectopic ureters is achieved with the same array of diagnostic studies that are available for other types of ectopic ureters. In bilateral cases, the diagnosis of ectopia usually requires an IVP and VCUG.[24, 46] Radiological findings on the VCUG include a small bladder and an open bladder neck. If the ureter drains into the urethra, VUR is commonly observed on the VCUG.

The treatment of patients with bilateral single ectopic ureters is dictated by their bladder capacities. When the bladder capacity is adequate, ureteral reimplantations with a concomitant bladder neck reconstructive procedure are sufficient. When the bladder capacity is small, the appropriate intervention requires a bladder neck reconstruction in conjunction with a bladder augmentation that uses bowel to create a low-pressure, capacious reservoir. The ureters are reimplanted in the reservoir in an antirefluxing fashion. Drainage of the reservoir is then usually accomplished with clean, intermittent catheterization.

The goal of bladder neck reconstructive procedures is to produce urinary continence by increasing bladder outlet resistance. One frequently performed technique is the Young-Dees-Leadbetter procedure,[47–50] which increases outlet resistance by tubularizing the posterior detrusor to lengthen the posterior urethra. This procedure entails an incision of the bladder along the anterior wall and reimplantations of the ureters to higher positions in the bladder to accommodate the creation of a long detrusor tube. A midline longitudinal strip of posterior bladder mucosa that is contiguous with the posterior urethra is marked out; this strip should be 4 to 5 cm long and 7 to 8 mm wide. After the bladder mucosa that is lateral to both sides of the strip is denuded, the mucosal strip is tubularized over a 5 to 8 French catheter with 4-0 polyglactic or polyglycolic acid stitches. The parts of the denuded detrusor wings that are immediately adjacent to the newly created tube are brought together in the midline with 3-0 polyglactic or polyglycolic acid stitches as a first layer to cover the tube. The remainder of the wings is then stitched with 3-0 polyglactic or polyglycolic acid sutures in the midline as a second layer. On the proximal end of this neourethra, a stitch of 2-0 polyglactic or polyglycolic acid is placed anteriorly into the detrusor layers and the mucosa on one side of the midline and out the mucosa and detrusor layers on the other side. The bladder is then closed. In our experience, the creation of a detrusor tube that is 8 French or smaller is crucial in effecting postoperative urinary continence. By adhering to this technique, we have been able to achieve complete continence in 92% of our patients.[51]

Another procedure to increase bladder outlet resistance involves the use of a pedicled strip of rectus fascia to suspend the posterior urethra either as a sling[52] or a cinch.[53] In this operation, a longitudinal strip of rectus fascia on one side of the midline is marked out. The size of this fascial strip varies according to the patient's size. For a sling a strip that is 2.5 cm wide and 10 cm long usually suffices, but for a cinch a strip at least 12 cm long is needed. The fascial strip is dissected free, but its attachments to the pubis and the pyramidal muscle are kept intact. An opening is made in the ipsilateral rectus

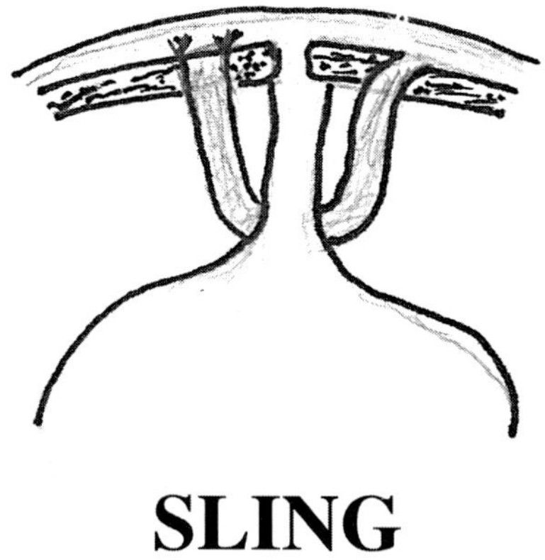

Figure 8–8 The rectus fascial sling: a pedicled strip of rectus fascia is passed beneath the posterior urethra and then tacked to the pubis. (Courtesy of Dr. M. K. Hanna.)

muscle through which the fascial strip is passed into the space of Retzius. The fascia is then either passed beneath the posterior urethra as a sling (Fig. 8–8) or wrapped around the posterior urethra as a cinch (Fig. 8–9). After this strip is brought out through the midline between the rectus bellies, it is pulled tight and tacked to the pubis using a nonabsorbable polypropylene stitch. In general, the sling usually provides an adequate increase in bladder outlet resistance to restore continence in girls. However, for boys, the cinch procedure is usually required to provide enough resistance to restore urinary continence.[53]

SUMMARY

The ectopic ureter is completely treatable surgically; therefore, prompt and proper diagnosis of this congenital anomaly is important. The ectopic ureter remains a diagnostic challenge because it can present in many different

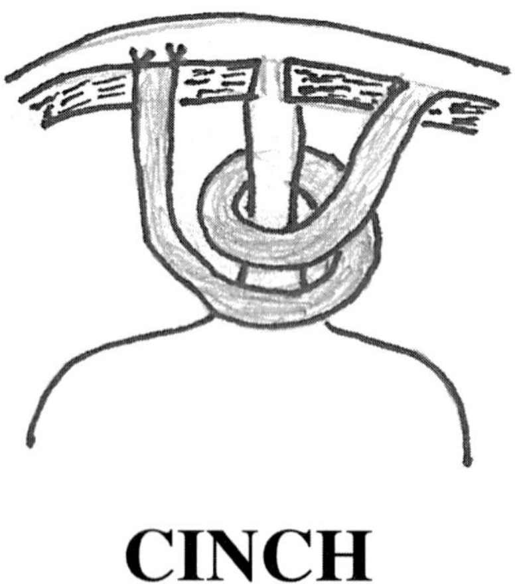

Figure 8–9 The rectus fascial cinch: a pedicled strip of rectus fascia is wrapped around the posterior urethra and then tacked to the pubis. (Courtesy of Dr. M. K. Hanna.)

ways depending on the site of the ectopia. This entity should always be considered in cases of urethral obstruction, urinary tract infection, epididymitis, and especially urinary incontinence.

REFERENCES

1. Ambrose SS, Nicolson WP III. The causes of vesicoureteral reflux in children. J Urol 87:688, 1962.
2. Stephens FD, Lenaghan D. The anatomical basis and dynamics of vesicoureteral reflux. J Urol 87:669, 1962.
3. Tanagho EA, Hutch JA. Primary reflux. J Urol 93:158, 1965.
4. Meyer R. Zur Anatomie und Entwicklungsgeschichte der Ureterverdoppelung. Virchows Arch [Pathol Ant] 187:408, 1907.
5. Weigert C. Ueber einige Bildungsfehler der Ureteren. Virchows Arch [Pathol Anat] 70:490, 1877.
6. Lund AJ. Uncrossed double ureter with rare intravesical orifice relationship: Case report with review of literature. J Urol 62:22, 1949.
7. Mackie GG, Stephens FD. Duplex kidneys: A correlation of renal dysplasia with position of the ureteral orifice. J Urol 114:274, 1975.
8. Kesavan P, Ramakrishnan MS, Fowler R. Ectopia in unduplicated ureters in children. Br J Urol 49:481, 1977.
9. Schulman CC. Les implantatins ectopiques de l'uretere. Acta Urol Belg 40:201, 1972.
10. Rognon L, Brueziere J, Soret JY, et al. Abouchement ectopique de l'uretere dans le tractus seminal: A propos de 10 cas. Chirurgie 99:741, 1973.
11. Campbell MF. Anomalies of the ureter. In Campbell MF, Harrison JH (eds), Urology, 3rd ed. Philadelphia: WB Saunders, 1970, p 1487.
12. Mandell J, Bauer SB, Colodny AH, et al. Ureteral ectopia in infants and children. J Urol 126:219, 1981.
13. Ellerker AG. The extravesical ectopic ureter. Br J Surg 45:344, 1958.
14. Schlussel RN, Retik AB. Ureteroceles and ectopic ureters. Monogr Urol 15:27, 1994.
15. Snyder H. Anomalies of the ureter. In Gillenwater JY, Grayhack JT, Howards SS, Duckett JW (eds), Adult and Pediatric Urology. Chicago: Mosby Yearbook, 1991, p 1851.
16. Johnston JH, Davenport TJ. The single ectopic ureter. Br J Urol 41:428, 1969.
17. Schulman CC. The single ectopic ureter. Eur Urol 2:64, 1976.
18. Gill B. Ureteric ectopy in children. Br J Urol 52:257, 1980.
19. Johnston JH. Problems in the diagnosis and management of ectopic ureters and ureteroceles. In Johnston JH, Scholtmeijer RJ (eds), Problems in Paediatric Urology. Amsterdam: Excerpta Medica, 1972, p 57.
20. Mogg RA. The single ectopic ureter. Br J Urol 46:3, 1974.
21. Ogawa A, Kakizawa Y, Akaza H. Ectopic ureter passing through the external urethral sphincter: Report of a case. J Urol 116:109, 1976.
22. Kjellberg SR, Ericsson NO, Rudhe U. The Lower Urinary Tract in Childhood: Some Correlated Clinical and Roentgenologic Observations. Chicago: Yearbook, 1968.
23. Wyly JB, Lebowitz RL. Refluxing ureteral ectopic ureters: Recognition by the cyclic voiding cystogram. AJR Am J Roentgenol 142:1263, 1984.
24. Vanhoutte JJ. Ureteral ectopia into a Wolffian duct remnant (Gartner's ducts or cysts) presenting as a urethral diverticulum in two girls. AJR Am J Roentgenol 110:540, 1970.
25. Uson AC, Schulman CC. Ectopic ureter emptying into the rectum: Report of a case. J Urol 108:156, 1972.
26. Malek RS, Kelalis PP, Stickler GB, et al. Observations on ureteral ectopy in children. J Urol 107:308, 1972.
27. DeWeerd JH, Litin RB. Ectopia or ureteral orifice (vestibular) without incontinence: Report of case. Mayo Clin Proc 33:81, 1958.
28. Davis DM. Urethral ectopic ureter in the female without incontinence. J Urol 23:463, 1930.
29. Childlow JH, Utz DC. Ureteral ectopia in vestibule of vagina with urinary incontinence. South Med J 63:423, 1970.
30. Vanhoutte JJ. Ureteral ectopia into a wolffian duct remnant (Gartner's ducts or cysts) presenting as a urethral diverticulum in two girls. Am J Roentgenol Radium Ther Nucl Med 110:540, 1970.
31. Uson AC, Womack CE, Berdon WE. Giant ectopic ureter presenting as an abdominal mass in a newborn infant. J Pediatr 80:473, 1972.
32. Finan B, Mollit DL, Golladay ES, et al. Giant ectopic ureter presenting as an abdominal mass in infant. J Urol 30:246, 1987.
33. Gordon HL, Kessler R. Ectopic ureter entering the seminal vesicle associated with renal dysplasia. J Urol 108:389, 1972.
34. Seitzman DM, Patton JF. Ureteral ectopia: Combined ureteral and vas deferens anomaly. J Urol 84:604, 1960.
35. Jona JZ, Glicklich M, Cohen RD. Ectopic single ureter and severe renal dysplasia: An unusual presentation. Urology 21:369, 1979.
36. Siegel A, Snyder HM, Duckett JW. Epididymitis in infants and boys: Underlying urogenital anomalies and efficacy of imaging modalities. J Urol 138:1100, 1987.
37. Bengmark S, Nilsson S, Romanus R. Ectopic ureter draining into a seminal megavesicle causing defecation troubles: Report of a case and review of the literature. Acta Chir Scand 123:471, 1962.
38. Williams DI, Royle M. Ectopic ureter in the male child. Br J Urol 41:421, 1969.
39. Weiss JP, Duckett JW, Snyder HM. Single unilateral vaginal ectopic ureter: Is it really a rarity? J Urol 132:1177, 1984.
40. Huisman TK, Kaplan GW, Brock WA, et al. Ipsilateral ureteroureterostomy and pyeloureterostomy: A review of 15 years of experience with 25 patients. J Urol 138:1207, 1987.
41. Culp OS: Heminephroureterectomy: Comparison of one-stage and two-stage operations. J Urol 83:369, 1960.
42. Cox CE, Hutch JA. Bilateral single ectopic ureter: A report of 2 cases and review of the literature. J Urol 95:493, 1966.
43. Williams DI, Lightwood RG. Bilateral single ectopic ureters. J Urol 44:267, 1972.
44. Noseworthy J, Persky L. Spectrum of bilateral ureteral ectopia. Urology 19:489, 1982.
45. Glenn JF. Agenesis of the bladder. JAMA 169:2016, 1959.
46. Prewitt LH Jr, Lebowitz RL. The single ectopic ureter. AJR Am J Roentgenol 127:941, 1976.
47. Young HH. An operation for the cure of incontinence of urine. Surg Gynecol Obstet 28:84, 1919.
48. Young HH. An operation for the cure of incontinence associated with epispadias. J Urol 7:1, 1922.
49. Dees JE. Congenital epispadias with incontinence. J Urol 62:513, 1949.
50. Leadbetter GW Jr. Surgical correction of total urinary incontinence. J Urol 91:261, 1964.
51. Franco I, Kolligan M, Reda EF, Levitt SB. The importance of catheter size in the achievement of urinary continence in patients undergoing a Young-Dees-Leadbetter procedure. J Urol 152:710, 1994.
52. Millin T. Retropubic Urinary Surgery. Baltimore: Williams & Wilkins, 1947, p 184.
53. Hanna MK. Results of Millin's pedicled fascial sling for urinary incontinence due to sphincter incompetence (abstract no. 16). Paper presented at the annual meeting of the American Academy of Pediatrics (Section on Urology), San Francisco, Oct, 1995.

PART IV
The Bladder

9

JOHN P. GEARHART & JACOB BEN-CHAIM

Exstrophy and Epispadias

The surgical reconstruction of the infant born with bladder exstrophy is one of the most challenging efforts in pediatric urology. An initial successful closure is clearly the key to later urinary continence when the child is older. The staged approach to the reconstruction of bladder exstrophy has been very successful over the last several years.[1, 2] Our current plan of treatment consists of bladder closure with or without penile lengthening and pelvic osteotomy as soon after birth as possible. After successful initial closure, the epispadias repair is accomplished at about 2 years of age for the outlet effect of the urethroplasty to increase the bladder capacity. Bladder neck reconstruction along with an antireflux procedure is usually performed at about 4 to 5 years of age after satisfactory bladder capacity has been achieved and if the child is ready to accept toilet training.

In this chapter, the techniques for managing the initial closure, epispadias repair, and bladder neck reconstruction in the child with classic bladder exstrophy is discussed, and the results of these efforts are summarized. Last, a brief discussion of failure in the exstrophy patient and the options available for management is presented.

INCIDENCE AND GENETICS

Exstrophy of the bladder is rare, and the incidence of bladder exstrophy is calculated to be 1 per 50,000 to 100,000 live births. The male to female ratio ranges from 1.5 to 5:1.[3]

Some evidence exists indicating that there is a genetic predisposition for exstrophy and epispadias. The risk for recurrence of exstrophy or epispadias in a given family is 1 of 275 births.[4] The likelihood of an exstrophic parent producing a newborn with epispadias or exstrophy is one in 70, or 500 times the risk of the general population.[5]

PRENATAL DIAGNOSIS

Formerly, exstrophy of the bladder was rarely diagnosed prenatally. However, in a retrospective review of 43 prenatal ultrasound studies from 25 pregnancies resulting in live delivery of an infant with classic bladder exstrophy, five criteria associated with classic bladder exstrophy were identified[6]: (1) a bladder never seen on ultrasonogram was noted in 71% of cases, (2) a lower abdominal bulge that represents the exstrophied bladder was found in 47% (Fig. 9–1), (3) a small penis with anteriorly displaced scrotum was detected in 57% of males, (4) a low-set umbilical insertion was found in 29% of patients, and (5) abnormal widening of the iliac crests was found in 18% (see Fig. 9–1*A*, *B*). Because the fetal bladder can be seen on prenatal ultrasonogram after 14 weeks of gestation, the prenatal diagnosis of bladder exstrophy should be considered seriously when the bladder is not demonstrated or when any of the just-mentioned findings are noted.[6–8]

INITIAL EVALUATION AND MANAGEMENT

Shortly after birth, the exposed bladder needs to be protected from surface trauma (Fig. 9–2). The best form of management is to cover the bladder immediately with a sheet of plastic wrap to allow urine to escape while establishing a barrier between the outside environment and the fragile bladder mucosa. Old urine, mucus, and any detritus should be washed from the surface of the bladder with body temperature sterile saline at each diaper change or even more frequently.

At birth the umbilical cord should be ligated with 2-0 silk to avoid bladder mucosal damage from an umbilical clamp. After ligation of the umbilical stump and covering with plastic wrap, prophylactic antibiotics are begun. After these maneuvers, the parents should be extensively counseled about the full nature of the condition: that it is possible to correct the urinary storage problem and reconstruct the genitalia so that sexuality and function approach normal. A thorough general and cardiovascular assessment should be completed because major surgery in the neonatal period is anticipated. The urinary tract should be evaluated by ultrasonogram or a nuclear scan to assess for the presence of upper tract anomalies.

Referral to a surgical team experienced in the treat-

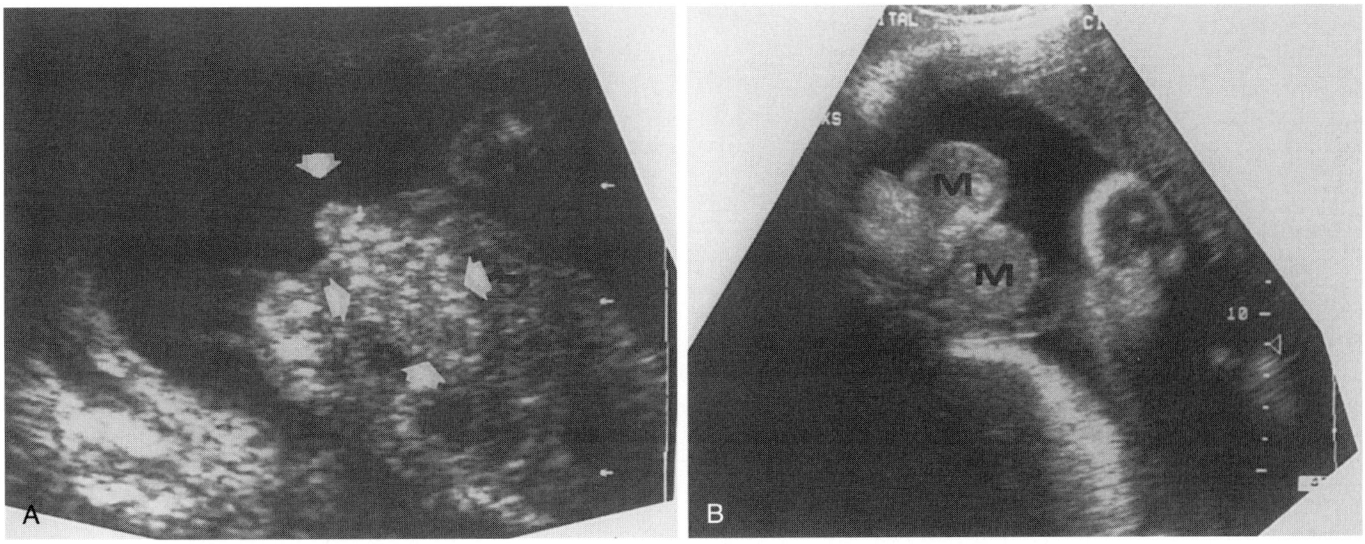

Figure 9–1 *A,* Coronal anterior view of an exstrophy mass in a male fetus with bladder exstrophy. Exstrophy mass can be seen in the anterior aspect of the abdomen as an anterior bulge *(arrows)*. *B,* Supine anterior sagittal view of a male fetus with exstrophy. A bilobed mass (M)—the bladder exstrophy—arises immediately inferiorly to the cord insertion. The anterior surface of the abdomen superior to the cord insertion can be seen.

ment of bladder exstrophy should be arranged. This will allow the parents to be realistically counseled about this major birth defect and the complexities of reconstruction. The best mode of therapy can then be determined.

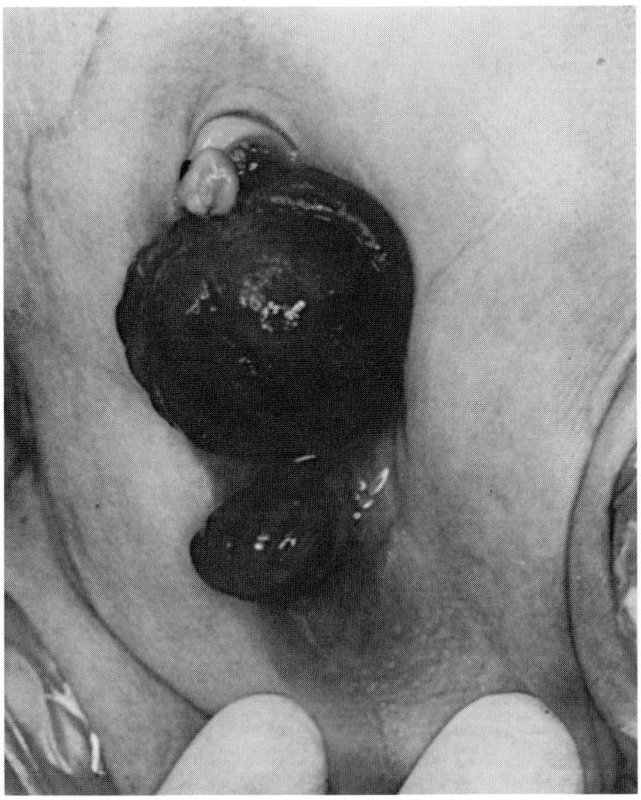

Figure 9–2 Newborn male with classic bladder exstrophy.

INITIAL EXSTROPHY CLOSURE

At the time of the initial exstrophy closure, preoperative antibiotics are given in the form of ampicillin and gentamicin, which are routinely administered for 10 days after bladder closure. Appropriate antibiotic administration is an important component of a successful bladder closure because all exstrophied bladders and surrounding tissues are contaminated areas. The entire abdominal and genital areas are liberally washed and cleaned with povidone-iodine (Betadine) along with liberal soaking of the bladder, its interstices, and the umbilical area. The actual wound preparation includes the area from the nipples to the knees anteriorly and from the base of the scapula to the popliteal fossa posteriorly. Because only anterior osteotomies are performed in our institution, the only time the posterior field is encountered is when the pelvic ring and hips are rotated medially at the time of pubic closure. However, the entire prepared area is draped into the operative field at the time of surgery. A small gauze sponge soaked in povidone-iodine is placed in the anal verge and covered with a clear surgical adhesive dressing to prevent stool contamination during the procedure.

The bladder often appears much smaller than expected for the gestational age of the child, so that bladder size can only be judged adequately under anesthesia. A bladder that appeared small in the newborn nursery may demonstrate an acceptable capacity, indenting easily into the pelvis when pushed inward by a gloved sterile finger. Also the presence of hamartomatous surface polyps may actually prevent the examiner from realizing the true size of the bladder. Once these are excised from the bladder surface, the true size of the bladder template may be ascertained. If the initial bladder capacity is believed to be 5 mL or more after closure, one can expect the bladder to develop a useful size and capacity after a successful closure. Once irritation and surface trauma are prevented, the bladder should gradually increase in capacity over time.

INITIAL BLADDER CLOSURE: USE OF OSTEOTOMY

Formerly, many exstrophy patients underwent closure in early life without osteotomy. However, studies have clearly shown the valuable adjunctive use of osteotomy at the time of initial closure.[9–11] When the closure is carried out within the first 72 hours of life, the newborn is still under the effect of the maternal hormone relaxin. The relaxing effect of this hormone on the pelvis may allow the ring to be brought together without the use of osteotomy.[1] This determination should only be made by careful examination under anesthesia. If there is any doubt on the part of the surgeon about the need for osteotomy, it is better to err on the conservative side and perform an osteotomy. If the pubic separation is very wide, the surgery may be performed at an older age. If it is a reclosure, osteotomy is essential to achieve good closure of the pelvic ring.[11, 12]

The osteotomy should be performed at the same time as bladder closure because it reduces the tension on the abdominal wound and helps secure the closure. In addition, the osteotomies help to restore the pelvic anatomy, may increase the chances of eventual continence, and may reduce the likelihood of later uterine and rectal prolapse.

Our current preference for osteotomy is a combined anterior innominate and vertical iliac osteotomy, which involves dividing the innominate bones just above the acetabulum. Using this osteotomy for either initial or failed closures of bladder exstrophy gives superior results over posterior iliac osteotomy because there is (1) no need to turn the patient intraoperatively, (2) less blood loss, (3) better apposition and mobility of the pubic rami at the time of closure, and (4) more secure external fixation.[10] Although external fixator devices are used even in those younger than 6 months, the intrafragmentary pins do not hold as well in younger patients because of the lack of cancellous bone. Therefore, the fixator cannot be brought together as snugly in these younger patients.[10]

This new combined anterior innominate and vertical iliac osteotomy is done within the periosteum through the same skin incision for better pelvic correction (Fig. 9–3). We have had experience with 36 of these combined osteotomies over the last 3 years in 32 patients with classic exstrophy and 4 patients with cloacal exstrophy. There was only one minor prolapse in a patient with cloacal exstrophy. In the rest of the group, which included patients who underwent both primary and secondary closures, there were no instances of prolapse or dehiscence.[10]

In all patients undergoing exstrophy closure both with or without osteotomy, some manner of postoperative traction or fixation must be used. The authors do not used any "mermaid" or "mummy wrap"–type dressings because they do not sufficiently immobilize the patient and can result in dehisence.[12] In those patients who undergo closure without an osteotomy, modified Bryant's traction is used for 4 weeks. If a combined osteotomy is utilized, an external fixation device is used for 4 weeks along with light Buck's traction (Fig. 9–4), with the legs supported on one pillow for 4 weeks. In a reclosure patient, fixation and traction are maintained for 6 weeks in younger patients and for up to 8 weeks in older patients.[11, 12]

INITIAL BLADDER CLOSURE

The technique for initial primary bladder closure is described and diagrammed in Figure 9–5*A* to *K*. The initial

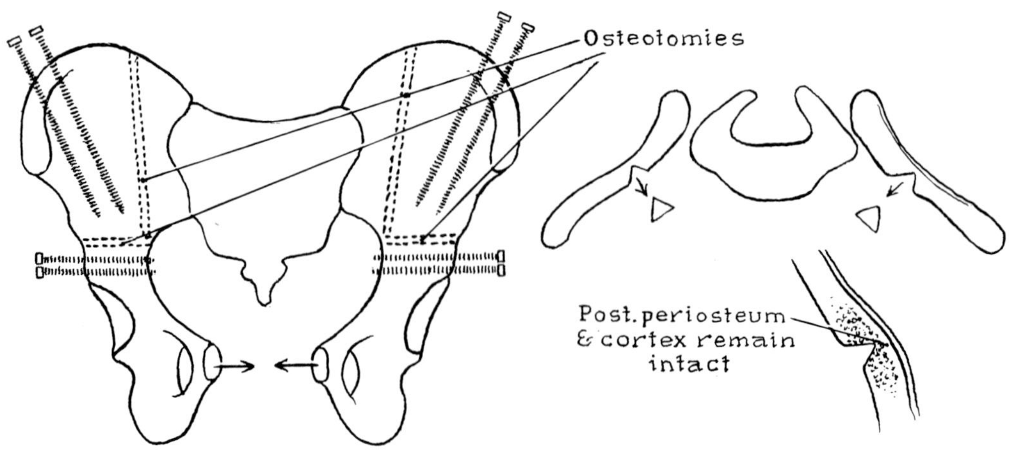

Figure 9–3 The combined anterior innominate and posterior vertical osteotomies for closure of bladder exstrophy.

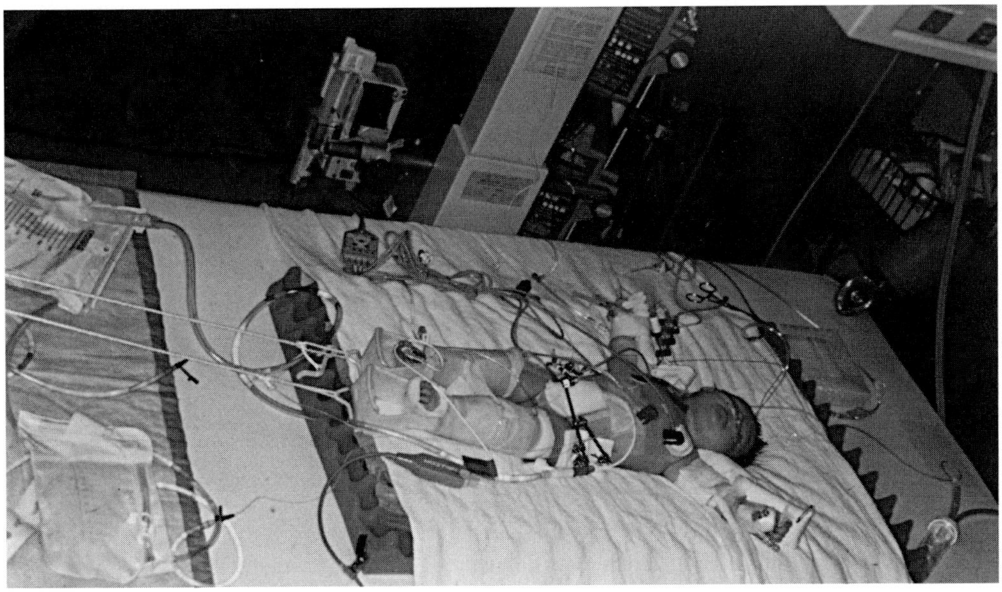

Figure 9–4 Fixator pins and drains after exstrophy closure along with modified Buck's traction.

procedure is closure of the bladder, displacement of the bladder to a posterior position deep within the pelvis, approximation of the pubic symphysis, and provision for free urethral drainage (Fig. 9–5*A*). For later reconstruction and eventual production of continence, it is important to place the bladder and bladder neck within the pelvic ring so that the urethra can exit and drain within a well-closed pubic arch. Placing the posterior urethra and bladder neck area within the pelvic ring allows the pelvic musculature to act upon the posterior urethra and bladder neck area and, one hopes, aid eventual continence. Later tailoring and narrowing of the bladder neck area during a Young-Dees-Leadbetter procedure are more easily achieved when the bladder neck area is within the pelvic ring.

The bladder closure starts with dissection and excision of the umbilicus (Fig. 9–5*B*). All umbilical vessels are ligated so the bladder can be placed deep into the pelvis and not tethered superiorly by any remaining umbilical vessels. We have reoperated on a number of failed exstrophy closures and found the vessels to be intact in a number of these patients.[3] Although some have tried to preserve the umbilicus, we believe it is a potential source of wound infection and should be excised. Mitchell and Sumfest, Hanna, and others described excellent techniques of umbilical reconstruction.[13, 14] If paraexstrophy skin flaps are required to lengthen the posterior urethra, the operation proceeds as in Figure 9–5*C1* to *C3*. In most cases, however, the urethral plate can remain intact as in Figure 9–5*C* and *D*.

The bladder muscle is freed from the rectus sheath on each side (Fig. 9–5*E*). The peritoneum is exposed and swept from the dome of the bladder. After the peritoneum is retracted superiorly, the dissection proceeds under the ligated umbilical vessels and into the retropubic space on each side of the bladder (see Fig. 9–5). As the dissection moves caudally, the wide band of fibers representing the remnants of the urogenital diaphragm is encountered. These fibers attach the lateral aspect of the posterior urethra to the pubic ramus bilaterally. These fibers must be detached subperiosteally from the pubis on both sides down to the inferior ramus (Fig. 9–5*F*). In a number of reoperative cases, we have found these fibers to be still intact. If these fibers are not adequately detached, the posterior urethra and bladder neck will be displaced anteriorly when the pubis is joined and be more prone to prolapse or dehiscence should pubic separation or wound complications ensue.

At this juncture, the caudal extension of the rectus fascia is followed laterally to the pubic ramus. Because of the high probability of inguinal hernia, the area lateral to the ramus is spread gently, exposing the inguinal canal. Bilateral inguinal exploration is then performed and the hernias are repaired.

At the same time as the urogenital diaphragm is sectioned, the remnants of the suspensory ligaments of the penis and the anterior attachments of the corpora cavernosa to the anterior ramus of the pubis are incised. This allows the penis to gain length, corrects a good deal of the dorsal chordee, and allows the penis to assume a more dependent angle (Fig. 9–5*G*). If significant chordee remains after these maneuvers, the posterior urethra must be lengthened. This is accomplished by incising the mucosal urethral groove distal to the verumontanum (Fig. 9–5C1–C3) and allowing the posterior urethra and bladder to retract back into the pelvis. The gap produced is usually filled with paraexstrophy rotation skin flaps (Fig. 9–5C1–C3). If paraexstrophy flaps are selected, it is very important to follow established plastic surgical procedures to ensure viability of these flaps. In the newborn

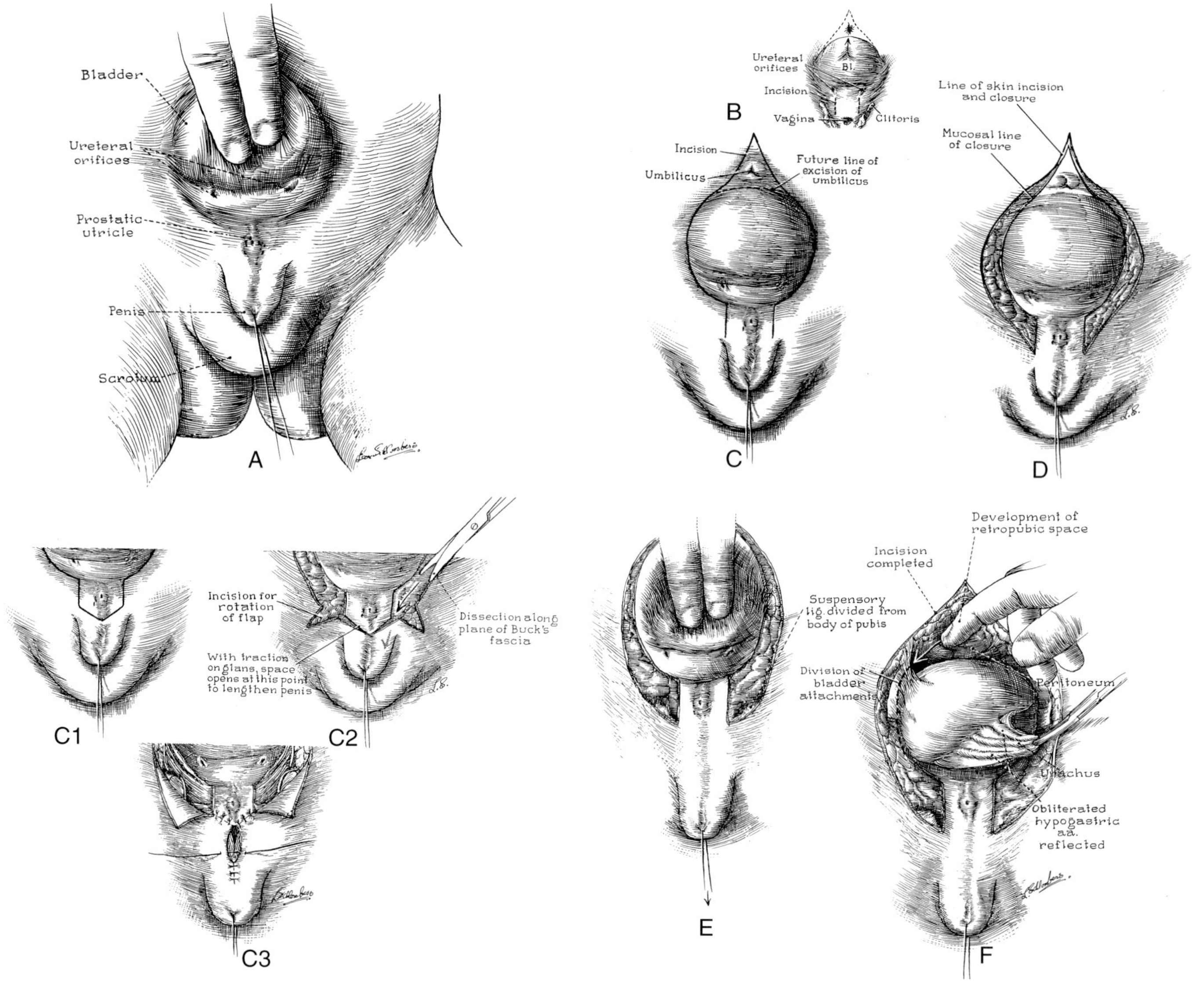

Figure 9–5 *A–K,* Steps in primary bladder closure with or without osteotomy. *B, C,* and *D,* The incision line around the umbilicus and bladder down to the urethral plate. *C1–C3,* The incision line only if urethral lengthening is needed to facilitate the closure. *E* and *F,* Development of the retropubic space from below the area of the umbilical dissection to facilitate separation of the bladder from the rectus sheath and muscle.

infant who has a straight penis and a deep urethral groove, the urethral mucosa should be maintained, thus reserving these tissues for later Cantwell-Ransley epispadias repair.[15] Formerly, if division of the urethral plate was performed, an attempt was made to bring the corpora together at their cephalad divergence. However, with the later Cantwell-Ransley procedure, this is no longer necessary because the entire urethral plate is later brought below the corporal bodies. Thus, there is no need for their apposition at the time of initial exstrophy closure.[15, 16]

The bladder is then closed in the midline using 3-0 polyglycolic acid sutures in two layers (Fig. 9–5*H–J*). Before bladder closure, a suprapubic cystostomy tube and two ureteral stents are brought out through the bladder wall. These tubes are brought out cephalad to the bladder through the neoumbilicus (Fig. 9–5*I*).

The urethral opening should provide enough resistance to stimulate bladder growth and prevent bladder prolapse but not be so tight as to cause outlet obstruction and dilatation of the upper tracts. The urethra is not stented to avoid pressure necrosis, especially in the presence of paraexstrophy flaps, and also to prevent accumulation of infected secretions. Husmann and colleagues have shown that the incidence of prolapse and dehiscence increases when urinary drainage tubes exit the

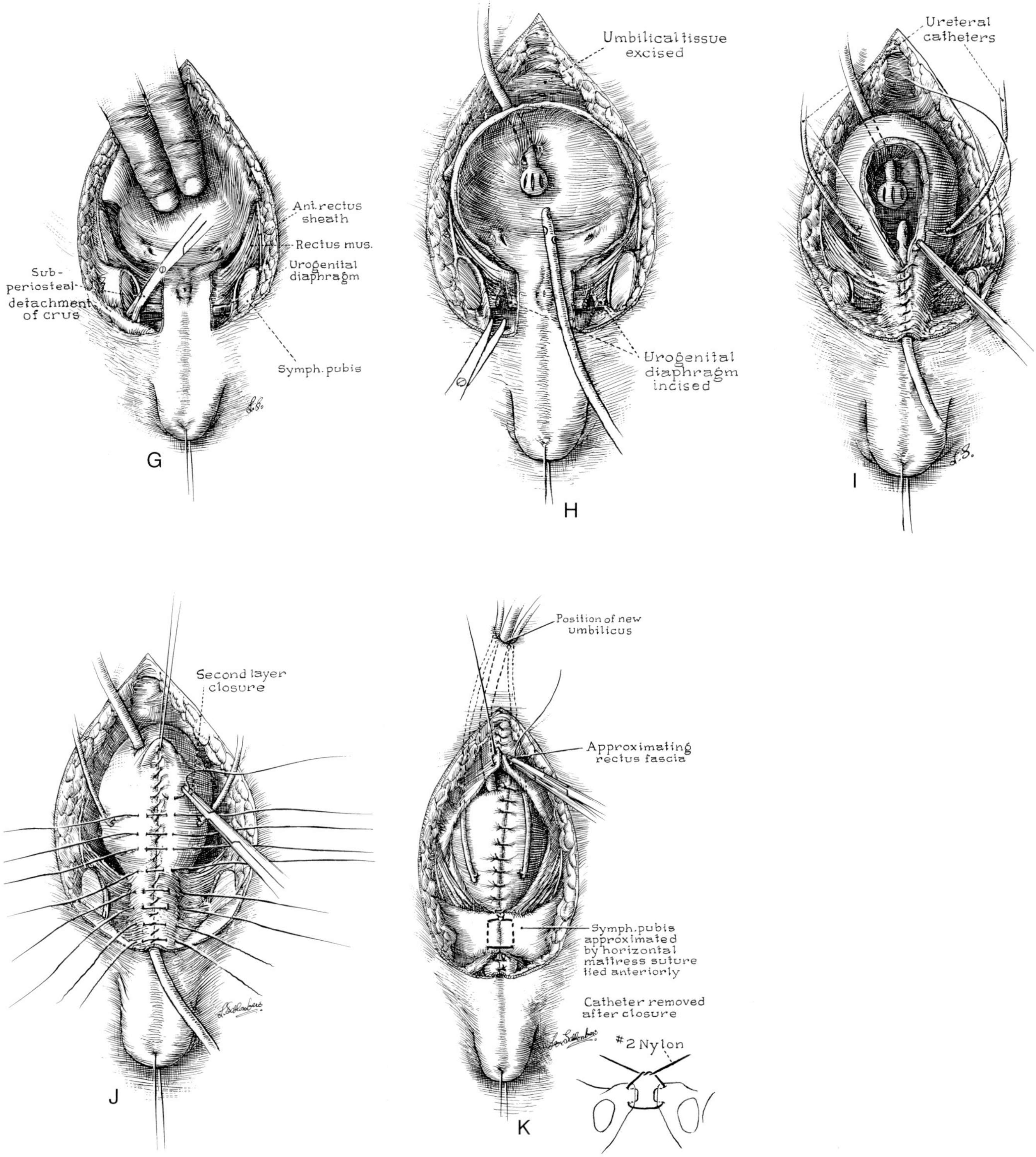

Figure 9–5 *Continued* *G,* The medial fan of erectus fascia attaching behind the prostate to the urogenital diaphragm. The urogenital diaphragm and anterior corpus are freed from the pubis in a subperiosteal plane. *H,* The urogenital diaphragm is incised. *I* and *J,* Ureteral stents and a suprapubic tube are left to drain the bladder, and the bladder and posterior urethra are closed in two layers. *K,* Closure is completed by approximation of the symphysis pubis and reconstruction of a new umbilicus.

neourethra, and we agree.[2] Because of the risk of occurrence of latex allergy in exstrophy patients, only nonlatex tubes are used in these patients.

After the bladder and urethra are closed and all drainage tubes are placed, the pelvis is closed by medial rotation of the greater trochanters. One assistant cradles the infant's gluteal folds with his or her hands and then rotates the greater trochanters medially. While this is being done, the surgeon ties a stitch of number 2 nylon, which has previously been placed in the pubis as a horizontal mattress (Fig. 9–5*K*). Approximating the pubis in this manner places the knot away from the posterior urethral closure. With a well-done osteotomy and excellent rotation of the inferior bony fragments, another heavy nylon suture can often be placed in the lowermost rectus fascia for added security.

After the pubic bones are closed, the posterior urethra is calibrated to be sure it accepts a number 14 French sound, and abdominal wall closure is begun. The midline rectus fascia is closed with interrupted sutures of 2-0 polyglycolic acid. A nonlatex drain is then placed in the prevesical space and brought through the neoumbilicus. The subcutaneous tissues are closed with 4-0 polyglycolic acid sutures and the skin with interrupted sutures of 5-0 nylon. A gauze dressing is placed over the area of the exit of the suprapubic tube, stents, and drain.

POSTOPERATIVE MANAGEMENT AFTER NEWBORN CLOSURE

The factors that are important for achieving successful primary closure have been previously documented and include use of osteotomy, avoidance of urethral drainage tubes and abdominal distention, the use of postoperative antibiotics, pelvic immobilization and fixation, ureteral stenting catheters, and appropriate control of pain, movement, and bladder spasms.[17]

The pediatric feeding tubes used as ureteral stents are commonly left indwelling for 10 to 14 days or longer if they continue to drain and keep the wound dry. The stents, along with the suprapubic catheter, are irrigated at regular intervals to ensure patency. The bladder outlet is calibrated with a urethral sound after the child is removed from traction. If the outlet is judged to be adequate, the suprapubic tube is clamped. If the residual urines are low, the suprapubic tube is removed. A sonogram is performed before discharge from the hospital and again in 4 months. The upper tracts should then be examined at least twice yearly afterward. Prophylactic antibacterials are continued because almost all of these children exhibit vesicoureteral reflux at this stage.

At the time of discharge, the parents are cautioned about potential complications, including urinary tract infections and retention of urine. They are warned to be very suspicious of dry diapers in the months after the initial closure, which could indicate outlet obstruction. If the parents notice dry diapers, the child should have an immediate bladder and renal ultrasonogram. If hydronephrosis exists or significant urine in the bladder is noted, the bladder outlet should be checked by catheterization.

At about 2 years of age, a cystoscopy and gravity cystogram under anesthesia are performed to assess bladder growth. A 10 French Foley catheter is inserted into the bladder and the bladder is filled by gravity while maintaining the catheter on traction to prevent bladder neck leakage. Vesicoureteral reflux is seen in almost 100% of these cases. Occasional patients will experience recurrent pyelonephritis without bladder outlet obstruction. In this instance, we proceed to ureteral reimplantation before bladder neck reconstruction. If uncontrollable hydronephrosis develops, revision of the bladder outlet is performed. On rare occasions, a child will require urinary diversion either to a nonrefluxing colon conduit or a single-stage reconstruction with bladder augmentation and continent diversion to protect renal function.

EPISPADIAS REPAIR

The goals of penile reconstruction in exstrophy patients are reconstruction of the urethra and glans penis, release of potential length, correction of dorsal chordee, and achievement of adequate skin coverage. Another goal of urethral reconstruction is an increase in bladder capacity.[18] Prior studies have shown that, after repairing the epispadias, there is an increase in bladder capacity. In the exstrophy group, this increase has been a median of 54 mL during the follow-up period. Although there are several approaches to reconstruction of the penis in exstrophy, we have adopted the Cantwell-Ransley repair as the procedure of choice for penile and urethral reconstruction.[15, 16] Preoperatively, the very diminutive penis of these boys is stimulated with testosterone enanthate, 2 mg/kg intramuscularly, 5 weeks and 2 weeks before the repair.

Our adaption of the Cantwell-Ransley procedure is depicted in Figure 9–6*A* to *K*. A ventral circumcising incision is made and the ventral skin degloved from the shaft. An incision is made in either side of the urethral plate, leaving an adequate width for tubularization (15 mm) (Fig. 9–6*A*, *B*). The area corresponding to the neourethral meatus has a dorsal orientation and must be advanced to the end of the urethral plate by making a vertical incision in the midline of the plate and closing it horizontally, using interrupted 7-0 polyglycolic acid sutures (Fig. 9–6*C*, *D*). During degloving of the ventral skin, care must be taken to preserve the central mesentery of vascular tissue, which runs dorsally to provide the blood supply to the urethral plate. The base of this mesentery is usually found just where the corporal bodies diverge on the ventral aspect of the corpora (Fig. 9–6*E*).

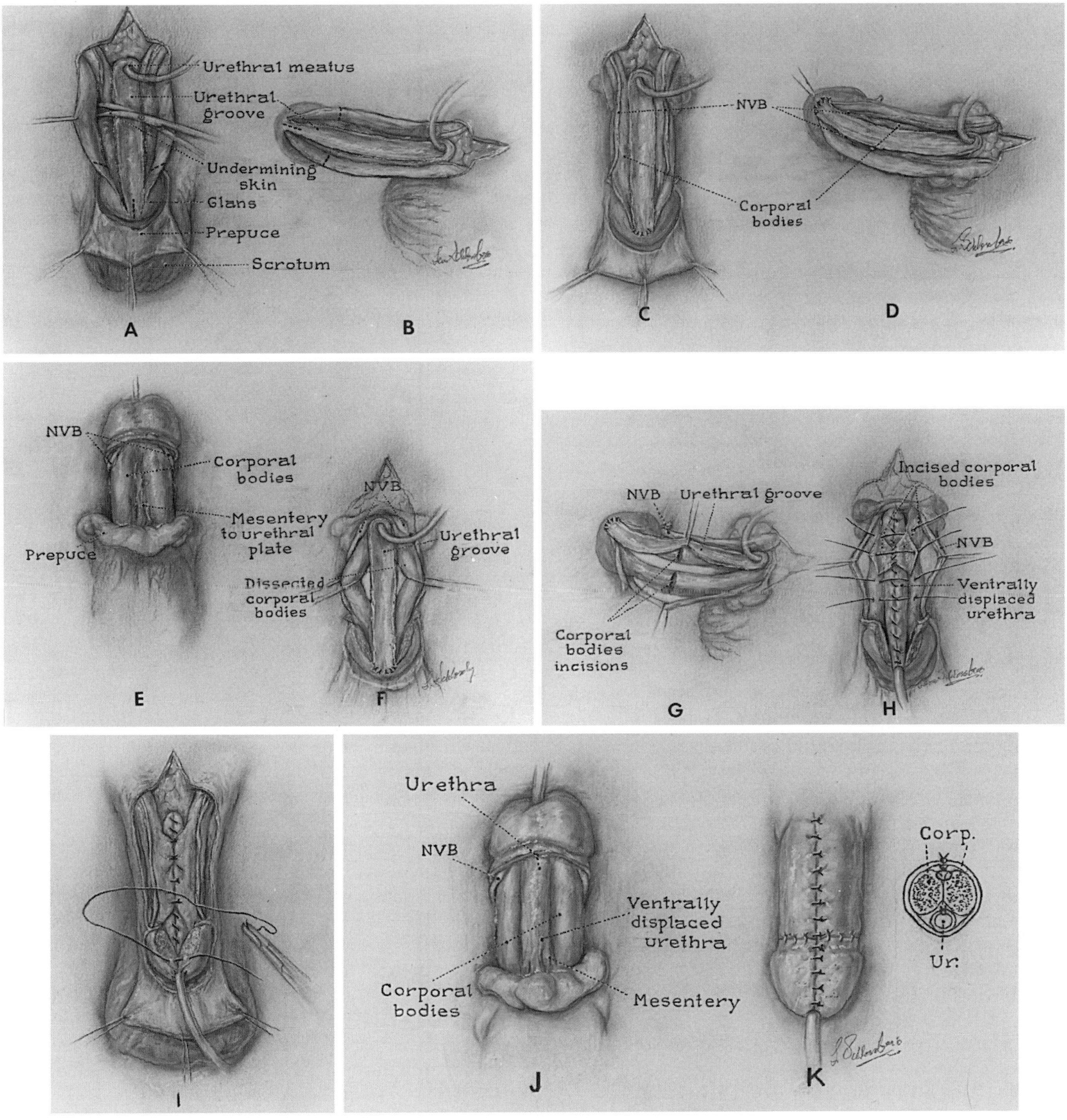

Figure 9–6 *A–K,* Steps in the modified Cantwell-Ransley epispadias repair. *A* and *B,* An incision is made on the urethral groove and the penile skin is mobilized. *C* and *D,* Meatal advancement is performed, and the neurovascular bundles (NVB) are identified and exposed. *E* and *F,* Separation of the urethral groove from the corporal bodies with dissection initially started from below and continued above. *G* and *H,* Mobilization of the neurovascular bundles if necessary from the corporal bodies and incision of the corporal body if severe chordee exists. The urethral groove is closed to the tip of the penis and the corporal incision is closed (if necessary), displacing the urethra ventrally. Further sutures are placed distally to further bury the urethra under the corporal bodies. *I,* The corpora are closed over the ventrally displaced urethra, and the glans is closed. *J* and *K,* The completed repair with urethra (Ur.) below the corporal bodies and closure of the penile skin.

The urethral plate is then approached from below (Fig. 9–6*F*). The dissection proceeds in a circumferential fashion around the corpora. Once the dissection is almost completed around the corpus, the dissection is begun from the top just under the urethral plate. If the dissection from below has been adequate, these two incisions are easily joined. A similar dissection is then accomplished on the contralateral side. Once this circumferential plane has been developed and a vessel loop passed, the dissection proceeds in a cephalad manner, separating the urethral plate from the dorsal aspect of the corpora (Fig. 9–6*G*). After the urethral plate is dissected completely from the corpora, a decision can be made concerning whether corporal incisions will be required to lengthen the corpora further and correct any remaining chordee. If so, the neurovascular bundles are then dissected from the corpora bilaterally and suspended with additional vessel loops (Fig. 9–6*G*). The urethral plate is then tubularized over a 10 French soft silicone (Firlit) stent, and the entire urethral plate is closed using continuous 6-0 polyglycolic suture (Fig. 9–6*H*). The corpora are then joined with 5-0 polydioxanone sutures to close the corporal incision and lengthen the dorsal corpora. If the decision is made not to perform the corporotomy incisions, the corpora are simply brought over the tubularized urethral plate and sewn to each other with 5-0 polydioxanone or polyglycolic acid suture (Fig. 9–6*H*). The point at which the urethra emerges from between the corpora is the area where fistulas most commonly occur.[15] It is very important to obtain as much soft tissue coverage as possible in this area. In children with very little subcutaneous tissue, we have used a tunica vaginalis flap in a "reversed Snow" approach with excellent results.[19]

The glans is then closed in three layers with 5-0 polyglycolic acid suture for the inner layers and 6-0 or 7-0 polyglycolic acid suture for the glanular epithelium (Fig. 9–6*I*). The shaft of the penis is then recovered with skin that may be obtained from the unrolled ventral prepuce, which is then transferred to the dorsum, or by primary closure of the local skin on the dorsal aspect of the penis (Fig. 9–6*J–K*).

POSTOPERATIVE CARE OF THE EPISPADIAS PATIENT

The urethral stent is left indwelling for 10 to 14 days. A penile dressing of adhesive plastic is left on the penis for 5 to 7 days and then soaked off in the bath. Broad-spectrum antibiotics are continued as long as the urethral stent is in place. As soon as the stent is removed, prophylactic antibacterials are begun and the broad-spectrum antibiotics are discontinued. Liberal anticholinergic and analgesic medications are used while the stent is in place because the bladders associated with exstrophy at this stage of repair are often small and prone to spasms, with associated pain and the attendant risk of fistula formation.

BLADDER NECK RECONSTRUCTION

The purpose of bladder neck reconstruction is to allow for voluntary voiding with resulting urinary continence. Several criteria must be met in order for a child to be a candidate for bladder neck reconstruction, including the ability of the child to communicate, the desire to be continent of urine, and a minimal bladder capacity of 60 mL. The optimum time for bladder neck repair is about 4 to 5 years of age when the child is mature enough to cooperate with toilet training. All children will have had their bladder capacity determined under anesthesia before bladder neck repair.

Because all closed exstrophy patients have vesicoureteral reflux, an antireflux procedure is required at the time of bladder neck reconstruction. Also if there is a persistently wide pubic diastasis or soft intrapubic bar, initial or repeat osteotomy may be required. We have used this technique along with bladder neck reconstruction in more than 12 patients; however, whether this actually adds to improvement in eventual continence is unknown.

The bladder is exposed and opened using a midline or lower transverse incision, and the bladder neck is dissected free of surrounding structures (Fig. 9–7*A*). If this maneuver is not performed, the bladder neck muscle will not roll into a tight tube and will be difficult to suspend to the rectus fascia at the end of the repair. If needed, the intrasymphyseal bar can be incised vertically to enhance visualization and operative exposure. The ureters are then reimplanted in the manner of Cohen in either a transtrigonal or cephalotrigonal direction, depending on their distance from the bladder neck (Fig. 9–7*B*, *C*).[20]

After ureteral reimplantation, a 15-mm wide mucosal strip extending from the midtrigone to the prostatic urethra with a length of 3 cm is outlined (Fig. 9–7*D*). Lateral to the mucosal strip, triangles of bladder wall are then denuded of mucosa. After demucosalization, 1/200,000 epinephrine–soaked sponges are held against the denuded bladder wall for a few minutes to control bleeding (Fig. 9–7*E*). After this maneuver, pinpoint cautery is used to stop any persistent bleeding from the lateral muscle flaps.

The previously outlined mucosal strip is rolled into a tube over a 8 French urethral catheter using interrupted 4-0 polyglycolic acid sutures (Fig. 9–7*F*). The denuded muscle flaps are overlapped tightly and sutured in place with 3-0 polyglycolic acid sutures to reinforce the bladder neck (Fig. 9–7*G*). These final sutures in the superficial detrusor are left long so that the bladder neck can be suspended for added outlet resistance (Fig. 9–7*H*, *I*). The suprapubic tube and ureteral stents are brought out through a stab wound in the bladder and then brought through the skin in the area of the old umbilical incision. The bladder is closed in two layers and a nonlatex drain placed in the prevesical space. Again, as in a primary bladder closure, no stents or catheters are brought out through the reconstructed bladder neck repair. The repair must heal for 3 weeks postoperatively before voiding trials begin.

POSTOPERATIVE MANAGEMENT AFTER BLADDER NECK REPAIR

Broad-spectrum antibiotics are continued for 7 to 10 days in the postoperative period. Postoperative bladder spasms and pain are controlled with the use of continuous caudal epidural catheters, anticholinergics, nonsteroidal anti-inflamatory agents, narcotics, and benzodiazepines. The stents are left in place for 2 to 3 weeks, as long as they are draining significant amounts of urine. At 3 weeks postoperatively, a soft 8 French catheter is passed through the urethra and bladder neck for calibration, and the suprapubic tube is then clamped before removal to ensure adequate voiding. If the child cannot void and a catheter cannot be passed, a gentle cystoscopy with an infant cystoscope and placement of a urethral catheter are required. This may require cystoscopic placement of a guide wire to pass the catheter into the bladder. The catheter is then left indwelling for 2 to 5 days. After removal of the catheter, voiding trials are then begun. We have seen patients who have required up to two or three catheter placements to achieve proper voiding. After removal of the tube, it is expected that there will be only a short dry interval. At first, the bladder capacity will be quite small, and the patients are not familiar with the sensation of bladder filling or detrusor contractions. Therefore, it usually takes several months of readjustment before a reasonable dry interval is obtained. If in the first month or so there is a dry interval of 15 minutes or more, no continuous urethral dribbling, and no stress incontinence, then eventual total urinary continence is expected. Complete day and night continence should be achieved by 1 year postoperatively. A few will gain continence in the second year, but this development is rare in our experience.

Before discharge from the hospital, a renal ultrasonogram is obtained. Four months after bladder neck plasty, another ultrasonogram or limited intravenous pyelogram is obtained. If possible, a cystogram is also obtained. These studies are performed to ensure freedom from reflux and satisfactory drainage of the upper urinary tract. Patients are maintained on suppressive antibiotics until regular complete bladder emptying occurs and there is no evidence of vesicoureteral reflux.

RESULTS AND COMPLICATIONS OF BLADDER EXSTROPHY TREATMENT

The results of functional bladder closure can be expected to be as high as a 75 to 85% continence rate with preservation of renal function as documented by several large series.[1, 2] The success of the initial bladder closure impacts in a major way on the child's eventual ability to achieve continence through spontaneous voiding without the adjunctive use of intermittent catheterization and bladder augmentation. The main complications of initial closure are bladder prolapse, outlet obstruction, bladder calculi, renal calculi, and wound dehiscence. However, our recent results suggest a significant decline in these complications.

Cases involving children who have a bladder prolapse or dehiscence must be classified as failed closure attempts. Bladder prolapse usually results from either a partial wound separation or the failure to create a satisfactory bladder outlet, which allows unimpeded egress of urine but prevents prolapse. Dehiscence of the wound and extrusion of the bladder can occur as a result of infection or more commonly a result of pubic separation because of inadequate fixation of the pelvis before healing of the abdominal wound. If the size of the bladder template is adequate, a second closure of the bladder should be performed within 4 to 6 months of the initial attempt.[12] Repeat closure should be attempted with the aid of an osteotomy and external fixation.[10, 11]

The importance of a successful initial bladder closure becomes more apparent when one sees that after two prior closures only 40% of patients achieve enough capacity for bladder neck plasty and barely 50% of these achieve continence, so that actually only 20% are voiding spontaneously and continent of urine.[12]

With the introduction of the Cantwell-Ransley epispadias repair, better functional and cosmetic results can be obtained than with the older Young urethroplasty. The Cantwell-Ransley repair achieves better cosmesis, an easily negotiable urethra, better correction of chordee, and a lower incidence of urethrocutaneous fistulas.[15, 16]

Urinary continence, defined as a 3-hour dry interval during the day and dry at night, is usually achieved within 1 year of bladder neck reconstruction. In our experience, those patients who fail to develop a 3-hour dry interval within 1 to 2 years after bladder neck plasty are unlikely to do so. Previously, it was suggested that puberty and its resultant prostatic growth may improve continence in those with less than perfect dryness. However, Gearhart and colleagues, in a study of prostatic size and configuration in the exstrophy population, found that no anatomic basis for a significant contribution to the outlet resistance by the postpubertal enlarged prostate.[21]

If the patient remains wet after an appropriate observation period, other choices remain to achieve dryness. If the bladder neck is patulous and the bladder capacity

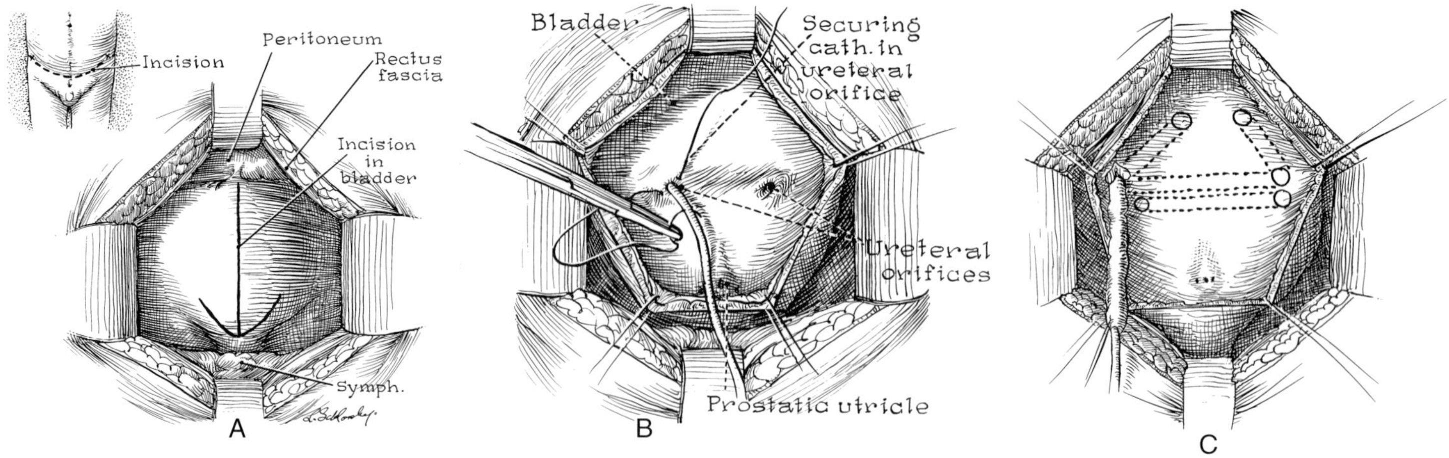

Figure 9–7 *A–I,* Steps in Young-Dees-Leadbetter bladder neck reconstruction for continence. *A,* Midline incision in the bladder. *B* and *C,* Ureteral mobilization with either transtrigonal or cephalotrigonal course for ureteral reimplantation.

remains reasonable, reoperative bladder neck plasty offers a very acceptable option to gain continence.[22] However, many patients in whom bladder neck repair fails will have a marginal or inadequate bladder capacity and require bladder augmentation, another outlet procedure (bladder neck repair, artificial urinary sphincter, or bladder neck closure), with or without a continent urinary stoma, to become dry.[22, 23] In 1995, Ben-Chaim and others reported moderate success with injection of bovine cross-linked collagen into the bladder neck in those patients with an inadequate dry interval or significant stress incontinence after bladder neck repair.[24]

MANAGEMENT OF THE FAILED EXSTROPHY RECONSTRUCTION

The small bladder after initial exstrophy reconstruction is one of the greatest problems to face the reconstructive urologist. If the bladder capacity remains small by gravity cystogram under anesthesia at age 2, one should proceed to epispadias repair. Significant increases in bladder capacity can be achieved with this maneuver. If the bladder capacity remains small after urethroplasty, other procedures to increase outlet resistance may be tried, but one must understand that the potential for the bladder to gain enough capacity for primary bladder neck repair is markedly decreased. Caione and coworkers reported significant increases in bladder capacity after bladder neck collagen injection.[25]

If the bladder capacity remains small after the procedures just discussed, the main therapeutic alternative is enhancement of the bladder capacity with bowel segments. In addition to increasing capacity, attention must be given to increasing the bladder outlet resistance. Our choice in this situation is Young-Dees-Leadbetter bladder neck repair, but others have used the artificial urinary sphincter or even closure of the bladder neck.[26, 27] Also reliable intermittent catheterization through the reconstructed urethra and bladder neck may be difficult, and a continent urinary stoma will need to be constructed to allow easy, reliable catheter passage.[23]

With failed bladder neck reconstructions, the just-mentioned principles of bladder reconstruction still apply. Because only those patients with adequate bladder capacities are candidates for reoperative bladder neck repair, most will require augmentation with or without continent stoma construction and bladder outlet enhancement.

Reconstruction of the penis and urethra in the patient with a failed epispadias repair is a formidable task in these difficult patients. However, with modern reconstructive techniques, the majority of patients will have a functional penis that is cosmetically acceptable without chordee and allows satisfactory sexual function. Three significant problems with the external genitalia may be seen at the time of puberty: desire for additional penile length, prominent scars from previous repairs, and residual dorsal chordee. The goals in the female exstrophy patient are the same: cosmetically acceptable genitalia and adequate sexual function.

Modern techniques of plastic repair of the penis, including lower abdominal flaps, dorsal corporal grafts, and ventral corporal rotation, may be helpful in those with unsatisfactory external genitalia.[28–31] If the urethra is found to contribute to the continuing dorsal chordee, then it will need to be divided and reconstructed with one of several substitutes available.

ALTERNATIVES FOR FUNCTIONAL EXSTROPHY RECONSTRUCTION

Even with modern reconstructive techniques, not all children born with classic bladder exstrophy will be candi-

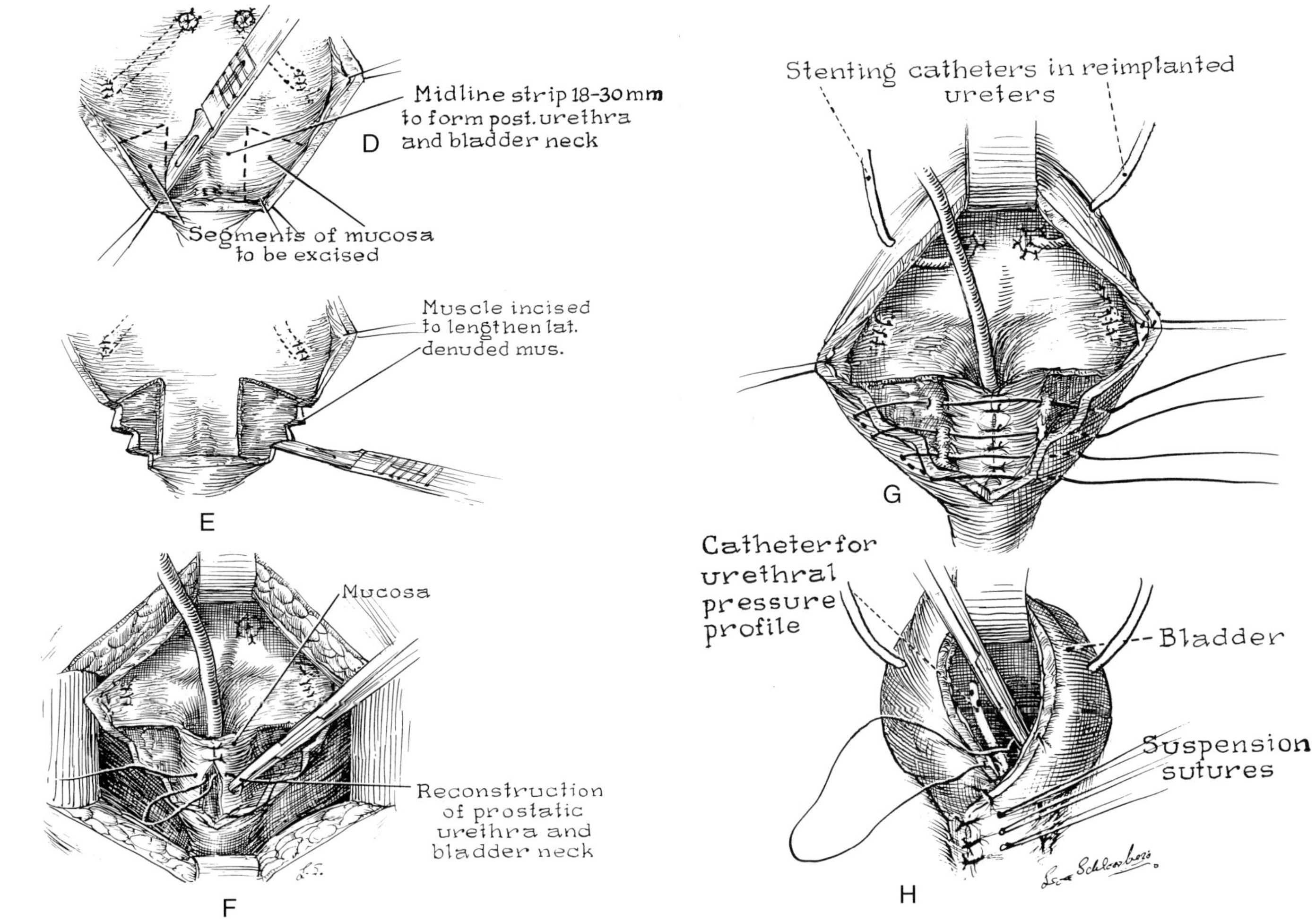

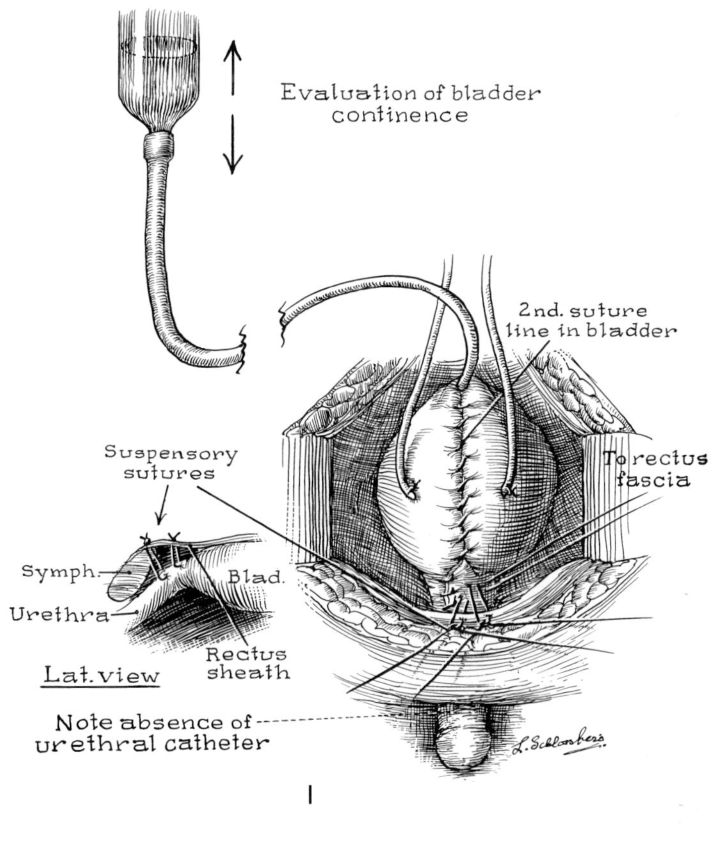

Figure 9–7 *Continued* *D,* Mucosal strip of trigone to form bladder neck and prostatic urethra. *E* and *F,* Lateral denuded muscle triangles are lengthened by several small incisions to allow tailoring and funneling of the bladder neck reconstruction and initial mucosal closure of posterior urethra and bladder neck. *G* and *H,* The denuded muscle flaps are closed above the previously closed mucosal strip. *I,* Bladder neck suspension is performed; the bladder neck and urethra are unstented. Drainage is by ureteral catheters and suprapubic tube. Bladder outlet resistance can be estimated by the use of a water manometer intraoperatively.

dates for functional bladder reconstruction. Formerly, ureterosigmoidostomy was a popular choice in this situation.[32] However, long-term concerns, especially with later development of malignancy, have decreased its popularity.[33, 34]

Ileal conduit urinary diversion formerly enjoyed widespread usage in the exstrophy population. Long-term complications have also decreased its popularity. Currently, this method of diversion is not considered acceptable in children.[35] In the newborn with exstrophy and a bladder too small for functional reconstruction, our approach is a nonrefluxing colonic conduit, which will be converted to part of a continent urinary diversion at an older age or anastomosed to the rectosigmoid after the child achieves anal continence.[36]

CONCLUSION

Modern techniques of exstrophy reconstruction allow the preservation of renal function, achievement of functional and cosmetically pleasing external genitalia, and attainment of urinary continence in the vast majority of cases. With the use of staged functional reconstruction, most patients can achieve these goals and void spontaneously. However, those who are not candidates for this type of reconstruction or those with failed exstrophy repairs can still attain these goals through clean intermittent catheterization and associated bladder augmentation, continent diversion, or bladder replacement.

REFERENCES

1. Gearhart JP, Jeffs RD. Management of the exstrophy-epispadias complex and urachal anomalies. In Walsh PC, Retik AB, Stamey TA (eds), Campbell's Urology. 6th ed, Philadelphia: WB Saunders, 1992, pp 1772–1821.
2. Husmann DA, McLorie GA, Churchill BM. Closure of the exstrophic bladder: An evaluation of the factors leading to its success and its importance on urinary continence. J Urol 142:522, 1989.
3. Lancaster PAL. Epidemiology of bladder exstrophy and epispadias: A communication from the International Clearinghouse for Birth Defects Monitoring System. Teratology 36:221, 1987.
4. Ives E, Coffey R, Carter CO. A family study of bladder exstrophy. J Med Genet 17:139, 1980.
5. Shapiro E, Lepor H., Jeffs RD. The inheritance of exstrophy-epispadias complex. J Urol 132:308, 1980.
6. Gearhart JP, Ben-Chaim J, Jeffs RD, Sanders R. Criteria for prenatal diagnosis of classic bladder exstrophy. Obstet Gynecol 85:961, 1995.
7. Jaffe R, Schoenfeld A, Ovadia J. Sonographic findings in the prenatal diagnosis of bladder exstrophy. Am J Obstet Gynecol 162:675, 1990.
8. Barth RA, Filly RA, Sondheimer FK. Prenatal sonographic findings in bladder exstrophy. J Ultrasound Med 9:359, 1990.
9. Sponseller PD, Gearhart JP, Jeffs RD. Anterior innominate osteotomies for failure or late closure of bladder exstrophy. J Urol 146:137, 1991.
10. Gearhart JP, Forschner DC, Sponseller PD, Jeffs RD. A new combined vertical and horizontal pelvic osteotomy approach for the initial and secondary repair of bladder exstrophy. J Urol 155:689, 1996.
11. Gearhart JP, Peppas DS, Jeffs RD. The failed exstrophy closure: Strategy for management. Br J Urol 71:217, 1993.
12. Gearhart JP, Ben-Chaim J, Sciortino C, et al. The multiple failed exstrophy closure: What affects the bladder? Urology 47:240, 1996.
13. Sumfest JM, Mitchell M. Reconstruction of the umbilicus in exstrophy. J Urol 151:453, 1994.
14. Hanna MK, Ansong K. Reconstruction of the umbilicus in bladder exstrophy. Urology 24:324, 1984.
15. Gearhart JP, Leonard MP, Burgers JK, Jeffs RD. The Cantwell-Ransley technique for repair of epispadias. J Urol 148:851, 1992.
16. Gearhart JP, Sciortino C, Ben-Chaim J, Jeffs RD. The Cantwell-Ransley epispadias repair: Lessons learned. Urology 46:92, 1995.
17. Jeffs RD, Guice SL, Oesch I. The factors in successful exstrophy closure. J Urol 127:974, 1982.
18. Gearhart JP, Jeffs RD. Bladder exstrophy: Increase in capacity following epispadias repair. J Urol 142:525, 1989.
19. Snow BW. Use of tunica vaginalis to prevent fistulas in hypospadias surgery. J Urol 136:861, 1986.
20. Canning DA, Gearhart JP, Peppas DS, Jeffs RD. The cephalotrigonal reimplant in bladder neck reconstruction for patients with exstrophy or epispadias. J Urol 150:156, 1993.
21. Gearhart JP, Yang A, Leonard MP, et al. Prostate size and configuration in adults with bladder exstrophy. J Urol 149:308, 1993.
22. Gearhart JP, Canning DA, Jeffs RD. Failed bladder neck reconstruction: Options for management. J Urol 146:1082, 1991.
23. Gearhart JP, Peppas DS, Jeffs RD. The application of continent urinary stomas to bladder augmentation or replacement in the failed exstrophy reconstruction. Br J Urol 75:87, 1995.
24. Ben-Chaim J, Jeffs RD, Peppas DS, Gearhart JP. Submucosal bladder neck injections of glutaraldehyde cross-linked bovine collagen for treatment of urinary incontinence in patients with the exstrophy-epispadias complex. J Urol 154:862, 1995.
25. Caione P, Lais A de GM, Capozza NP. Glutaraldehyde cross-linked bovine collagen in exstrophy/epispadias complex. J Urol 150:631, 1993.
26. Decter RM, Roth DR, Fishman IJ, et al. Use of the AS800 device in exstrophy and epispadias. J Urol 140:1202, 1988.
27. Hanna MK. Artificial urinary sphincter for continence in children. Urology 18:370, 1981.
28. Mesrobian HG, Kelalis PP, Kramer SA. Long-term follow up of cosmetic appearance and genital function in boys with exstrophy: Review of 53 patients. J Urol 136:256, 1986.
29. Kramer SA, Jackson IT. Bilateral rhomboid flaps for reconstruction of the external genitalia in epispadias-exstrophy. Plast Reconstr Surg 77:621, 1986.
30. Woodhouse CR. Reconstruction of the epispadiac penis in adolescents. Prog Pediatr Surg. 23:165, 1989.
31. Koff SA, Eakins M. The treatment of penile chordee using corporeal rotation. J Urol 131:931, 1984.
32. Stockle M, Becht E, Voges G, et al. Ureterosigmoidostomy: An outdated approach to bladder exstrophy? J Urol 143:770, 1990.
33. Strachan JR, Woodhouse CR. Malignancy following ureterosigmoidostomy in patients with exstrophy. Br J Surg 78:1216, 1991.
34. Gittes RF. Carcinogenesis in ureterosigmoidostomy. Urol Clin North Am 13:201, 1986.
35. Jeffs RD, Schwartz GR. Ileal conduit urinary diversion in children: Computer analysis follow up from 2 to 16 years. J Urol 114:285, 1975.
36. Hendren WH. Exstrophy of the bladder: An alternative method of management. J Urol 115:195, 1976.

MARTIN KAEFER & STUART BAUER

10

The Surgical Correction of Incontinence in Myelodysplastic Children

Abnormal spinal column development represents the most common cause of neuropathic bladder dysfunction in children. Myelodysplasia is an all-inclusive term used to describe abnormal vertebral column development with associated injury to and alterations in spinal cord function. Three major types of neurospinal dysraphisms exist. A meningocele occurs when the dural envelope surrounding the spinal cord herniates beyond the confines of the vertebral column without any neural elements contained within it. A myelomeningocele, which accounts for the majority of all open spinal dysraphisms (90%),[1] implies that neural tissue accompanies the everted meningeal sac. A lipomyelomeningocele denotes a myelomeningocele with associated fatty tissue. Most of these spinal defects occur at the level of the lumbar vertebrae, with the sacral, thoracic, and cervical areas affected in decreasing order.[2] In the majority of cases, the meninges lie intact over the spinal cord, but they may be breached and leaking cerebrospinal fluid. Congenital abnormalities of the spinal column also can occur in the absence of an open vertebral column. These lesions, referred to as occult spinal dysraphisms, may be very subtle in presentation. A high index of suspicion, coupled with a careful inspection for a cutaneous abnormality overlying the lower spine (present in more than 90% of these occult lesions), is required to identify these children.

Immediate postpartum care of an open spinal dysraphism consists of urgent repair of the defect to reduce the chance of cerebrospinal infection. Additionally, early assessment for the presence of the Arnold-Chiari malformation is imperative. In the Arnold-Chiari malformation, the cerebellar tonsils herniate through the foramen magnum, effectively obstructing the fourth ventricle and preventing cerebrospinal fluid from entering the vertebral space. These children (85% of the myelodysplastic population) will require ventriculoperitoneal shunting to prevent the deleterious effects of hydrocephalus.

The neurologic lesion resulting from spinal dysraphism is dependent on which neural elements, if any, have everted into the meningocele sac. It is important to recognize that the bony abnormality will often give little indication as to the level, symmetry, or completeness of the neurologic deficit. Up to 20% of these children will have an intraspinal defect, which can further affect neural function. Not only can the deficit extend higher than the observed vertebral column abnormality, but cord function can remain largely unaffected for up to three vertebral levels below the bony lesion.[2] Finally, children with thoracic and cervical vertebral defects can demonstrate a complete reconstitution of their spine at the sacral level. These individuals will frequently have intact sacral function in the absence of brain stem or cortical control.[3]

Thus, the neurologic lesion produced by the spinal dysraphism, particularly as it relates to genitourinary function, cannot be fully assessed by means of a simple physical examination of the back or neurologic function of the lower extremities. Rather, it is imperative that urodynamic assessment of the neonate with neurospinal dysraphism (or in older children when the diagnosis is made) be carried out as part of a full evaluation in every child.

NEWBORN ASSESSMENT AND MEDICAL MANAGEMENT

After delivery, renal ultrasonography and evaluation of residual urine are performed as a means of ensuring adequate urinary drainage. For infants who cannot empty their bladder to completion (e.g., postvoid residual > 5 mL) after a spontaneous void or with Credé's maneuver, clean, intermittent catheterization (CIC) is instituted. Antibiotics are begun after the urine has been collected for urinalysis and culture and are continued until the child can be properly assessed for vesicoureteral reflux.

After the spinal closure has healed sufficiently to warrant safe and infection-free investigational testing, either intravenous pyelography or renal sonography combined with a nuclear medicine scan is performed to reassess upper urinary tract architecture and function. Following this, voiding cystourethrography and urodynamic evaluation are conducted. These studies serve as a baseline to monitor future changes in upper and lower urinary tract function. In addition, they provide important information used to proactively treat infants at risk of future deterioration.

Children at particularly high risk for upper urinary tract deterioration include those with detrusor hypertonicity or outflow obstruction from detrusor sphincter dyssynergia. CIC alone or in combination with anticholinergic agents can considerably reduce the risk of upper tract deterioration in these individuals.[4] We prefer the use of oxybutynin hydrochloride, 1.0 mg per year of age every 12 hours, to lower detrusor filling pressure. When a hyper-reflexic or hypertonic bladder fails to respond to these conservative measures, a cutaneous vesicostomy may be used as a temporizing measure. Alternatively, definitive surgical treatment may be undertaken to improve the bladder's storage capacity.

Complete radiological and urodynamic evaluation of the neonate serves as a baseline from which to assess future alterations in genitourinary function. The neurogenic injury affecting the lower urinary tract can be a highly dynamic lesion, with alterations in neurologic function occurring most frequently when axial growth is the greatest (e.g., early childhood). As a result, yearly urodynamic and radiographic testing is recommended beginning in the newborn period and continuing until 5 years of age. The information obtained from these sequential evaluations provides the means for early detection, thus offering the hope that timely neurosurgical intervention may help to arrest or reverse a pathologic process.

SURGICAL CORRECTION OF INCONTINENCE

The attainment of socially acceptable urinary continence significantly impacts on the quality of life of patients with myelodysplasia. The majority of these children can be successfully treated with conservative nonsurgical management.[5] However, despite an array of pharmacologic agents and widespread acceptance of CIC in the management of children with neurogenic bladders, a significant number of patients will eventually require surgical intervention to correct vesicoureteral reflux, inadequate bladder outlet resistance, and poor bladder compliance.

Because the neurogenic lesion is a dynamic process in children with myelodysplasia, the potential to undergo changes in detrusor compliance, outlet resistance, and detrusor-sphincter coordination necessitates an individualized and often changing management strategy for each child with spinal dysraphism. Alterations in micturition physiology, identified by periodic uroradiographic and urodynamic assessment, should prompt the physician to assess the central nervous system for a surgically correctable cause. Acquired lesions, which may result in altered bladder dynamics, include spinal cord tethering, a syrinx of the cord, ventriculoperitoneal (VP) shunt malfunction, or cerebellar herniation through the foramen magnum.

Two primary and often interdependent objectives exist in managing the urinary tract of these children: preservation of renal function and attainment of diurnal continence. To achieve these two primary goals, the clinician must ascertain that the patient has a compliant large-capacity reservoir, competent ureterovesical and bladder neck mechanisms, and a reliable mechanism for effectively emptying the bladder. Before embarking on any surgical intervention, careful consideration must be given to the pathophysiology of the entire urinary tract, including renal function, ureteral dynamics, detrusor function, and detrusor-sphincter synergy.

INCONTINENCE SECONDARY TO A DYSFUNCTIONAL RESERVOIR

The low-pressure storage of urine is dependent on the compliant properties of the bladder wall. Effective modulation of bladder pressure is also dependent on intact peripheral and spinal cord neural pathways. In the absence of appropriate modulation of bladder reflex activity (i.e., upper motor neuron lesion), the patient with spinal dysraphism will experience hypertonicity or hyper-reflexia or both. Elevated detrusor storage pressures will, in turn, impact on ureteral drainage, challenge the competency of the ureterovesical junction, and often result in incontinence by overwhelming the bladder neck–urethral closure mechanism. The concept of pressure-specific bladder volume (the volume that a bladder can accommodate at a specific pressure)[6] provides a functional measure for determining the adequacy of the storage reservoir.

Initial attempts at improving bladder capacity should include the use of anticholinergics and direct smooth muscle relaxants. The poorly compliant, stiff bladder that is unresponsive to these medications is best managed by either augmentation cystoplasty or autoaugmentation. A variety of gastrointestinal segments singly and in combinations thereof have been used for bladder augmentation.[7–9] In deciding which segments to use, the pathophysiology of the entire gastrointestinal and urinary tracts must be considered. First, it must be determined which bowel segments may be used without adversely affecting gastrointestinal function. Myelodysplastic children are highly dependent on controlled constipation for fecal continence. Removal of the ileocecal segment in this population can lead to intractable chronic diarrhea,[10] thereby trading urinary for fecal incontinence. With many alternative methods for reconstruction available, we now avoid using the ileocecal segment in these individuals.

Metabolic considerations are equally as important in determining the segment of bowel to incorporate into the storage reservoir. The potentially adverse metabolic consequences of placing small bowel or colon in contact with urine are well established.[11] In patients with renal acidosis, incorporation of small or large bowel into the urinary tract will lead to an increase in absorbed chloride that subsequently overwhelms an impaired kidney's ability to maintain an adequate acid-base balance. Stomach, on the other hand, is preferable in patients with poor renal function who cannot tolerate an increase in acid solute load. The secretory nature of the gastric epithelium not only clears some of the acid load but also prevents infection, limits mucus, and makes stone formation less likely.

Although it is the optimal choice from a metabolic standpoint, we believe there are situations in which the use of stomach is not the correct choice in patients with renal failure. Children with low-output renal failure or those whose kidneys are likely to be removed will be left with a relatively dry anastomotic site that is chronically exposed to an acidic milieu. With minimal urine available to dilute the secreted acid load, these patients may have an increased propensity to experience gastric ulceration and hematuria. This may increase the likelihood of perforation.[12]

PREOPERATIVE PREPARATION

Although a select group of patients will be able to empty the bladder spontaneously after augmentation cystoplasty, the majority will require CIC to achieve this goal. Therefore, it is imperative that before augmenting the bladder the caregiver and child thoroughly understand the lifelong commitment to CIC. Although situations may arise in which very young children can benefit from augmentation cystoplasty (i.e., persistent hydroureteronephrosis secondary to a bladder that is unresponsive to anticholinergic medication), it is our policy to wait until patients have reached an age at which social continence would be normally obtained and comprehension of the importance of CIC demonstrated when it is necessary for continence.

Many factors determine which bowel segment is optimally suited for a given patient; the final decision is often made at the time of laparotomy. Therefore, although the use of certain bowel segments may require less bowel preparation than others (e.g., stomach), every patient receives a standard mechanical and antibiotic bowel cleansing so as not to limit one's options at the time of exploration.

The preoperative preparation begins with a low-residue diet 5 days before surgery and then a clear-liquid diet 48 hours before surgery. On the day before surgery, a cathartic (GoLYTELY) is administered per nasogastric tube. Normal saline enemas followed by bisacodyl suppositories aid in evacuating any remaining fecal residue. Antibiotic prophylaxis is provided in the form of neomycin and erythromycin base (50 mg/kg) divided into three oral doses after the oral cathartic. In addition, a single intravenous dose of a broad-spectrum antibiotic (e.g., cefoxitin) is administered 1 hour before surgery. Intravenous hydration is started the night before surgery to maintain adequate fluid status during mechanical bowel preparation.

TECHNICAL CONSIDERATIONS

General

Nearly all children with neurogenic bladders have had extensive exposure to latex products (e.g., gloves, catheters), resulting in sensitivity to the latex protein. Although only a portion of this population will subsequently experience an anaphylactic reaction when exposed to the latex, it is our policy to maintain the strictest of latex precautions during all of our operative procedures on these children.[13] Ensuring the availability of latex-free gloves, suprapubic tubes, ureteral stents, nephrostomy tubes, tape, and other surgical items is imperative. Failure to ensure a latex-free environment can lead to a latex allergy in those at risk or can be catastrophic in those already sensitized.[14]

Intestinocystoplasty is frequently performed in conjunction with procedures designed to correct vesicoureteral reflux or increase bladder outlet resistance. Because of their increased body surface area–body mass ratio, children, especially toddlers, are exquisitely sensitive to heat loss during these extensive operations. By delaying entry into the peritoneum until all extraperitoneal portions of the procedure (i.e., ureteral reimplantation) are performed, one can reduce heat and fluid loss through an exposed peritoneal surface. Delayed entry into the peritoneum also helps maintain optimal exposure when operating in the true pelvis.

Adequate exposure of the entire gastrointestinal tract is achieved through a midline incision. After the planned bladder and ureteral surgery, the peritoneum is entered and the abdominal contents are examined. If the patient has a VP shunt, the tubing is identified, wrapped in an antibiotic-soaked gauze sponge, and placed in one of the upper quadrants. Every precaution should be taken to avoid contaminating the VP shunt while performing the enterocystoplasty. It has not been our practice to exteriorize the shunt at the time of augmentation cystoplasty.

Before isolating the gastrointestinal segment, the bladder is opened in preparation to receive the augmentation. Just before making the cystotomy, the peritoneum overlying the dome is dissected free of the bladder. This will later serve to "re-retroperitonealize" the augmented bladder. A midline vertical cystotomy is made from anterior to posterior surfaces over the dome of the bladder. It is best not to extend this incision any more caudally than necessary. This will reduce potential tension at the anastomotic site in cases in which there is limited mobility of the intestinal patch down into the pelvis. A bladder that is particularly thick and contracted may fail to provide an adequately wide base after simply bivalving it. In such cases, an additional vertical incision down each lateral wall will allow the opened bladder to form a more suitable wide-mouthed base to receive the augmentation.

As our experience with augmentation has increased, so has the understanding of basic physical principles that determine the behavior of the augmented bladder. Size and configuration of the segment used for augmentation play key roles in determining ultimate reservoir capacity and resting pressures. The first aim in reconfiguration of the bowel segment is to achieve a spherical storage reservoir. This will provide the most volume for the least surface area.[15] By opening and reconfiguring cylindrical segments of bowel (ileum or colon), the volume is increased by the square of the radius. Stomach, with its diamond-shaped patch, creates the optimal globular shape to the bladder without requiring this reconfiguration.[7] Early experience with continent urinary reconstruction demonstrated that closed intact bowel was also capable of generating pressures of greater than 100 cm H_2O. Opening the bowel along its antimesenteric border so as to disrupt the continuity of the circular musculature (detubularization) reduces the ability of the bowel wall to generate such high pressures. Nevertheless, in the case of sigmoid colon, contractions may persist. These contractions can at times be intractable, can be unresponsive to all medications, and can lead to incontinence. In such cases, the patient may require a second augmentation to act as a pressure sink for these contractions.

Finally, we do not now advocate incidental appendectomy, a common operation in the past. The potential use of the appendix as a catheterizable urinary stoma or the provision of anterograde continent enemas (ACEs) underscores the importance of preserving this structure.[16]

Ileocystoplasty (Fig. 10–1)

A segment of ileum measuring approximately 15 to 20 cm in length with adequate mobility of the mesentery to reach the bladder is identified. To avoid vascular compromise of the cecum and terminal ileum, the distal extent should be approximately 15 cm from the ileocecal valve, thus preserving the ileocolic artery. This is also done to avoid isolating the very terminal portion of ileum, which has several important absorptive functions. Proximal and distal windows are developed through avascular segments of the mesentery, and the proposed segment is isolated with moist towels. Residual intraluminal contents are "milked" from the ileum, atraumatic bowel clamps are placed, and the ileum is divided. After a hand-sewn, two-layer end-to-end ileoileostomy is performed, the ileal segment is irrigated clear with a neomycin saline solution and opened along its antimesenteric border using Bovie cautery. The detubularized ileum is reconfigured into a U-shape patch using two layers of running interlocking Vicryl suture. The patch is folded over, and the lateral edges are sewn together. It is then anastomosed to the bivalved bladder using the same two-layer closure. A suprapubic tube and any necessary ureteral drainage stents are brought through the bladder wall. A perivesical

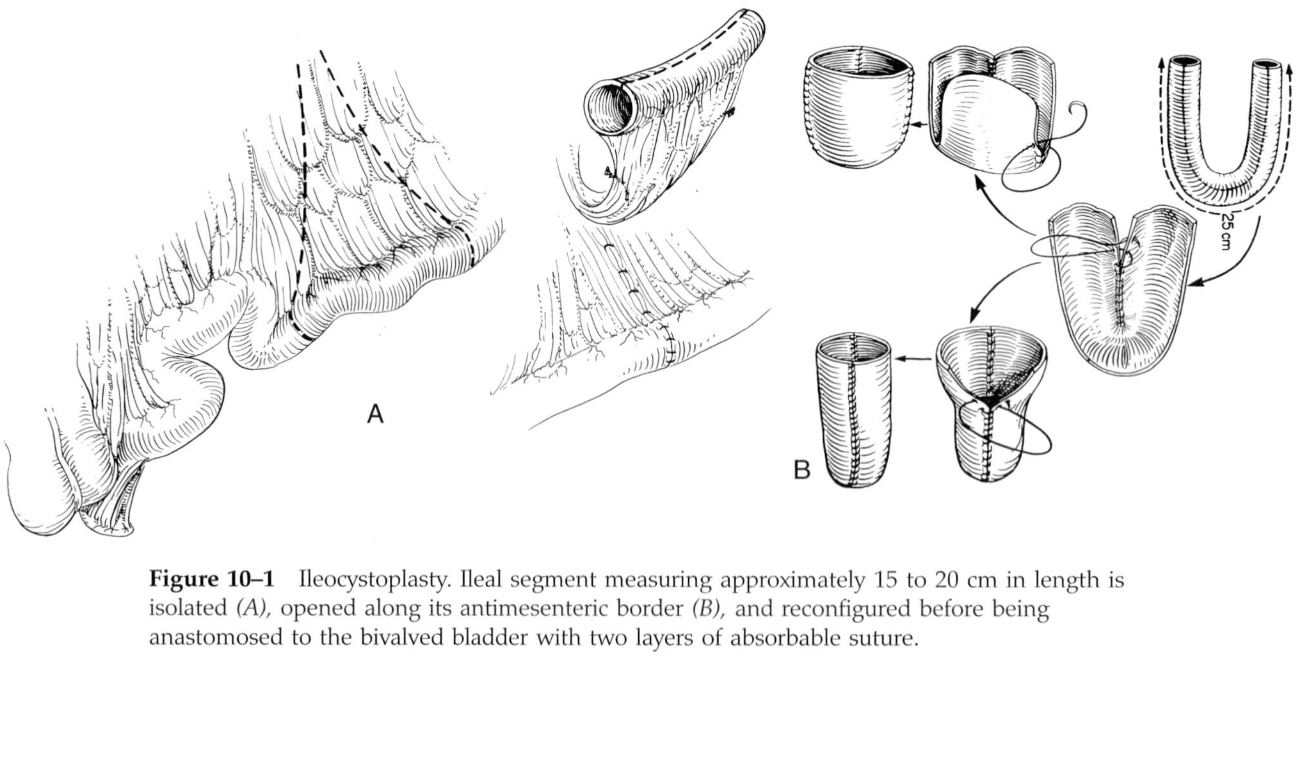

Figure 10–1 Ileocystoplasty. Ileal segment measuring approximately 15 to 20 cm in length is isolated *(A)*, opened along its antimesenteric border *(B)*, and reconfigured before being anastomosed to the bivalved bladder with two layers of absorbable suture.

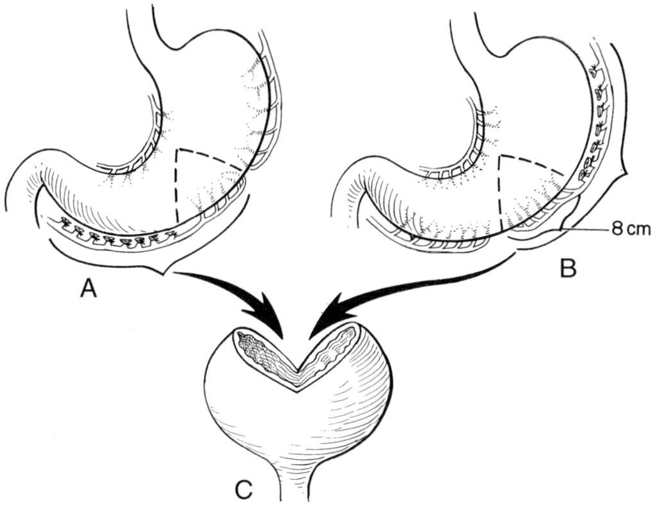

Figure 10–2 Gastrocystoplasty. An 8-cm-long wedge of the gastric fundus is resected without impinging on the vasculature of the lesser curvature. This can either be based on the right *(A)* or left *(B)* gastroepiploic circulation. *C,* A two-layer anastomosis of the wedge to the bivalved bladder is completed (not shown).

drain is left in the pelvic location; and, by bringing previously mobilized peritoneum over the augmented segment, the completed reservoir is effectively isolated in a retroperitoneal location.

Gastrocystoplasty (Fig. 10–2)

The stomach is an excellent organ for bladder augmentation because in children it is rarely in the field of radiation or affected by intrinsic disease. Gastric flaps are highly mobile and can be based on either the left or right gastroepiploic vessels. Although we prefer a right-sided pedicle, the decision is based in part on where the right and left gastroepiploic vessels attenuate or end. In harvesting a wedge of stomach, it is desirable to take a primarily parietal cell–rich segment (corpus) to optimize the acid secretion. Gastrocystoplasty is begun by identifying a wedge of stomach with its base measuring 7 to 8 cm along the greater curvature, with radii extending to within 2 to 3 cm of the lesser curvature, thus ending beneath the lesser curvature perforating vessels. When basing the pedicle on the right gastroepiploic vasculature, the short gastric vessels may be ligated to the level of the pyloric junction to improve mobility. After excising the wedge, the gastric wall is closed in two layers: an outer layer of interrupted silk and an inner running locking layer of absorbable suture. After this closure, one must ensure that the tip of the nasogastric tube is situated distal to the anastomotic site. The isolated segment is then brought through both the transverse mesocolon and the small bowel mesenteries. This leaves the blood supply to the augmentation in a reliable retroperitoneal location and limits the potential for kinking or entrapment of the small bowel. The two openings in the mesentery are approximated with absorbable suture to reduce the potential for bowel herniation through either site. The globular shape of the gastric wedge is then anastomosed to the previously bivalved bladder using two layers of absorbable suture.

Sigmoid Cystoplasty (Fig. 10–3)

Because of the close proximity of the descending colon and the bladder, the sigmoid colon has also been used for bladder augmentation. Additional advantages include its large lumen and thick wall. However, because of the higher resting pressures, intractable contractions despite

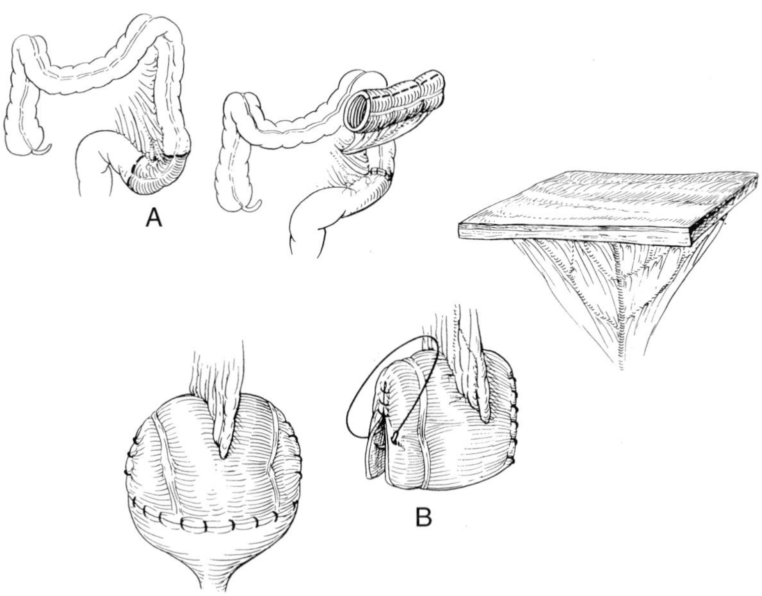

Figure 10–3 Sigmoid cystoplasty. *A,* Sigmoid segment measuring approximately 10 cm in length is isolated and opened along its antimesenteric border (dotted line). *B,* A two-layer anastomosis of the reconfigured segment to the bivalved bladder is fashioned.

detubularization, and increased mucus production exhibited by sigmoid segments, this location has typically been our last choice of a segment for augmentation. The sigmoid might be chosen in the patient with extensive peritoneal reaction secondary to the presence of a VP shunt. As a result of the largely retroperitoneal position of the colon, the sigmoid will often be spared from this inflammatory process. The sigmoid colon may also be the optimal choice in someone with a previous partial small bowel resection.

After entry into the peritoneal cavity, the sigmoid is mobilized by incising along the white line of Toldt. The sigmoid is then mobilized from its lateral and posterior attachments as far as the sacral promontory medially and the inferior mesenteric artery superiorly. A 10-cm-long segment is identified and mesenteric windows are developed. Crossing mesenteric vessels are individually divided and ligated. In general, these windows may be kept quite small because of the close proximity to the bladder. The segment is then subtracted from the remaining descending colon and isolated with towels to prevent contamination of the peritoneal cavity. After a two-layer colocolostomy (as outlined for small bowel), the sigmoid segment is irrigated with neomycin solution, detubularized, and anastomosed to the bivalved bladder using two layers of absorbable suture. As with ileal and gastric augmentation, all drainage tubes exit through the native bladder wall.

ALTERNATIVE METHODS FOR INCREASING BLADDER CAPACITY

Because of problems that can arise after enterocystoplasty, alternative methods to increase bladder capacity have been sought. Structures lined with transitional epithelium may, by avoiding electrolyte imbalances and the formation of mucus, provide the ideal substitute for bladder augmentation. Two clinically applied methods for providing a urothelium-lined augmentation have been explored: ureteral augmentation and autoaugmentation.

Ureteral Augmentation (Fig. 10–4)

In the occasional patient who has an abnormally dilated ureter subserving a nonfunctional renal moiety, augmentation using ureter may achieve increased storage capacity.[17] Similarly, ureteral bladder augmentation can be performed with a dilated lower pole or upper pole ureter in a duplicated system.[18] Excellent improvement in functional storage capacity has been realized while avoiding the metabolic complications associated with various bowel segments.[17]

The patient receives a full bowel preparation in case the ureter cannot be used for this purpose and intestinal augmentation is necessary. As when operating on a massive megaloureter, we prefer the exposure that a midline

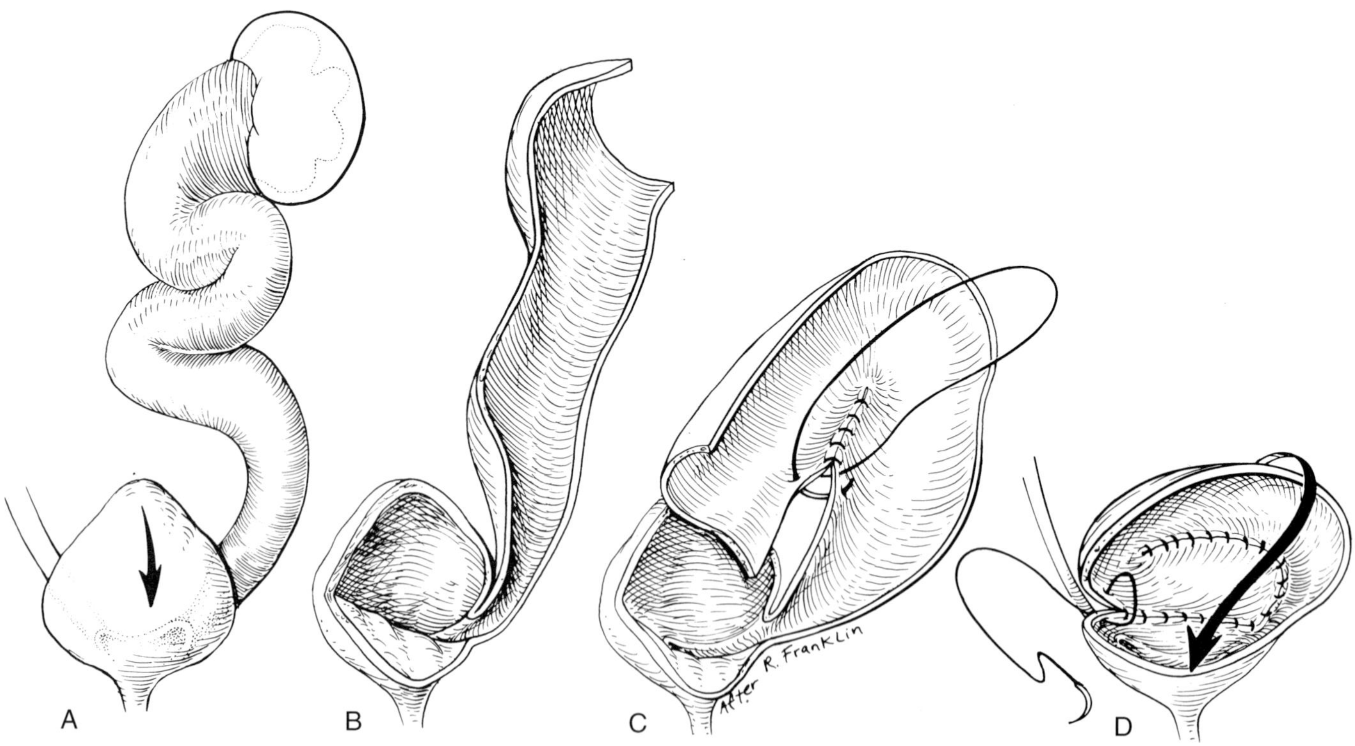

Figure 10–4 Ureteral cystoplasty. *A,* Dilated ureter subtending a nonfunctional kidney. The dilated ureter is detubularized longitudinally following nephrectomy *(B),* reconfigured as a U-shaped patch *(C),* and anastomosed to the bladder *(D).*

incision provides. Dissection is performed extraperitoneally. An extraperitoneal approach through a Pfannenstiel incision is also possible. After nephrectomy or transureteroureterostomy, the ureter is mobilized, taking great care to preserve its vascular supply. The ureter is detubularized longitudinally along its anterior wall from the renal pelvis (or upper end of the ureter) caudally through the intramural segment. The ureter is reconfigured as a U-shaped patch and anastomosed to the bladder in a similar fashion as that for an ileal augmentation. A suprapubic catheter is brought out through the native bladder wall to ensure optimal postoperative drainage.

Autoaugmentation (Fig. 10–5)

In performing an autoaugmentation of the bladder, a large, well-draining diverticulum is created that, in theory, should increase storage capacity.[19] Advantages of this technique over standard enterocystoplasty include avoidance of electrolyte imbalances, an extraperitoneal approach, and absence of suture lines.

A Foley catheter is inserted transurethrally at the beginning of the procedure, and the bladder is distended to aid in dissection during the seromyotomy. The bladder is exposed through a Pfannenstiel incision, and the peritoneum is swept off the dome and posterior aspect of the bladder to keep the procedure completely extraperitoneal. The muscle of the distended bladder is incised almost to the mucosa in a vertical midline plane over the dome in a posterior to anterior direction. The remaining few muscle fibers are teased apart with a hemostat to reveal the underlying bluish mucosa. A plane is developed laterally between the detrusor muscle and the underlying mucosa, taking great care not to violate the mucosal layer. Maintaining mucosal continuity may be especially difficult in a markedly hypertrophied and trabeculated bladder with numerous cellules. Should perforation of the mucosal layer occur, the site is oversewn with fine absorbable suture. Adequate mobilization of the muscle layer has been achieved when a wide-mouthed diverticulum is appreciated. The muscle flaps are excised, and the remaining detrusor muscle remains open by performing bilateral psoas hitches with absorbable suture. Postoperatively, the patient is left with a urethral catheter. Irrigation fluid is instilled into the bladder, beginning on the first postoperative day, as a means of keeping the neodiverticulum expanded.

Other authors have found that simple midline seromyotomy provides comparable results to seromyotomy and excision of the detrusor muscle.[20] Autoaugmentation has likewise been performed laparoscopically through both transabdominal and extraperitoneal approaches.[21, 22] Although initial results demonstrated improved capacity and compliance, reduced capacity seen with longer follow-up has tempered our enthusiasm for this procedure.[23] Many authors now reserve this procedure for the infrequent patient who has a poorly compliant bladder with an adequate preoperative capacity.[24]

Postoperative Management

Postoperative management principles common to all augmentation cystoplasties include meticulous attention to postoperative fluid shifts, secure dependable drainage, and early irrigation of the augmentation to clear mucous secretions. The ileocystoplasty or colocystoplasty is irri-

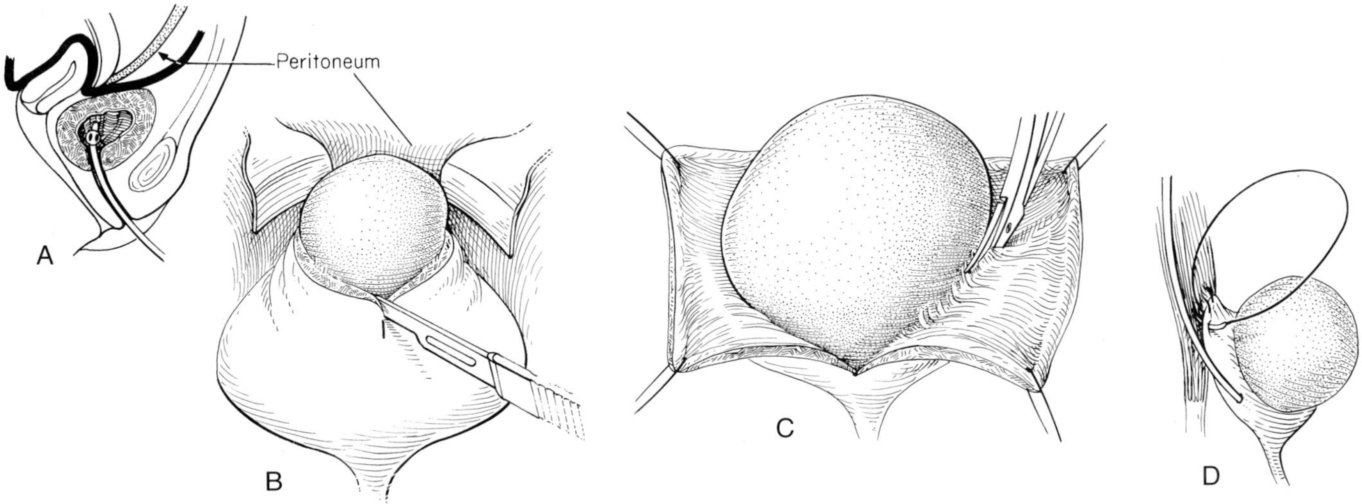

Figure 10–5 Autoaugmentation. *A,* The peritoneum is swept off the dome and posterior aspect of the bladder. *B,* The bladder is incised almost to the mucosa in the vertical midline, and *(C)* the muscularis is resected laterally leaving a large-mouthed diverticulum. *D,* Bilateral psoas hitches are performed with absorbable suture to keep the bladder base fixed in position.

gated three times a day with normal saline. A gastric augmentation is irrigated on the same schedule but with 500 mEq $NaHCO_3$/liter of normal saline to neutralize secreted acid. Further steps taken to reduce exposure of the suture line to stomach acid include the administration of histamine receptor antagonists (e.g., cimetidine). Initially administered parenterally, these medications are subsequently taken orally and continued until 6 months postoperatively. Urine pH is measured to ensure that an optimal buffering effect is achieved. The maintenance of a neutral pH is most important when urine is diverted from the reconstructed bladder during the early postoperative period. Failure to do so has been associated with a perforation in the early weeks after surgery.

Patients are discharged to home once they resume a regular diet. The reconstructed bladder is studied radiographically 3 weeks postoperatively with a cystogram.

INCONTINENCE SECONDARY TO LOW OUTLET RESISTANCE

General

Although augmentation cystoplasty reliably provides a compliant storage reservoir for urine, not all procedures to correct bladder neck incompetence have enjoyed the same success. In patients who are incontinent secondary to a low leak point pressure (less than 30 cm H_2O), restoration of urethral outlet resistance may take many forms, including conventional bladder neck tubularization, creation of a flap-valve mechanism, elevation-compression of the urethrovesical unit with a fascial sling, and the utilization of artificial materials to narrow the urethral lumen. If outlet resistance cannot be reliably restored or the patient is unable to successfully catheterize the urethra, construction of a continent efferent limb (e.g., Mitrofanoff principle)[25] or a continent cystostomy has proven to be a versatile and reliable solution.

BLADDER NECK TUBULARIZATION AND URETHRAL LENGTHENING

The concept of improving outlet resistance by increasing the functional length of the urethra was first proposed by Young in 1907.[26] Bilateral triangular reduction of the vesical neck was introduced by Dees as a means to add mechanical support to the lengthened urethra.[27] Leadbetter further modified this operation by demonstrating that proximal reimplantation of the ureters and full-thickness wrapping of bladder neck musculature would allow for improved reconstruction of the trigonal tube.[28] The primary advantage of this and other urethral lengthening procedures is the avoidance of artificial materials or nonorthotopic tissue in the reconstruction. The primary disadvantage is the necessity for ureteral reimplantation as well as the resultant reduction in bladder capacity. Success with this procedure depends on the availability of healthy tissue at the bladder neck. In boys who achieve only partial continence after this surgery, maturation of the prostate during puberty may provide the necessary increase in outlet resistance to achieve socially acceptable continence.[29]

Young-Dees-Leadbetter Procedure (Fig. 10–6)

The patient is placed in a supine position, and the perivesical space is exposed through either a Pfannenstiel or midline incision (if a concomitant augmentation cystoplasty is performed). The vesical neck and urethra are dissected free from surrounding tissue. Posterior mobilization is avoided so as not to risk injury to vagina, bowel, or pelvic neurovascular bundles. The bladder is opened in the vertical midline plane, and proximal reimplantation of the ureters is performed to allow more cephalad tubularization of the trigone. Reimplantation is typically achieved using the transtrigonal technique. A posterior strip of bladder measuring 14 mm in width by 4 cm in length is outlined. The triangular segment of mucosa on either side of this central mucosa strip is denuded using fine-needle cautery. The muscular triangles are incised transversely along their cephalad border. A running 4-0 chromic suture is used to create the mucosal layer of the neourethra over an 8 French feeding tube. A second layer of 4-0 Vicryl is placed to reinforce this first suture line. The lateral musculature is then closed over the newly formed urethral tube in a pants-over-vest fashion with interrupted 3-0 Vicryl suture. In doing so, the more mobile flap is wrapped first. It is sutured to the junction between the neourethra and the opposite muscle flap. The second flap is then wrapped over the first as tightly as possible. Postoperative drainage consists of a suprapubic tube, and the neourethra is left stented with an 8 French feeding tube for 3 weeks. The stent is removed, and once successful catheterization can be performed the suprapubic tube is removed.

Two procedures are designed to increase bladder outlet resistance by combining the principle of urethral lengthening and flap-valve dynamics. In the Kropp procedure,[30] a tube created from a full-thickness strip of anterior bladder wall is tunneled under the posterior bladder wall mucosa (Fig. 10–7). As the bladder fills the tunnel is compressed, preventing anterograde passage of urine. Although this is quite successful in achieving continence, frequent difficulties with catheterization have reduced the enthusiasm for this technique. Building on the same mechanical principles for increasing resistance, Pippi Salle and colleagues proposed a "flip-flap" technique to lengthen the urethra.[31]

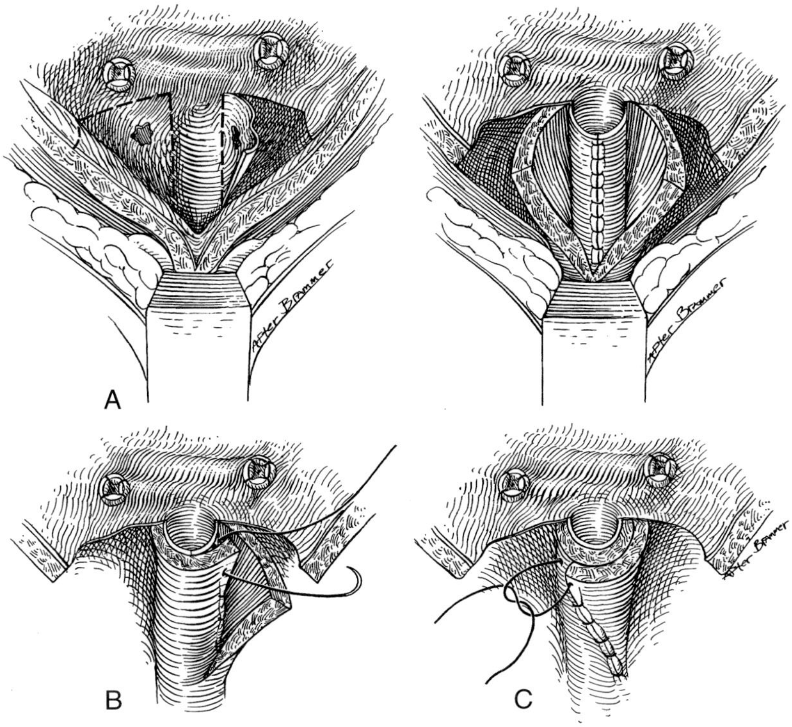

Figure 10–6 Leadbetter procedure. *A,* The full-thickness posterior wall of the bladder is incised down to the old bladder neck, and the mucosa is tubularized with a running suture over an 8 or 10 French catheter (not shown). *B* and *C,* Lateral flaps of the bladder neck are placed over the neourethra in a pants-over-vest fashion, creating a three-layer closure.

The Pippi Salle Procedure (Fig. 10–8)

The perivesical space is developed through either a Pfannenstiel or midline incision. With the bladder partially filled, a 7-cm long anterior flap is outlined. The flap is 2.5 cm wide at its base and tapers down to 1.5 cm at the most cephalad extent. A 3-mm edge of mucosa is removed from the lateral edges of the flap, and an excess is left at the cephalad extent to aid in later maturation of the stoma. Next, a posterior bladder mucosal strip measuring 7 cm long × 1 cm wide is developed. Once the ureters are reimplanted in a more cephalad position, the mucosa is elevated on either side of the posterior bladder wall flap. They should be freed up enough so that the mucosal edges can be brought together in the midline without tension (typically beyond the old hiatus). The mucosa of the anterior bladder wall flap is sutured to the posteriorly outlined strip using a running subcuticular 4-0 Vicryl suture. Uniform tubularization is made easier by progressing simultaneously with both the left and right suture lines. The muscle layer of the flap is sewn to the exposed posterior trigonal muscle on either side of the mucosal strip using interrupted 4-0 Vicryl suture. Care is taken not to make this closure too tight to avoid injuring the blood supply of the flap. Once ease of catheterization is demonstrated, a submucosal tunnel is constructed from the previously mobilized lateral mucosal flaps. These flaps should cover the entire intravesical urethra down to the level of the bladder neck. The extra mucosa that has been left with the cephalad extent of the flap is sutured to the reapproximated lateral trigonal mucosal flaps to effectively mature the new "bladder neck." A two-layer closure of the bladder is performed, allowing a pocket of bladder neck to extend down to the base of the neourethra. The bladder wall is sutured to the serosal surface of the flap as far inferiorly as possible to effectively elongate the tunnel and the bladder base. As this narrow pouch of bladder neck fills with fluid, it will compress the newly created flap-valve mechanism and provide continence. Postoperative drainage consists of a suprapubic catheter, bilateral ureteral stents, and an 8 French feeding tube left across the neourethra. As with other urethral lengthening procedures, the urethral stent is removed 3 weeks postoperatively and the patient is started on CIC.

BLADDER NECK SUSPENSION

Another method that improves outlet resistance while keeping the bladder outlet intact is a rectus fascial sling. By elevating and maintaining the urethrovesical unit in a more intra-abdominal position, this technique both compresses the urethral lumen and improves transmission of sudden increases in abdominal pressure to the bladder outlet.[32, 33] The procedure is technically straightforward, can be performed after other types of failed bladder neck operations, and avoids the use of artificial materials.[34] Although this procedure has been performed successfully in both females and males,[35] concern remains over the ability to adequately raise and compress the

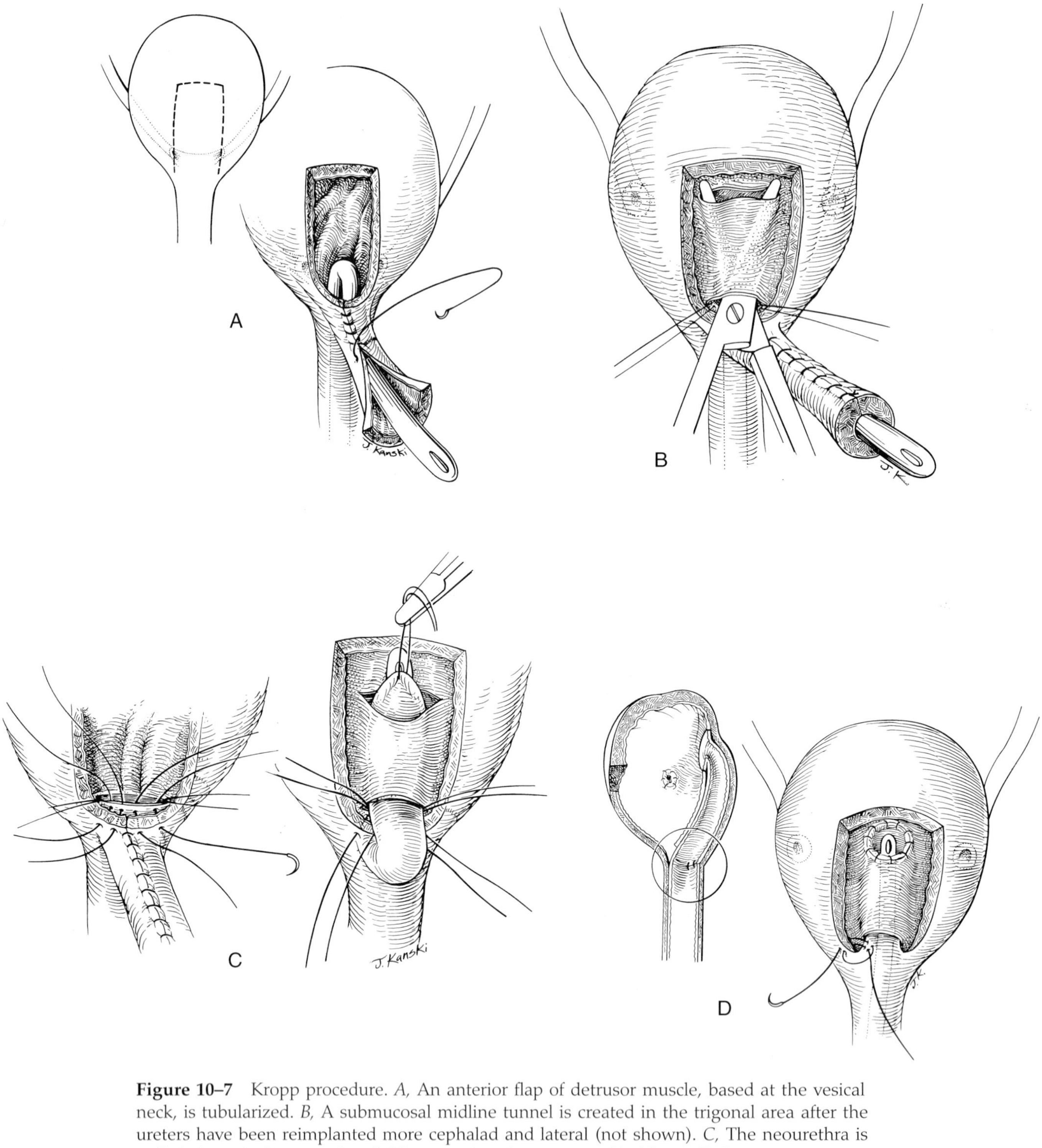

Figure 10–7 Kropp procedure. *A,* An anterior flap of detrusor muscle, based at the vesical neck, is tubularized. *B,* A submucosal midline tunnel is created in the trigonal area after the ureters have been reimplanted more cephalad and lateral (not shown). *C,* The neourethra is pulled through this tunnel and *(D)* sutured to the posterior bladder wall. Strategic sutures are placed to fix the base of the tube to the posterior bladder wall.

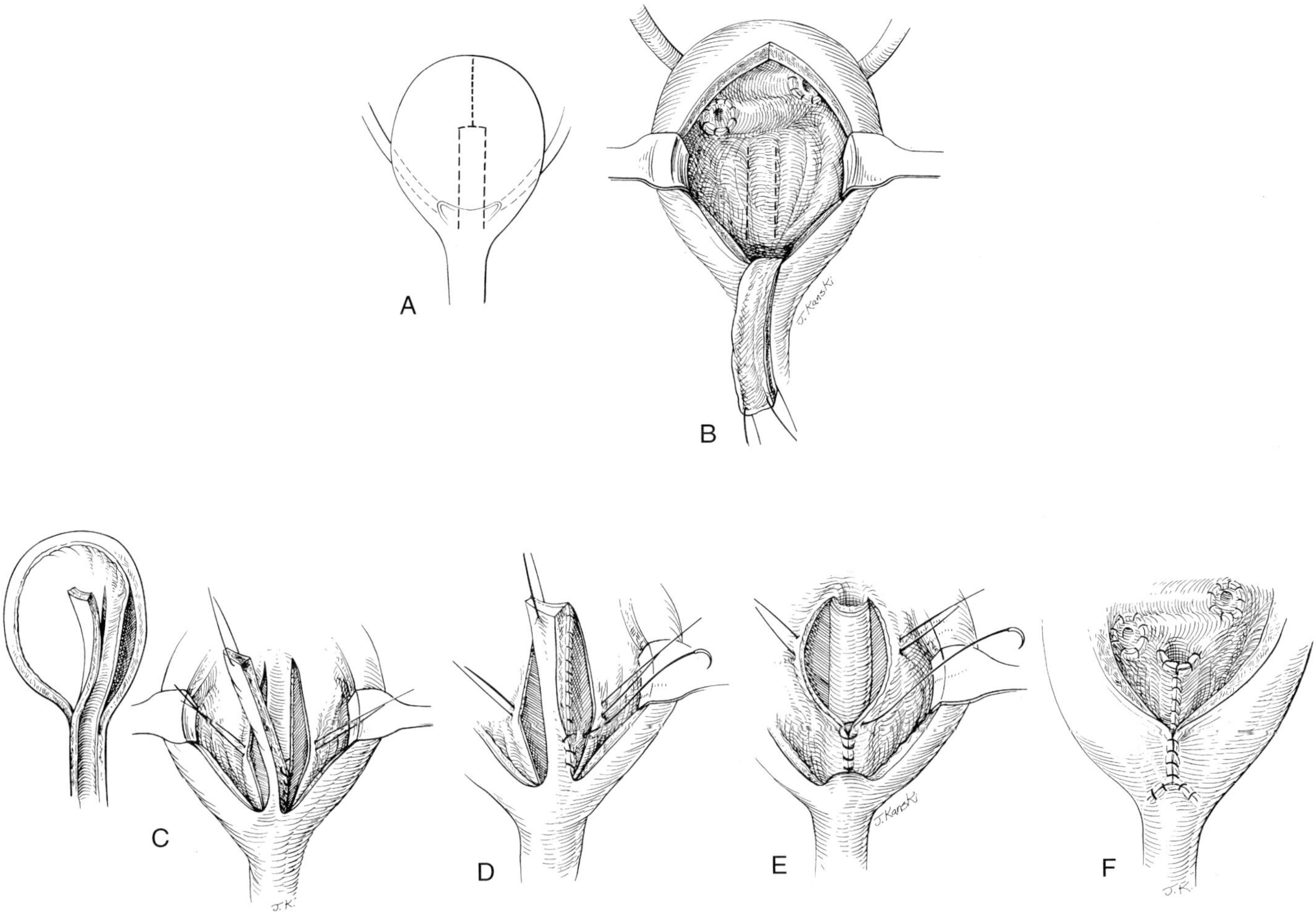

Figure 10–8 Pippi Salle procedure. *A,* With the bladder partially filled, a 7-cm-long anterior flap is developed. *B,* Once the ureters are reimplanted in a more cephalad position, a posterior bladder mucosal strip measuring 7 cm long × 1 cm wide is developed. *C,* The mucosa of the anterior bladder wall flap is sutured to the posteriorly outlined strip using a running subcuticular suture. *D,* The muscle is then sutured to the posterior bladder wall musculature, and *(E)* a submucosal tunnel is constructed from the previously mobilized lateral mucosal flaps to create a flap valve mechanism. *F,* Completed anastomosis with maturing of the neourethral meatus.

prostatic urethra against the anterior abdominal wall in postpubertal boys.[34]

The Rectus Fascial Sling

Preoperatively, an enema is used in male patients to evacuate stool from the rectum. Postpubertal females receive a vaginal povidone-iodine (Betadine) douche. Sterility of the urine is documented, and all patients receive perioperative parenteral prophylactic antibiotics. At surgery, patients are placed in either a frog-legged (prepubertal girls and boys) or lithotomy (postpubertal females) position. A vaginal preparation is performed in females, and a povidone-iodine–soaked sponge is placed per rectum in all males. A suprapubic approach through a Pfannenstiel incision provides excellent exposure to harvest rectus fascia and dissect around the bladder neck. A 12- to 14-cm-long and 1.5-cm-wide strip of rectus fascia is harvested in either the transverse or vertical direction. A significantly smaller strip of rectus fascia, on the order of 3 × 4 cm, is required when using the vaginal approach. In both cases, the harvested strip is prepared by placing Prolene sutures in all four corners and then placing the tissue in a saline-soaked sponge while the bladder neck is prepared.

Suprapubic Approach (Fig. 10–9)

When using the suprapubic approach, the vesical neck is cleared of surrounding loose connective tissue. Incising the endopelvic fascia provides access to the plane between the urethra and vagina in females or the urethra and rectum in males. Care must be taken in developing this plane. Dissection too close to the urethra can result

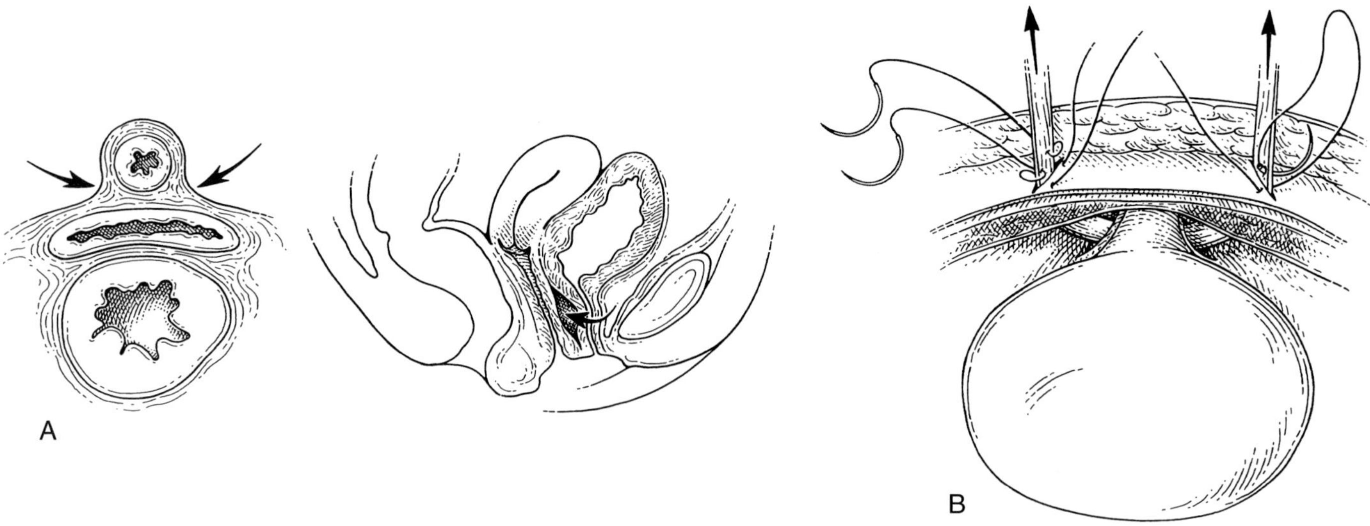

Figure 10–9 Rectus fascial sling (suprapubic approach). *A,* After adequate suprapubic exposure of the space of Retzius, the plane between either the urethra and vagina (girls) or urethra and rectum (boys) is developed *(arrows). B,* After a 7 × 2-cm segment of anterior rectus fascia has been harvested, it is placed around the urethra. The ends of the strip are brought through the anterior abdominal wall and secured to the rectus sheath at each lateral edge before being tied over one another on top of the midline rectus sheath.

in violation of the urethral wall, and a more lateral dissection around the urethra can lead to injury to the rectum, vagina, or neurovascular bundles. For prepubertal girls in whom the vaginal wall can be quite thin, insertion of a separately gloved finger into the vagina may help in properly identifying this plane. Gentle tension to snug the Foley balloon catheter up against the bladder neck may also prove helpful in defining the posterior wall of the urethra. Once this plane is properly developed, the sling is brought around the bladder neck and through the rectus fascia as close to the pubic bone as possible. The ends are tied over the rectus fascia in a crisscross manner so as to leave the sling fitting snugly under the urethrovesical junction. It is important to avoid applying too much upward force in securing the sling because this might make catheterization difficult or impossible.

Vaginal Approach (Fig. 10–10)

When performing a sling procedure in the postpubertal sexually active female, the vaginal approach with its capacious channel facilitates exposure to the bladder neck for placement of the fascial patch. Exposure is optimized by tacking the labia laterally with silk sutures and placing a weighted speculum in the vagina. An inverted U-shaped incision is made in the vaginal mucosa with the apex at the level of the midurethra. The vaginal flap is raised and the glistening white periurethral fascia identified. Lateral and superior dissection of the anterior vagina is continued to the level of the bladder neck. With a Metzenbaum scissors placed against the pubic bone and directed toward the ipsilateral shoulder, the endopelvic fascia is opened. Using an index finger, the remaining endopelvic fascia is swept posteriorly from the pubic bone, thereby mobilizing the urethra and vagina. A double-ligature carrier is introduced through a small Pfannenstiel incision, dissected down to the rectus fascia, and placed onto the surgeon's index finger that has been positioned retropubically through the vaginal incision. The sutures are transferred suprapubically, and cystoscopy is performed to ensure there has been no perforation of the bladder or urethra. Methylene blue is given to test patency of the ureters. The midpoint of the strip is now secured in the midline with a fine absorbable suture, and the vaginal incision is closed. The sutures of the sling are tied snugly over the rectus fascia, and an antibiotic-soaked vaginal packing is placed to conclude the procedure.

PROSTHETIC MECHANICAL COMPRESSION

Increasing urethral resistance using prosthetic materials is available by two methods: placement of an artificial urethral sphincter (AUS)[36] or injection of periurethral bulking agents (Teflon, collagen, autologous chondrocytes).[37–39] After the initial description of the artificial urethral sphincter by Scott and coworkers in 1973, numerous improvements in biomaterials and product design helped it gain acceptance.

The incontinent child with myelodysplasia who potentially benefits the most from an AUS should have a

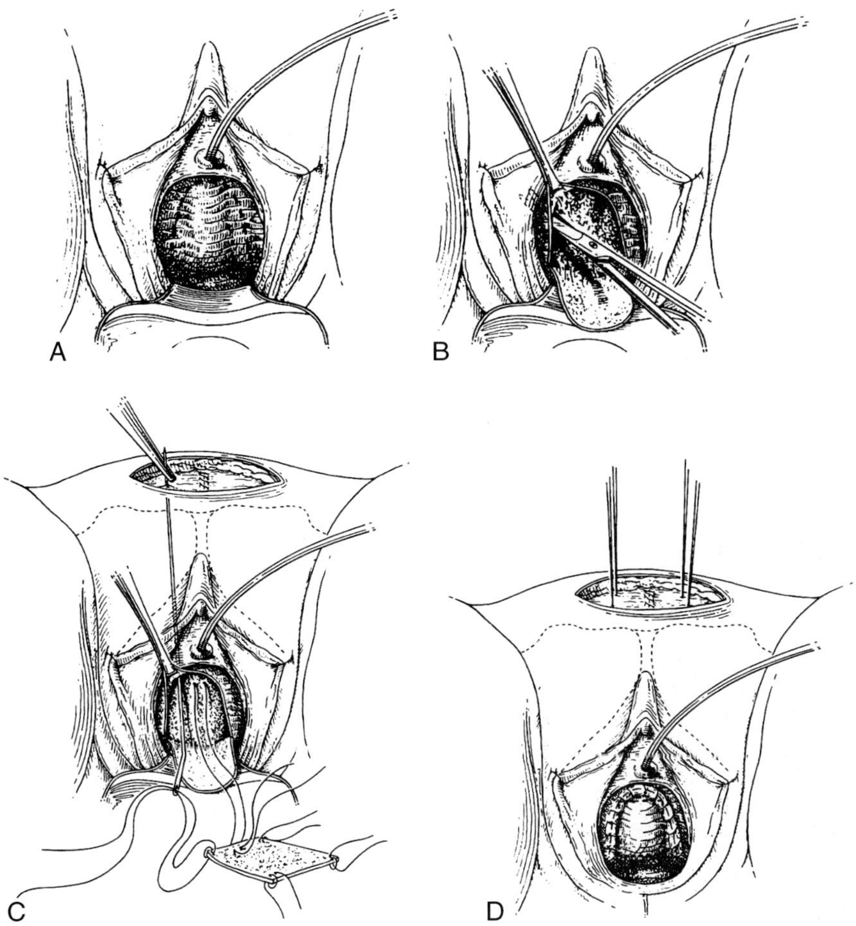

Figure 10–10 Pubovaginal sling (vaginal approach). *A,* An inverted U flap is created, *(B)* exposing the endopelvic fascia along the bladder neck. *C,* Sutures are then passed from the corners of a 3 × 4-cm rectus fascial patch to the anterior rectus sheath. *D,* After proper positioning of the flap against the urethra and bladder neck, the vaginal incision is closed. Sutures are subsequently tied over the intact rectus fascia.

large-capacity, highly compliant bladder and be able to void spontaneously. Patients with a low-capacity, poorly compliant reservoir who have had prior augmentation and can still demonstrate the ability to void to completion with abdominal straining are also considered appropriate candidates. Only 5% of myelodysplastic patients fit into this category. The advantage of the AUS is that it provides adequate outlet resistance that can be episodically lowered. Artificial sphincter placement does not preclude the use of CIC in those children who cannot empty their bladders by Valsalva or Crede's maneuver. Despite a high initial success rate, enthusiasm has been tempered somewhat by its modest complication rate and the need for periodic revision.[40–42]

Technique of AUS (Fig. 10–11)

As with any artificial device, if the AUS becomes infected it will require immediate removal. Therefore, before implantation of this device, it is imperative that sterility of the urine be documented. Patients receive a Fleet's enema and a bisacodyl (Dulcolax) suppository to empty the rectum. A povidone-iodine–soaked sponge in the rectum in the male or in the vagina in the female aids in identification of the plane surrounding the urethra.

The perivesical space is entered through either a midline or transverse abdominal incision. After correction of any upper urinary tract disease (e.g., vesicoureteral reflux, ureterovesical junction obstruction), the bladder neck is cleared of surrounding soft tissue, the endopelvic fascia incised, and the plane between the urethra and vagina (rectum in boys) developed. The sphincter cuff sizer is then placed snugly around the urethra to determine the appropriate length of the cuff. Tubing from the cuff leads to the pump that is placed in the hemiscrotum opposite the child's dominant handedness. The reservoir is placed into a pouch below the rectus fascia outside of the peritoneum on the same side as the pump. We try to choose a balloon pressure that is below the diastolic pressure. Higher reservoir pressures have been shown to have a significantly higher rate of erosion.[43] The tubing from the reservoir is then brought through the rectus fascia and connected to the pump. All tubing from each component is kept on one side of the midline in case nonprosthetic surgery is required in the future (this avoids exposure of any portion of the device as long as the surgeon remains in the midline). Postoperatively, the sphincter is left deactivated (in the open position) for 10 to 12 weeks to allow for healing of tissues beneath the cuff and in the scrotum.

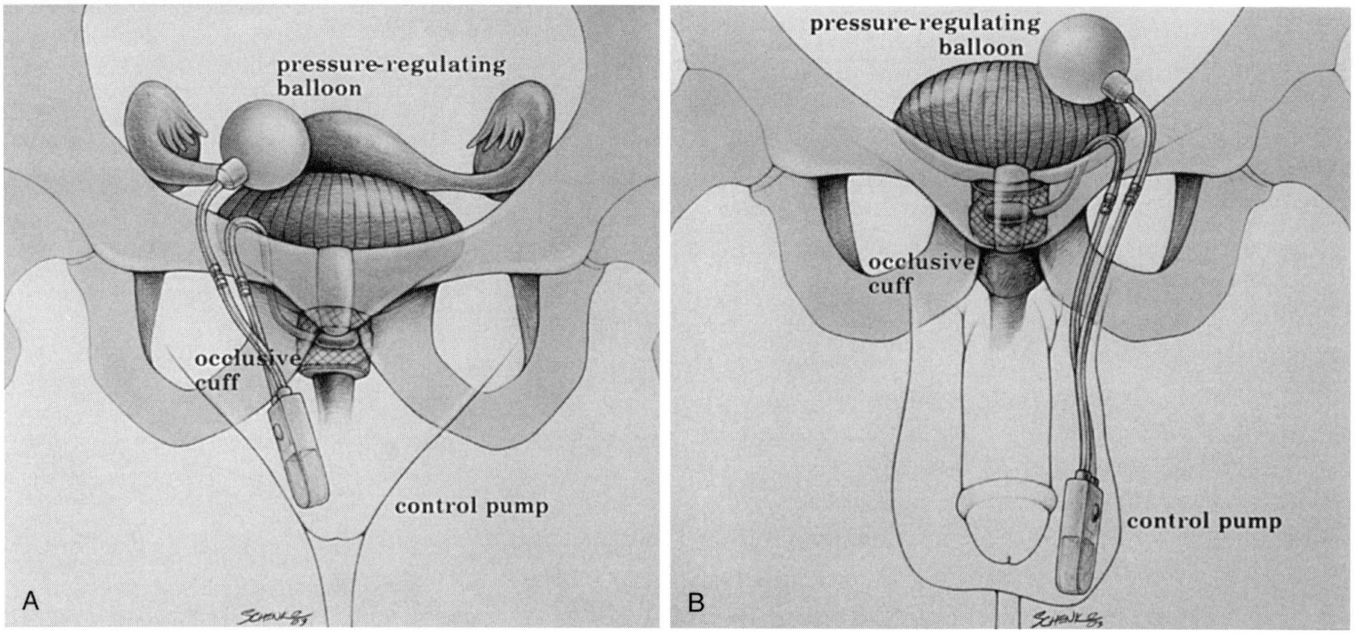

Figure 10–11 Artificial urinary sphincter (AUS). The connected AUS in place with the cuff at the bladder neck and the pump in either the *(A)* labia majora or (B) dependent scrotum (bulbar placement is not recommended in the prepubertal male).

In the older male, the sphincter cuff may be placed around the bulbous urethra. Although this approach is technically easier to perform than the perivesical approach, this location should not be used in the prepubertal boy because the tissue of the immature bulb is thin and the risk of erosion is high.

Technique of Periurethral Collagen Injection

The concept of injecting an exogenous substance in a periurethral location to coapt the urethral lumen and thereby increase urethral resistance was introduced in the 1960s. Polytetrauroethylene was the first widely applied substance for this purpose. Although improvement in continence in both adult and pediatric patients was realized, enthusiasm waned as reports of particle migration into vital structures (e.g., brain, liver) appeared in the literature.[44] The early favorable results from this minimally invasive procedure spurned interest in identifying biologically compatible substances that could achieve the same end. Many such alternative substances have been proposed, with glutaraldehyde cross-linked collagen having had the greatest application and longest follow-up thus far.

Potential candidates receive an intradermal injection of 0.1 mL glutaraldehyde cross-linked bovine collagen to rule out hypersensitivity. Children with a negative skin test and a negative urine culture are suitable candidates for the procedure. Procedures in children are carried out under general anesthesia in the dorsal lithotomy position. Prophylactic antibiotics are provided, and a suprapubic tube is placed to avoid postoperative catheterization with its potential to deform the collagen bleb. Two techniques exist for delivery of injectable collagen. In males the transurethral approach is preferred. Through the working channel of a cystoscope, a 5-gauge needle is inserted beneath the urothelial surface with injections at the 3 and 9 o'clock positions just distal to the bladder neck. The epithelium is elevated until visual occlusion of the urethral lumen is achieved. A periurethral approach for delivery is preferred in girls because of the shorter urethra. With the cystoscope positioned just distal to the bladder neck, a 22-gauge spinal needle is introduced into the periurethral tissue. Once movement of the needle tip can be identified below the surface of the epithelium, collagen is injected until visual occlusion of the urethra is achieved. After the injection, the cystoscope is not introduced into the bladder so as to avoid deforming the collagen bleb.

The advantage of periurethral injection therapy lies in its ease and the ability to perform the injections on an outpatient basis. Perez and colleagues showed that, after a single injection, 20% become dry and an additional 28% are improved.[45] Bomalaski and others reported improved continence in the neurogenic population in up to 70% of cases, with an average follow-up of 2.1 years.[46] Multiple injections were needed in the majority of these children to maintain this success.

Periurethral injections may be successful in myelomeningocele patients who suffer from low outlet resistance and who have stress urinary incontinence. Although periurethral collagen injections have been reported not to increase the difficulty of subsequent urethral lengthening or sling procedures, we prefer not to use this method as first-line therapy. We reserve the use of collagen injections to improve residual incontinence in patients who have undergone a partially successful open procedure and who have minimal residual leakage.

CONTINENT URINARY DIVERSION

Surgical procedures at the bladder neck may fail to provide the necessary increase in outlet resistance to keep the child dry. Patients with severe neurologic disorders and those who have undergone multiple surgical procedures at the bladder neck may benefit from bladder neck closure and creation of a catheterizable stoma. Patients who demonstrate difficulty catheterizing via the normal urethra may likewise benefit from the Mitrofanoff procedure. Reliable bladder neck closure requires complete disruption of epithelial continuity and meticulous multiple-layer closure with interposition of vascularized tissue (i.e., omentum) to avoid fistula formation. Optimal exposure is achieved with the bladder open so the bladder neck can be viewed under direct vision.

Numerous techniques have been devised to provide a continent catheterizable stoma when the native bladder neck is considered inadequate for continent reconstruction.[47, 48] We believe that the flap-valve principle is the most versatile and reliable method by which to achieve this end.

The flap-valve principle, commonly referred to as the Mitrofanoff principle, is a recapitulation of the nonrefluxing intramural ureter. Pressure elevation within the reservoir is effectively transmitted to a supple, small-diameter conduit positioned in a submucosal location, thus compressing its lumen.[49] Structures that have been used as the catheterizable conduit include the appendix,[25] ureter,[25] tapered ileum,[50] stomach,[51, 52] cecum,[53] fallopian tube,[54] and even preputial skin.[55] In patients with a large-capacity bladder, a detrusor tube can also function as a flap-valve mechanism.[56] The wide range of potential segments from which one can construct this narrow-gauge conduit underscores its versatility. We prefer using the appendix when available. This sentiment is borne out after conduit pressure profilometric findings of 20 children with catheterizable urinary conduits in which appendiceal segments were found to have the longest functional profile length.[57] Other authors have cited higher complication rates[58] and greater discomfort with catheterization[50] when incorporating ureter in the efferent limb. When other segments are used, it is imperative that a functional Mitrofanoff profile length of greater than 2.0 cm be created. Care is required in establishing an adequate tunnel length, especially when ureter is tunneled into bowel.[57] If a refluxing distal ureter is chosen as the conduit, an extravesical type of reimplantation (i.e., Lich-Gregoir[59]) should be used so as to preserve its distal blood supply.

Appendicocystostomy (Fig. 10–12)

All patients undergo a mechanical and antibiotic bowel preparation and receive broad-spectrum intravenous antibiotics before proceeding to the operating room. Through a midline laparotomy, the appendix is identified and isolated from the cecum, taking care to preserve the appendiceal blood supply. If the appendix is not of adequate length, a segment of cecum may be taken with the appendix and tubularized to extend the proximal end of the conduit. After the cecum is closed and appendix irrigated free of any fecaliths, a catheter is placed through the appendiceal lumen to ensure an adequate diameter and no obstruction. The proximal end of the appendix is implanted into the bladder to create a flap-valve continence mechanism. The distal end of the appendix is brought through the abdominal wall stoma site or umbilicus and sutured at both the level of the fascia and skin. To prevent stomal stenosis, a U-shaped skin flap is advanced into the spatulated end of the appendix. Finally, PDS suture is used to fix the bladder to the anterior abdominal wall at the site where the appendix traverses the rectus fascia. This will help support the appendix, prevent kinking, and facilitate catheterization.

The Continent Cystotomy (Fig. 10–13)

The patient who possesses a highly compliant large-capacity bladder (i.e., lower motor neuron lesion) but does not have the ability to empty the bladder completely is typically maintained on CIC. Although CIC is an excellent means of emptying the bladder efficiently, several factors may make CIC through the native urethra difficult: poor manual dexterity, obesity, bracing, posture, urethral stricture, or previously failed bladder neck surgery. In these individuals, a catheterizable tube based on the Mitrofanoff flap-valve mechanism may be constructed from the bladder itself.[56] This technique allows one to use bladder tissue for both the continence mechanism and the stoma.

The bladder is exposed through a Pfannenstiel incision and the peritoneum is swept off the dome and posterior aspect of the bladder wall. A bladder flap measuring 7 cm in length and 2 cm in width is marked out just lateral to midline. Electrocautery is used to incise the flap down through the mucosa. The strip is rotated cephalad and the incisions are advanced an additional 3 cm distally through the intact bladder mucosa only at the base of the flap. The mucosa on either side of the additional incisions is elevated for later construction of a submucosal tunnel. The flap is tubularized over a 10 French feeding tube by approximating the mucosa along its entire 10-cm length with a running 4-0 Vicryl suture (see Fig. 10–13). The 10 French feeding tube is replaced by an 8 French feeding tube, and the muscle portion of the flap is closed with a running 3-0 Vicryl suture. The

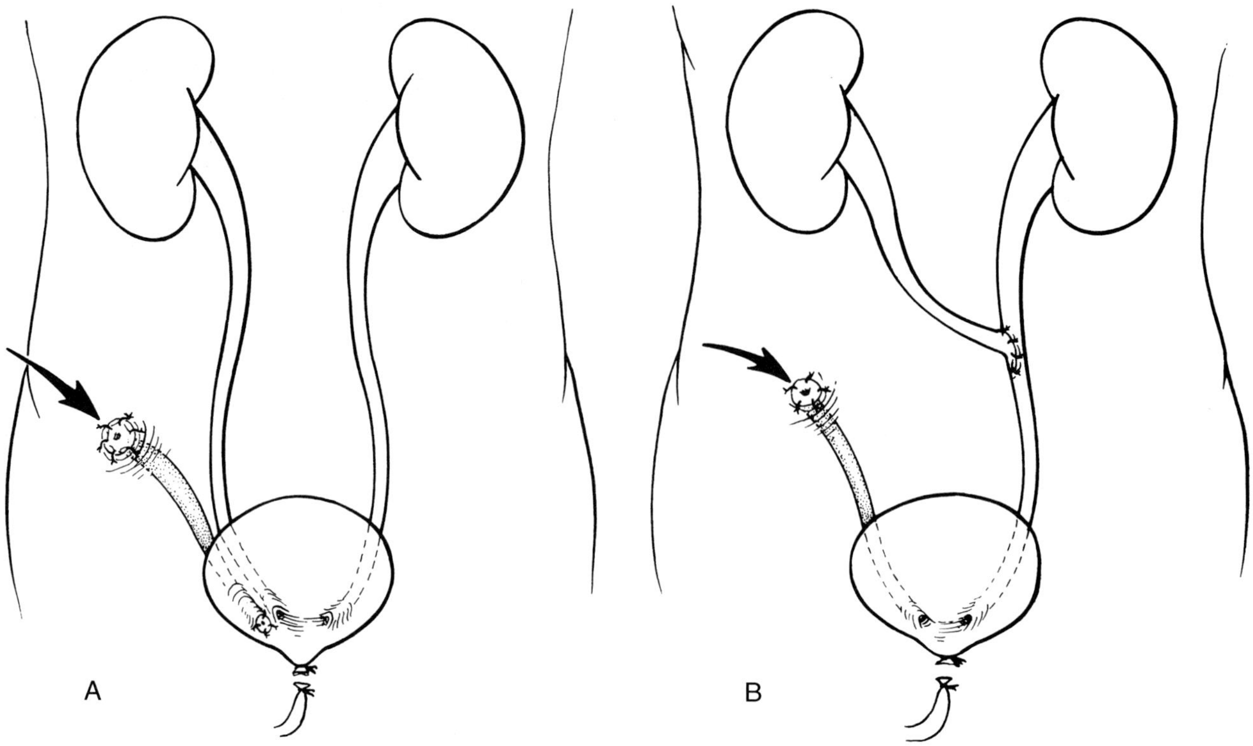

Figure 10–12 Mitrofanoff principle. A nonrefluxing flap valve mechanism is created from appendix *(A)* or distal ureter *(B)*.

bladder mucosa lateral to the 3-cm extension of the tube is approximated to provide a continent submucosal tunnel. The anterior bladder wall is closed in two layers using running 3-0 Vicryl suture. The distal end of the tube is brought through the anterior abdominal wall at the site of the proposed stoma. A wide-based triangular skin flap is interposed into the stomal end of the tube to provide a better cosmetic result and to prevent stomal stenosis. At the completion of the procedure, the bladder is filled through a urethral catheter to test the continence mechanism. As with other Mitrofanoff catheterizable stomas constructed from intestinal segments, multiple passes of a catheter across the tube are performed to ensure ease of catheterization. This is performed with the bladder both partially and completely full to guarantee reliable emptying at different bladder capacities. An 8 French feeding tube is left in place in the conduit and the bladder drained with a suprapubic tube. Catheterization through the stoma is begun 3 weeks postoperatively.

MANAGEMENT OF VESICOURETERAL REFLUX

Vesicoureteral reflux is present in 3 to 5% of newborns with myelodysplasia and increases to 30 to 40% by 5 years in children with detrusor hypertonicity and/or dyssynergia. A substantial number of these individuals will experience spontaneous resolution of their reflux if provided with low-pressure urinary storage and a means of timely evacuation. Patients with detrusor hypertonicity are treated with anticholinergic medication (e.g., oxybutynin chloride) to lower intravesical pressure and thereby ensure upper urinary tract decompression. CIC is instituted whenever complete bladder emptying cannot be achieved spontaneously. As with primary reflux, these children are kept on continuous antibiotic prophylaxis to prevent recurrent pyelonephritis.

Indications for antireflux surgery mirror those used for the care of primary reflux in the non-neurogenic population. Once low-pressure storage and reliable emptying are achieved, the indications for surgery include recurrent symptomatic urinary tract infections, persistent hydroureteronephrosis, severe reflux with an anatomic abnormality (i.e., Hutch diverticulum), progressive scarring or failure of renal growth, and reflux persisting into puberty. Antireflux surgery is also undertaken if one is considering a procedure to increase bladder outlet resistance. Ureters can be reliably implanted in a nonrefluxing fashion into either native bladder, the tenia of the colon,[60] or the wall of a gastric patch.[61]

MANAGEMENT OF FECAL INCONTINENCE

Although much attention has been given to achieving urinary continence in the myelodysplastic child, fecal con-

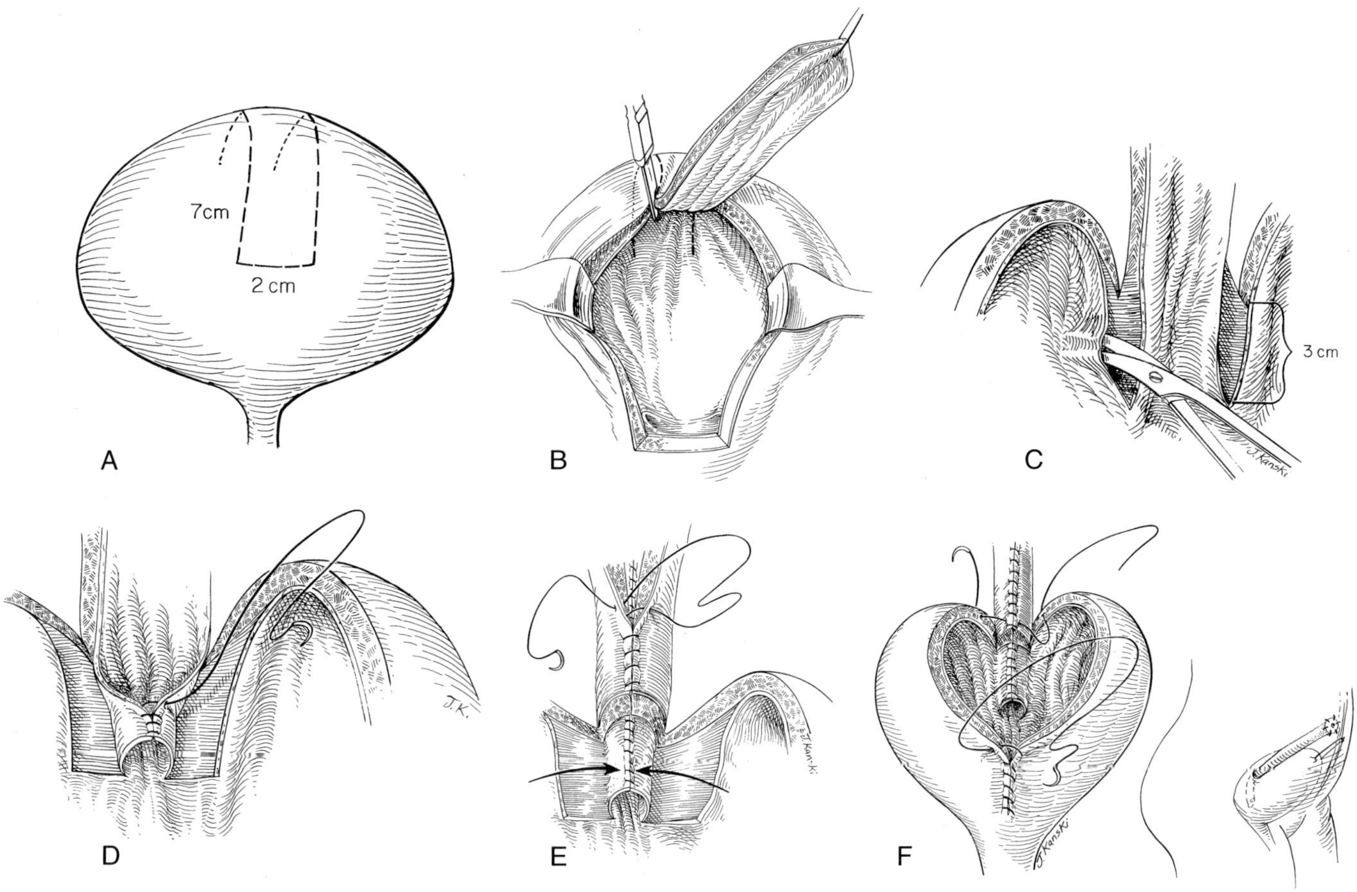

Figure 10–13 Continent cystotomy. *A,* An anterior flap of detrusor muscle based on the posterior bladder wall is outlined and *(B)* mobilized. *C,* The strip is rotated cephalad, and the incisions are advanced an additional 3 cm distally through the intact bladder mucosa at the base of the flap. *D,* The flap is tubularized over a 10 French tube by approximating the mucosa along its entire 10-cm length (catheter not shown). *E,* The muscle portion of the flap is closed with a running suture. The bladder mucosa lateral to the 3-cm extension of the tube is approximated to provide a continent submucosal tunnel *(arrows). F,* The tube is brought out to an abdominal wall stoma, and the anterior bladder wall is affixed, via pexis, to the posterior rectus sheath to prevent kinking of the conduit.

tinence has historically gone unaddressed by the urologist. Fecal soiling is a particularly important issue to consider because nearly 80% of these children will have abnormal bowel control.[5] Often, this is the only reason why many children remain in diapers. Conservative management to achieve fecal continence is typically based on a paradigm of controlled constipation with periodic evacuation. Specific measures to establish a regular bowel habit includes control of stool consistency through diet and drugs followed by purgatives or enemas to induce periodic colonic emptying. Although this regimen can be highly successful, a small segment of the spina bifida population remains incontinent.

In 1990, Malone and coworkers described a novel surgical technique to facilitate the maintenance of fecal continence.[62] On the basis of the principles set forth by Mitrofanoff, a nonrefluxing catheterizable channel is created with an appendiceal conduit tunneled into the cecum. Administration of anterograde washouts allows for reliable and complete evacuation of stool and a highly successful ability to achieve fecal continence.

The ACE Procedure (Fig. 10–14)

The patient undergoes a preoperative mechanical and antibiotic bowel cleansing. If the procedure is performed in conjunction with an augmentation cystoplasty or continent diversion, a midline laparotomy is the incision of choice. If plans include only the creation of an appendicocecostomy, then a right lower quadrant incision will suffice. After the appendix is identified, it can be either resected with an elongated cuff of cecum or left attached to the cecum if in situ implantation is anticipated. Care is taken in maintaining the appendiceal blood supply.

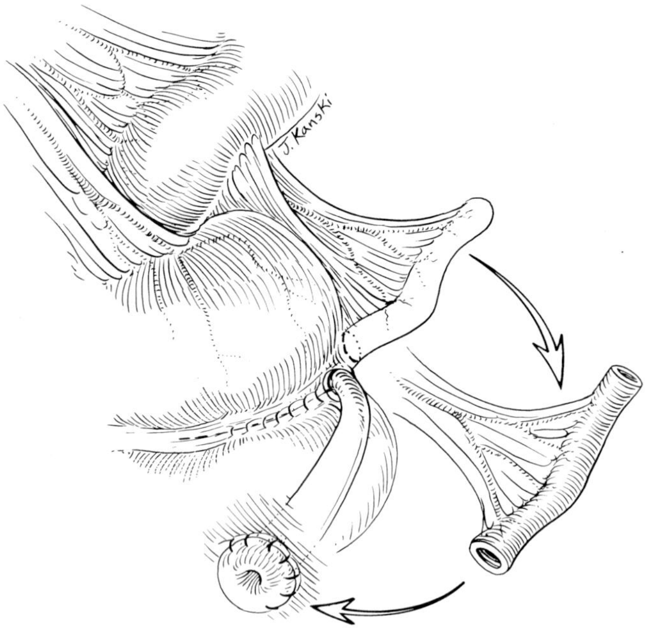

Figure 10–14 Anterograde continent enema (ACE) procedure. The base of the appendix is transected at the level of the cecum, taking great care to preserve its blood supply, after which the appendix is tunneled into the tenia of the colon and brought out as an umbilical stoma.

The distal end of the appendix is amputated, the lumen irrigated to remove any fecal residue, and the patency checked with a catheter.

For in situ implantation the appendix is placed into a submucosal tunnel in the tenia of the cecum. The distal end of the appendix is brought through the proposed stomal site and the cecum is anchored circumferentially to the anterior abdominal wall. The stoma is fashioned by sewing a broad-based U-shaped skin flap down to the appendiceal lumen. This technique serves to bury the appendix, minimize discharge onto the anterior abdominal wall, and prevent stomal stenosis.

COMPLICATIONS

The astute surgeon or clinician should be aware of and able to treat postoperative complications when performing urinary reconstruction in patients with neurogenic bladder dysfunction. These complications include bladder perforation, the formation of bladder calculi, metabolic disturbances, and difficulty with catheterization.

Perforation of the augmented bladder is usually manifest by abdominal distension, abdominal pain, decreased urine output, tachycardia, sepsis, and hypotension. In the neurogenic population, bladder perforation may be insidious in its onset and symptomatology (because of reduced peritoneal and bladder sensation), resulting in a substantial delay in diagnosis. Evaluation of these children requires an increased level of awareness that this condition may exist in order to detect this potentially life-threatening complication. Reduced urinary output, bloody drainage, and fever may well precede the significant signs of peritoneal irritation and sepsis. When perforation is suspected, a catheter is placed into the bladder and a fluoroscopically monitored cystogram is performed, with anteroposterior, oblique, and lateral films taken as the bladder is slowly filled to capacity and then emptied.[63] If the cystogram fails to reveal a perforation, computed tomography may aid in identifying a leak.

The presence of retained mucus, coupled with bacterial colonization of the reservoir, may result in the formation of urinary calculi. Adequate fluid intake, with a sustained diuresis, is of paramount importance in reducing the accumulation of lithogenic mucus. Stone formation is largely due to an inability to empty the augmented bladder completely. When a catheterizable stoma is used, it is more difficult to remove secretions and urine that pool in the dependent portion of the bladder. Although colonization is nearly impossible to avoid, daily irrigations with saline or an antibiotic solution followed by aspiration of the catheter will likely reduce the incidence of this menacing complication. Reservoirs consisting of gastric segments have the advantage of producing less mucus and maintaining a bacteriostatic (acidic) environment.[9] In our experience, stones or pyelonephritis developed in very few of the reservoirs that contain a segment of stomach. Finally, the presence of a foreign body may be responsible for the formation of bladder calculi. These may include nonabsorbable sutures, staples, and pubic hairs introduced during catheterization.

When stones do occur, it is important to evacuate all fragments because infectious stones will quickly reaccumulate if not completely cleared. Percutaneous methods can be applied if the stone burden is low.[64] In cases in which the stone burden is relatively great, open removal is simple, effective, and less time consuming and is the treatment of choice.

When incorporated into the urinary tract, each type of bowel segment can create its own potential metabolic alterations. If the ileum or colon is used, a hyperchloremic metabolic acidosis may ensue. Fortunately, the acidosis that develops is usually minor and does not result in any acute decompensation for most individuals with normal renal function. Long-term implications of chronic acidosis can, however, be quite significant. With persistent acidosis, the protons are buffered by release of calcium from bone. This has resulted in a reduction in mineralized bone in some patients with ileal or colonic cystoplasties.[65] We are presently monitoring bone mineralization in our patients with augmented bladders. Should profound acidosis be encountered, treatment includes the administration of oral alkalinizing agents.

Patients who have augmentations constructed from stomach may typically experience a hypochloremic metabolic alkalosis.[66] Treatment of subacute episodes primarily consists of oral histamine receptor antagonists. Severe episodes are frequently preceded by a gastrointestinal illness with associated diarrhea and vomiting. Despite the loss of hydrochloride from the gut, the gastric segment continues to secrete acid independently from the physiologic state, resulting in a profound metabolic derangement. Resuscitation with intravenous sodium chloride, potassium chloride, arginine hydrochloride, and histamine receptor antagonists should remedy the acute situation. If the metabolic derangement persists and proves resistant to available medical therapy, the patient may benefit from the addition of an absorptive surface (ileal patch) to the previously augmented bladder.[9]

Difficulty with catheterization can be encountered with each of the procedures used to increase outlet resistance. The highest incidence of problems with catheterization occurs with neotubularization techniques. This can prove especially deleterious in patients possessing an outlet configuration that depends on the flap-valve principle. As the bladder fills, the resistance to emptying progressively increases, and this can ultimately precipitate a perforation of the bladder. Difficulty with catheterization in all of these techniques can be minimized by creating a well-vascularized tube with a uniform diameter and smooth course. In the case of the Mitrofanoff catheterizable abdominal stoma and the continent cystostomy, transfixing the reservoir to the undersurface of the anterior abdominal wall or pelvic floor will also prevent angulation of the conduit at the point where it assumes an intramural course. Stenosis and subsequent difficulties with catheterization are minimized by preserving optimal vascular supply to the efferent segment. Finally, the advent of a U flap of abdominal skin connected to a spatulated conduit has proven to be an excellent method for avoiding stomal stenosis when creating an abdominal stoma.[67]

CONCLUSION

Many options exist for reconstructing the genitourinary tract of the myelodysplastic patient with neurogenic bladder. Rational surgical choices, close follow-up, and awareness of potential complications will ensure optimal results in these children.

REFERENCES

1. Stark G. Spina bifida: Problems and management. Oxford, England: Blackwell Scientific, 1977.
2. Bauer S, Labib K, Dieppa R, et al. Urodynamic evaluation in a boy with myelodysplasia and incontinence. Urology 10:354, 1977.
3. Pontari M, Keating M, Kelly M, et al. Retained sacral function in children with high level myelodysplasia. J Urol 154:775, 1995.
4. Bauer S, Hallet M, Khoshbin S, et al. The predictive value of urodynamic evaluation in the newborn with myelodysplasia. JAMA 152:650, 1984.
5. Hilwa N, Perlmutter AD. The role of adjunctive drug therapy for intermittent catheterization and self-catheterization for children with vesical dysfunction. J Urol 119:551, 1978.
6. Landau EH, Churchill BM, Jayanthi VR, et al. The sensitivity of pressure specific bladder volume versus total bladder capacity as a measure of bladder storage dysfunction. J Urol 152:1578, 1994.
7. Atala A, Bauer SB, Hendren WH, Retik AB. The effect of gastric augmentation on bladder function. J Urol 149:1099, 1993.
8. Hendren WH, Hendren RB. Bladder augmentation: Experience with 129 children and young adults. J Urol 144:445, 1990.
9. McLaughlin KP, Rink RC, Adams MC, Keating MA. Stomach in combination with other intestinal segments in pediatric lower urinary tract reconstruction. J Urol 154:1162, 1995.
10. Roth S, Semjonow A, Waldner M, Hertle L. Risk of bowel dysfunction with diarrhea after continent urinary diversion with ileal and ileocecal segmants. J Urol 154:1969, 1995.
11. Koch MO, McDougal WS. The pathophysiology of hyperchloremic metabolic acidosis after urinary diversion through intestinal segments. Surgery 98:561, 1985.
12. Reinberg Y, Manivel JC, Froemming C, Gonzalez R. Perforation of the gastric segment of an augmented bladder secondary to peptic ulcer disease. J Urol 148:369, 1992.
13. Kelly KJ, Pearson ML, Kurup VP, et al. A cluster of anaphylactic reactions in children with spina bifida during general anesthesia: Epidemiologic features, risk factors, and latex hypersensitivity. J Allergy Clin Immunol 94:53, 1994.
14. Merguerian PA, Klein RB, Graven MA, Rozycki AA. Intraoperative anaphylactic reaction due to latex hypersensitivity. Urology 38:301, 1991.
15. Hinman FJ. Selection of intestinal segments for bladder substitution: Physical and physiological characteristics. J Urol 139:519, 1988.
16. Wheeler RA, Malone PS. Use of the appendix in reconstructive surgery: A case against incidental appendicectomy (review). Br J Surg 78:1283, 1991.
17. Churchill BM, Aliabadi H, Landau EH, et al. Ureteral bladder augmentation. J Urol 150:716, 1993.
18. Ben-chaim J, Partin AW, Jeffs RD. Ureteral bladder augmentation using the lower pole ureter of a duplicated system. Urology 47:135, 1996.
19. Cartwright PC, Snow BW. Bladder autoaugmentation: Early clinical experience. J Urol 142:505, 1989.
20. Stothers L, Johnson H, Arnold W, et al. Bladder autoaugmentation by vesicomyotomy in the pediatric neurogenic bladder. Urology 44:110, 1994.
21. McDougal EM, Clayman RV, Figenshau RS, Pearle MS. Laparoscopic retropubic auto-augmentation of the bladder. J Urol 153:123, 1995.
22. Ehrlich RM, Gershman A. Laparoscopic seromyotomy (auto-augmentation) for non-neurogenic neurogenic bladder in a child: Initial case report. Urology 42:175, 1993.
23. Landa HM, Moorhead JD. Detrusorectomy. Probl Urol 8:404, 1994.
24. Rink RC. Choice of material for bladder augmentation. Curr Opin Urol 5:300, 1995.
25. Mitrofanoff P. Cystostomie continent trans-appendiculaire dans le traitement des vessies neurologiques. Chir Pediatr 21:297, 1980.
26. Young HH. Suture of the urethral and vesical sphincters for the cure of incontinence of urine, with a report of a case. Trans South Surg Gynecol Assoc 20:210, 1907.
27. Dees JE. Congenital epispadias with incontinence. J Urol 62:513, 1949.
28. Leadbetter GWJ. Surgical correction of total urinary incontinence. J Urol 91:261, 1964.

29. Kramer SA, Kelalis PP. Vesical neck reconstruction in patients with epispadias-exstrophy. J Urol 139:1278, 1988.
30. Kropp KA, Angwafo FF. Urethral lengthening and reimplantation for neurogenic incontinence in children. J Urol 135:533, 1986.
31. Pippi Salle JL, deFraga JCS, Amarante A, et al. Urethral lengthening with anterior bladder wall flap for urinary incontinence: A new approach. J Urol 152:803, 1994.
32. Woodside JR, Borden TA. Pubovaginal sling procedure for the management of urinary incontinence is a myelodysplastic girl. J Urol 127:744, 1982.
33. McGuire EJ, Wang CC, Usitalo H, Savastano J. Modified pubovaginal sling in girls with myelodysplasia. J Urol 135:94, 1986.
34. Bauer SB, Peters CA, Colodny AH, et al. The use of rectus fascia to manage urinary incontinence. J Urol 142:516, 1989.
35. Raz S, McGuire EJ, Ehrlich RM, et al. Fascial sling to correct male neurogenic sphincter incompetence. The McGuire/Raz approach. J Urol 139:528, 1988.
36. Scott FB, Bradley WE, Timm GW, Kothari D. Treatment of incontinence secondary to myelodysplasia by an implantable prosthetic urinary sphincter. South Med J 66:987, 1973.
37. Atala A, Cima LG, Kim W, et al. Injectable alginate seeded with chondrocytes as a potential treatment for vesicoureteral reflux. J Urol 150:745, 1993.
38. Berg S. Polytef augmentation urethroplasty. Correction of surgically incurable urinary incontinence by injection technique. Arch Surg 107:379, 1973.
39. Leonard MP, Canning DA, Peters CA, et al. Endoscopic injection of glutaraldehyde cross-linked bovine dermal collagen for correction of vesicoureteral reflux. J Urol 142:115, 1991.
40. Bauer SB, Reda EF, Colodny AH, Retik AB. Detrusor instability: A delayed complication in association with the artificial sphincter. J Urol 135:1212, 1986.
41. Light JK, Pietro T. Alteration in detrusor behavior and the effect on renal function following insertion of the artificial urinary sphincter. J Urol 136:632, 1986.
42. Roth DR, Vyas PR, Kroovand RL, Perlmutter AD. Urinary tract deterioration associated with the artificial urinary sphincter. J Urol 135:528, 1986.
43. Bosco PJ, Bauer SB, Colodny AH, et al. The long-term results of artificial sphincters in children. J Urol 146:396, 1991.
44. Malizia AA Jr, Reiman HM, Myers RP, et al. Migration and granulomatous reaction after periurethral injection of polytef (Telfon). JAMA 251:3277, 1984.
45. Perez L, Smith E, Parrott T, et al. Submucosal bladder neck injection of bovine dermal collagen for stress urinary incontinence in the pediatric population. J Urol 156:633, 1996.
46. Bomalaski MD, Bloom DA, McGuire EJ, Panzl A. Glutaraldehyde cross-linked collagen in the treatment of urinary incontinence in children. J Urol 155:699, 1996.
47. Benchekroun A, Essakalli N, Faik M, et al. Continent urostomy with hydraulic ileal valve in 136 patients: 13 years of experience. J Urol 142:46, 1989.
48. Hendren WH. Ileal nipple for continence in cloacal exstrophy. J Urol 148:372, 1992.
49. Hinman F Jr. Functional classification of conduits for continent diversion. J Urol 144:27, 1990.
50. Duckett JW, Snyder HMD. Continent urinary diversion: Variations on the Mitrofanoff principle. J Urol 136:58, 1986.
51. Bihrle R, Klee LW, Adams MC, Foster RS. The clinical experience with the transverse colon-gastric tube continent urinary reservoir. J Urol 146:751, 1991.
52. Gosalbez R, Padron OF, Singla AK, et al. The gastric augment single pedicle tube catheterizable stoma: A useful adjunct to reconstruction of the urinary tract. J Urol 152:2005, 1994.
53. Cromie WJ, Barada JH, Weingarten JL. Cecal tubularization: Lengthening technique for creation of catheterizable conduit. Urology 37:41, 1991.
54. Woodhouse CR, MacNeily AE. The Mitrofanoff principle: Expanding upon a versatile technique. Br J Urol 74:447, 1994.
55. Krstic ZD. Preputial continent vesicostomy: Preliminary report of a new technique. J Urol 154:1160, 1995.
56. Casale AJ. Continent vesicostomy: A new method utilizing only bladder tissue (abstract 72). Paper presented at the 60th Annual Meeting of the American Academy of Pediatrics, New Orleans, 1991.
57. Watson HS, Bauer SB, Peters CA, et al. Comparative urodynamics of appendiceal and ureteral Mitrofanoff conduits in children. J Urol 154:878, 1995.
58. Sumfest JM, Burns MW, Mitchell ME. The Mitrofanoff principle in urinary reconstruction. J Urol 150:1875, 1993.
59. Gregoir W. Le traitement chirurgical du reflux vesico-ureteral congenital. Acta Chir Belg 63:431, 1964.
60. Leadbetter WF, Clarke BG: Five years' experience with uretero-enterostomy by the "combined" technique. J Urol 73:67, 1954.
61. Adams MC, Mitchell ME, Rink RC. Gastrocytoplasty: An alternative solution to the problem of urological reconstruction in the severely compromised patient. J Urol 140:1152, 1988.
62. Malone PS, Ransley PG, Kiely EM. Preliminary report: The antegrade continence enema. Lancet 336:1217, 1990.
63. Bauer SB, Hendren WH, Kozakewich H, et al. Perforation of the augmented bladder. J Urol 148:699, 1992.
64. Roth S, Van Ahlen H, Semjonow A, et al. percutaneous pouch lithotripsy in continent urinary diversions with narrowed Mitrofanoff conduit. Br J Urol 73:316, 1994.
65. Mundy AR, Nurse DE. Calcium balance, growth and skeletal mineralisation in patients with cystoplasties. Br J Urol 69:257, 1992.
66. Gosalbez RJ, Woodard JR, Broecker BH, Warshaw B. Metabolic complications of the use of stomach for urinary reconstruction. J Urol 150:710, 1993.
67. Shapiro SR, Johnston JH. The results of conservative management of neurogenic vesical dysfunction in children. Prog Pediatr Surg 10:185, 1977.

DOUGLAS CANNING

11

Continent Urinary Diversion

Continent urinary diversion dates to Gilchrist and colleagues,[1] who initially described a catheterizable urinary pouch in which the cecum and ascending colon, plus a segment of terminal ileum, were separated from the intestinal tract. The ureters were then implanted, and the ileourethra was brought out to the right lower quadrant (Fig. 11–1). With this procedure, continence was excellent; however, some of the initial problems that would continue to plague the urologist throughout the next five decades became apparent. The pouch was often difficult to catheterize, probably because of the ileal segment, which was not plicated. In addition, the colon segment was not reconfigured and, therefore, was subject to intermittent high pressures. As a result of the difficulties with this early pouch, Bricker's operation,[2] the ileal conduit became more popular for use after pelvic exenteration. In children, the ureterosigmoidostomy[3, 4] was widely used in children with bladder exstrophy, and most children with neuropathic bladder, like adults after cystectomy, underwent ileal conduit.

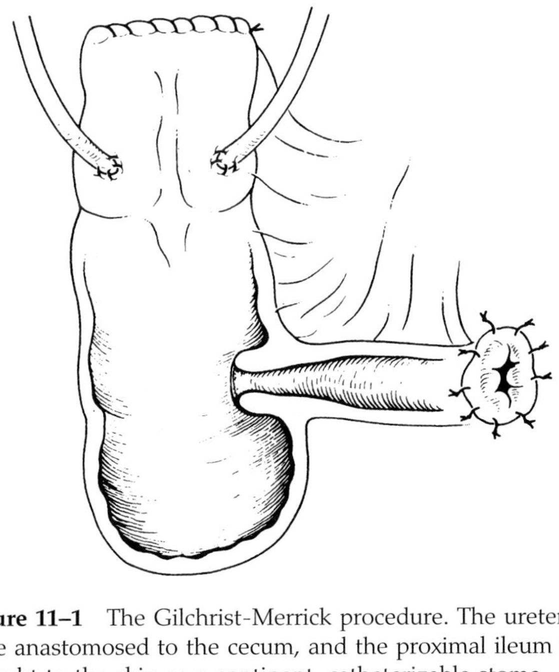

Figure 11–1 The Gilchrist-Merrick procedure. The ureters were anastomosed to the cecum, and the proximal ileum was brought to the skin as a continent, catheterizable stoma. Difficulty with catheterization occurred probably because the patulous ileum prevented funneling of the junction of the ileum with the colonic pouch. The colon was not reconfigured, resulting in intermittent high pressures within the pouch. From Ashken MH. Urinary reservoirs. In Ashken MH (ed), Urinary Diversion. New York: Springer-Verlag, 1982. Used with permission.

The long-term complications of both ureterosigmoidostomy (tumor)[5] and ileal conduit (renal deterioration)[6] became apparent within the next 25 years, and the idea of using substitute urinary reservoirs was rekindled beginning in the early 1970s under the leadership of Hendren.[7] Meanwhile, Lapides and colleagues began to promote the idea of clean, intermittent self-catheterization as a means of emptying the continent pouch.[8] This, along with the initiation of low-dose prophylactic antibiotics, allowed the urologist a simple solution providing for safe storage of urine without infection at low pressure.

CONCEPTS

A tremendous number of techniques have been designed to enlarge or replace the bladder to provide low-pressure storage. In this chapter, we offer an overview of the principles of reconstruction, which will allow the urologist to combine aspects of a number of different approaches. No one technique is acceptable for each patient.

The ideal continent urinary reservoir maintains a consistent low pressure, is easy to catheterize, is free from infection, and is easy to empty via a stoma placed in a convenient, cosmetically pleasing location. A few children will have a functional pelvic diaphragm that will allow spontaneous bladder (or pouch) emptying. If the bladder outlet is normal and it is possible to reduce the pressure gradient between the interior of the bladder and the distal end of the urethra to a very low level, then the bladder will passively empty. Children undergoing exenterative surgery for tumor are an illustrative group. Most will require clean, intermittent catheterization. Unfortunately, in pediatrics, most of our patients are children who have congenital (bladder exstrophy) or acquired (neuropathic bladder in spinal dysraphism) anomalies of both the outlet and the detrusor. This has led us to pursue a low-pressure reservoir that provides adequate capacity to enable 4 to 6 hours of urine collection without the development of pressures in excess of 35 to 40 cm H_2O. Chronic pressures in excess of 40 cm H_2O result in a much higher risk of vesicoureteric reflux and hydronephrosis in patients with neuropathic bladder.[9]

CHOICE OF BOWEL SEGMENT

The reservoir should be made with an intestinal segment that results in minimal metabolic consequences of absorption of urinary metabolites. The only bowel segment that is almost never used is the jejunum. If the jejunum, particularly the proximal jejunum, is used, electrolyte changes occur, including hyponatremia, hypochloremia, hyperkalemia, azotemia, and metabolic acidosis. This results from increased secretion of sodium and chloride with an increased reabsorption of potassium and hydrogen ions. Loss of sodium and chloride carries with it water, resulting in hypovolemia and thus stimulating renin secretion and aldosterone production.[10] Aldosterone stimulates potassium secretion and sodium reabsorption by the kidney with resultant production of a sodium-depleted, potassium-rich urine to the jejunal pouch, causing even further increased reabsorption of potassium and thus perpetuating the abnormalities. These changes result in symptoms of lethargy, nausea, vomiting, muscle weakness, and further dehydration. Death may ensue if no action is taken.

The ileum and colon have had the widest use in the creation of an intestinal urinary reservoir.[11, 12] The absorptive characteristics of the ileum and colon are not significantly different. The characteristic electrolyte abnormality after ileal or colonic cystoplasty is a hyperchloremic metabolic acidosis, like that of the jejunal segment but to a much lesser degree. The length of the segment affects the degree of electrolyte disturbance. Short segments rarely result in severe acidosis; patients undergoing reconstruction with longer segments may require bicarbonate replacement. Of patients undergoing Mainz pouches in which a total of 40 cm of ileum and 10 cm of colon are used, 65% require bicarbonate to maintain normal acid-base balance.[13]

Impaired renal function will also reduce the patient's ability to maintain electrolyte homeostasis. The amount of renal function required depends on the length and type of bowel segment used as well as the length of time the urine will be exposed to the intestinal mucosa. Better renal function will be needed in patients who will undergo creation of a reservoir than, for example, an ileal conduit. In general, adults with a serum creatinine above 2.0[14] or children with a creatinine clearance of less than 30 mL/min will need careful study before consideration for bowel augmentation or bladder replacement. A nomogram (Fig. 11–2*A*) or formula (Fig. 11–2*B*) such as that provided by Traub and Johnson[15] is helpful in estimating renal function in these children.

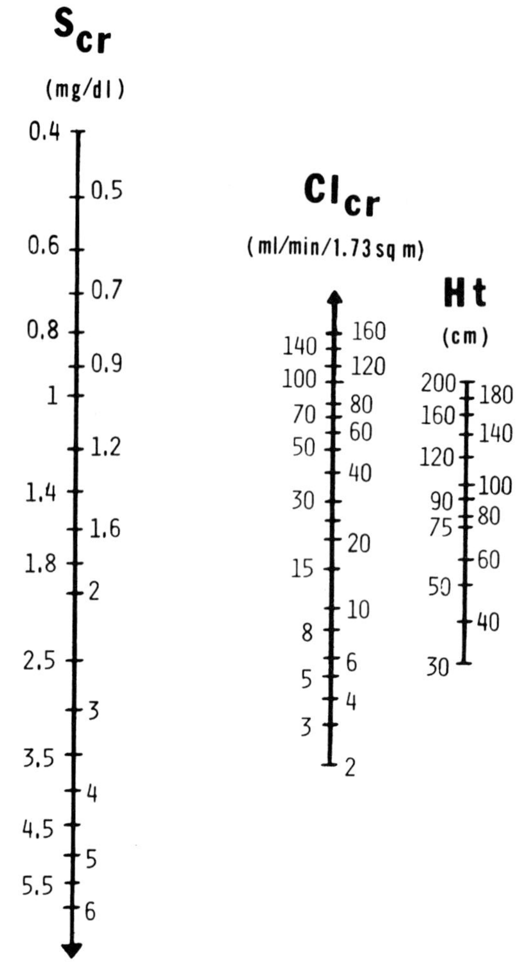

A

$$C_{Cr} = \frac{0.48\,(\text{height})}{Cr_s}$$

B

Figure 11–2 *A,* Nomogram for rapid estimation of creatinine clearance in patients 1 to 18 years of age. A ruler used to connect the child's serum creatinine value (S_{cr}) and height (Ht) will intersect the center line at a value approximating creatinine clearance (Cl_{cr}). If Cl_{cr} is less than 30, careful consideration of bowel segment type must be made before augmentation cystoplasty or bladder replacement. From Traub SL, Johnson CE. Comparison of methods of estimating creatinine clearance in children. Am J Hosp Pharm 37:195, 1980. Used with permission. *B,* Traub's formula for estimating creatinine clearance (C_{cr}) from the patient's height (in centimeters) and the serum creatinine (Cr_s).

In addition to electrolyte abnormalities associated with small bowel and colonic pouches, short bowel and nutritional problems may occur. In a patient with significant loss of ileum, vitamin B_{12} malabsorption has been reported with resultant anemia and neurologic abnormalities. Vitamin B_{12} deficiency has been reported in as many as 10 of 41 patients after radical cystectomy and ileal conduit who had been previously radiated.[16] In this study it was thought that preoperative radiation therapy had disabled the enterohepatic circulation. However, others have reported vitamin B_{12} deficiency in as many as 25% of patients after ileocolic cystoplasty following radical cystectomy[17] in patients who have *not* been previously radiated. The studies to date in children have not identified problems with vitamin B_{12} deficiency in relatively short-term follow-up, but careful monitoring is probably in order in patients in whom large segments of the terminal ileum, particularly the ileocecal junction, are incorporated into the urinary tract.[18]

Mitchell and coworkers began to introduce gastric segments into the urinary tract in the mid-1980s. The gastric segment is attractive because it provides an advantage to the patient with limited renal reserve and metabolic acidosis who cannot re-excrete the increased acid absorption when the ileum or colon is in contact with urine. The stomach patch becomes attractive as well in patients who can spare very little ileum or colon; for example, the child with cloacal exstrophy with the short-gut syndrome. Clinically significant hyponatremic, hypochloremic, hypokalemic metabolic acidosis has been noted in a few patients with renal insufficiency[19] and even in a few when renal function is normal.[20] The pathophysiology of this electrolyte pattern appears to be related to continued secretion of hydrogen and chloride into the urinary tract by the gastric segment, accompanied by the obligate intravascular secretion of bicarbonate. With renal insufficiency the ability of the kidney to excrete bicarbonate can be exceeded, resulting in systemic alkalosis. This has led some authors to recommend against use of gastric segments in patients in whom metabolic acidosis does not exist.[21] The secretion of acid from the gastric patch also results in dysuria and hematuria in a few patients.[22] This problem is generally mild in severity and appears to affect about one third of patients, particularly those with a sensate urethra and those in whom renal function is particularly poor. The problem is usually amenable to treatment with omeprazole, which inhibits the hydrogen-potassium pump and results in decreased secretion of acid.

To reduce the effect of the gastric segment on acid secretion and to try to provide a more homeostatic pouch, stomach has been combined with sigmoid or ileum.[23] This has the advantage of allowing some secretion of acid from the stomach to counteract the absorption of the ileum.[24] A few patients in whom hypochloremic, hyponatremic, hypokalemic metabolic acidosis has developed have been salvaged in this way.[20] This pouch is somewhat more difficult to prepare in that it requires two bowel anastomoses and two sets of mesenteric segments to fashion. Nevertheless, in some patients, it may provide an excellent solution when stomach, ileum, or colon alone seems inappropriate.

In addition to augmentation with gastrointestinal segments, Cartwright and Snow introduced *autoaugmentation*.[25] In this procedure, the detrusor muscle is excised or incised, creating a large bladder diverticulum through which the small bladder expands. This provides increased capacity at low pressure and reduces the tendency of the bladder to develop uninhibited contractions. Autoaugmentation can be particularly effective in a bladder that has a marginal volume but that develops relatively high pressures early in filling.[26] Because the bladder can be enlarged without the addition of bowel and the ensuing inherent complications, autoaugmentation is often the first choice in a patient who requires improved compliance but not a significant increase in bladder volume. The main advantage is that no intestinal mucosa is used; as a result, there are no associated side effects from secretion or absorption of urinary metabolites. Dewan and Byard attempted a modification of autoaugmentation in which a diverticulum is created and then stabilized with demucosalized stomach.[27] Initially used in sheep, this technique has been shown to be effective in humans.[28] However, three of five of Dewan and Byard's patients experienced early satiety and lost weight, which may limit the applicability of this technique. Gonzalez and colleagues incorporated the concept of adding intestinal backing to the exterior of the diverticulum by removing the mucosa from a segment of sigmoid colon and adding it to the diverticulum.[29] This has been accomplished in animals and humans without significant complication. The major shortcoming with this procedure appears to be the relative small increase in bladder volume afforded by this procedure compared with enterocystoplasty and also the presence of some colonic mucosa in the bladder.[30]

In *ureterocystoplasty*, a dilated ureter or segment of a dilated ureter is used to provide additional bladder volume.[31] Depending on the size of the ureter, excellent increased volume and compliance can be achieved with the use of ureter. Unfortunately, few patients who require augmentation can spare a ureter to increase bladder size. In some cases, transureteral ureterostomy with augmentation of the bladder using the ipsilateral distal ureter can be very effective. These excellent results have led others to experiment with transureteral ureterostomy even in nondilated cases with *progressive hydrodilation* of the distal stump.[32]

The potential difficulties associated with augmentation of the bladder with any gastrointestinal segment combined with the relatively few patients who can donate ureter for ureterocystoplasty has stimulated researchers to attempt to grow uroepithelium on a matrix template. Atala and associates used a biodegradable polyglactin mesh onto which urothelial cells are introduced. These

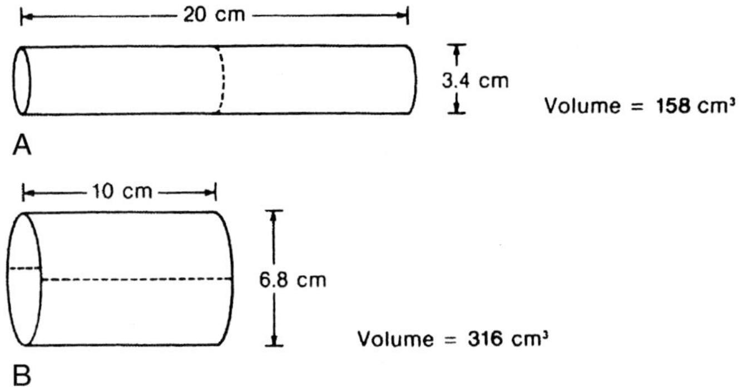

Figure 11–3 Hinman reminds us that the volume of a cylinder ($V = r^2h$, where h is the height of the cylinder and r is the radius) increases exponentially with radius. Obviously, to maximize pouch volume, for a given length of intestine the lumenal diameter (2r) of the pouch should be maximized to make the pouch as spherical as possible. From Hinman F Jr. Selection of intestinal segments for bladder substitution: Physical and physiological characteristics. J Urol 139:519, 1988. Used with permission.

cells have been shown to survive and proliferate in athymic mice.[33] Similarly harvested cells were successfully expanded in vitro, suggesting that strips or patches of native urothelium could potentially be bioengineered and transplanted to augment the small or noncompliant bladder.[34] Kropp and colleagues, in a series of novel experiments,[35–37] developed a technique in which small intestinal submucosa (SIS) is harvested from porcine jejunum and separated from its mucosa. This results in a separation of the superficial tunica mucosa from the deeper stratum compactum. The serosa and muscularis are then removed from the outer surface, leaving a thin graft membrane, which is then sterilized. This graft is then introduced as a patch into the bivalved bladder. In 19 dogs monitored from 1 to 15 months, complete regeneration of detrusor muscle, transitional epithelium, and serosa occurred with no contraction of the SIS patch.[38] These remarkable results may result in an augmentation substrate that is readily available and easy to use with no metabolic consequences. It is unclear, however, whether the augmented patch will provide improved compliance when it is applied to the neuropathic bladder. Through a series of bioengineering procedures, both researchers have been able to grow uroepithelium. Obviously, if enough uroepithelium could be produced to provide a large enough patch for augmentation, the potential risks of absorption of urinary metabolites could be minimized.

Regardless of the augmentation type, the goals of surgery are the same: to provide a large-capacity pouch that will fill at low pressures and provide 4 to 6 hours of urine storage before high pressures are realized. Without low-pressure storage, no efferent valve will maintain continence without risking deterioration of renal function.

Creation of the Pouch

Hinman reminded us that, when creating a continent pouch or augmenting the bladder, the most effective use of a given segment of intestine will be gained when the segment of intestine (cylinder) is converted into as spherical a shape as possible. Because the volume of a sphere increases exponentially with the radius, the larger the radius that can be provided for a given length of intestine, the greater is the volume provided per centimeter of intestine removed from the gastrointestinal tract (Fig. 11–3). The bladder should be widely opened in such a fashion as to prevent an hourglass contraction at the site of the intestinal anastomosis. In addition, the law of LaPlace—$T = Pr$ (where T = wall tension, P = lumenal pressure, and r = radius of the cylinder or sphere)—can be applied to reconstructive bladder surgery (Fig. 11–4). If one converts the formula to $P = T/r$, it is easily seen that, for a given wall tension, the larger the radius, the lower is the intraluminal pressure.[39]

Once the pouch is configured, it should be carefully arranged in such a way that the mesenteric lines do not cross. The wall that will accept the flap valve should be located so that good backing of the valve is ensured and the catheter may be directed away from the trigone to ensure comfortable intermittent catheterization.

Closure of the Bladder Neck

We try to avoid closure of the bladder neck to preserve the urethral pop-off mechanism. In most cases, additional resistance at the bladder neck can be achieved by tubu-

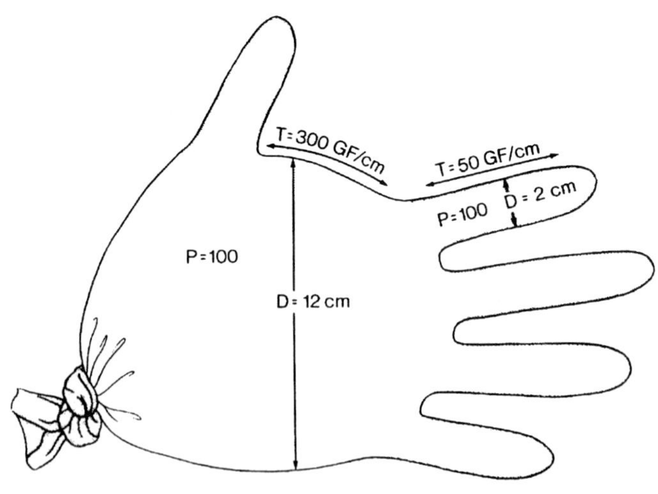

Figure 11–4 Pascal's law as illustrated by Hinman. Inflated surgeon's glove illustrates LaPlace's relationship. Although the pressure (P) is equal throughout, tension (T) is greater in the portion of the glove with the greater diameter. From Hinman F Jr. Selection of intestinal segments for bladder substitution. Physical and physiological characteristics. J Urol 139:519, 1988. Used with permission.

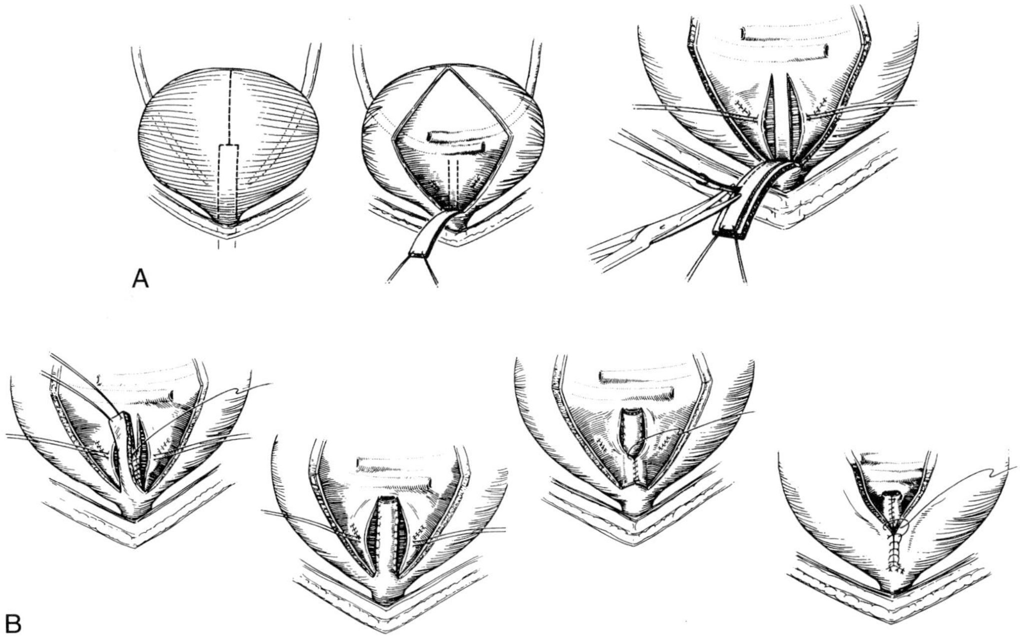

Figure 11–5 *A,* The Salle urethral onlay: Salle modified Kropp's procedure to provide a flap valve at the bladder neck. Left: In this procedure, a 1- × 4-cm anterior bladder wall flap based on the urethra is outlined; the bladder is opened superiorly to the flap in the midline. Center: Two parallel incisions 0.5 cm in width are made on the posterior bladder wall. The ureters are reimplanted superiorly or transversely above the incisions. Right: The incisions are made through the mucosa only. The mucosa is elevated lateral to the incisions. The midline mucosal strip remains intact. The mucosa of the flap is excised laterally to leave a 5- to 7-mm strip. *B,* The Salle procedure. Left: The mucosa of the flap is anastomosed to the posterior bladder mucosa over an 8 French catheter. Center, left: The anterior flap musculature is secured to the exposed trigone musculature. Center, right: The mucosa lateral to the new urethra is mobilized and sutured over the new tube. Right: The anterior bladder wall is secured at the base of the new tube and the bladder is closed. From Rink RC, Adams MC, Keating MA. The flip-flap technique to lengthen the urethra (Salle procedure) for treatment of neurogenic urinary incontinence. J Urol 152:799, 1994. Used with permission.

larization or by creation of a second flap valve. In the past, we have used the Young-Dees-Leadbetter bladder neck plasty or a urethral suspension with a fascial sling.[40] More recently, we have been using a modification of the Kropp procedure.[41, 42] This procedure was developed by Salle[43] (Fig. 11–5) and uses an anterior bladder flap, which is sutured to the posterior wall to provide a flap valve, another modification of the Mitrofanoff procedure. Using an onlay technique rather than a tunneled tube seems to provide improved ease of catheterization. Continence rates have been good in limited experience so far.

In patients in whom scarring precludes bladder neck plasty, a sling, or urethral flap procedure, closure of the bladder neck remains an option. In general, we believe that it is important to preserve the ability to catheterize the urethra in case catheterization of the abdominal stoma becomes difficult. In addition, we like to preserve the urethral pop-off in case patients become less compulsive in frequency of catheterization. In some cases, however, closure of the bladder neck provides the only real hope for dryness. If bladder neck closure is deemed necessary, the bladder neck should be totally transected and the urethra and bladder neck each closed in two layers. We often interpose fat, omentum, or even a flap of rectus muscle in the space between the bladder neck and the urethra to prevent leakage.[44]

Types of Continence Mechanisms

Three main types of continence mechanisms exist: the tube valve, the nipple valve, and the flap valve. A continence mechanism dependent purely on hydraulic resistance is typified by the Young-Dees-Leadbetter type of detrusor tubularization[45–47] (Fig. 11–6). Resistance to leakage in this form of valve is provided by lengthening and narrowing the urethra, bladder neck, and trigone to increase resistance to flow based on the simple hydraulic principle: resistance approximates length ÷ diameter × tension in the wall. Although this can be an effective method of providing continence, one disadvantage is that

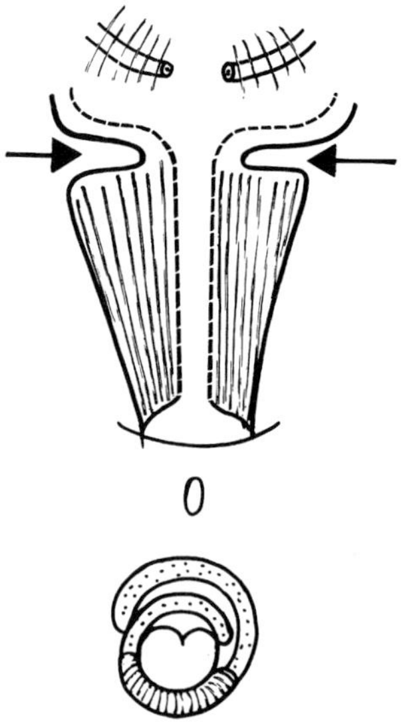

Figure 11–6 The Young-Dees-Leadbetter bladder neck plasty. This is a typical tube valve. The resistance to leakage is approximated by the formula: resistance ~ (length/diameter) × wall tension. Tube valves tend to leak as soon as the reservoir pressure exceeds the resistance intrinsic to the tube. From Mollard P. Exstrophies et epispades. In Precis d'Urologie de l'Enfant. Paris: Masson, 1984, p 226. Used with permission.

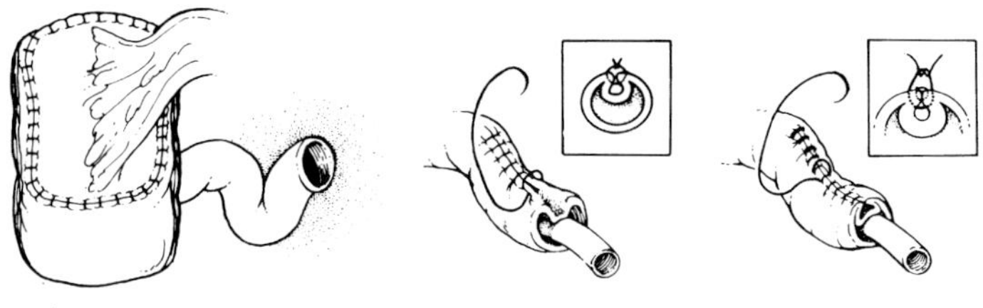

Figure 11–7 The Indiana continent urinary reservoir. Another example of a tube valve; the continence is dependent on the hydraulic resistance from the plicated terminal ileum. From Rowland RG, Mitchell ME, Bihrle R, et al. Indiana continent urinary reservoir. J Urol 137:1136, 1987. Used with permission.

the hydraulic resistance does not increase with the rising pressure within the bladder or urinary reservoir. Once the threshold resistance to flow is overcome, leakage will occur. This results in a tendency toward stress urinary incontinence, particularly in patients in whom the reservoir is marginally large and in patients who tend to use Valsalva during mobility movement (e.g., patients with spina bifida who walk with crutches).

On the other hand, a pop-off mechanism as provided by the urethra following a Young-Dees-Leadbetter procedure, or the efferent ileal limb in an Indiana continent urinary reservoir[48] may be beneficial (Fig. 11–7). These pressure-dependent leaks provide a means of egress of urine, which will tend to lower the pressure within the lumen of the reconstructed reservoir and probably reduce the risk of bladder perforation from infrequent catheterization. The leakage may act as a reminder to the patient who is beginning to get wet that it is time to catheterize.

Nipple valves depend on pressure within the reservoir to compress the nipple (Fig. 11–8). The Gilchrist-Merrick procedure[1] from which the Indiana pouch evolved is an example of an early nipple valve. The nipple valve depends on pressure from within the reservoir to compress the lumen of the nipple to prevent leakage. The major flaw with this system is that the same forces that tend to compress the nipple and provide continence

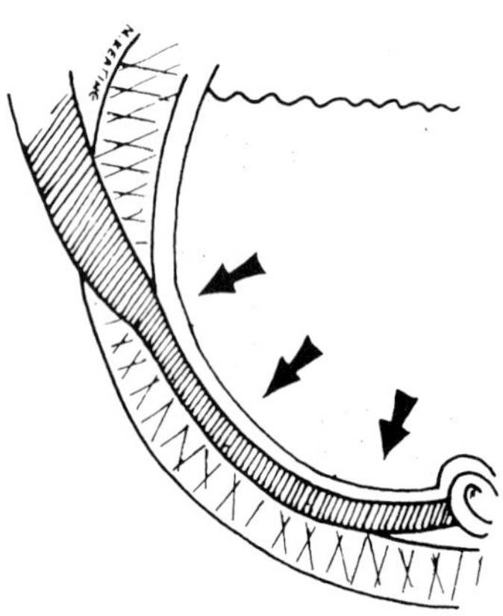

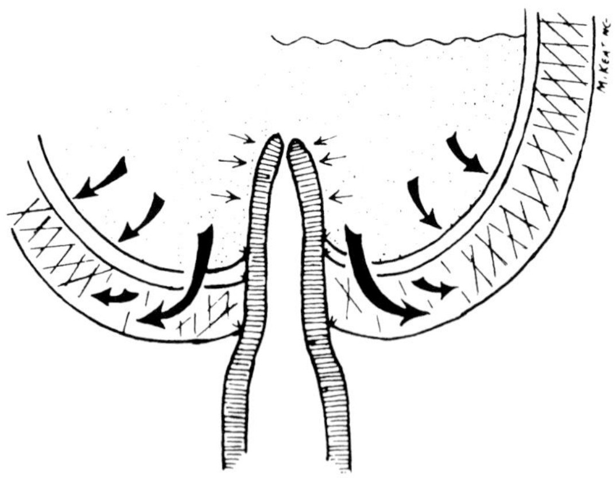

Figure 11–8 Flap valves versus nipple valves. A nipple valve produces continence by the effect of the interior pouch pressure, which compresses the nipple. Unfortunately, this same pressure also produces lateral displacement of the wall of the reservoir, causing gradual effacement of the nipple and loss of continence. A flap valve results in continence by having the catheterizable tube supported in a fixed position on the inner wall of the reservoir, which is similar to the reimplanted ureter.

also tend to evert the nipple, causing loss of intussusception or flattening and inversion of the nipple with loss of continence.

The Gilchrist-Merrick operation has not provided consistently good continence over long-term follow-up. Most patients have required additional techniques to try to shore up the nipple valve with further intussusception[49] or by formation of a wrap of cecum around the distal ileum.[50] Despite all efforts at nipple stabilization, most of these have required reoperation because of loss of the effective valve.[50, 51] These problems with the nipple valve led to attachment of the intussuscepted ileal nipple against the inner wall of the cecum. This fixed the intussuscepted nipple valve against the inner wall of the cecum, thus stabilizing the nipple and effectively creating a flap valve (Fig. 11–9).[52]

The Mitrofanoff technique uses a flap-valve mechanism for continence. Nearly all current techniques for continent reservoirs use this concept. A small-diameter tube is placed into the reservoir by tunneling through the bladder or intestinal wall to place a significant portion of the tunnel beneath the submucosa. As the reservoir fills, pressure is exerted along the length of the tube in such a way as to close the lumen and, therefore, increase the resistance to retrograde flow. An advantage of the flap valve is that it provides increasing resistance as the pressure within the reservoir increases, thereby providing predictable continence over time without compromising the ability to catheterize the stoma.

For the same reason that a flap valve provides excellent continence, it is also potentially dangerous in that, unless the patient is committed to catheterizing at regular intervals with frequent emptying, the pouch can increase pressure to the point that ischemia along the reconstructed suture line results in perforation. Thus, a flap-valve mechanism for continent reconstruction leads to very successful outcomes but also requires meticulous compliance on the patient's part for safety.[41]

Because of these risks, preoperative evaluation is essential. We currently require a period of intermittent catheterization to be performed optimally by the child or by the parents at 4-hour intervals. During this period, the family keeps a record of the time and volume obtained at each catheterization. Compliance with preoperative visits with the record must be meticulous before the patient is considered for creation of a catheterizable stoma. Renal function must be carefully assessed, with particular attention paid to acid-base balance, before introducing an intestinal segment into the urinary tract. Incorporation of colon or ileum results in increased tendency toward metabolic acidosis.

BLADDER AUGMENTATION OR BLADDER SUBSTITUTION?

In general, if the trigone is functional, it is generally better to use it as a template from which to build a storage reservoir than to remove the bladder base. In children, bladder malignancies are rare. We are only rarely required to replace the trigone and can usually augment rather than replace the bladder. Augmentation, by preserving the trigone, reduces the risks of ureteral anastomotic complications. Most of our bladder replacements have been in children who underwent previous diversion. We are performing fewer undiversions and more augmentations because primary diversion is becom-

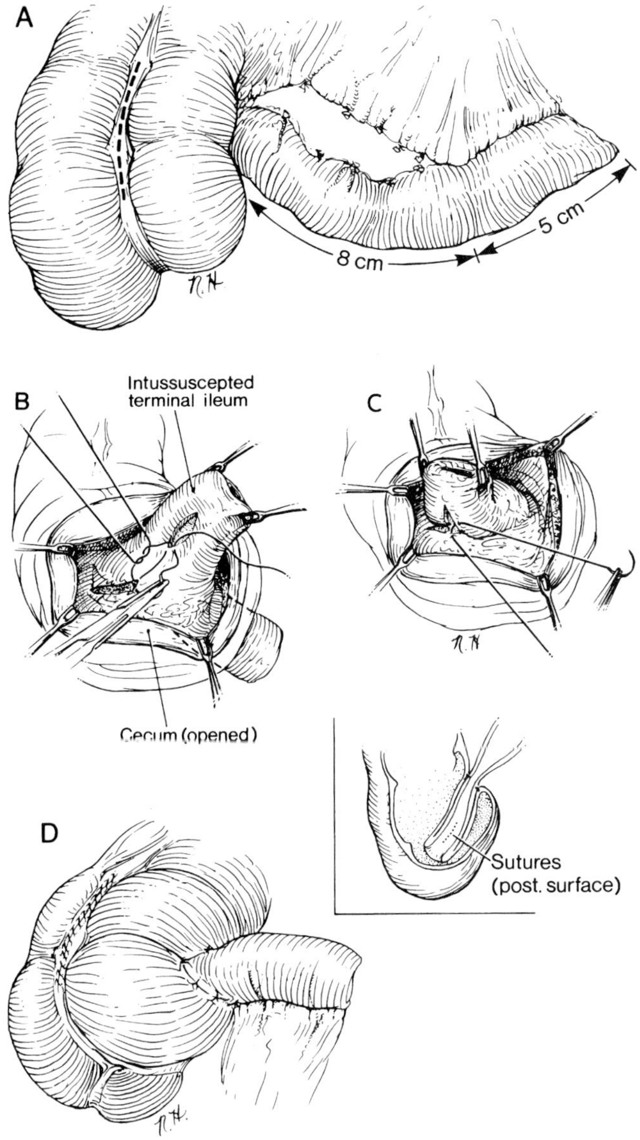

Figure 11–9 *A–D,* Converted nipple valve: King's modification of the nipple valve to a flap valve. Ileocecal intussusception with fixation of the nipple to the side wall of the cecum with an incision through the mucosal surface to secure the valve and prevent effacement of the nipple. From King LR, Robertson CN, Bertram RA. A new technique for the prevention of reflux in those undergoing bladder substitution or undiversion using bowel segments. World J Urol 3:195, 1985. Used with permission.

ing more and more uncommon, except in patients with poor renal function. Even in patients with diversion, the bladder can be cycled to improve compliance. In general, if the previous diversion was performed in the context of infection, the bladder is often very small when undiversion is contemplated. On the other hand, if the diversion was performed for obstruction or incontinence not associated with chronic infection, the bladder can usually be salvaged but rarely can be used alone without augmentation. So many variations of technique now exist that I have chosen only a few that are widely used to illustrate the principles necessary to provide success.

FLAP-VALVE CONTINENCE MECHANISMS

The Mitrofanoff Principle

The Mitrofanoff principle[53] uses a very small–diameter tube implanted on the inner wall of the continent catheterizable reservoir in such a way as to provide a 5:1 ratio between tunnel length and luminal diameter, analogous to the normal intravesical ureter. In this way continence is ensured. We have found this technique to be consistently successful with few associated complications.[54, 55] Mitrofanoff first described the procedure using the appendix as the catheterizable tube. The techniques described, however, hold for the ureter, narrowed intestine or modeled gastric segment, and even the fallopian tube. We tend to think of the procedure as involving three parts: (1) harvest of the appendix, (2) creation of the stoma, and (3) implantation of the appendix. This technique is nearly always used in conjunction with enlargement of the urinary reservoir. In most cases bladder neck resistance must be increased to prevent postoperative leakage through the urethra.

Harvesting the Appendix

The appendicular artery is the terminal branch of the superior mesenteric artery (Fig. 11–10). The appendix can be moved virtually anywhere in the abdomen if one mobilizes the root of the mesentery to expose the retroperitoneum as one would in beginning a retroperitoneal lymph node dissection. Although this maneuver is not always necessary, we find it helpful because it enables the surgeon to bring the appendix easily to the umbilicus without separating the appendix from the cecum except for a very short distance. The cecum and the appendix are, therefore, moved as a unit rather than separately. Planning the dissection in this way prevents compromise of the appendiceal blood supply, which might otherwise result in stenosis of the lumen of the appendix. It is logical to think that one must examine the appendix before embarking on its use, and we do routinely identify and cannulate the appendix before proceeding. In most

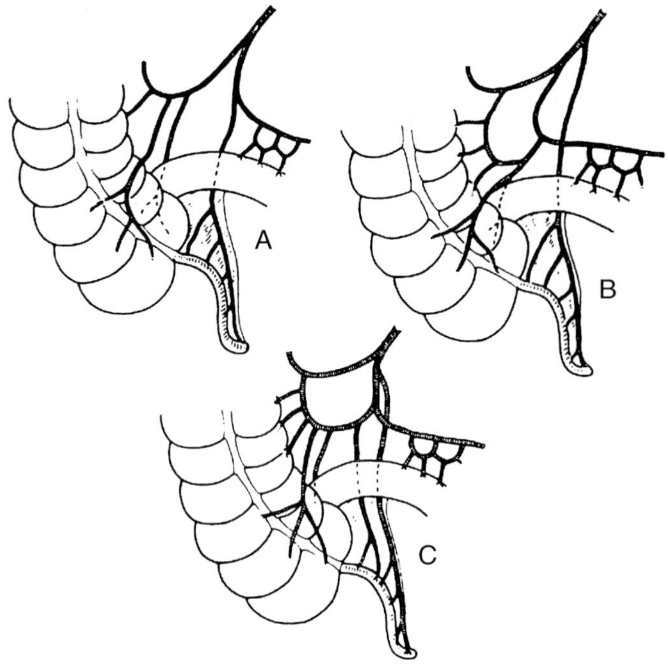

Figure 11–10 Variations of appendiceal vasculature. The appendiceal artery is usually the terminal branch of the superior mesenteric artery *(A)*, but can originate more proximally from the ileocolic *(B)* or from two separate branches from the anterior or the posterior cecal artery or from the ileal branch of the ileocolic artery *(C)*. If the appendix and the cecum are both moved as a unit, the appendiceal pedicle will not be injured regardless of the arterial anatomy.

cases, however, even a very short appendix can be lengthened by harvesting a cuff of adjacent cecum and only rarely is the appendix not suitable for use (Fig. 11–11). A small cuff of the cecum is routinely included to provide a wider skin-to-appendix stoma. We believe this results in fewer cases of stenosis at the skin level.

Creation of the stoma is straightforward. We now use the umbilicus almost exclusively for three reasons. First, cosmetically, the appendix can be hidden in the depths of the umbilicus, making it virtually invisible. Second, the skin at the umbilicus is fixed to the midline fascia, avoiding the need for any length of appendix to traverse a thick pannus of fat, which might be the case if the stoma was placed elsewhere on the abdomen. This is particularly important in patients with spina bifida, who often become heavier as they lose mobility later in life and become wheelchair bound. Third, the umbilicus can be catheterized blindly. We use a semicircular incision from about the 3 o'clock to the 9 o'clock position along the umbilical fold. This results in a superiorly based umbilical flap, which will be used to provide a spatulated appendiceal-umbilical suture line. The appendix should be recessed within the umbilicus to provide posterior displacement of the lumen, thereby hiding the stoma and providing an optimum cosmetic appearance. The

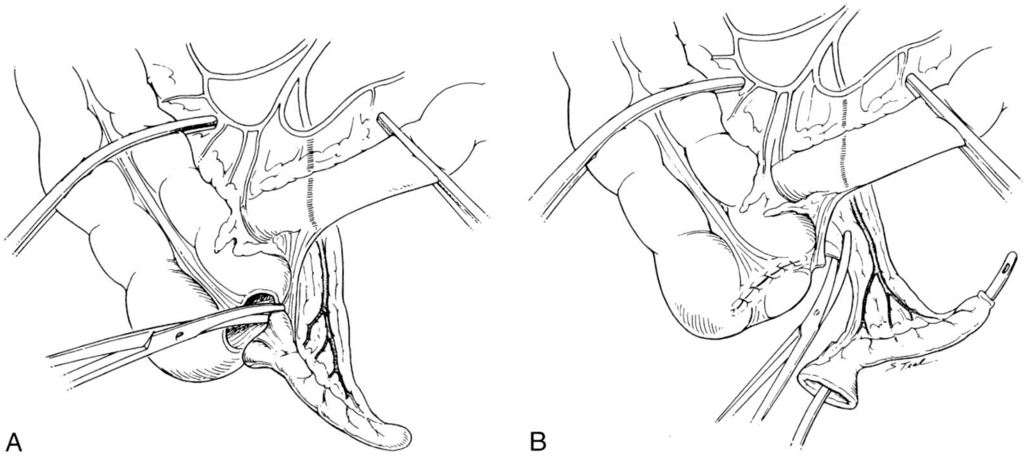

Figure 11–11 Harvest of the appendix. *A,* Dissection begins at the cecum. A short appendix can be lengthened by taking a larger cuff of cecum and narrowing the cecal cuff for a short distance. *B,* Only a short length of mesoappendix need be mobilized. From Keating MA, Rink RC, Adams MC. Appendicovesicostomy: A useful adjunct to continent reconstruction of the bladder. J Urol 149:1091, 1993. Used with permission.

superior-based flap ensures that when the catheter is introduced it strikes the tough umbilical skin and is directed into the appendix with minimal trauma to the appendiceal mucosa.

A generous fascial opening beneath the skin incision must be made and should be adequate to permit the passage of an index finger. A large opening is important because it prevents constriction of the blood supply to the appendix. A large fascial opening also prevents angling or kinking of the appendix as it traverses the fascia. Despite the large fascial opening, we have not had problems with parastomal hernias.

The appendix is drawn through the fascial and umbilical incision and spatulated. The umbilical flap is sutured to the spatulated side of the appendix (Fig. 11–12). The suture line is carried around the stoma site. With this completed, the appendix can be drawn inferiorly before implantation into the bladder or pouch. In this way, the stoma is well hidden within the umbilicus. The stoma is always created before implantation of the tube into the bladder. We find this is best in providing a recessed stoma and a straight passage of the appendix. We carefully take solid bites of appendiceal wall when drawing the umbilical skin flap into the spatulation.

Implantation of the Appendix

The appendix is then drawn inferiorly, and the pouch or bladder is brought up and supported on the inner wall of the reservoir. The bladder, usually close to the dome, is pushed up against the interior fascia of the abdominal wall. After estimating the final location and orientation of the pouch in relationship to the appendix, the tunnel, or more commonly the trough, for the appendix is created. If a submucosal tunnel is used, the lumen must be generous to avoid constriction of the appendiceal blood supply. If a mucosal trough technique is to be used, the appendix is carefully fixed to the back wall of the trough. Before passage of the appendix into the trough or tunnel, the tip of the appendix is amputated and the lumen rinsed. The superior wall of the pouch is attached to the rectus fascia with nonabsorbable suture, taking care to prevent passage of the suture through the wall of the pouch. In this way, the entire unit is fixed to provide straight, easy passage of the catheter through the appendix. The purpose of the careful attachment of the pouch to the abdominal wall is to minimize any angulation or unsupported distance the appendix might traverse before entering its intravesical tunnel. If the appendix is allowed

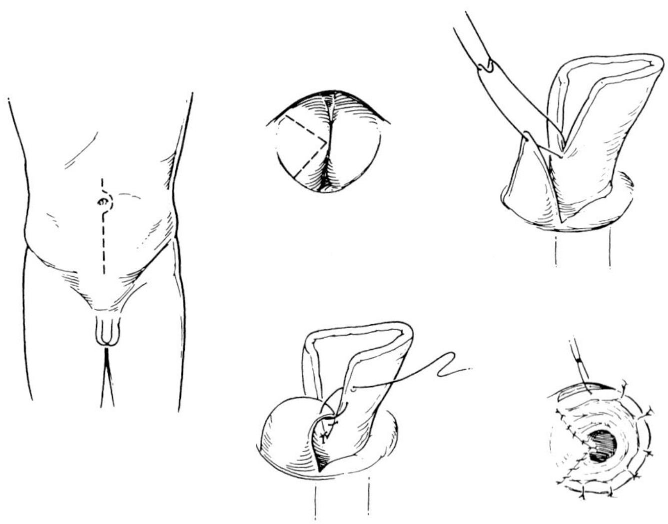

Figure 11–12 The umbilical stoma: A superior based flap of umbilical skin is made by making a semicircular incision along the inferior margin of the umbilicus from the 3 to 9 o'clock positions. Eversion of the appendix and the umbilical skin makes the anastomosis easier to perform. The anastomosis is carried around the cut edge of the umbilicus. From Keating MA, Rink RC, Adams MC. Appendicovesicostomy: A useful adjunct to continent reconstruction of the bladder. J Urol 149:1091, 1993. Used with permission.

to kink at the junction of the outer wall of the bladder, there will be gradual dilation of the appendix at that point as the catheter continually traumatizes that area. Ultimately, catheterization will become impossible. We usually use 2-0 or 3-0 monofilament nylon sutures, placing three to four carefully with the surgeon's finger within the bladder to ensure that the mucosa is not transgressed (Fig. 11–13). Additional sutures are placed to complete the fixation of the bladder against the interior abdominal wall circumferentially, except at the point at which the appendiceal mesentery enters the bladder (Fig. 11–14). These maneuvers are carried out before fixing the appendix in the trough.

The appendix is kept on gentle traction as the distal end is anchored to the detrusor or intestinal reservoir with absorbable suture. We spatulate the appendix on its intravesical wall upward over a distance of approximately 1 cm before completing the maturation of the appendix to the bladder mucosa. This reduces the risk of circumferential contracture at the appendiceal meatus, which would result in stenosis of the appendix at its junction with the bladder. We select the course for the appendix through the bladder depending on how it seems to lie comfortably. In patients with a sensate bladder, however, we believe it is important to direct the catheter away from the trigone, which might otherwise result in passage across the most sensitive part of the bladder and result in uncomfortable catheterization for the patient. The proximal end of the appendix is matured with interrupted chromic sutures, taking care to avoid leaving a lip at the junction of the appendix with the bladder or reservoir.

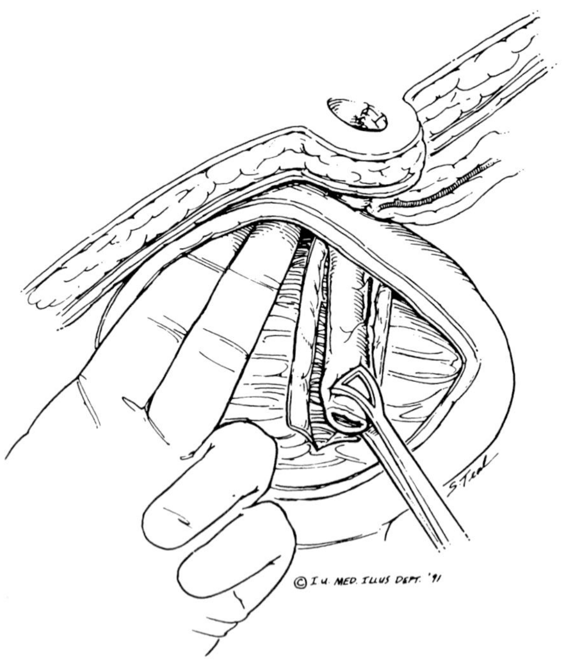

Figure 11–13 Attachment of the pouch to the abdominal wall. The surgeon's fingers approximate the reservoir to the abdominal wall as the pexing sutures are placed. The distal appendix is drawn into the pouch, which recesses the stoma. From Keating MA, Rink RC, Adams MC. Appendicovesicostomy: A useful adjunct to continent reconstruction of the bladder. J Urol 149:1091, 1993. Used with permission.

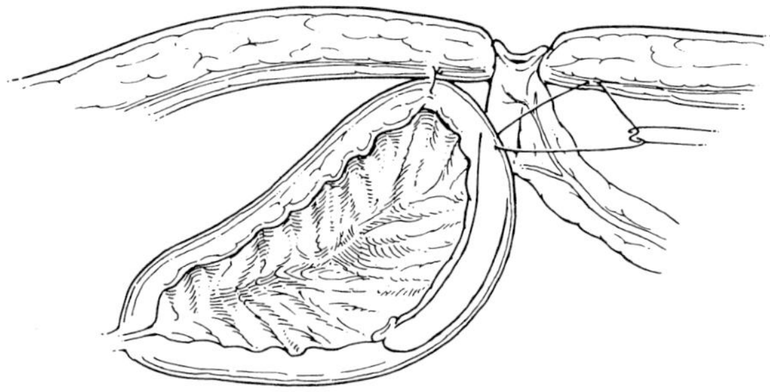

Figure 11–14 Pouch attached: suitable attachment ensures ease of catheterization by minimizing the risk of angulation and false passage of the catheter. From Keating MA, Rink RC, Adams MC. Appendicovesicostomy: A useful adjunct to continent reconstruction of the bladder. J Urol 149:1091, 1993. Used with permission.

When planning a surgical procedure when both an appendicocystostomy and an enterocystoplasty are anticipated, we generally perform the appendicocystostomy first to create a fixed bladder to which the augmenting segment of intestine or stomach can be sutured as a last step.

Care is taken to practice catheterization of the appendix before closure of the pouch. If there is any difficulty with passage of the catheter, the system must be reexamined and reconstructed to ensure easy catheterization. We try to position the appendix to provide good dependent drainage of the pouch without the catheter passing over the trigone. This provides easy emptying without much discomfort.

The pouch or bladder is closed carefully to prevent leakage. A 20 to 22 French Malecot catheter is left in place. We are still searching for the ideal latex-free catheter to be used in patients with exstrophy or myelomeningocele. We are currently using a 22 French Silastic Malecot (Cook Urological, Inc., Spencer, IN). We usually divert the urine with ureteral stents even if the ureters were not reimplanted. We use small-caliber infant feeding tubes, which are brought out through the bladder wall at a site remote from the position of the Malecot catheter. A meticulous bladder closure must be performed to minimize extravasation of urine. After placement of the catheter, the pouch is tested for leakage. Any leaks are repaired. An 8 to 10 French Silastic Foley catheter is left through the appendix.

In patients who have functioning ventricular peritoneal shunts, we leave closed system Jackson-Pratt drains for 48 hours regardless of output. Broad-spectrum antibiotics are continued until the drain is removed. In all other patients, we leave Penrose-type drains that we fashion from latex-free gloves.

Postoperative Care

The ureteral stents are left in place for 7 to 10 days unless ureteral tapering was necessary. If the ureters were tapered, the stents are left for at least 2 weeks. Before removal, contrast is injected through the stents. If good drainage occurs around the stent, then the stents are removed.

The suprapubic tube is left on straight drainage. If an intestinal augmentation has been done, daily irrigation to remove mucus is carried out. After 3 postoperative weeks, the child is brought back to the office for a cystogram. The cystogram is performed before initiation of intermittent catheterization. If no leaks are present, a trial of catheterization of the appendicocystostomy by the parents and the patient is undertaken. Gentle catheterization with plenty of water-soluble lubricant is stressed. We like to use a 12 French straight polyethylene catheter because it has a more rounded and less sharp tip than other smaller caliber tubes. During the time that the patient is learning to catheterize, the suprapubic tube is left in place. If the intermittent catheterization goes smoothly, the suprapubic tube can be clamped during the day and then opened at night while bladder capacity is improving. During this time, we continue to irrigate the bladder to cycle the augment and also to remove mucus. Both parent and patient should be able to remove the mucus through the appendicocystostomy. We continually emphasize the importance of frequent catheterization and daily irrigation to keep the pouch from becoming overdistended and to minimize late mucous build-up as well as to reduce stone formation. We have learned the hard way that any difficulty with catheterization needs to be brought to the surgeon's attention promptly. If one makes the mistake of moving to a smaller and smaller catheter to facilitate passage, one may end up without the ability to pass a catheter at all. It is better to resolve a catheterization problem early before a simple problem becomes one that necessitates a total revision of the appendicocystostomy. The suprapubic tube is removed only when the patient can be dry overnight without discomfort with the suprapubic tube clamped.

We assess the pouch volume and look for vesicoureteral reflux at 3 months with an additional cystogram. The prophylactic antibacterials initiated after surgery may be discontinued if reflux is not present and if the pouch is of adequate size. We also carefully monitor for hyperchloremic acidosis if a significant length of intestine is used in the augmentation. We arrange for a Medic-Alert bracelet for each patient, because they will require continued lifetime follow-up. We check a periodic ultrasonogram initially at 6 months after surgery and then every 12 months.

VARIATIONS IN THE MITROFANOFF PRINCIPLE

When the appendix is not available, the ureter, tapered or plicated small intestine, and even the fallopian tube have been used as an efferent limb.

In our experience, a cutaneous ureterostomy has often been used when the appendix is not available. In the case of a previous loop cutaneous ureterostomy, it is obvious that the lower end will often make an attractive efferent limb after separation from the proximal ureter and subsequent reimplantation into the bladder.

Even if the bladder has been removed and an end cutaneous ureterostomy created, the distal ureter will obtain a supportive blood supply through its cutaneous anastomosis. Ashcraft and Dennis[56] have shown experimentally in the dog that this effect may take place over as short a period as 6 weeks. The blood supply to the distal ureter derived from the skin permits division of the ureter. The distal ureter is implanted as a continent catheterizable channel with a submucosal tunnel into the continent reservoir (Fig. 11–15). A high transureteroureterostomy to the opposite ureter, which is longer and implanted submucosally in the continent reservoir, completes the reconstruction. Gentle handling of the ureter

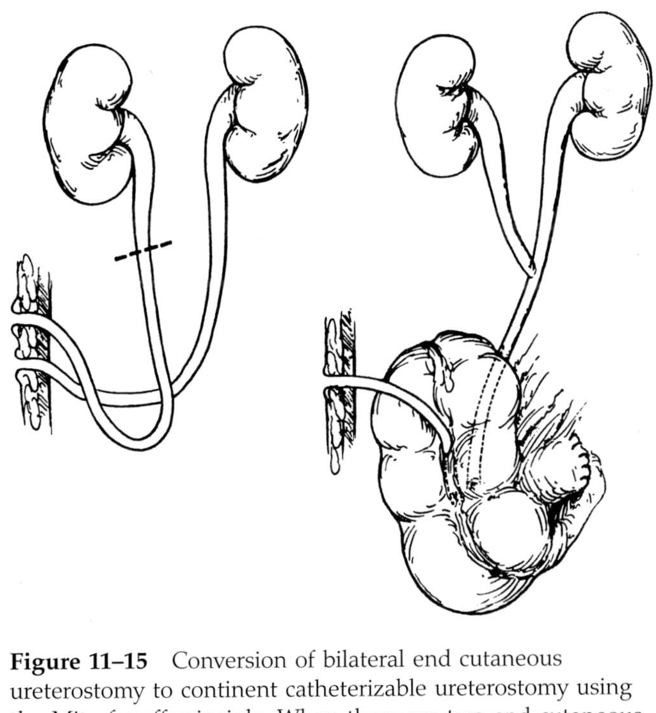

Figure 11–15 Conversion of bilateral end cutaneous ureterostomy to continent catheterizable ureterostomy using the Mitrofanoff principle. When there are two end cutaneous ureterostomies, one distal ureter can be supported by its stomal blood supply, permitting the construction of a submucosal, catheterizable, continent flap valve attachment to an intestinal reservoir. A high transureteroureterostomy completes the repair. From Duckett JW, Snyder HM. Use of the Mitrofanoff principle in urinary reconstruction. World J Urol 3:191, 1985. Used with permission.

is stressed to avoid injuring its intrinsic blood supply. The segment of ureter draining the kidney and its joining transureteroureterostomy is easily diverted with internal ureteral stents until a contrast study shows good healing, no extravasation, and free drainage.

When a loop cutaneous ureterostomy has previously been used or when the kidneys are being removed in patients awaiting renal transplant surgery, the ureter, if refluxing, can be reimplanted at the bladder end using the Lich-Gregoir technique, the Hutch reimplant,[57] or the Gil-Vernet technique.[58] In this case (Fig. 11–16), the distal blood supply is from the trigone and must be carefully preserved. Accordingly, if the antireflux mechanism must be rebuilt, a technique such as the Lich-Gregoir[59] that does not disturb the anastomosis of the ureter with the trigone is used. Postoperatively, these patients are managed similarly to those with appendicocystostomy.

A tubularized small intestinal segment can be tapered and used as another alternative to the appendix. A 10- to 12-cm segment of distal ileum is separated from the gastrointestinal tract and tailored along the antimesenteric border to approximately a 10 to 12 French intraluminal diameter. The anastomosis along the longitudinal plane is made with 4-0 polyglycolic acid (PGA) suture. Extreme care is taken to make the tapering uniform to provide for ease of catheterization. This technique is readily applicable to conversion of an ileal conduit. The ileal conduit can be preserved and tapered as the catheterizable stoma.[60] In addition to the appendix, ureter, and plicated small intestine, fallopian tube has been used as well.[61] Plicated stomach has also been described.[62] We have not been particularly pleased with the use of either of these two options. Fallopian tube is rarely redundant, and the plicated stomach, in our experience, resulted in significant excoriation at the stomal site, making its long-term use impractical.

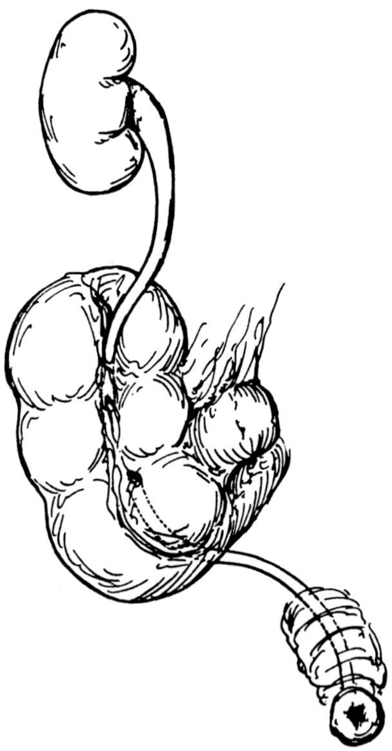

Figure 11–16 In the case of a solitary kidney, when the appendix is not available, the ureter can be divided more distally. The distal ureter is left with the attachment to the bladder remnant and reimplanted with a Lich-Gregoir or Gil-Vernet technique, if necessary. The proximal ureter is reimplanted into the pouch. From Duckett JW, Snyder HM. Use of the Mitrofanoff principle in urinary reconstruction. World J Urol 3:191, 1985. Used with permission.

RESULTS

Results following creation of the Mitrofanoff stoma have been largely satisfying. The vast majority of patients can be made dry, with the principal failures occurring because of high bladder pressures, which resulted in some stomal leakage in the few patients who have had the Mitrofanoff stoma made without augmentation of the bladder.[63] Patient acceptance is excellent with most patients who have the ability to catheterize both the bladder and the urethra choosing to catheterize the abdominal stoma over the urethra.[64] For boys with a sensate urethra, it clearly provides a more comfortable route for catheterization. For girls with spinal bifida confined to a wheelchair, it provides a much more accessible stoma than does the urethra. Complications, however, do occur.

Complications can be divided into two groups: those involving the efferent limb and those involving the pouch. Complications of the efferent limb include leakage, kinking, and stenosis. Complications of the pouch include stone formation, perforation, and infection.

Complications of the efferent limb occur in about 10 to 30% in most large series.[55, 61, 65] Most of these complications should be preventable. Leakage seems to be rare. A watertight valve can be made with as little as 2 cm of tunnel within the lumen of the bladder (P. Mitrofanoff, personal communication, May 1995). The functional continence length seems to rely on the type of tube and the type of backing. Ureters seem to leak more readily than the appendix, and the bowel wall seems to require a longer tunnel than does detrusor.[66] Kinking of the efferent limb is best prevented and usually requires revision when it occurs. Creation of the stoma and appendiceal-detrusor anastomosis to minimize length and provide a straight passage the entire length of the conduit is essential. Stomal stenosis occurs not infrequently, usually in about 10% of patients.[55] This can sometimes be corrected with careful revision of the stoma. More proximal narrowing of the tube usually requires more extensive revision.[61]

Complications of the pouch—infection, perforation,

and stone formation—are also preventable but require a firm commitment from the patient. Few patients who are emptying the pouch every 4 to 6 hours and irrigating to remove mucus have problems. However, not all patients continue to catheterize as frequently and become complacent in pouch management as they become more comfortable with the new bladder. Stasis and chronic distension can result in failure of the best surgical endeavor.

Colonization of the pouch with bacteria is common, and asymptomatic bacteriuria requires no treatment.[67] However, chronic infection and distension are the common denominators that lead to perforation. Any patient who experiences abdominal discomfort, especially with associated fever, should be treated on an emergency basis and undergo careful evaluation for signs of perforation. Ultrasonography and cystography will sometimes show evidence of extravasation on the drainage film. Perforations, however, are often not detectable radiologically. Failure to recognize and treat bladder perforation promptly results in significant morbidity[68] and even death.[69]

Reservoir or bladder stones are common in all types of reservoirs. The combination of infection, especially with *Proteus mirabilis,* mucus formation, and urinary stasis results in a stone formation rate that can be as high as 40%.[55] In Blyth and coworkers' review,[70] 26 of 87 patients with reservoirs experienced stones, with 23 of these in the reservoir. Most were triple-phosphate stones. Upper tract stones were managed successfully with extracorporeal shock wave lithotripsy. Stones located in the reservoirs were most effectively removed with open rather than endoscopic technique. Attempts at electrohydraulic lithotripsy or endoscopic litholapaxy usually resulted in incomplete extraction and recurrence. We much prefer to approach a reservoir stone or a collection of stones through a small suprapubic incision.

Loss of dependent drainage and incomplete irrigation results in accumulation of mucus, which acts as a foreign body nidus for stone formation. Bushman and Howards[71] described the effectiveness of nightly irrigation with a urea solution to prevent stones in augmented patients. To avoid stones, we have our patients irrigate with 300 mL of tap water each night to clear mucus. If compliance with this routine is good, few stones will develop; as a consequence, we have not used urea or other substances in the irrigant.

Appendicocystostomy with the common augmentation cystoplasty or creation of a continent pouch requires a considerable commitment from the surgeon, the patient, and the family. It is not for everyone. For selected patients, however, the ability to stay dry without long-term deterioration of the kidneys is a tremendous benefit.

AUGMENTED NIPPLE VALVES

In 1969 Kock developed a continent ileostomy reservoir for patients after total proctocolectomy.[72] The principle of the intussuscepted nipple and pouch of ileum was then used in 1975 for continent urinary diversion.[73] In this ileal pouch, the mechanism for continence as well as for prevention of ureteral reflux is based on an ileal intussusception valve devised initially to prevent intestinal regurgitation.[74, 75] This was first put to use in the urinary tract in dogs by Smith and Hinman to create a continent ileocystostomy through which the dogs could be catheterized. After the initial report by Kock in 12 patients,[76] Skinner popularized the procedure and continues to be its strongest advocate.[77–80] Numerous modifications from Skinner's group have helped bring this pouch into widespread use in the adult population. The Kock pouch is complicated and requires the use of a large (>70 cm) segment of ileum in the adolescent. Marginally smaller segments can be used in smaller children. Simpler pouches, however, continue to be more widely used in pediatric patients largely because of the uncertain long-term metabolic complications of such long bowel segments and the somewhat inconsistent catheterizable nipple, which may not stand up to repeated instrumentation by the child. Because of the technical difficulties with the Kock pouch, techniques that use the ileocecal junction are more common. Most of the children who require augmentation or continent diversion are myelodysplastic and have bowel motility problems and poorly tolerate loss of a substantial small bowel segment from the intestinal tract. A few examples of alternatives to the innovative Kock pouch that may be more appropriate for children follow.

MAINZ POUCH

The Mainz (mixed augmentation ileum and cecum) represented the evolution of the nipple valve from Gilchrist's cecal pouch, which used the ileocecal valve as a continence mechanism.[1] Portions of Kock's and Skinner's modifications of the ileal reservoir and Benchekroun's reversed intussusception of the ileum[81, 82] led to the development of this technique. Mansson and Sundin began using an intussuscepted loop of small intestine into the cecum, which failed because of difficulties with persistence of the intussuscepted limb.[83]

Beginning in 1983, the Mainz group began experimenting with a new reservoir that used several of the concepts of the Kock pouch but incorporated the use of cecum.[84] The concept is applicable to both bladder augmentation and bladder replacement.

Surgical Technique

For bladder augmentation, 10 to 15 cm of cecum and ascending colon and two segments of the adjacent terminal ileum are isolated with stay sutures. As in the Mitrofanoff procedure, it is often helpful to generously mobilize

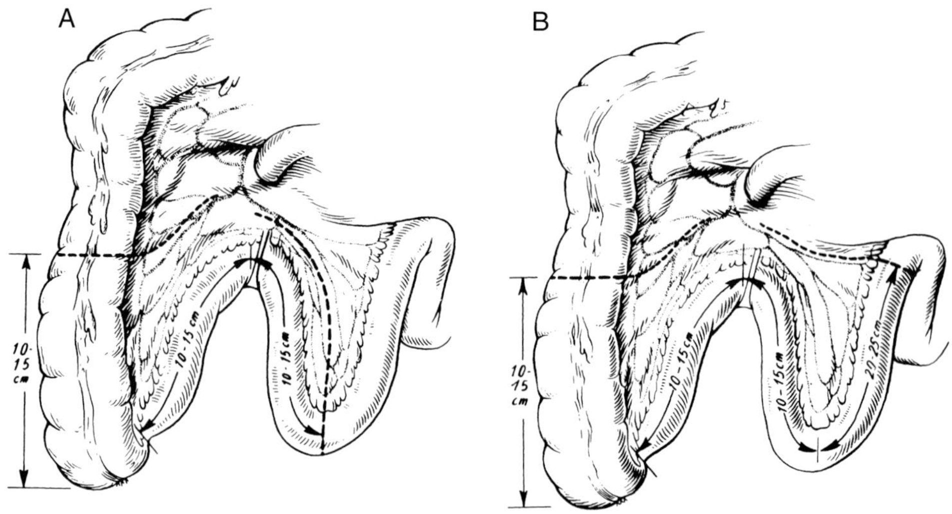

Figure 11–17 Mainz pouch ileal colonic segments: *A,* Segments needed for augmentation cystoplasty. *B,* Segments needed for continent urinary diversion. From Thuroff JW, Alken P, Riedmiller H, et al. The Mainz pouch (mixed augmentation ileum and cecum) for bladder augmentation and continent diversion. J Urol 136:17, 1986. Used with permission.

the ascending, transverse, and descending colon to provide for good mobility of the pouch. For continent urinary diversion, the same segments are used to fashion the pouch, but 20 to 25 cm of ileum must be isolated for ileoileal intussusception (Fig. 11–17). After isolation of the segment, the proximal ileum is reanastomosed to the distal colon superior to the isolated segments using either a stapled or sewn anastomosis. The mesenteric gap is

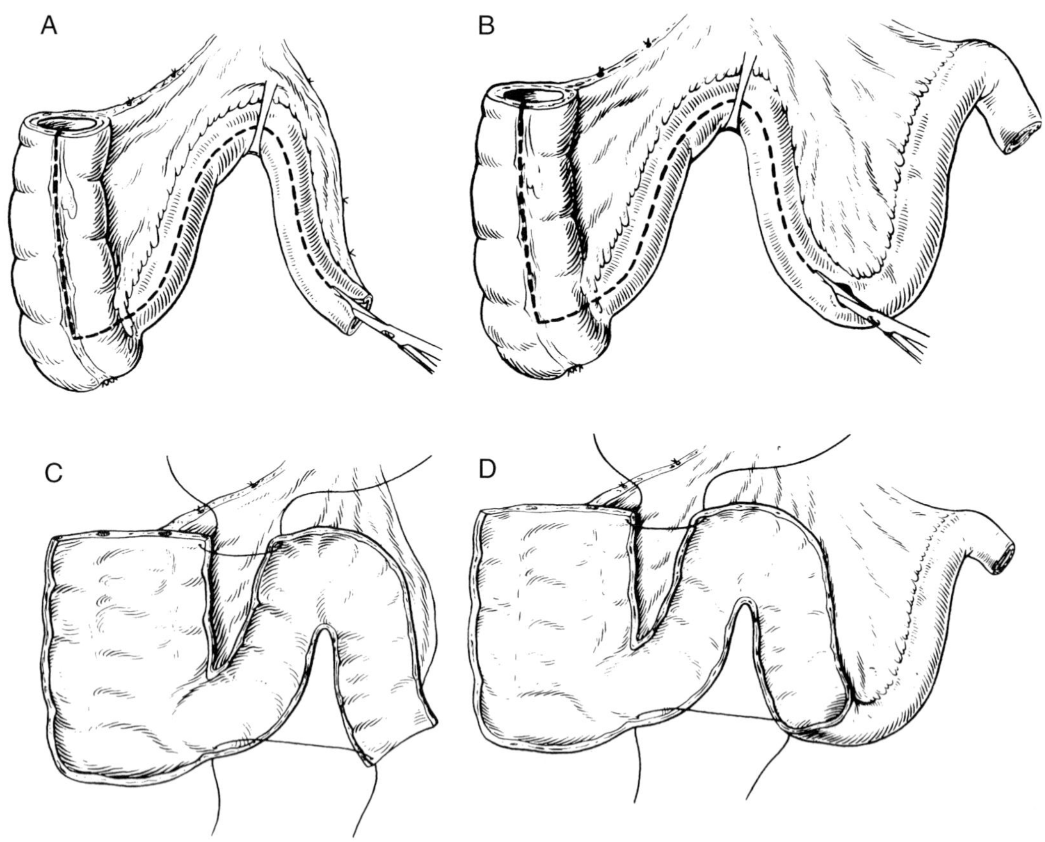

Figure 11–18 Mainz pouch segments. *A,* For augmentation. *B,* For continent urinary diversion. *C,* Segments opened. *D,* Note the proximal ileal segment to be used for intussusception in the case of bladder replacement. From Thuroff JW, Alken P, Riedmiller H, et al. The Mainz pouch (mixed augmentation ileum and cecum) for bladder augmentation and continent diversion. J Urol 136:17, 1986. Used with permission.

closed with interrupted sutures. The isolated segments are then opened along the antimesenteric border into an inverted-N shape. The two arms of the "N" are then closed with 4-0 absorbable PGA suture, providing a double reconfiguration of the segment (Fig. 11–18). The bladder is then prepared to accept the augmentation, usually by widely bivalving the bladder wall with incisions extending nearly to the trigone. The ureters may be reimplanted into the bladder base (preferable if they are still in situ in the bladder) or into the colonic segment (if previously diverted). We prefer, if possible, to implant the ureters as inferiorly on the pouch or bladder base as possible to prevent kinking of the ureters, which would likely occur as the pouch fills. If the implantation must be made on the superior portion of the pouch as shown (Fig. 11–19), the pouch itself must be fixed at the point of ureteral insertion. The pouch is then sewn to the bladder base with running 4-0 PGA suture. The ureteral

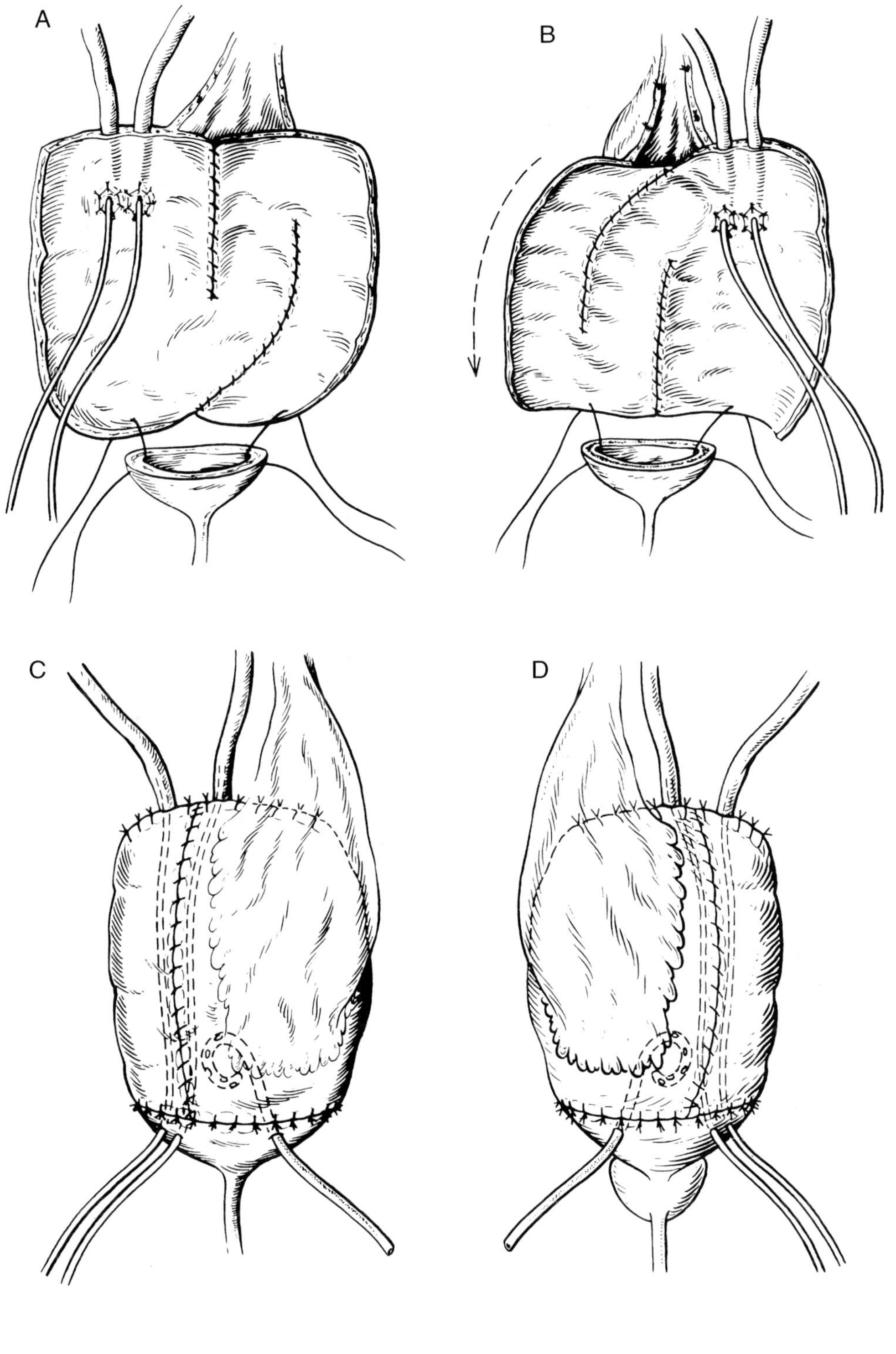

Figure 11–19 Mainz pouch anastomosis to bivalved bladder. *A*, With good colonic mobilization, rotation of the pouch as shown in *B* and *D* is unnecessary. *C*, Pouch sewn into place with ureteral stents taken through the bladder to drain percutaneously. I prefer a Malecot catheter rather than the pigtail catheter shown here for drainage. From Thuroff JW, Alken P, Riedmiller H, et al. The Mainz pouch (mixed augmentation ileum and cecum) for bladder augmentation and continent diversion. J Urol 136:17, 1986. Used with permission.

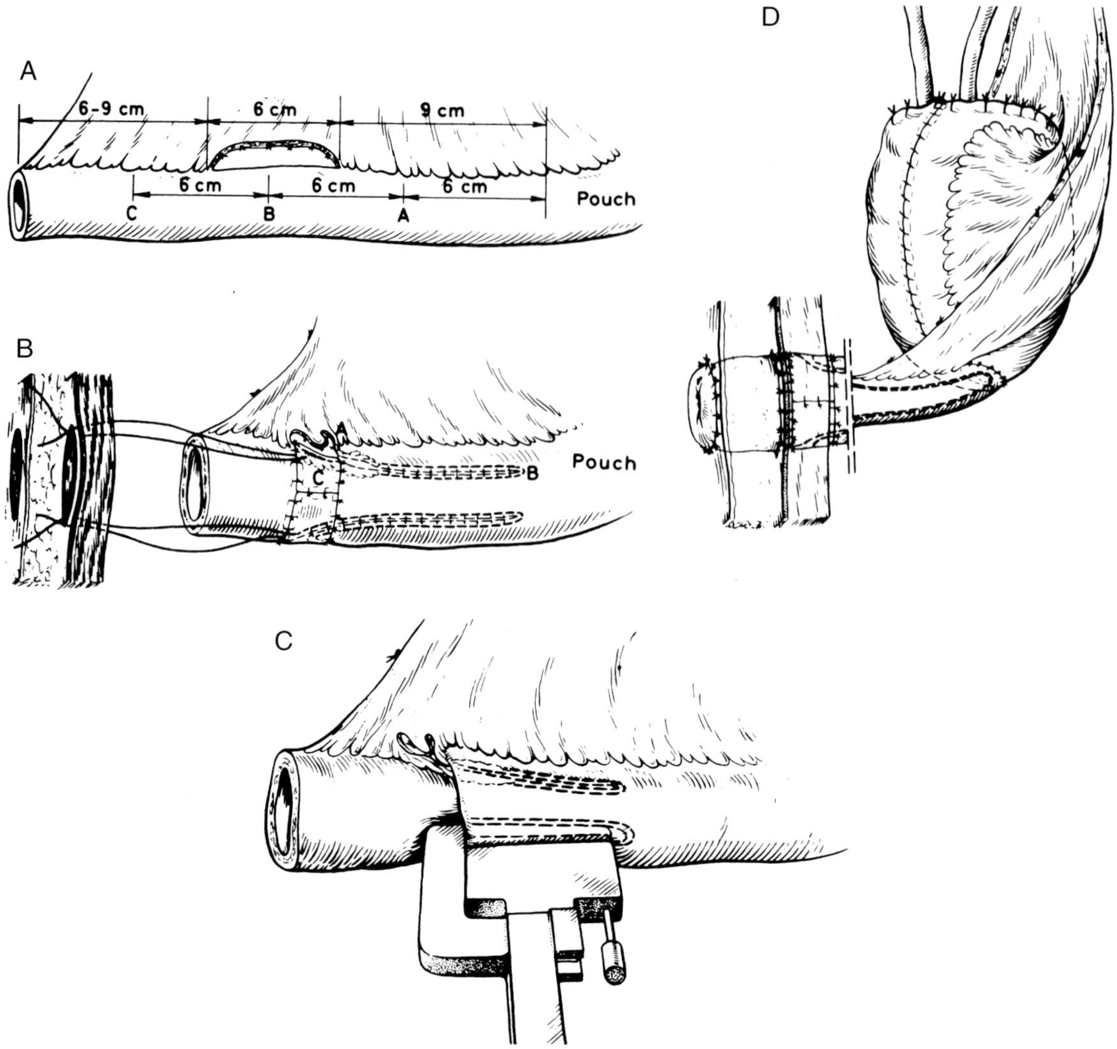

Figure 11–20 Mainz pouch efferent nipple. *A,* Outline of the segment to be intussuscepted. The mesentery of 6 cm of ileum is dissected off the bowel, leaving room for about 3 cm of intussusception. *B,* Completed intussusception. *C,* Nipple is secured with four rows of staples using the TA55 device. *D,* Completed stoma. The stoma is sutured with 5-6 interrupted sutures of 3-0 polyglycolic acid. From Thuroff JW, Alken P, Riedmiller H, et al. The Mainz pouch (mixed augmentation ileum and cecum) for bladder augmentation and continent diversion. J Urol 136:17, 1986. Used with permission.

stents are left for 10 days and the cystostomy tube (usually a 20 to 24 French Silastic Malecot catheter) is left for 3 weeks and clamped before removing, as in the Mitrofanoff procedure.

In the case of bladder replacement or if catheterization per urethra is not feasible (the majority of wheelchair-bound spina bifida patients), an efferent nipple is fashioned from the proximal 25-cm segment (Fig. 11–20).

Complications

Complications from the Mainz pouch are similar to those of other pouches with a few additions. The staples used in fashioning the ileal intussusception are prone to erosion and subsequent stone formation. Because of the complex nipple technique, the nipple, even when bolstered with the staples as described, is prone to disintussusception. This complication results in difficulty with catheterization and incontinence. For this reason we have been more pleased with the Mitrofanoff technique. The Mainz group adapted their pouch to incorporate the use of the appendix folded back and buried into a tenia instead of using the ileal nipple. This maneuver, when the appendix is in place, uses less intestine and is probably more dependable.

INDIANA POUCH

In an effort to simplify the efferent nipple further, the Indiana group developed another ileocecal pouch that plicated the ileal segment[85] rather than using it to create a nipple. In so doing, the surgery became simpler and contributed to the widespread use of continent urinary diversion. As mentioned, the plicated nipple uses the narrowed ileal segment to provide continence. Continence is not as reliable as with a flap valve or nipple valve, but this mechanism is easier to construct than the nipple and seems to hold up longer than the nipple to the trauma of catheterization. The pouch must be made large enough, rather too large than too small, because the plicated segment usually leaks at high pressures. This feature may in some cases provide an advantage if compliance is an issue, because leakage from the pouch will serve as a reminder to the patient that it is time to catheterize. As a result of this tendency for the efferent limb to "pop off" and drain, perforation may be less common with this pouch.

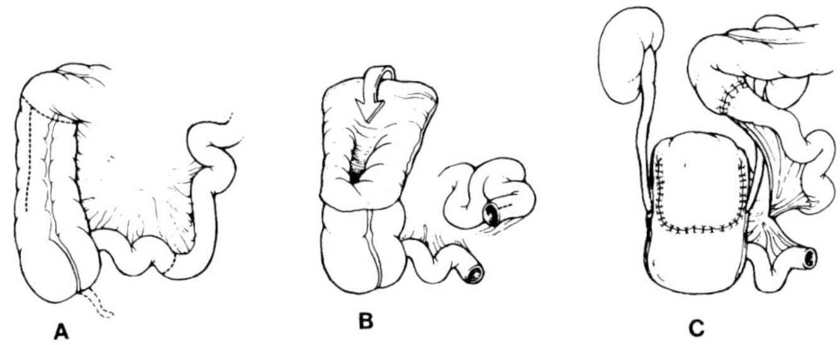

Figure 11–22 Indiana pouch, reconfigured technique. *A,* A slightly larger colonic segment is selected and opened. *B,* The distal colon is folded over the proximal cecum to increase the radius of the pouch. *C,* Completed pouch. From Rowland RG, Mitchell ME, Bihrle R, et al. Indiana continent urinary reservoir. J Urol 137:1136, 1987. Used with permission.

Surgical Technique

The ascending colon and intestine are mobilized as previously described for the Mainz pouch. Twenty centimeters of cecum and ascending colon are taken along with 15 to 18 cm of terminal ileum (Fig. 11–21*A*). A 12- to 15-cm segment of the terminal ileum is also divided to create a patch along the antimesenteric border of the spatulated end of the cecal segment (Fig. 11–21*B* and *C*). Alternatively, the cecum can be reconfigured as shown (Fig. 11–22).

After creation of the pouch, the ureters may be implanted along a tenia as originally described by the Indiana group (Fig. 11–23) or within the bladder if the pouch is used as an augmentation. As mentioned in the section on the Mainz pouch, if the ureters are reimplanted directly into the posterior portion of the colon, that portion of the pouch must be immobilized to prevent kinking of the ureter as the pouch fills.

The continent efferent limb is created by plicating the terminal ileum over a 12 French catheter (Fig. 11–24). Originally, the Indiana group described a hand-sewn plication. This was done in two layers, the first a series of 3-0 silk Lembert sutures about 8 to 10 mm apart beginning at the ileocecal valve and extending to the end of the ileal segment. After the plication is completed, the 12 French catheter is replaced with a 14 to 16 French

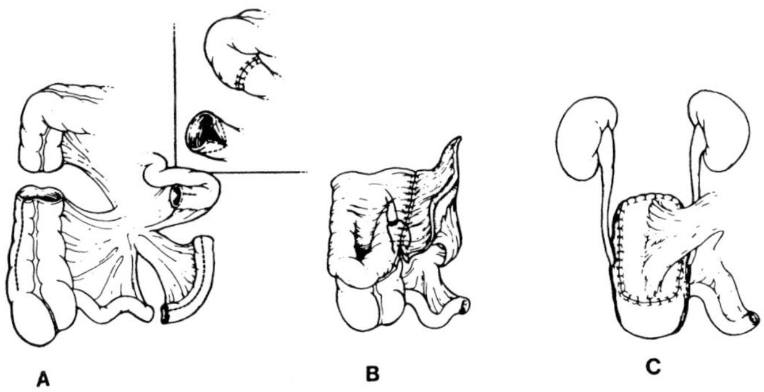

Figure 11–21 Indiana pouch. *A,* Ileocecal segment and adjacent ileal segment are mobilized, and the proximal ileum is anastomosed to the distal ascending or proximal transverse colon. *B,* The colon and ileum are opened along the antimesenteric border, and the ileum is sewn to the colon to reconfigure the segments. *C,* Completed pouch before plication. This technique is particularly attractive in cases in which an ileal conduit is present before undiversion. In practice, the plication of the ileum and ureteral reimplantation are completed before the closure of the pouch. Sigmoid may be substituted for ileum in cases in which an ileal conduit did not exist before undiversion. From Rowland RG, Mitchell ME, Bihrle R, et al. Indiana continent urinary reservoir. J Urol 137:1136, 1987. Used with permission.

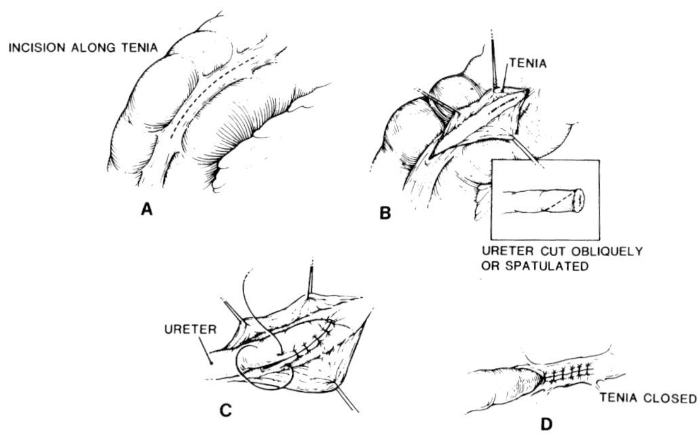

Figure 11–23 Indiana pouch: ureteral anastomosis. *A,* The tenia is opened along the dashed line. *B,* The colonic mucosa is opened for the ureteral anastomosis and spatulated along as shown in the inset. *C,* The ureter is anastomosed to the colonic mucosa with interrupted sutures of 5-0 or 6-0 polyglycolic acid suture. *D,* The tenia is then closed to create a tunnel to support the ureter and prevent vesicoureteric reflux. From Rowland RG, Mitchell ME, Bihrle R, et al. Indiana continent urinary reservoir. J Urol 137:1136, 1987. Used with permission.

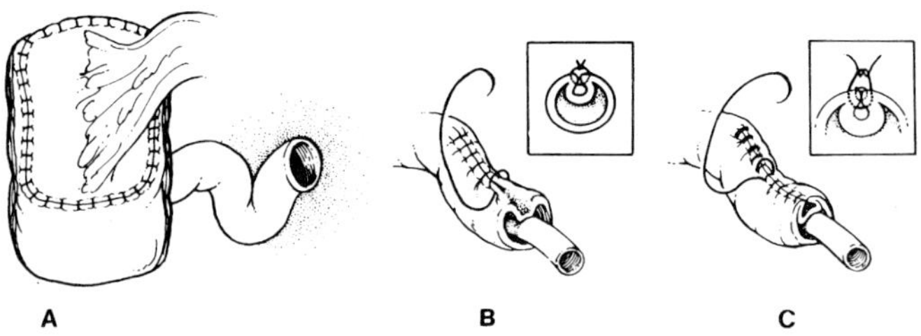

Figure 11–24 Indiana pouch: creation of the efferent limb. *A,* Pouch before plication (better to plicate before closing the pouch). *B,* The segment is plicated over a 12 French catheter with 3-0 Lembert sutures 8 to 10 mm apart, extending from the ileocecal valve to the end of the ileal segment. Modification to include stapling over the catheter would now be used. *C,* Second layer of reinforcing sutures can be placed over the stapled or sewn plication to improve continence or ease of catheterization. From Rowland RG, Mitchell ME, Bihrle R, et al. Indiana continent urinary reservoir. J Urol 137:1136, 1987. Used with permission.

catheter. If the larger catheter passes easily, the pouch is closed and filled with 300 to 400 mL of saline and catheterization is repeated. After the catheter is removed, the pouch is compressed to test continence. If there is leakage of saline through the efferent limb, additional sutures of 3-0 silk are placed. The catheter must then again be passed to ensure patency, ease of catheterization, and continence.

Modifications of the pouch—including a stapled, rather than plicated, efferent limb, tunneled ureteral reimplants, and plication of the ileocecal valve—have resulted in improved continence and reduced operative time.[48] The major problem with this pouch is in the concept of a tube valve rather than a flap valve and the lower leak pressure with this system.

MODIFIED URETEROSIGMOIDOSTOMIES

Ureterosigmoidostomy (USO) is the oldest form of urinary diversion, dating to 1852.[86] In traditional USO, the ureters are implanted into the sigmoid colon and continence is provided by the levator group. USO was applied nearly universally for the treatment of incontinence associated with exstrophy before 1970. Beginning at that time, reports of malignancy associated with ureteral colonic anastomosis began to become more common[87–90] and ultimately the risk of colon neoplasia was estimated at about 5 to 10%. This finding, along with the annoyingly common problem of night-time incontinence of urine and stool, combined to result in the demise of USO as an option for continent diversion in most centers.

MAINZ II POUCH

Despite USO's fall from popularity in the United States, Hohenfellner[91] in the Mainz group continued to use USO in the treatment of exstrophy. His attention to close follow-up seems to be effective in controlling the risk of malignancy. His modification of traditional USO to include a reconfiguration of the sigmoid loop to provide a pouch, which prevents propagation of colonic peristalsis, results in day and night-time dryness in nearly all patients.[91–94] These results have caused a resurgence in the use of USO,[95] which, I believe, restores it to its proper position as an effective tool in cases of failed primary bladder reconstruction in exstrophy.[96] Patients must be carefully selected. Those patients with encopresis or stool retention are not candidates for these procedures.

Surgical Technique[97]

Diverticulosis or polyps of the sigmoid colon, if suspected, are ruled out with lower intestinal radiography. Contraindications to Mainz pouch II include an incompetent anal sphincter, sigmoid diverticulosis, prior or planned radiotherapy, or intestinal polyps.

The colon is opened along the tinea at the junction between the sigmoid colon and rectum for a distance of 10 to 12 cm distal and proximal to create an inverted V shape, with the apex of the "V" based at the sigmorectal junction (Fig. 11–25). The hiatus for the ureter is created by incision of a segment of rectal wall as well as mucosa to prevent narrowing of the hiatus and ureteral obstruction as healing progresses. The ureters may be implanted along the tinea,[3] or using an open technique,[98] or in an open-ended technique, which is effective especially if the ureters are dilated. The ureters are sutured in place with interrupted 5-0 and 6-0 absorbable suture and stented for 8 to 10 days. The ureteral hiatus is closed gently on each side with 4-0 absorbable suture. The ureteral stents are led out through the rectum.

The pouch is then fixed to the sacral promontory (Fig. 11–26) to prevent migration or kinking of the ureters as the pouch fills. A rectal tube is left in place for 5 days. The rectal tube should be a single-lumen tube of wide caliber that is watched vigilantly for obstruction and irrigated often to prevent distension of the pouch.

Because of the risk of tumor after USO, careful monitoring with sigmoidoscopy is needed to identify tumors early in those at risk. The shortest reported time from USO to tumor in Husmann and Spence's large series was 3 years (juvenile polyp) and the longest period from surgery to initial tumor was 53 years (malignancy).[99] It seems logical that biannual sigmoidoscopies should begin about 6 years after diversion and continue indefinitely. Attention should be directed to the location of the ureterocolonic anastomosis.

ILEOCECAL URETEROSIGMOIDOSTOMY

When a previous ileal conduit has been performed, or as an alternative to the Mainz pouch II, a nonrefluxing ileal

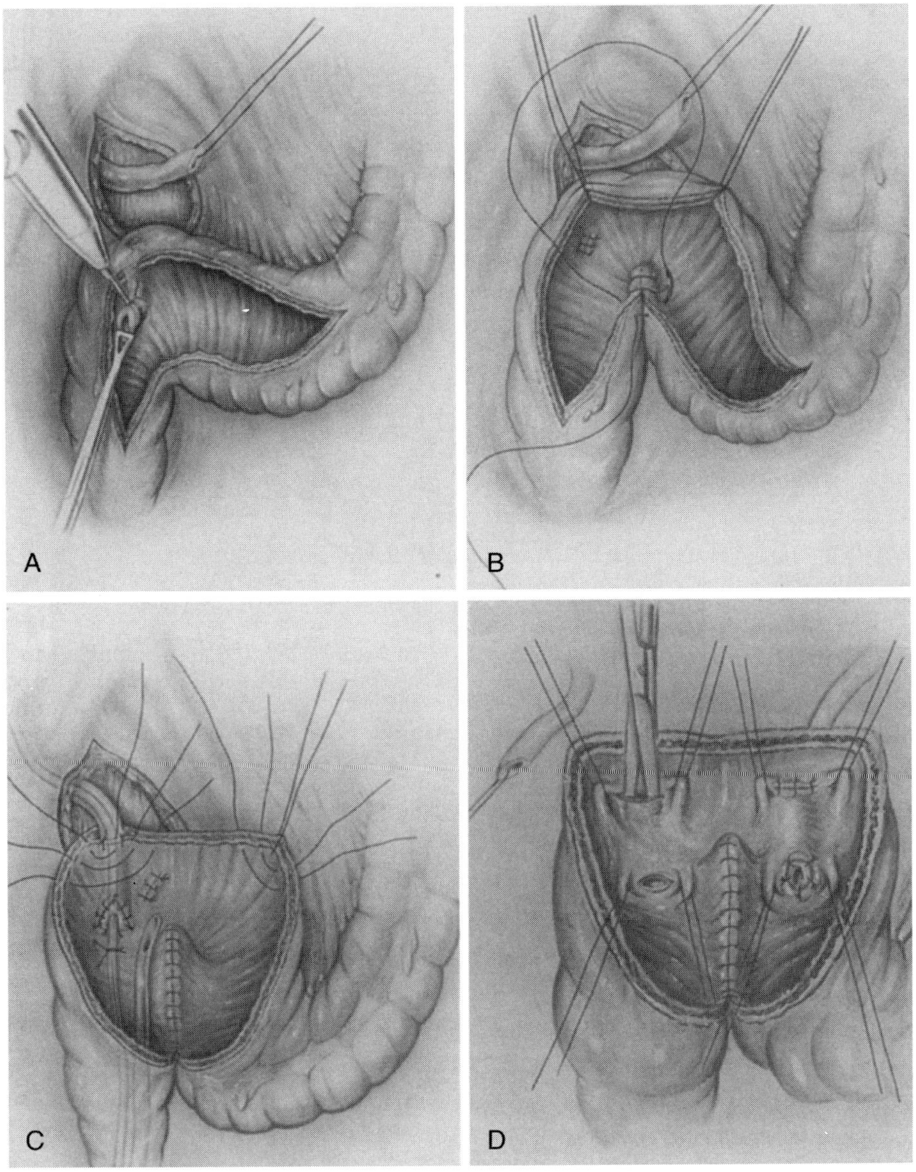

Figure 11–25 Mainz pouch II: creation of the pouch. *A,* After the ureter is transected at the ureterovesical junction, the anterior wall of the sigmoid is opened 12 cm proximal and 12 cm distal to the sigmorectal junction, creating the appearance of an inverted V. *B,* The ureter is divided at the ureterovesical junction (in cases of primary diversion) or mobilized from the previous ureterosigmoidostomy site (in cases in which a ureterosigmoidostomy is to be converted to a Mainz pouch II. The posterior wall of the sigmoid is then closed with a running suture of 4-0 Vicryl. *C,* The right ureter is brought in through the back wall as an open-ended technique (for dilated ureters) or *(D)* tunneled (for normal caliber ureters). From Fisch M, Wammach R, Muller S, Hohenfellner R. The Mainz pouch II (sigma rectum pouch). J Urol 149:258, 1993. Used with permission.

conduit has been fashioned that is taken down onto the sigmoid. This modification could theoretically reduce the risk of cancer by eliminating the combination of stool, urine, and a ureteral-colonic anastomosis, which has been implicated as the necessary setting for colonic tumor after ureterosigmoidostomy.[100] Rink and Retik devised this technique and used it in five patients as a staged approach.[101] Kim, Susskind, and King then reported five subsequent patients with exstrophy and one with epispadias in whom a one-stage ileocecal ureterosigmoidostomy was performed.[102]

Surgical Technique

The ascending colon and distal ileum are mobilized, and a short segment of cecum and 15 cm of terminal ileum are selected (Fig. 11–27*A*). The proximal ileum is anastomosed to the ascending colon as in the Indiana and Mainz pouches. A 4- to 5-cm long nipple is fashioned from the distal 6- to 7-cm segment of ileum from which the mesentery has been separated. An incision is made through the full thickness of the outer wall of the intussusception. The cecal mucosa is stripped from the muscle of the cecal wall to provide a surface on which the ileal serosa will scar to stabilize the nipple (Fig. 11–27*B*). Interrupted 2-0 chromic suture is used to suture the exposed ileal muscle to the exposed cecal muscle. In this way, staples and the inherent complication of stone formation are avoided in the construction of the nipple. By suturing the nipple to the side wall of the cecum, the nipple valve is converted to a flap valve, which further reduces the tendency for disintussusception. The ureters are then anastomosed to the ileal segment proximal to the nipple, which prevents reflux from the pouch to the

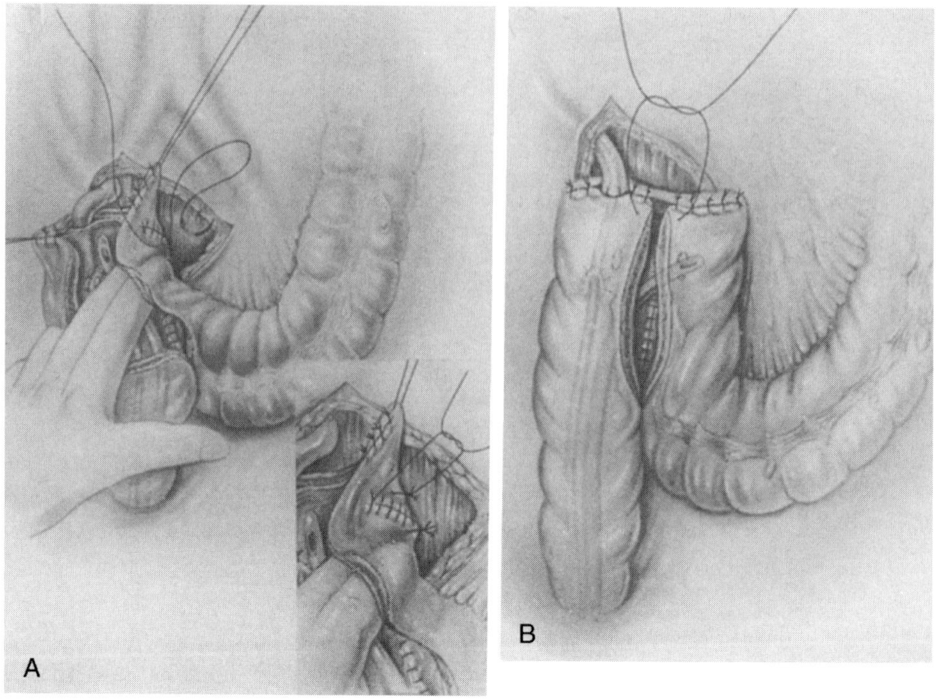

Figure 11–26 Mainz pouch II: fixation and closure. *A,* The pouch is then fixed to the sacral promontory, taking care to prevent compromise of the sigmoid mesentery. Sutures are placed lateral to the mesentery on each side. These sutures may be absorbable if a window has been made in the posterior parietal peritoneum. *B,* The anterior wall is closed with two layers of 4-0 absorbable sutures. The rectal tube is left for 3 to 5 days. The ureteral stents are left for 8 to 10 days. From Fisch M, Wammach R, Muller S, Hohenfellner R. The Mainz pouch II (sigma rectum pouch). J Urol 149:258, 1993. Used with permission.

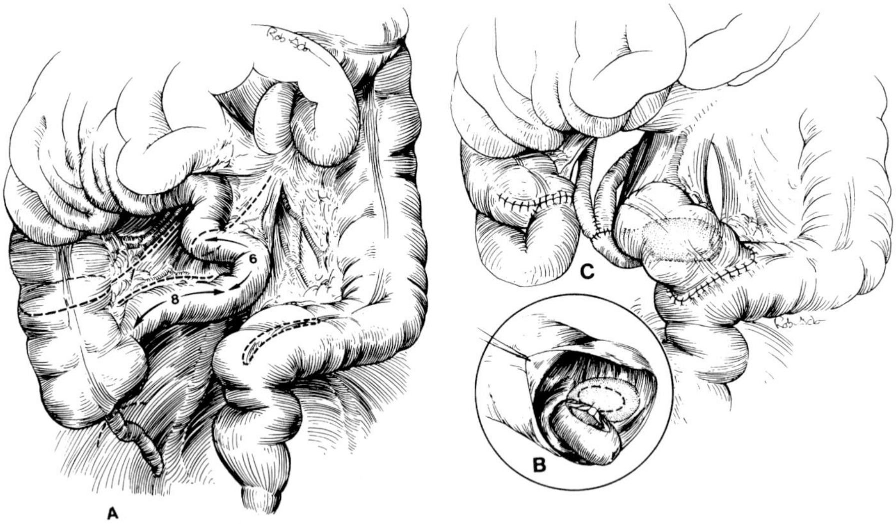

Figure 11–27 Ileocecal ureterosigmoidostomy (King). *A,* Segments selected: 12 cm of terminal ileum and enough cecum to carry the stabilized ileal intussusception to the sigmoid are marked. The proximal ileum is anastomosed to the ascending colon. *B,* The nipple is created and stabilized with a muscle-to-muscle anastomosis, which converts the nipple to a flap valve, providing a stable intussusception. *C,* The ureters are sutured to the ileal segment proximal to the nipple. From Kim KS, Susskind MR, King LR. Ileocecal ureterosigmoidostomy: An alternative to conventional ureterosigmoidostomy. J Urol 140:1494, 1988. Used with permission.

ureter (Fig. 11–27C). The anastomosis of the ureter to the ileum rather than the sigmoid breaks the triad known to be associated with adenocarcinoma of the colon.[103]

Complications of Modified Ureterosigmoidostomy

Short-term complications include anastomotic leak, which can be hazardous because of the risk of infection after dissemination of enteral bacteria within the pelvis and intraperitoneal space. With the advent of the antirefluxing ureteral anastomosis, the reconfigured pouch, and the widespread use of prophylactic antibiotics after the surgery, the risks of pyelonephritis have become minimal. Hyperchloremic metabolic acidosis, normally mild in patients with good renal function, can be dangerous, particularly if emptying is infrequent. Some patients will require exogenous bicarbonate to keep the serum level above 20 mg/dL. Dehydration resulting from diarrhea (not just urinary tract infection) can be particularly dangerous in this group of patients. The combination of fever, increased urinary concentration, and infrequent emptying combine to worsen the acidosis and may require hospital admission for intravenous fluids and rectal drainage with a large-bore single-lumen tube.

SUMMARY

This short review of selected techniques applicable to continent urinary diversion or bladder augmentation is designed to provide a series of tools to be used in patients desiring reconstructive surgery to become dry. No single technique will serve every patient, nor are any of the operations described commonly performed without some sort of modification to suit the individual patient. These are complicated procedures that should not be undertaken without a thorough understanding of the principles of the procedures. If performed on the incompletely prepared patient or family, the surgeon may risk trading incontinence, which is a social problem, for a difficult medical handicap. Continent urinary diversion should never be performed on a child without careful consultation that has grown out of a long-standing relationship with the patient and family. Well performed and well scrutinized pre- and postoperatively, these techniques and their variations will serve carefully chosen patients well and provide them an opportunity to live a much more normal life.

REFERENCES

1. Gilchrist RK, Merrick JW, Hamlin HH, Rieger IT. Construction of a substitute bladder and urethra. Surg Gynecol Obstet 90:752, 1950.
2. Bricker EM. Bladder substitution after pelvic evisceration. Surg Clin North Am 30:1511, 1950.
3. Leadbetter W. Consideration of problems incident to performance of uretero-enterostomy: Report of a technique. J Urol 65:818, 1951.
4. Coffey R. Transplantation of the ureters into the large intestine in the absence of a functioning urinary bladder. Surg Gynecol Obstet 32:383, 1921.
5. Spence HM, Hoffman WW, Fosmire GP. Tumour of the colon as a late complication of ureterosigmoidostomy for exstrophy of the bladder. Br J Urol 51:466, 1979.
6. Schwarz GR, Jeffs RD. Ileal conduit urinary diversion in children: Computer analysis of followup from 2 to 16 years. J Urol 114:285, 1975.
7. Hendren WH. Exstrophy of the bladder: Alternative method of management. J Urol 115:195, 1976.
8. Lapides J, Diokno AC, Gould FR, et al. Clean intermittent self-catheterization in the treatment of urinary tract disease. J Urol 107:458, 1972.
9. McGuire EJ, Woodside JR, Borden TA, Weiss, RM, et al. Prognostic value of urodynamic testing in myelodysplastic patients. J Urol 126:205, 1981.
10. Golimbu M, Morales P. Jejunal conduits, technique and complications. J Urol 113:787, 1975.
11. Mitchell ME, Rink RC. Pediatric urinary diversion and undiversion. Pediatr Clin North Am 34:1319, 1987.
12. Kass EJ, Koff SA. Bladder augmentation in the pediatric neuropathic bladder. J Urol 129:552, 1983.
13. Thuroff JW, Alken P, Riedmiller H, et al. The Mainz pouch for augmentation or substitution of the bladder and continent diversion. Semin Urol 5:69, 1987.
14. McDougal W. Use of intestinal segments in the urinary tract: Basic principles. In Walsh P, Retik A, Stamey T, Vaughan EJ. (eds), Campbell's Urology. Philadelphia: WB Saunders, 1992, p 2619.
15. Traub S, Johnson C. Comparison of methods of estimating creatinine clearance in children. Am J Hosp Pharm 37:195, 1980.
16. Kinn AC, Lantz B. Vitamin B12 deficiency after irradiation for bladder carcinoma. J Urol 131:888, 1984.
17. Steiner MS, Morton RA, Marshall FF. Vitamin B12 deficiency in patients with ileocolic neobladders. J Urol 149:255, 1993.
18. Canning DA, Perman JA, Jeffs RD, Gearhart JP. Nutritional consequences of bowel segments in the lower urinary tract. J Urol 142:509, 1989.
19. Adams MC, Mitchell ME, Rink RC. Gastrocystoplasty: An alternative solution to the problem of urological reconstruction in the severely compromised patient. J Urol 140:1152, 1988.
20. Gosalbez R Jr, Woodard JR, Broecker BH, Warshaw B. Metabolic complications of the use of stomach for urinary reconstruction. J Urol 150:710, 1993.
21. Plawker MW, Rabinowitz SS, Etwaru DJ, Glassberg KI. Hypergastrinemia, dysuria-hematuria and metabolic alkalosis: Complications associated with gastrocystoplasty. J Urol 154:546, 1995.
22. Nguyen DH, Bain MA, Salmonson KL, et al. The syndrome of dysuria and hematuria in pediatric urinary reconstruction with stomach [see comments]. J Urol 150:707, 1993.
23. Lockhart JL, Davies R, Cox C, et al. The gastroileoileal pouch: An alternative continent urinary reservoir for patients with short bowel, acidosis and/or extensive pelvic radiation. J Urol 150:46, 1993.
24. Lockhart JL, Davies R, Persky L, et al. Acid-base changes following urinary tract reconstruction for continent diversion and orthotopic bladder replacement. J Urol 152:338, 1994.
25. Cartwright PC, Snow BW. Bladder autoaugmentation: Partial detrusor excision to augment the bladder without use of bowel. J Urol 142:1050, 1989.

26. Cartwright PC, Snow BW. Bladder autoaugmentation: Early clinical experience. J Urol 142:505, 1989.
27. Dewan PA, Byard RW. Autoaugmentation gastrocystoplasty in a sheep model. Br J Urol 72:56, 1993.
28. Dewan PA, Stefanek W. Autoaugmentation gastrocystoplasty: Early clinical results. Br J Urol 74:460, 1994.
29. Buson H, Manivel JC, Dayanc M, et al. Seromuscular colocystoplasty lined with urothelium: Experimental study. Urology 44:743, 1994.
30. Gonzalez R, Buson H, Reid C, Reinberg Y. Seromuscular colocystoplasty lined with urothelium: Experience with 16 patients [see comments]. Urology 45:124, 1995.
31. Bellinger MF. Ureterocystoplasty: A unique method for vesical augmentation in children. J Urol 149:811, 1993.
32. Lailas NG, Cilento B, Atala A. Progressive ureteral dilation for subsequent ureterocystoplasty. J Urol 156:1151, 1996.
33. Atala A, Freeman MR, Vacanti JP, et al. Implantation in vivo and retrieval of artificial structures consisting of rabbit and human urothelium and human bladder muscle. J Urol 150:608, 1993.
34. Cilento BG, Freeman MR, Schneck FX, et al. Phenotypic and cytogenetic characterization of human bladder urothelia expanded in vitro. J Urol 152:665, 1994.
35. Vaught JD, Kropp BP, Sawyer BD, et al. Detrusor regeneration in the rat using porcine small intestinal submucosal grafts: Functional innervation and receptor expression. J Urol 155:374, 1996.
36. Kropp BP, Eppley BL, Prevel CD, et al. Experimental assessment of small intestinal submucosa as a bladder wall substitute. Urology 46:396, 1995.
37. Kropp BP, Badylak S, Thor KB. Regenerative bladder augmentation: A review of the initial preclinical studies with porcine small intestinal submucosa. Adv Exp Med Biol 385:229, 1995.
38. Kropp BP, Rippy MK, Badylak SF, et al. Regenerative urinary bladder augmentation using small intestinal submucosa: Urodynamic and histopathologic assessment in long-term canine bladder augmentations. J Urol 155:2098, 1996.
39. Hinman F Jr. Selection of intestinal segments for bladder substitution: Physical and physiological characteristics. J Urol 139:519, 1988.
40. Elder JS. Periurethral and puboprostatic sling repair for incontinence in patients with myelodysplasia. J Urol 144:434, 1990.
41. Kropp KA, Angwafo FF. Urethral lengthening and reimplantation for neurogenic incontinence in children. J Urol 135:533, 1986.
42. Nill TG, Peller PA, Kropp KA. Management of urinary incontinence by bladder tube urethral lengthening and submucosal reimplantation. J Urol 144:559, 1990.
43. Salle JL, de Fraga JC, Amarante A, et al. Urethral lengthening with anterior bladder wall flap for urinary incontinence: A new approach. J Urol 152:803, 1994.
44. Hensle TW, Kirsch AJ, Kennedy W II, Reiley EA. Bladder neck closure in association with continent urinary diversion. J Urol 154:883, 1995.
45. Dees JE. Congenital epispadias with incontinence. J Urol 62:513, 1949.
46. Leadbetter GWJ. Surgical correction of total urinary incontinence. J Urol 91:261, 1964.
47. Young HH. An operation for the cure of incontinence of urine. Surg Gynecol Obstet 28L:84, 1919.
48. Rowland RG, Kropp BP. Evolution of the Indiana continent urinary reservoir. J Urol 152:2247, 1994.
49. Hendren WH. Reoperative ureteral reimplantation: Management of the difficult case. J Pediatr Surg 15:770, 1980.
50. Zinman L, Libertino JA. Right coloplasty for bladder replacement. Urol Clin North Am 13:321, 1986.
51. Mitchell ME, Rink RC. Urinary diversion and undiversion. Urol Clin North Am 12:111, 1985.
52. King LR, Robertson CN, Bertram RA. A new technique for the prevention of reflux in those undergoing bladder substitution or undiversion using bowel segments. World J Urol 3:194, 1985.
53. Mitrofanoff P. Cystostomie continente trans-appendendiculaire dans le traitement des vessies neurologiques. Chir Pediatr 21:297, 1980.
54. Duckett JW, Snyder HM. Continent urinary diversion: Variations on the Mitrofanoff principle. J Urol 135:58, 1986.
55. Duckett JW, Lotfi AH. Appendicovesicostomy (and variations) in bladder reconstruction. J Urol 149:567, 1993.
56. Ashcraft KW, Dennis PA. The reimplanted ureter as a catheterizing stoma. J Pediatr Surg 21:1042, 1986.
57. Hutch JA. Vesicoureteral reflux in the paraplegic: Cause and correction. J Urol 68:457, 1952.
58. Gil-Vernet JM. A new technique for surgical correction of vesicoureteral reflux. J Urol 131:456, 1984.
59. Lich-Gregoir W. Le traitement chirurgical du reflux vesico-ureteral congenital. Acta Chir Belg 63:431, 1964.
60. Lobe TE. Conversion of an ileal conduit into a neourethral entero-plication for urinary continence: Tips in its proper construction. J Pediatr Surg 21:1040, 1986.
61. Woodhouse CR, MacNeily AE. The Mitrofanoff principle: Expanding upon a versatile technique. Br J Urol 74:447, 1994.
62. Gosalbez R, Padron OF, Singla AK, et al. The gastric augment single pedicle tube catheterizable stoma: A useful adjunct to reconstruction of the urinary tract. J Urol 152:2005, 1994.
63. Jayanthi VR, Churchill BM, McLorie GA, Khoury AE. Concomitant bladder neck closure and Mitrofanoff diversion for the management of intractable urinary incontinence. J Urol 154:886, 1995.
64. Horowitz M, Kuhr CS, Mitchell ME. The Mitrofanoff catheterizable channel: Patient acceptance. J Urol 153:771, 1995.
65. Hasan ST, Marshall C, Neal DE. Continent urinary diversion using the Mitrofanoff principle. Br J Urol 74:454, 1994.
66. Watson HS, Bauer SB, Peters CA, et al. Comparative urodynamics of appendiceal and ureteral Mitrofanoff conduits in children. J Urol 154:878, 1995.
67. Akerlund S, Campanello M, Kaijser B, Jonsson O. Bacteriuria in patients with a continent ileal reservoir for urinary diversion does not regularly require antibiotic treatment. Br J Urol 74:177, 1994.
68. Elder JS, Snyder HM, Hulbert WC, Duckett JW. Perforation of the augmented bladder in patients undergoing clean intermittent catheterization. J Urol 140:1159, 1988.
69. Braverman RM, Lebowitz RL. Perforation of the augmented urinary bladder in nine children and adolescents: Importance of cystography. AJR Am J Roentgenol 157:1059, 1991.
70. Blyth B, Ewalt D, Duckett J, Snyder H. Lithogenic properties of enterocystoplasty. J Urol 148:457, 1992.
71. Bushman W, Howards S. The use of urea for dissolution of urinary mucus in urinary tract reconstruction. J Urol 151:1036, 1994.
72. Kock NG. Intra-abdominal "reservoir" in patients with permanent ileostomy. Preliminary observations on a procedure resulting in fecal "continence" in five ileostomy patients. Arch Surg 99:223, 1969.
73. Kock NG, Nilson A, Norlen L, et al. Urinary diversion. Scand J Urol Nephrol 49:23, 1978.
74. Basso D. The efficacy and applicability of an intussuscepted conical valve in preventing regurgitation and leakage of intestinal contents. Ann Surg 133:477, 1951.
75. Perl J. Intussuscepted conical valve formation in jejunostomies. Surgery 25:297, 1949.
76. Kock NG, Nilson AE, Nilsson LO, et al. Urinary diversion via a continent ileal reservoir: Clinical results in 12 patients. J Urol 128:469, 1982.

77. Skinner DG. The Kock pouch for continent urinary reconstruction focusing on the afferent segment and the reservoir. Scand J Urol Nephrol Suppl 142:77, 1992.
78. Skinner DG, Lieskovsky G, Boyd S. The continent ileal reservoir as an alternative to cutaneous urinary diversion. Nippon Hinyokika Gakkai Zasshi 77:1928, 1986.
79. Skinner DG, Boyd SD, Lieskovsky G. Clinical experience with the Kock continent ileal reservoir for urinary diversion. J Urol 132:1101, 1984.
80. Skinner DG, Lieskovsky G, Boyd SD. Technique of creation of a continent internal ileal reservoir (Kock pouch) for urinary diversion. Urol Clin North Am 11:741, 1984.
81. Benchekroun A. Continent caecal bladder. Eur Urol 3:248, 1977.
82. Benchekroun A. Continent caecal bladder. Br J Urol 54:505, 1982.
83. Mansson W, Sundin T. The continent caecal reservoir for urine. Thesis. Scand J Urol Nephrol 48:4, 1978.
84. Thuroff JW, Alken P, Riedmiller H, et al. The Mainz pouch (mixed augmentation ileum and cecum) for bladder augmentation and continent diversion. J Urol 136:17, 1986.
85. Rowland RG, Mitchell ME, Bihrle R, et al. Indiana continent urinary reservoir. J Urol 137:1136, 1987.
86. Simon J. Ectopia vesicae (absence of the anterior wall of the bladder and pubic abdominal parietes): Operation for directing the orifices of the ureters into the rectum; temporary success; subsequent death. Lancet 2:568, 1852.
87. Richter RM, Ginsberg SA. Late development of colonic carcinoma complicating ureterosigmoidostomy. Am J Surg 113:843, 1967.
88. Kozak JA, Watkins WE, Jewell WR. Neoplastic stomal obstruction: A complication of ureterosigmoidostomy. J Urol 96:691, 1966.
89. Oetjen L Jr, Campbell JL, Thomley MW, Parsons RL. Carcinoma of the colon following ureterosigmoidostomy: Report of a case. J Urol 104:536, 1970.
90. Myers JW. Carcinoma of the colon associated with ureterosigmoidostomy: Report of an unusual case. Mich Med 72:285, 1973.
91. Altwein JE, Jonas U, Hohenfellner R. Long-term followup of children with colon conduit urinary diversion and ureterosigmoidostomy. J Urol 118:832, 1977.
92. Fisch M, Wammack R, Muller SC, Hohenfellner R. The Mainz pouch II. Eur Urol 25:7, 1994.
93. Fisch M, Wammack R, Steinbach F, et al. Sigma-rectum pouch (Mainz pouch II). Urol Clin North Am 20:561, 1993.
94. Fisch M, Wammack R, Hohenfellner R. Seven years experience with the Mainz pouch procedure. Arch Esp Urol 45:175, 1992.
95. Hohenfellner R. Ureterosigmoidostomy: Past, present and future. Scand J Urol Nephrol Suppl 142:86, 1992.
96. Canning D. Bladder exstrophy: The case for primary reconstruction. Urology 48:831, 1996.
97. Fisch M, Wammach R, Muller S, Hohenfellner R. The Mainz pouch II (sigma rectum pouch). J Urol 149:258, 1993.
98. Goodwin WE, Scardino PT. Ureterosigmoidostomy. J Urol 118:169, 1977.
99. Husmann DA, Spence HM. Current status of tumor of the bowel following ureterosigmoidostomy: A review. J Urol 144:607, 1990.
100. Gittes RF. Carcinogenesis in ureterosigmoidostomy. Urol Clin North Am 13:201, 1986.
101. Rink R, Retik A. Ureteroileocecal sigmoidostomy (ileal ureterosigmoidostomy) and avoidance of carcinoma of the colon. In King L, Stone A, Webster G (eds), Bladder Reconstruction and Continent Urinary Diversion. Chicago: Year Book, 1987, p 172.
102. Kim KS, Susskind MR, King LR. Ileocecal ureterosigmoidostomy: An alternative to conventional ureterosigmoidostomy. J Urol 140:1494, 1988.
103. Crissey MM, Steele GD, Gittes RF. Rat model for carcinogenesis in ureterosigmoidostomy. Science 207:1079, 1980.

ALAN B. RETIK

12

Comments on Ureteroileocecal Sigmoidostomy—An Alternative Method of Urinary Diversion

For many years ureterosigmoidostomy was the most popular form of urinary diversion. Multiple modifications of the technique were devised to prevent the complications associated with coloureteral reflux and ureteral obstruction (e.g., pyelonephritis, formation of calculi, and ultimate impairment of renal function). In the early 1900s, Coffey[1] described a long tunnel for entry of ureter into the colon. Nesbit[2] and Cordonnier[3] suggested a direct ureteral mucosa–colonic mucosa anastomosis and in 1953, Mathisen[4] reported the creation of an intraluminal ureteral nipple. Goodwin,[5, 6] at the same time, described the open transcolonic ureterocolonic anastomosis. One year later, Leadbetter and Clarke[7] reported a technique combining Coffey's tunnel and Nesbit's direct elliptical anastomosis to prevent reflux and obstruction. Hendren modified this technique further.[8–10] The newer techniques have reduced the complication rate. However, hyperchloremic acidosis with hypokalemia, pyelonephritis, calculi, ureteral obstruction, and incontinence still pose problems in some patients.

The ileal conduit, introduced by Bricker[11] in 1950, was used widely in adults and children with an initial low complication rate. However, the high long-term complication rate has virtually eliminated its use in children.[12–14]

During the past decade, there has been increased interest in continent urinary diversion with better management of metabolic acidosis and the ability to create an antireflux ureteral-colonic anastomosis with continence provided by the patient's own sphincteric muscles. Thus, ureterosigmoidostomy has enjoyed somewhat of a revival. A number of investigators regard ureterosigmoidostomy as the preferred method of management in children with exstrophy of the bladder if primary reconstruction is not possible.[9, 15, 16]

A major complication of ureterosigmoidostomy that has evolved with long-term follow-up has been the development of neoplasia of the colon. Some of the tumors are benign adenomatous polyps, but most are malignant; adenocarcinoma is the primary type.[17] The mortality rate in the adenocarcinoma group has been approximately 50%. Hamer[18] in 1929 first reported this complication, and by the early 1980s more than 85 cases had been reported. The average lag time from ureterosigmoidostomy to tumor occurrence has been 25 years. The overall latency period has varied from 7 to 50 years in the group that underwent diversion for benign disease. The incidence of tumor formation has been estimated at 550 times that of the population at large with a 7000-fold increase among patients younger than 25 years. Therefore, there is approximately a 5% overall risk that a patient with a ureterosigmoidostomy will subsequently experience adenocarcinoma of the colon. The tumor occurs most often at the site of implantation of the ureter into the sigmoid colon.[19] Several tumors have occurred at the ureterosigmoid anastomotic stump left in situ many years after the diversion of urine to an ileal conduit or ipsilateral nephrectomy. Adenocarcinoma at the ureteral stump developed in one patient more than 20 years after conversion to an ileal conduit after the ureterosigmoidostomy had been in place for only 9 months.[20–22]

A number of theories exist regarding the cause of colonic tumors after ureterosigmoidostomy. The most impressive study was performed by Crissey,[23] who in a rat model found that adenocarcinoma occurred only if feces and urine were admixed after ureterosigmoidostomy. It was believed that the carcinogen was probably formed by the conversion of urinary nitrates to nitroamines by fecal bacteria. However, this internal form of diversion, which provides both continence and an antireflux mechanism, remains attractive enough to encourage us to use alternatives that may avoid or decrease the possibility of carcinogenesis. From the experimental model, it appears that all efforts should be made to avoid mixing urine and feces and to control infection. In those patients in whom diversion by ureterosigmoidostomy seems appropriate, we have elected to perform ureteroileocecal sigmoidostomy as a one- or two-stage procedure. The patients to whom we are referring are usually those with bladder exstrophy in whom the bladder is nonreconstructible (e.g., small, fibrotic patch) and who have normal anal sphincter tone and innervation. This procedure is an alternative to other types of reconstructive procedures that would invariably require clean intermittent catheterization. Initially, we performed the procedure in two stages; the first stage was a nonrefluxing ileocecal conduit with the ureters anastomosed to the ilium. Later, at the second stage, when we were certain that the ileocecal nipple was competent, we anastomosed the ileocecal conduit to the sigmoid (Fig. 12–1). We have also performed this in one operative procedure. The advantage of this procedure is that there is no anastomosis of the ureter to the sigmoid and no urine-feces admixture at the site of ureteroileal anastomosis. The intussuscepted ileocecal valve protects the ureteroileal anastomosis from contact with feces. In a small number of patients (6) with limited follow-up (longest follow-up, 15 years), no neoplasm has occurred.

TECHNIQUE

After the cecum, right colon, and hepatic flexure are mobilized, the ileocecal vessels, which are constant, are identified. The ileum is then divided 15 cm proximal to the ileocecal valve, and the right colon is divided proximal to the right colic artery. After the ileal colonic bowel anastomosis is completed and the mesenteric windows are closed, the ileal mesentery is removed from the ileum for about 8 cm just proximal to the ileocecal junction to allow intussusception of the long nipple of ilium into the cecum (Fig. 12–2*A–I*). The ilium is then grasped with a Babcock clamp from within the cecum and inverted. The intussuscepted nipple has been secured using a technique described by Hendren. Three rows of GIA staples at the 12, 3, and 9 o'clock positions are placed. The mucosa of the ileum and facing cecum along the 6 o'clock quadrant is incised and the submucosa approximated with interrupted fine Vicryl sutures. The serosa of the ileum and cecum is also fixed at several points around the base of the intussusception with fine Prolene. This serves as the antireflux mechanism and should be continent to at least 50 cm H_2O. After the left ureter is brought under the sigmoid mesentery and through an opening in the posterior peritoneum, it is spatulated and anastomosed to the right ureter. The conjoint ureters are then anastomosed to the ileum using the Wallace technique. A standard stoma is then placed in the right lower quadrant. On occasion, the cecum may be tapered if a smaller stoma is desired.

After x-ray films demonstrate a nonobstructed upper urinary tract and no reflux, the second stage is performed by excising the cecal stoma and performing an end-to-side colocolostomy (Fig. 12–3). A rectal tube is left in place for several days.

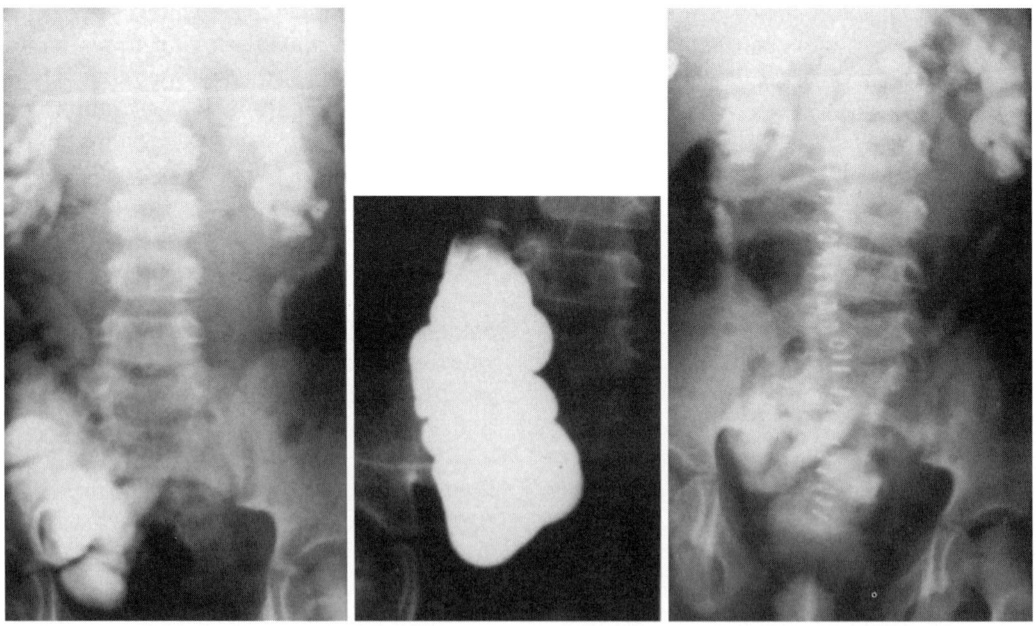

Figure 12–1 Excretory urogram in a 6-year-old boy with exstrophy of the bladder, which was not reconstructible after numerous procedures (left). Conduitogram reveals no evidence of reflux (center). Excretory urogram after the second stage, that is, anastomosis of the ileocecal segment to the intact sigmoid colon (right). From King LR, Stone A, Webster G (eds), Bladder Reconstruction and Continent Urinary Diversion, 2nd ed. St. Louis: CV Mosby, 1987, used with permission.

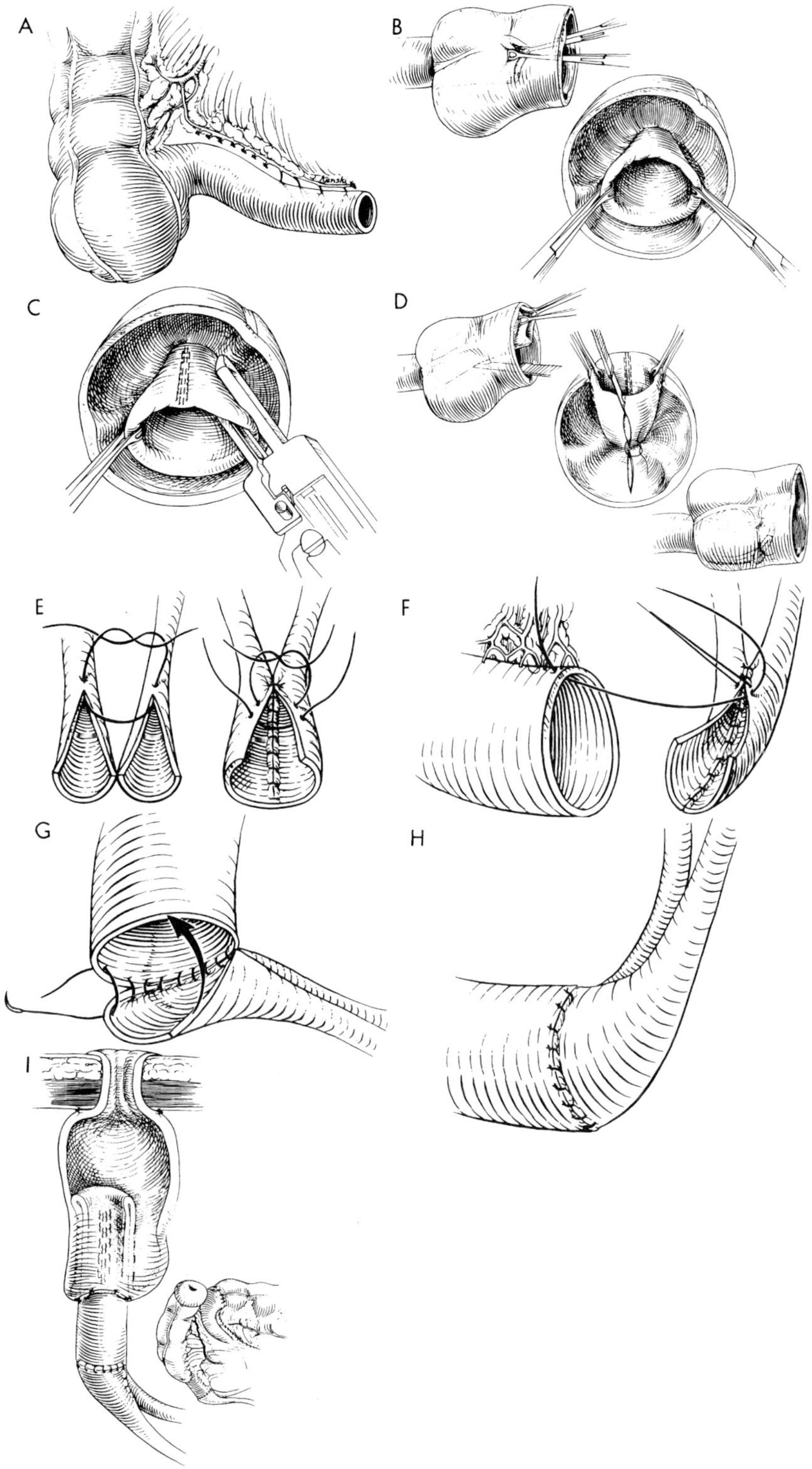

Figure 12–2 *A,* Ileocecal segment is isolated on the ileocolic vessels. The ileal mesentery is detached from the terminal ileum over a distance of 8 cm. *B,* Ileum is intussuscepted into the cecum by grasping the ileum with Babcock clamps from within the cecum. *C,* Three rows of quadrant staples are placed with the GIA stapler. *D,* Ileal and facing cecal mucosa are incised in the fourth quadrant. A submucosal anastomosis is then performed. *E,* Spatulated ureters are anastomosed side to side with fine chromic catgut. *F* and *G,* Combined ureters are then sutured end to end to the ileum. *H,* Completed ureteroileal anastomosis. *I,* Ileal musculoserosa is secured to cecal musculoserosa layers, and cecum is sutured to the posterior abdominal wall. The stoma is created. The cecum may be tapered if desired to create a smaller stoma. From King LR, Stone A, Webster G (eds), Bladder Reconstruction and Continent Urinary Diversion, 2nd ed. St. Louis: CV Mosby, 1987, used with permission.

Although many patients with existing conventional ureterosigmoidostomies do well, we must inform them of the malignant risk with this type of diversion. If a decision is made to convert electively to another type of diversion, it is probably important to excise the segment of colon containing the ureterocolonic anastomosis with 6 cm of bowel both proximal and distal to the anastomosis. However, many patients are very pleased with their internal diversion and opt to keep their ureterosigmoidostomy intact. Therefore, in this particular group, they must examine their stool on a regular basis for occult blood and obtain serial electrolytes, hemograms, and carcinoembry-

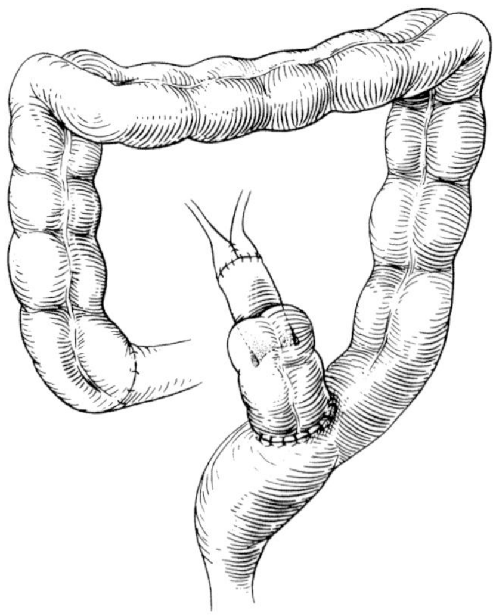

Figure 12–3 The previous ileocecal conduit is taken down, the abdominal wall at the previous stomal site is closed, and the conduit is anastomosed end to side to the sigmoid colon. From King LR, Stone A, Webster G (eds), Bladder Reconstruction and Continent Urinary Diversion, 2nd ed. St. Louis: CV Mosby, 1987, used with permission.

onic antigen determinations. Renal ultrasonography is performed annually, and starting 7 years after the surgery colonoscopy is also performed, with biopsy of the anastomotic site if indicated.

The most common complication of the procedure is for the ileal nipple to become undone. Securing it to the back wall of the cecum has minimized this complication. Ureteral obstruction is very unlikely using the Wallace technique.

In conclusion, because the incidence of colon carcinoma in patients undergoing ureterosigmoidostomy is increased, we have offered a select group of patients, usually those with nonreconstructible exstrophy of the bladder, the option of a one- or two-stage ureteroileocecal sigmoidostomy. Follow-up has ranged from 6 to 15 years in a group of six patients. Obviously, long-term follow-up is necessary to determine in this group whether there actually will be a reduced incidence of adenocarcinoma of the colon.

REFERENCES

1. Coffey RC. Transplantation of the ureters into the large intestine. Surg Gynecol Obstet 47:593, 1928.
2. Nesbit RM. Ureterosigmoid anastomosis by direct elliptical connection: A preliminary report. J Urol 6:728, 1949.
3. Cordonnier JJ. Ureterosigmoid anastomosis. Surg Gynecol Obstet 88:441, 1949.
4. Mathisen W. A new method for ureterointestinal anastomosis: A preliminary report. Surg Gynecol Obstet 96:255, 1953.
5. Goodwin WE. Ureterosigmoidostomy: Pros and cons. Dial Pediatr Urol 5:2, 1982.
6. Goodwin WE, Harris AP, Kaufman JJ, et al. Open transcolonic ureterointestinal anastomosis: A new approach. Surg Gynecol Obstet 97:295, 1953.
7. Leadbetter WF, Clarke BG. Five years experience with ureteroenterostomy by the "combined" technique. J Urol 73:67, 1954.
8. Hendren WH. Non-refluxing colon conduit for temporary or permanent urinary diversion in children. J Pediatr Surg 10:381, 1975.
9. Hendren WH. Exstrophy of the bladder: An alternative method of management. J Urol 115:195, 1976.
10. Hendren WH. Ureterocolic diversion of urine: Management of some difficult problems. J Urol 129:719, 1983.
11. Bricker EM. Bladder substitution after pelvic evisceration. Surg Clin North Am 30:1522, 1950.
12. Crooks KK, Enurile BG. Comparison of the ileal conduit and clean intermittent catheterization for myelomeningocele. Pediatrics 72:203, 1983.
13. Hendren WH, Radopoulous D. Complications of ileal loop and colon conduit urinary diversion. Urol Clin North Am 10:451, 1983.
14. Middleton AW, Hendren WH. Ileal conduits at the Massachusetts General Hospital from 1955 to 1970. J Urol 115:591, 1976.
15. Duckett JW. Ureterosigmoidostomy: The pros and cons. Dial Pediatr Urol 5:4, 1982.
16. Spence HM. Ureterosigmoidostomy: The pros and cons. Dial Pediatr Urol 5:3, 1982.
17. Spence HM, Hoffman WW, Fosmire GP. Tumor of the colon as a late complication of ureterosigmoidostomy for exstrophy of the bladder. Br J Urol 51:466, 1979.
18. Hamer E. Cancer du colon sigmoide dix ansa apres implantation des ureteres d'une vessie extrophiee. J Urol 28:260, 1929.
19. Parsons CD, Thomas MH, Garrett RA. Colonic adenocarcinoma: A delayed complication of ureterosigmoidostomy. J Urol 118:31, 1977.
20. Eraklis AJ, Folkman MJ. Adenocarcinoma at the site of ureterosigmoidostomies for exstrophy of the bladder. J Pediatr Surg 13:730, 1978.
21. Urdaneta LF, Duffel D, Creevy CD, et al. Late development of primary carcinoma of the colon following ureterosigmoidostomy. Ann Surg 164:503, 1966.
22. Schipper H, Decter A. Carcinoma of the colon arising at the ureteral implant sites despite early external diversion: Pathogenic and clinical implications. Cancer 47:2062, 1981.
23. Crissey MM, Steel GD, Gittes RF. Rat model for carcinogenesis in ureterosigmoidostomy. Science 207:1079, 1980.
24. Retik AB. Urinary diversion. Pediatr Urol 3:2, 1980.
25. Retik AB. Permanent urinary diversion. In Kelalis PP, King L, Belman AB (eds), Clinical Pediatric Urology. Philadelphia: WB Saunders, 1985, p 597.
26. Gittes RF. Ureterosigmoidostomy: Pros and cons. Dial Pediatr Urol 5:7, 1982.
27. Kim KS, Susskind M, King LR. Ileocecal ureterosigmoidostomy: An alternative to conventional ureterosigmoidostomy. J Urol 140:1494, 1988.
28. Mitchell ME, Rink RC. Urinary diversion and undiversion. Urol Clin North Am 12:111, 1985.
29. Orr JD, Shand JEG, Walters DAK, et al. Ileal conduit urinary diversion in children: An assessment of long-term results. Br J Urol 53:424, 1981.
30. Rabinowitz HH. Ureterosigmoidostomy in children: Revival or demise? J Urol 124:552, 1980.
31. Rink RC, Garrett RA, Mitchell ME. Adenocarcinoma of the colon following ureterosigmoidostomy. Soc Pediatr Urol Newslett May 17, 1983.
32. Rink RC, Retik AB. Current concepts of urinary diversion in

infants and children. In Retik AB, Cukier J (eds), Pediatric Urology: International Perspectives in Urology. Baltimore: Williams & Wilkins, 1987, p 384.

33. Schwartz GR, Jeffs RD. Ileal conduit urinary diversion in children: Computer analysis of follow up from 2 to 16 years. J Urol 114:285, 1975.
34. Simon J. Ectropia vesicae: Operation for directing the orifices of the ureters into the rectum: Temporary success, subsequent death, autopsy. Lancet 2:568, 1852.
35. Storer EH, Goldberg SM, Nivatvong S. Colon, rectum and anus. In Swartz SI, et al (eds), Principles of Surgery, 4th ed. New York: McGraw-Hill, 1984, p 1169.

KEVIN P. McLAUGHLIN & RICHARD C. RINK

13

Bladder and Prostate Rhabdomyosarcoma

Rhabdomyosarcoma (RMS) is an uncommon tumor that may arise virtually anywhere in the body that skeletal muscle is found. Among solid tumors in children, RMS ranks fifth after malignancies of the central nervous system, lymphoma, neuroblastoma, and Wilms' tumor,[1] accounting for 4 to 8% of childhood malignancies.[2] It comes to the attention of the urologist when the genitourinary tract is involved. These genitourinary tumors make up 20% of all RMSs. RMS occurs slightly more frequently in males than in females (1.4:1.0).[3] Syndromes or conditions associated with an increased incidence of RMS are listed in Table 13–1.

PATHOLOGY

The nomenclature and classification of soft tissue sarcomas have evolved over recent years. Currently, almost all cases of juvenile RMS are either alveolar or embryonal; a variant of embryonal is the well-described sarcoma botryoides. This variety often occurs in the hollow organs and in the genitourinary tract may affect the bladder or vagina. These pathologic designations have prognostic significance, as an alveolar pattern portends a poorer outcome. Only recently has consensus been reached regarding the exact criteria required to classify an individual tumor. This advance has improved the prognostic significance of tumor histology.[4, 5] In the second Intergroup Rhabdomyosarcoma Study (IRS), 57% of all patients eligible demonstrated embryonal (including 6% botryoidal) disease, whereas 21% had alveolar disease.[6] Among pelvic primaries, 90% are embryonal, 33% of which are botryoidal.[7] Pleomorphic and undifferentiated RMSs, which carry a worse prognosis, fortunately are uncommon in the pediatric age group. These may be anaplastic variants of the just noted types.[8]

Table 13–1
Syndromes and Conditions Associated with Rhabdomyosarcomas

Gorlin's nevoid basal cell carcinoma syndrome
Neurofibromatosis
Fetal alcohol syndrome
Rubenstein-Taybi syndrome
Roberts' syndrome
Li-Fraumeni syndrome
Siblings with other primary tumors

Optimal therapy for childhood RMS of any site is evolving largely because of the series of protocols begun by the IRS in 1972. By combining data from multiple institutions, larger numbers of patients were entered into protocols and more meaningful results obtained. The earlier clinical trials (IRS-I to IRS-III) chronicled improvement in survival in childhood RMS. Beginning in 1989, IRS-IV continues efforts to maximize survival while minimizing treatment-related morbidity by comparing varying chemotherapeutic and radiotherapeutic regimens while de-emphasizing the role of extirpative surgery as primary therapy. This is particularly true for tumors with a primary genitourinary site of origin. The Pediatric Oncology Group put together a handbook that outlines by site and stage of primary tumor the surgeon's responsibilities in the management of this tumor. Although improvements in survival have not been as great for childhood RMS as they have for Wilms' tumor, the multicenter, multidisciplinary approach that has been applied to the study of both these uncommon tumors has been a credible success.

PRESENTATION AND DIAGNOSIS

The presentation of pediatric genitourinary RMS varies depending on its site of origin. A tumor of the prostate frequently presents as a large, painless, solid mass in the pelvis of a boy typically younger than 4 years. Determining whether the tumor arises from the prostate or bladder neck may be quite difficult, particularly if there has been significant local invasion. If the predominant direction of growth is posterior and the rectal wall is invaded, constipation may be the presenting complaint. Growth toward the lumen of the bladder or urethra may result in obstructive voiding symptoms, increased residual urine, or even urinary tract infection. A take-home point here is that a digital rectal exam in a child complaining of constipation or difficulty voiding may suggest the diagnosis. Prostatic RMS has a greater tendency for lymphatic spread than do other genitourinary primary sites.

Tumors of the vagina affect a slightly younger group of girls, occurring at a mean age of less than 2 years.[9] Any vaginal discharge in this age group must elicit suspicion for RMS, although vaginal foreign bodies and ectopic ureters may share this presentation. Occasionally, a mass at the introitus or passage of tumor fragments may be the presenting sign. These tumors are commonly of the botryoid type, and their "bunch of grapes" appearance has been well described (Fig. 13–1). Vaginal discharge may also herald the diagnosis of a uterine RMS, although this organ tends to be affected during adolescence when a uterine primary tumor may present as an asymptomatic pelvic mass. Growth anteriorly may cause difficulty with voiding because of urethral compression or even bladder or urethral invasion. True invasion of the rectum is reportedly unusual conceivably because the rectovaginal septum provides a fairly effective barrier.

When the bladder is primarily involved, several factors affect the mode of presentation. If the tumor arises near the bladder neck, urethral obstruction is possible. Less commonly the tumor actually invades the urothelium, resulting in hematuria. A mass may be noted prolapsing at the meatus in girls or into the proximal urethra in boys. This tumor is also likely to have a botryoid pattern as it protrudes into the lumen of the bladder and may reach massive size before detection (Fig. 13–2). It is unusual after the age of 4 or 5 years. Interestingly, this tumor is almost twice as common in boys as in girls.

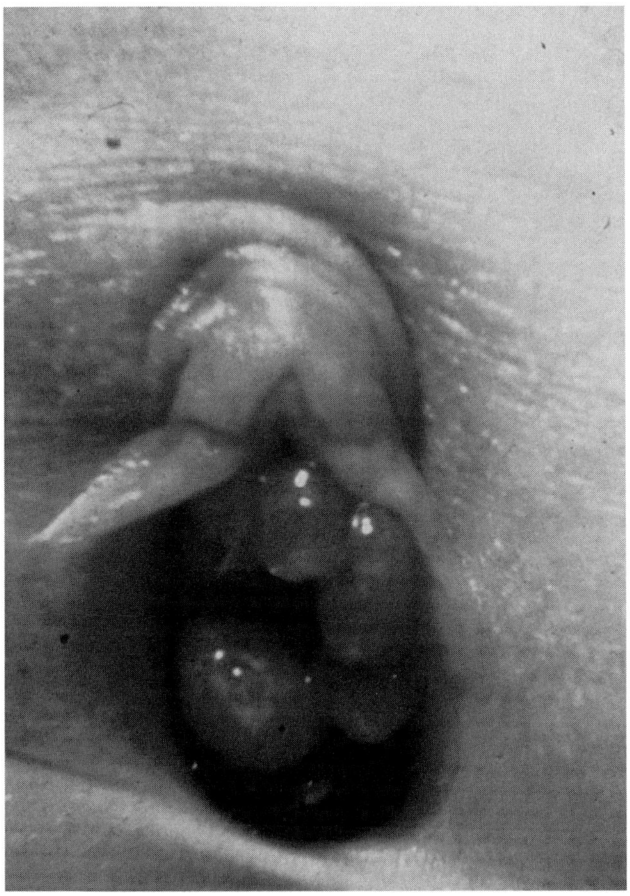

Figure 13–1 Botryoidal rhabdomyosarcoma of the vagina.

Rapid diagnosis of these tumors is facilitated by maintenance of a high index of suspicion. When a child of the appropriate age presents with the symptoms just described, the possibility of RMS must be entertained so that diagnosis is not delayed.

Initial diagnosis of bladder, prostate, vaginal, and uterine primary tumors, when large enough, may be made by needle biopsy, particularly when the tumor presents as a palpable pelvic mass. Open biopsy may be required, although most reports indicate that this is rarely necessary. Smaller genitourinary primary tumors lend themselves to endoscopic biopsy. Pediatric resectoscopes and cutting loops have been refined to the point that cystoscopy and vaginoscopy can be used to perform incisional or excisional biopsy of tumors in these sites. When coagulation artifact (because of the small size of the working elements in these instruments) renders specimens unsuitable, a cold cup biopsy forceps may be used to obtain tissue.

EVALUATION AND STAGING

Imaging of the child with a pelvic mass generally begins with sonography, which should provide fairly detailed anatomic information. Tumor size and organ involved can be assessed directly, and the presence of bladder outlet obstruction is inferred from an enlarged bladder capacity and large postvoid residual volume. Not surprisingly, the echo pattern of this tumor resembles that of skeletal muscle.[9] Computed tomographic (CT) scanning complements sonography, providing additional resolution to more accurately delineate tumor extent, organ involvement, and lymphatic spread. Necrotic areas may be easily seen. Despite this enhanced capacity, it remains difficult in occasional patients to define whether a large pelvic tumor arises primarily from the bladder, prostate (in males), or female genital tract. Magnetic resonance imaging (MRI) may provide additional information regarding local invasion. Sedation is sometimes required for those undergoing MRI because the scanner's tunnel may be quite intimidating to the pediatric patient. With the development of these technologies and the additional information they provide, use of the more conventional studies such as an intravenous pyelogram in evaluating a pelvic mass in children is seldom necessary. Voiding

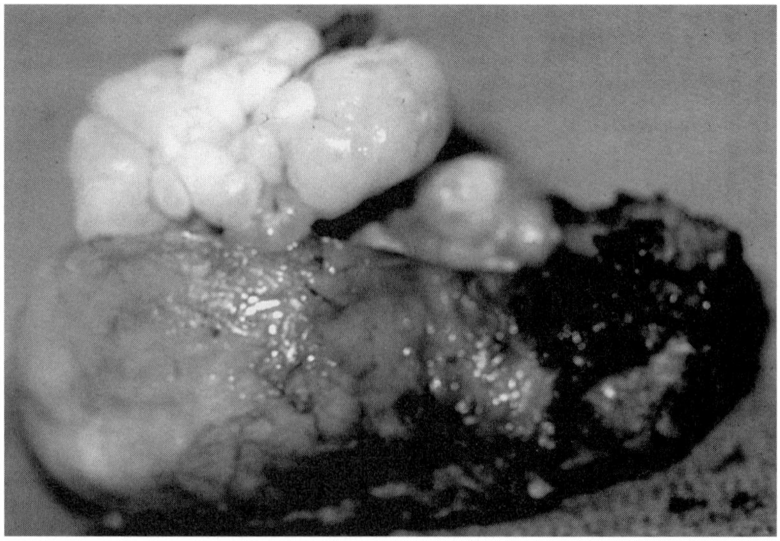

Figure 13–2 Cystoprostatectomy specimen with bulky tumor.

cystourethrography is at times helpful but is best done during the CT evaluation.

Once a tissue diagnosis has been made, the disease must be staged. RMS is primarily found to be locally invasive, but lymphatic spread is more common with GU tumors, particularly prostatic primary tumors, than in those arising elsewhere. Hematogenous spread to lung, bone, and liver occurs less commonly, but these areas must be evaluated. Local extent and nodal disease are assessed with CT or MRI if this has not been done during the initial evaluation. When CT is used for follow-up evaluation, it should be noted that its accuracy in predicting tumor recurrence is only 81%.[10] Radionuclide bone scan should be considered to rule out bony metastasis, and abnormalities noted should undergo biopsy. Analysis of a bone marrow aspirate is recommended.

Historically, staging has followed the IRS guidelines (Table 13–2). This system is based essentially on whether the tumor is initially completely resectable and on the status of the lymph nodes draining the organ of origin. A THNM system was introduced in IRS-II (Table 13–3)[11] and is being increasingly applied.

In addition to clinical group, several other factors indicate prognosis for a given tumor (Table 13–4). The issue of favorable versus unfavorable histology was specifically addressed in the protocol of IRS-III. Unfavorable histology, as might be anticipated, includes the anaplastic, alveolar, and monomorphous round cell types. Fortunately, these are all quite uncommon in pediatric genitourinary RMSs.

The management of pediatric genitourinary RMS has evolved considerably over the past quarter century; before this time patient outcome was quite poor. Although complete resection remains an attractive option, genitourinary tumors rarely, with the exception of paratesticular primary tumors, can be resected without considerable morbidity. Over the course of the three completed IRS protocols (I, 1972–1978; II, 1978–1984; III, 1984–1991), initial therapy has shifted away from radical extirpative surgery toward a multimodal approach in an effort to preserve the genitourinary tract intact. The alteration in lifestyle with an ostomy and infertility seemed too great. The successive protocols prospectively adjusted the dosage and pattern of chemotherapy administered, including assessing the impact of two- versus three-agent regimens, while measuring outcome compared with those of the earlier trials. Radiotherapy was similarly adjusted, added, or eliminated as well. Early on, aggressive radical surgery plus chemotherapy provided survival rates as high as 56% in genitourinary primary tumors.[12] Therefore, the principal therapeutic motive of late has been improvement in survival in children with RMS with attention to minimizing the often considerable morbidity associated with radical surgery and aggressive radiotherapy. No one institution has

Table 13–2
Intergroup Rhabdomyosarcoma Study Staging of Rhabdomyosarcoma

Group 1: localized, completely resected, no nodes involved
1. Confined to muscle/organ of origin only
2. Contiguous involvement beyond muscle/organ of origin
3. Microscopic confirmation of complete resection required

Group 2: grossly resected, evidence of regional spread
1. Complete *gross* resection, microscopic residual
2. Complete resection, regional nodes positive, no microscopic residual
3. Regional nodes positive, microscopic residual after complete *gross* resection or involvement of most distal regional node

Group 3: incomplete resection, gross residual
1. Biopsy only
2. Partial (>50%) resection

Group 4: distant metastases at diagnosis
1. Excludes regional nodes and contiguous organ involvement

Table 13–3
Pretreatment THNM Staging of Rhabdomyosarcomas

Tumor:	T1 site:	confined to site or tissue of origin
	1.	$<$ 5 cm
	2.	$>$ 5 cm
	T2 site:	contiguous tissue or organ involved
	1.	$<$ 5 cm
	2.	$>$ 5 cm
Histology:	H1:	favorable
	H2:	unfavorable
Regional nodes:	N0:	no clinical or radiologic involvement
	N1:	clinical or radiologic involvement present
Metastatic disease:	M0:	None
	M1 site:	Present

enough patients to answer the pressing therapeutic questions. The IRS reports have been an exemplary multicenter and multidisciplinary effort to improve survival and lifestyle.

The IRS-I trial differs from its successors in that it alone took a primarily surgical approach. Exenterative surgery was the initial therapy for the 62 patients with genitourinary RMS in this study. Most patients then received three-agent chemotherapy (vincristine, actinomycin D, and cyclophosphamide, or VAC); patients with bladder or prostate primary tumors received radiation. When patients presenting with Group 4 disease are excluded, survival from this trial was reasonably good at 75%. This did not come cheaply, however, because the bladder salvage rate was quite poor. Conclusions reached in IRS-I were that adding radiotherapy to standard VAC chemotherapy offered no advantage in Group I patients, 1 year of two-agent chemotherapy (VA) was as effective as the three-agent (VAC) regimen in Group 2 patients, and that the addition of doxorubicin to pulse-sequential VAC therapy offered no advantage in Group 3 and 4 patients. Also apparent from this trial was that recurrence carried a dismal prognosis.[13]

The concept of "special pelvic sites" was introduced in IRS-II and included bladder, prostate, vaginal, and uterine primary tumors. This trial of 109 patients differed markedly from IRS-I with respect to these tumors because it examined the ability of primary chemotherapy to reduce the frequency of cystectomy without compromising survival. Pelvic exenteration was still performed for relapse or lack of response to chemotherapy but was not randomized in this study. Most of the patients in this trial also underwent radiotherapy. Results, unfortunately, were disappointing; only eight patients survived with an intact bladder after chemotherapy alone. The overall combined therapy results with the IRS-I and IRS-II protocols were very similar. Furthermore, bladder salvage rates for IRS-I and IRS-II at 3 years were nearly identical at just less than 25%.[14] From this trial, investigators concluded that primary repetitive-pulse VAC therapy, although it did not compromise survival, did not result in improved long-term bladder salvage.[15] It appeared that primary surgery was still the most effective means of treatment.

While capitalizing on these earlier results, the IRS-III trial also recognized that the disease categories occupied by children with RMS represented a broad spectrum with a distinct prognosis for each tumor.[16] This trial explored the notion that tumors of different histology, although within the same clinical group, could be treated differently. Chemotherapeutic regimens were intensified, the timing of radiotherapy was formalized, and strategies for second-look surgery were fixed. The results were a dramatic improvement in bladder salvage to 60% at 4 years. The addition of partial cystectomy as a surgical option for tumors of selected sites (i.e., bladder dome) may have contributed to this success.[17] Survival in tumors of special pelvic sites improved as well, from 72% in IRS-II to 83% in IRS-III. Also recognized in IRS-III was the overall favorable prognosis for genitourinary RMS. Non-bladder–prostate genitourinary RMS ranked second and bladder-prostate genitourinary RMS third behind primary RMS of the orbit in overall survival.[16]

The protocol of IRS-IV was based on the results of IRS-II and includes the use of newer drugs in addition to continued modification of regimens using existing agents. Conventional radiation versus hyperfractionation radiation for Group 3 patients is also compared. Results from this study are limited at present. Some early data have suggested that aggressive primary chemotherapy may permit a less extensive surgical procedure in patients with uterine RMS. High treatment-associated mortality warrants further consideration in this setting.[18]

Table 13–4
Factors Affecting Prognosis in Rhabdomyosarcomas

Clinical grade
Primary site
Tumor histopathology (favorable vs. unfavorable)
Response to treatment
Age at diagnosis

LATE SEQUELAE

Of obvious concern in children is the long-term effect of therapy. This is particularly important in treatment of RMS, in which aggressive chemo- and radiotherapeutic regimens are used. Radiation is known to cause an obliterative endarteritis, which over time can result in fibrotic changes. When pelvic radiation is used, the bladder may be severely affected and bony pelvic growth may be retarded. Cyclophosphamide is notorious for causing hemorrhagic cystitis, which can develop years after the agent was given. The gonads suffer from both radiation and chemotherapy. They can occasionally be protected from radiation by shielding or surgical transposition to a thigh pouch if scrotal radiation is required, but the sterilizing effects of chemotherapy may be unavoidable.

It is important not only to look at bladder salvage rates when comparing various treatment modalities but also to assess how well the salvaged bladder functions. Incontinence, uncontrollable frequency and urgency, and pain are unacceptable results of therapy. A recent review of survivors of IRS-I and IRS-II with prostate and bladder primary tumors found an overall bladder salvage rate of 50%, but only 73% of these had satisfactory bladder function.[4] Further recommendations included follow-up of renal function and body growth and development.

THE ROLE OF SURGERY

The role of surgery for genitourinary RMSs has changed dramatically over the past 40 years. In the midportion of this century, radical surgery, usually total pelvic exenteration, was the mainstay of therapy, with survival rates of only 30%. This was the only option and because of local recurrence with segmental procedures, the thought was the bigger the operation, the better. Unfortunately, although total excision was possible, emotional and social debilitation were sometimes extreme.

With the advent of radiation therapy and multiagent chemotherapy, efforts have increased to salvage the genitourinary organs in hopes of preventing urinary diversion and maintaining fertility and sexual function. The thought process has come full circle in terms of surgery: the smaller the operation, the better. The obvious questions that arise from this type of therapy are: Can the same survival rates be achieved with less surgery? Does the preserved bladder following chemotherapy, radiation treatments, and biopsy or partial cystectomy maintain its normal function? What is the morbidity of aggressive chemotherapy and radiation?

The IRS group as well as others have tried to answer these questions. In IRS-1, 41 of 54 patients (76%) survived with a reported bladder salvage rate of 23%. In IRS-II, in which primary chemotherapy was given in an effort to lessen surgery, the survival rates were similar at 70%. Bladder salvage at 3 years, unfortunately, was no better in IRS-II, being 22%.

Partial cystectomy clearly has a role when conditions are right (i.e., complete tumor resection is achievable) (Fig. 13–3). The survival rate 3 years after partial cystectomy with multimodal therapy was 79%, which is obviously similar to those of more aggressive surgical management.[17]

The issue of the function of the preserved bladder was addressed by Raney and colleagues from the IRS-I and IRS-II groups. Of 54 patients with a preserved bladder for at least 5 years (10 underwent partial cystectomy), 38 (70%) had satisfactory bladder function, 9 (17%) were incontinent, 4 (7%) had frequency and nocturia, and 1 (2%) had frequency only.[19] Hematuria was seen in 20% of patients after treatment. Yeung and others[20] also reviewed bladder function after intensive chemotherapy and bladder-conserving surgery. Radiation therapy was given for nonresectability or incompletely resected tumors. Of 26 patients, 19 survived, 17 of whom had their bladder preserved. Eleven of these children were studied and 4 had a normal voiding pattern. Of the 7 with abnormal voiding, 3 were wet day and night and the other 4 had night-time wetting. Six had reduced functional bladder capacities.[20] It is clear that with aggressive multimodal therapy and conservative surgery bladder preservation can be achieved in a fairly high percentage of patients,

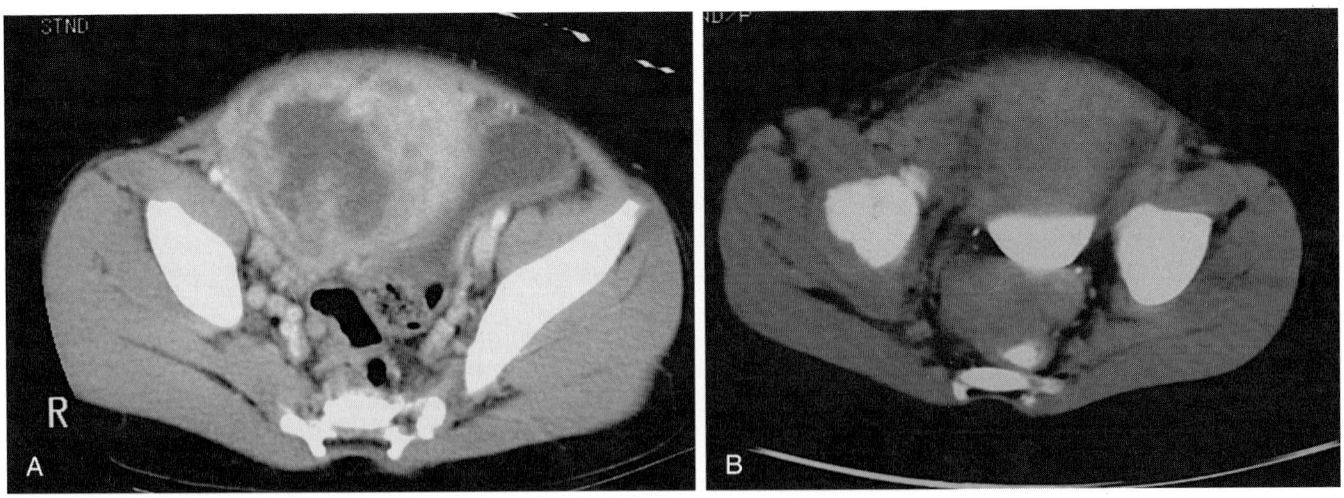

Figure 13–3 Post-chemotherapy computed tomographic scan of bladder dome rhabdomyosarcoma. *A*, Bladder displaced to left by right-sided tumor. *B*, More caudal section; trigone not involved by tumor.

but this retained bladder may not function normally. In those with an intact lower urinary tract, bladder function should be evaluated to protect the upper urinary tract and allow treatment of those suffering impaired function.

Raney and colleagues also looked at other sequelae such as long-term renal function, body growth, and development. The authors recognized as well the importance of psychosocial counseling as these patients mature.[19] Of major importance to older survivors after radical surgery is the effect of therapy on sexual development and function. This underscores the importance of frank discussions with patients not only as they undergo therapy but also long after it has concluded. Curing cancer should be the start of a long-term therapeutic relationship with these children, not the extent of it.

CURRENT SURGICAL RECOMMENDATIONS

Current surgical recommendations are set forth in the IRS-IV protocol, as are those for chemotherapy and radiation, based on the primary organ involved and disease stage. The approach is to treat initially with chemotherapy; surgery is generally limited to biopsy or tumorectomy. In the case of bladder RMS, partial cystectomy may be possible. Partial cystectomy is easily performed with complete tumor excision when it occurs away from the trigone. It becomes progressively more difficult to maintain a functioning bladder the closer the tumor is to the ureteral orifices and bladder neck. Some have tried submucosal resection of tumors in an effort to preserve the bladder.[10]

When radical surgery represents the only option for complete gross resection, anterior pelvic exenteration with sparing of the rectum is recommended in those patients with less than 50% response to primary chemotherapy who subsequently have biopsy-proven failure of complete response to radiotherapy. This will occur mainly in primary tumors of the prostate, bladder neck, or trigone. Augmentation cystoplasty may be required to maintain adequate functional capacity and has been used with success.[10] When cystoprostatectomy is carried out, urinary diversion can be accomplished by a variety of techniques, both noncontinent and continent. Although these latter procedures do not allow spontaneous voiding and are dependent on lifelong clean, intermittent catheterization, great advances have been made in these reconstructions. They are reliably continent and the abdominal wall can be free of any obvious stoma by hiding the catheterizable channel in the umbilicus. Continent urinary reservoirs (CUR) are covered elsewhere in this text. Occasionally, it is wise to perform a noncontinent diversion. These can easily be incorporated into a later continent diversion should the child and family so desire.

Organ preservation is also possible in tumors of the uterus and vagina, although anterior pelvic exenteration is occasionally necessary. Tumorectomy suits some uterine tumors, and hysterectomy alone without vaginectomy or oophorectomy may be appropriate for those involving only the uterine wall. Vaginectomy with uterine preservation for distal vaginal tumors may also be considered, but reconstruction is difficult.

NONCONTINENT URINARY DIVERSION

Although virtually any intestinal segment can be used to form a conduit, ileum and colon are most often chosen. Jejunal conduits are notorious for producing acidosis that is both hypochloremic and hyponatremic so these are used as a last resort only. Preoperative education is the key to a successful result and a satisfied patient, regardless of the segment chosen.

ILEAL CONDUIT

The ileal conduit (Fig. 13–4), although rarely selected today, is sometimes the optimal conduit choice, such as when the colon has been irradiated. The procedure actually begins a few days before the date of surgery when the patient is assessed for optimal stomal placement. A variety of opinions exist regarding where exactly "optimal" lies, but the key is to observe the patient in both the sitting and standing positions and to choose and mark a site that is not involved by skinfolds, scars from prior surgery, or the patient's clothing. Input from a specialized enterostomal therapist can help at this point. Although the patient's anatomy will ultimately dictate stomal location, it is difficult to select correctly with the patient supine on the operating table. Also, we prefer a full mechanical and antibiotic bowel cleansing before surgery.

With the patient supine and prepared from nipples to midthigh, a midline incision is made and carried down to enter the peritoneum sharply. Nasogastric suction is recommended. The ureters are identified bilaterally through the posterior peritoneum where they cross the iliac vessels. Either ureter can be approached directly through an incision in the posterior parietal peritoneum or by mobilizing the right and left colon medially. In the case of RMS, cystectomy or pelvic exenteration will have been performed, leaving the ureters already divided in the pelvis. Placement of feeding tubes secured with a traction stitch into the ureters eases their handling and minimizes tissue trauma. The left ureter should be mobilized proximally a distance of several centimeters so that it can cross the midline in the retroperitoneum anterior to the great vessels, taking care to preserve its adventitial blood supply. A similar but less lengthy mobilization of the right ureter is also done.

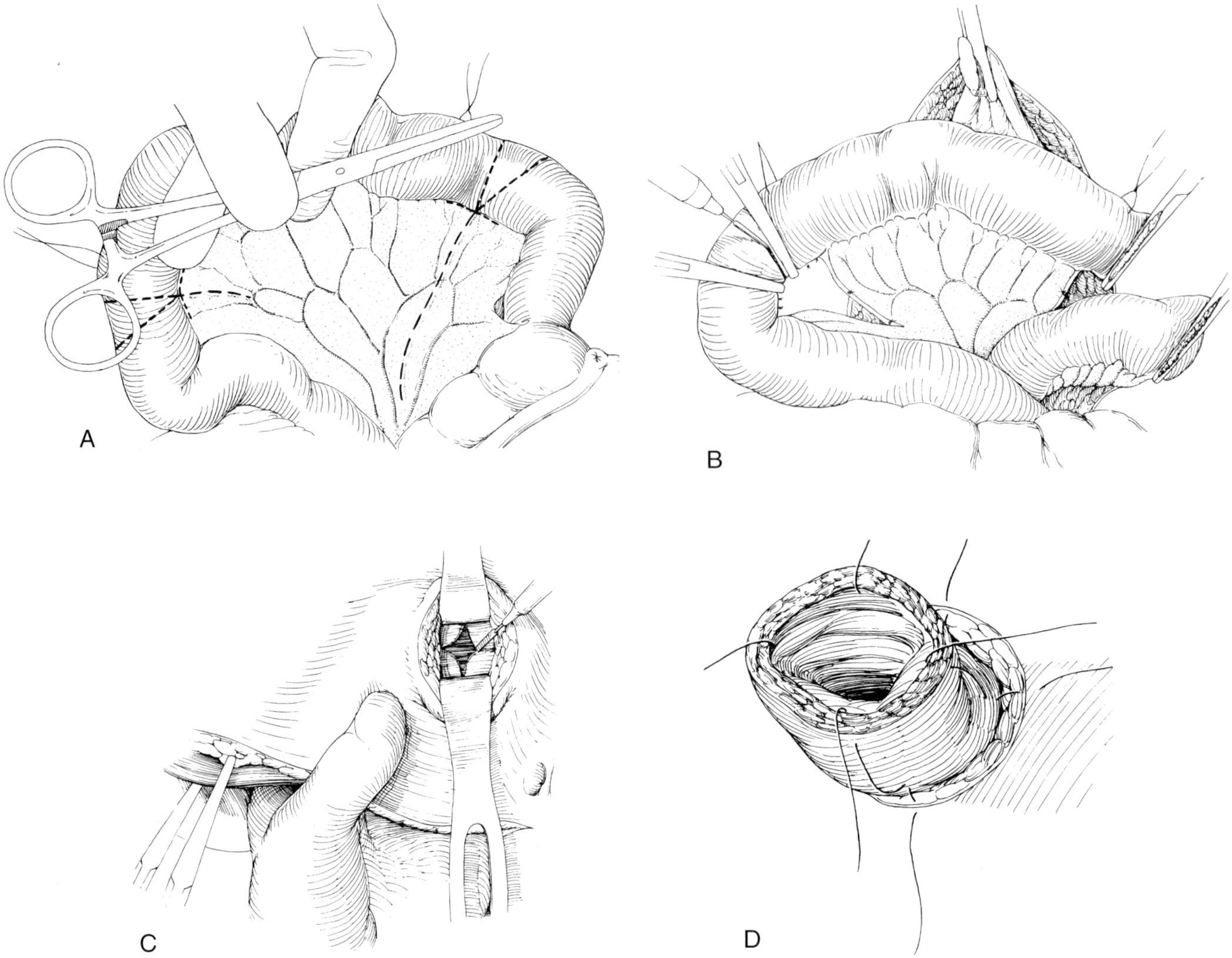

Figure 13–4 *A,* Ileal segment chosen based on vascular arcade. *B,* Mesenteric peritoneum is incised; mesentery is divided and cleaned off bowel wall for short distance. Bowel is divided between clamps (GIA stapler may be used). *C,* Cruciate incision in anterior fascia; muscle is split to permit passage of conduit. *D,* Creation of everted stoma is done first.

Selection of the appropriate segment of ileum approximately 12 cm in length is based on the distribution of the vascular arcade, which can be demonstrated by transilluminating the mesentery. Generally, we do not sacrifice the last 15 to 20 cm of ileum, preferring to preserve this segment within the gastrointestinal tract for its iron-absorbing capacity. Mark the ends of the conduit segment with suture and be sure the segment is long enough to reach from the sacral promontory to the abdominal wall. Dissect through the mesentery at two points below each of these sutures, one immediately beneath the bowel wall, and one 3 to 4 cm down the mesentery, taking care to avoid the vascular arcade. Place a Penrose or vessel loop through each of these four points. With gentle upward traction from the points closest to the bowel, carefully incise the mesenteric peritoneum between loops, perpendicular to the bowel. Clamp and divide any crossing vessels, ligating them with delicate silk ties. Leave the remaining vascular arcade intact. Clean the mesentery off the bowel wall for a short distance in both directions at both ends of the conduit segment. This facilitates the bowel anastomosis, stoma formation, and closure of the proximal end of the conduit.

In preparing to harvest this segment, keep in mind that orientation is important: the distal end becomes the stoma. It may help at this point to remove one of the marker stitches placed previously at both ends of the conduit, leaving the other for orientation. The segment can be divided in a variety of ways. We place atraumatic bowel clamps proximally and distally at each end of the segment and divide between the two sets. A GIA stapler can be used instead of bowel clamps. Once the segment is harvested, it is dropped into the pelvis and bowel continuity is re-established above it. Again, both hand-sewn

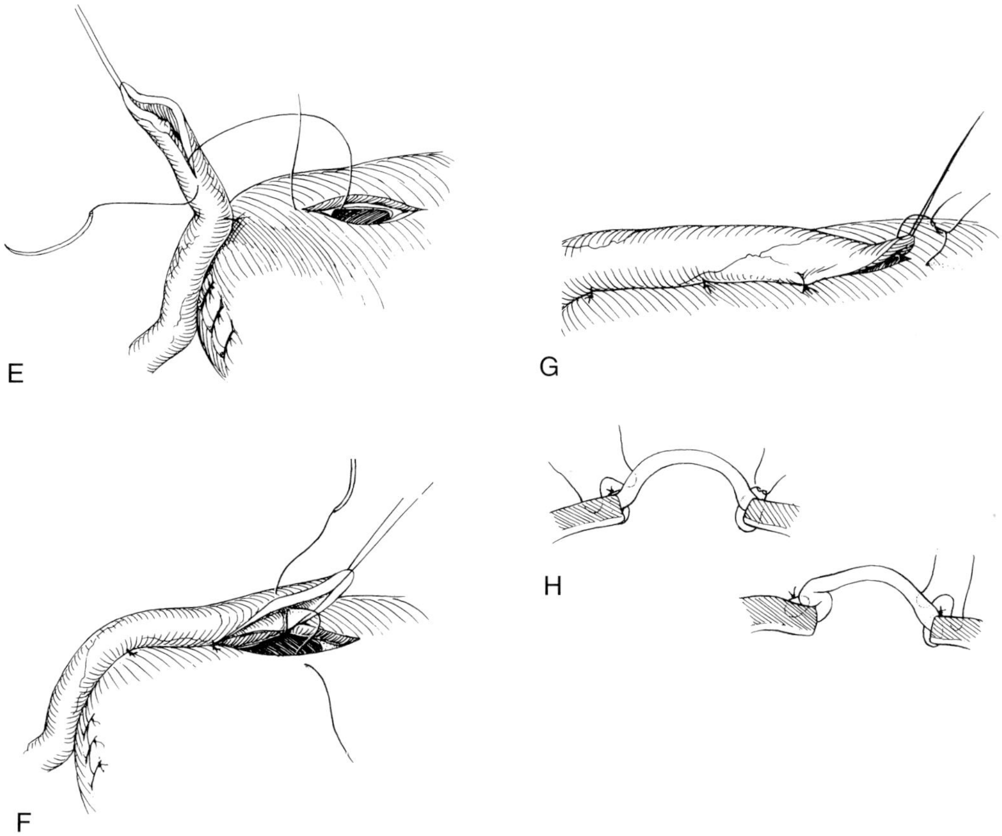

Figure 13–4 *Continued* *E–H,* Ureteroileal anastomosis follows.

and stapled anastomoses have proponents, although the stapled anastomosis may be performed more quickly. The mesenteric defect must be closed, approximating only the superficial peritoneum so as to avoid vessel injury.

At this point, the stoma is formed so that the ureteroileal anastomoses are in their final position. At the site marked preoperatively, a buttonhole of skin is removed in continuity with an underlying core of fat down to the fascia. A cruciate incision is made in the fascia, and the muscle below is split gently. It is rarely necessary to divide muscle. The posterior fascia and peritoneum are likewise incised in a cross, at which point a large sound or the index finger should pass easily through the entire abdominal wall. Medial traction on the fascial edge of the midline incision during these steps maintains the proper alignment. A Babcock clamp is passed from outside in to grasp the distal end of the conduit segment and gently draw it out where an everted stoma is formed. Careful suturing of the adventitia of the bowel to both the anterior fascia as well as the posterior fascia and peritoneum minimizes the risk of peristomal herniation. Avoid placing these latter stitches too close to the mesentery.

A number of ureteroileostomy techniques have been described. In the Wallace technique, after anterior ureteral spatulation, their medial walls are sewn together. The resulting large-mouthed double ureter is then anastomosed to the proximal end of the conduit. We generally prefer each ureter to be anastomosed separately to the ileum. An opening is made toward the proximal end of the ileum to expose the mucosa, which is buttonholed. Each ureter is brought from beneath to the anterior aspect of the conduit where it is spatulated and anastomosed with a mucosa-to-mucosa closure. With this technique, the proximal end of the conduit must subsequently be closed in two layers using an inverting stitch. The ureteroileal anastomoses are usually stented with specially designed diversion stents (or pediatric feeding tubes), which are brought out through the stoma.

It is our practice to run the entire bowel after any diversion to ensure that there are no missed bowel injuries or kinks that may later result in obstruction. The abdomen is then closed using a running absorbable monofilament suture to approximate the fascia.

Although losing popularity in the age of continent diversions, the ileal conduit is relatively simple and can be performed quickly when needed. It is also versatile in that it can later be incorporated into a continent diversion should the opportunity and patient inclination arise.

COLON CONDUIT

This technique of diversion (Fig. 13–5) shares many of the characteristics of the ileal conduit: It is noncontinent,

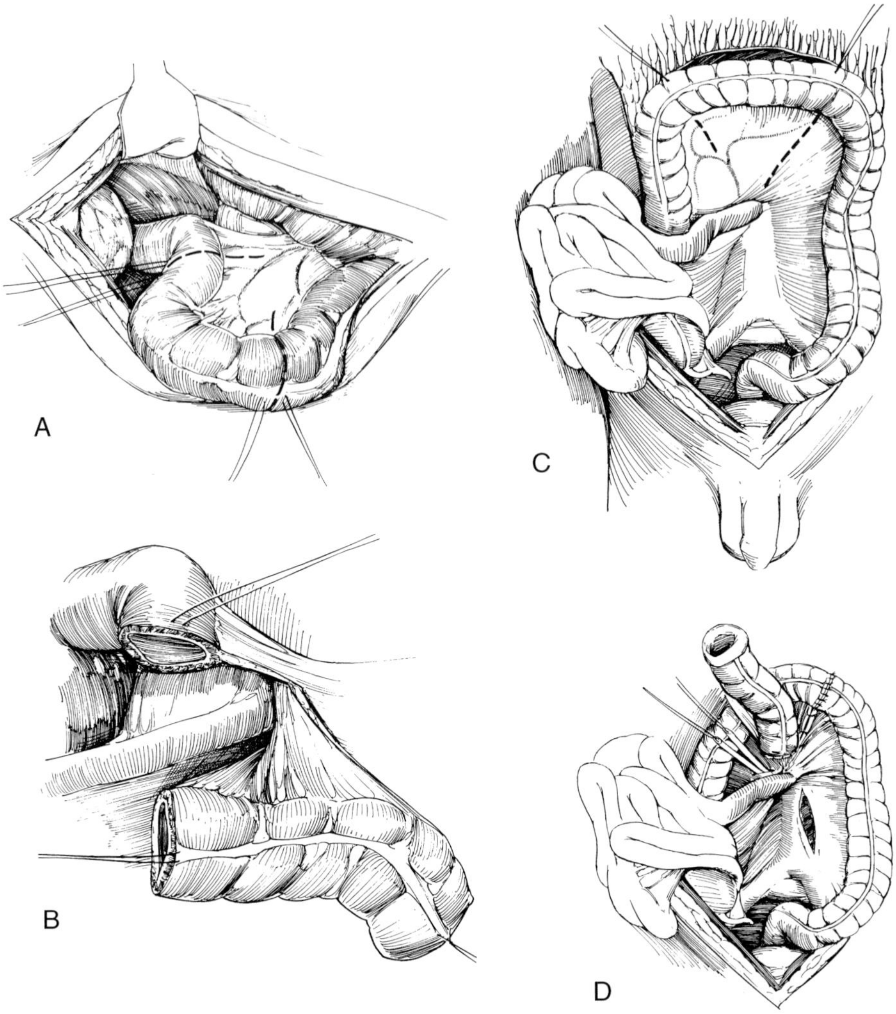

Figure 13–5 *A* and *B,* Sigmoid segment brought laterally after harvest. *C* and *D,* Transverse colon segment requires less ureteral length.

requiring a stomal appliance; it is not too difficult technically; the conduit can be harvested from virtually any segment of the colon, blood supply allowing; and, currently, it is not performed very often in children, given the current trend toward continent diversions. Its primary advantage is that the teniae of the large bowel permit a nonrefluxing ureteral anastomosis, lessening the incidence of upper tract deterioration. This is our choice of noncontinent diversion because of the antireflux mechanism and because it is easily incorporated into a later CUR without having to redo the ureteral anastomoses.

Preoperative bowel preparation and stomal site marking are carried out as described. The abdomen is prepared and draped widely, a midline incision made, and the peritoneum entered sharply. After inspection of the entire peritoneum and confirmation of correct nasogastric tube placement, the vascular arcade of the colon is inspected. Most often, a sigmoid colonic segment is chosen, but transverse colon may be used if the sigmoid has experienced radiation damage. The transverse colon can be convenient if ureteral length is lacking.

For the transverse colon, the omentum must be freed off the anterior surface of the bowel. The colonic segment is harvested in the same fashion as that described for the ileal conduit, although the distal mesenteric window does not need to be very long. Colonic segments often contract, and a somewhat longer segment should be selected. Bowel continuity is re-established by a two-layer closure or stapling. The conduit may be placed above or below this anastomosis for a transverse segment and either medial or lateral (usually lateral) when a sigmoid segment is used, depending on how it best lies. The proximal end of the conduit is closed. The stoma is constructed at the preoperatively determined site by excising a 3-cm circle of skin, fat, and fascia. A cruciate fascial incision is made, the muscle separated, and the posterior sheath opened. The bowel is brought through this opening, and an everted stoma is constructed. A single incision in the posterior peritoneum allows access to both ureters. To perform the ureterocolonic anastomosis, the teniae are identified and traction sutures are placed to allow the tunnels to be constructed easily. The proposed antireflux tenial tunnels are injected with saline, and the tenia is incised for 2 to 3 cm down to the level of the submucosa.

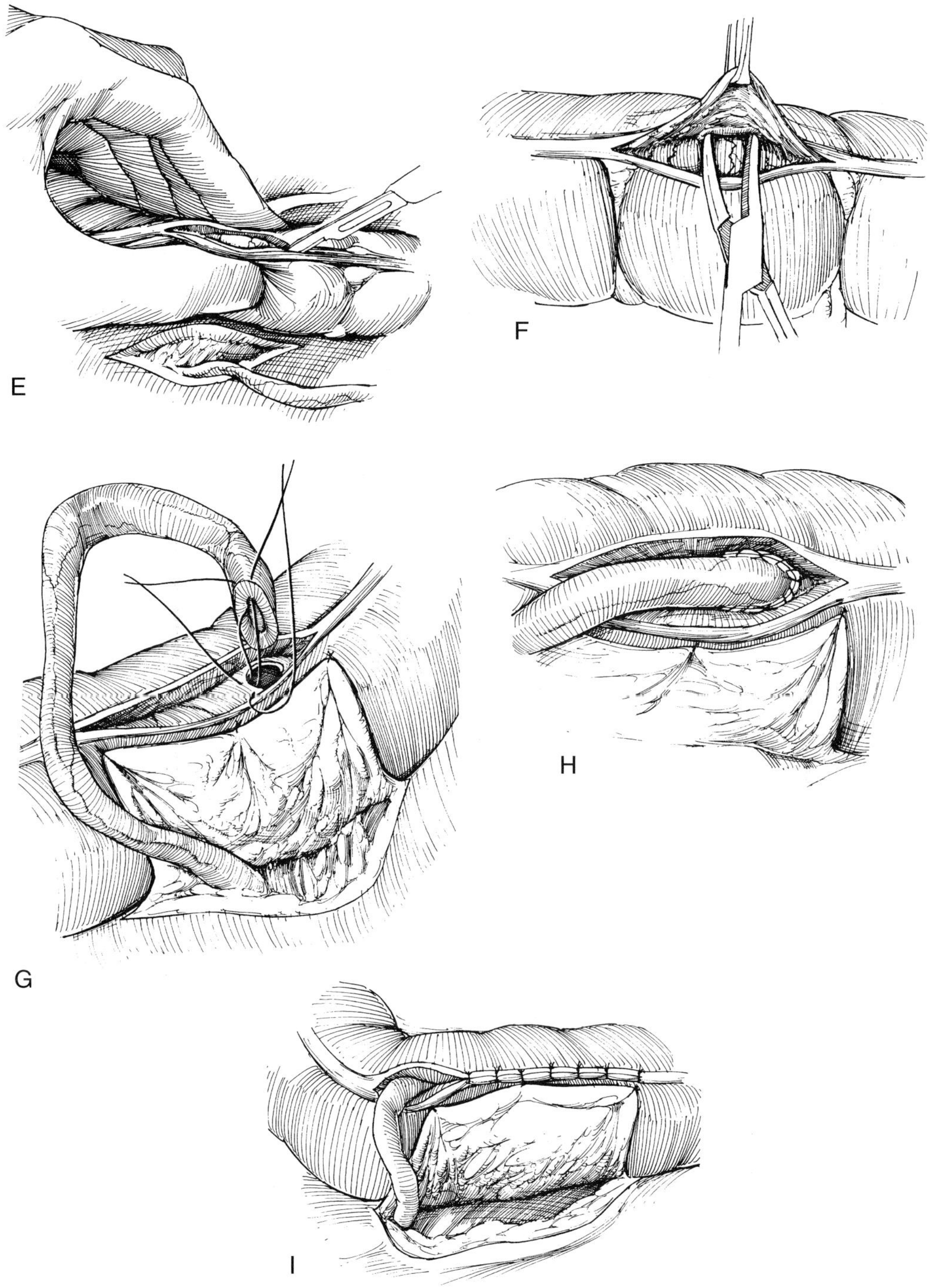

Figure 13–5 *Continued*
Ureteral anastomosis: *E,* Tenia is incised after injection of saline. *F,* Muscular wall is dissected laterally, preserving radial vessels. *G* and *H,* Direct urothelial-mucosal anastomosis is performed. *I,* Tenia is reapproximated over the ureter.

The submucosal tunnel is developed with gentle outward traction on the tenial walls. A nick is made in the mucosa at the distal end of this trough, the ureter spatulated, and a urothelial-to-mucosal anastomosis carried out with absorbable suture. The muscular tenia is then reapproximated over the ureter loosely, providing the firm backing needed to prevent reflux. Care is taken to avoid angulation or stenosis at the hiatus. Stenting of these anastomoses is recommended. The mesenteric defect is closed with permanent suture, and the proximal end of the conduit segment closed with two layers of absorbable suture.

COMPLICATIONS

As with any major abdominal surgery, several potential complications can occur after noncontinent diversion. Wound infection, fascial dehiscence, and intestinal obstruction or anastomotic leak are possible, although strict attention to technical detail can minimize their occurrence. We do prefer a full mechanical and antibiotic bowel preparation, especially when contemplating a colon conduit.

Complications more specifically associated with the conduit forms of urinary diversion are commonly discussed in terms of their timing after surgery. Those that occur in the early postoperative period include vascular compromise of the bowel segment and leak from the ureterointestinal anastomosis. Adequate bowel segment blood supply is ensured by careful preservation of a suitable vascular arcade during the harvest and then careful attention in positioning to avoid tension on the mesentery and prevent kinking of the vessels. Similarly, a tension-free, mucosal-to-urothelial anastomosis minimizes the risk of ureterointestinal leaks. We also strongly prefer to stent these with specially designed urinary diversion stents.

Dealing with these complications can be challenging. An ischemic ileal or colonic segment may require replacement. Percutaneous nephrostomy drainage may allow a leaking ureteral anastomosis to seal.

Later complications to these diversions are fairly common. Hydronephrosis and renal deterioration occur with both, particularly with the freely refluxing ileal conduit. This complication accounts for some of the waning enthusiasm to perform this procedure and its replacement in our minds by the colon conduit when noncontinent diversion is indicated. Stricture of the intestinal segment can occur, more commonly in ileal segments. A contrast loopogram will identify the problem and, if severe enough, should lead to replacement of the entire segment.

Stricture of the ureter may also develop later after diversion, usually from devascularization during mobilization. Fibrosis from a urine leak may also impair drainage, as can the effects of prior radiation. Endourologic approaches to these problems are under investigation, but open reanastomosis is often required. The occurrence of stomal stenosis or peristomal hernia formation can be minimized by ensuring an adequate blood supply as the segment is brought through the skin and by securing the intestinal adventitia to the abdominal wall fascia.

Chronic urinary tract infections may also occur. When stone-forming bacteria are the cause, urinary calculi can become a problem. Their management is also evolving in keeping with the rapid development of endourologic techniques.

SUMMARY

The consequences of RMS can be devastating in the child. Fortunately, it is a relatively rare tumor. This mandates a high index of suspicion in the appropriately aged child so that diagnosis is not delayed. Protocols have been established for the management of tumors involving the genitourinary tract. Although radical surgery is no longer recommended as initial therapy, it still has a role in tumors that fail to respond to multiagent chemotherapy and radiation. Improvements in both survival and quality of life in survivors of this disease are due in large part to the success of multi-institution trials such as the IRS. One hopes that as better understanding of all aspects of RMS is acquired further improvement in therapy and survival will occur.

REFERENCES

1. Young JL, Miller RW. Incidence of malignant tumors in U.S. children. J Pediatr 86:254, 1975.
2. Julian JC, Merguerian PA, Shortliffe LM. Pediatric genitourinary tumors. Curr Opin Oncol 7:265, 1995.
3. Mandell L. Ongoing progress in the treatment of childhood rhabdomyosarcoma. Oncology 7(1):71, 1993.
4. Raney RB, Hays DM, Tefft M, Triche TJ: Rhabdomyosarcoma and the undifferentiated sarcomas. In Pizzo PA, Poplack DG (eds), Principles and Practice of Pediatric Oncology, 2nd ed. Philadelphia, JB Lippincott, 1993, p 769.
5. Tsokos M. The diagnosis and classification of childhood rhabdomyosarcoma. Semin Diag Pathol 11:26, 1994.
6. Maurer HM, Gehan EA, Beltangady M, et al. The Intergroup Rhabdomyosarcoma Study-II. Cancer 71:1904, 1993.
7. Newton W, Soule EH, Hamoudi A, et al. Histopathology of childhood sarcomas: Intergroup Rhabdomyosarcoma Studies I and II. Clinicopathologic correlation. J Clin Oncol 6:67, 1988.
8. Kodet R, Newton WA, Hamoudi AB, et al. Childhood rhabdomyosarcoma with anaplastic (pleomorphic) features. Am J Surg Pathol 17:443, 1993.
9. Shapiro E, Strother D. Pediatric genitourinary rhabdomyosarcoma. J Urol 148:1761, 1992.
10. Atra A, Ward HC, Aitken K, et al. Conservative surgery in multimodal therapy for pelvic rhabdomyosarcoma in children. Br J Cancer 70:1004, 1994.
11. Lawrence W, Gehan EA, Hays DM, et al. Prognostic significance of staging factors of the UICC staging system in childhood rhabdomyosarcoma: A report from the Intergroup Rhabdomyosarcoma Study (IRS-II). J Clin Oncol 5:46, 1987.
12. Grosfeld JL, Weber TR, Weetman RM, Baehner RL. Rhabdomyosarcoma in childhood: Analysis of survival in 98 cases. J Pediatr Surg 18:141, 1983.
13. Hays DM, Raney RB, Lawrence W, et al. Bladder and prostatic tumors in the Intergroup Rhabdomyosarcoma Study (IRS-I). Cancer 90:1472, 1982.
14. Raney RB, Gehan EA, Hays DM, et al. Primary chemotherapy with or without radiation therapy and/or surgery for children with localized sarcoma of the bladder, prostate, vagina, uterus, and cervix. Cancer 66:2072, 1990.
15. Hays DM. Bladder/prostate rhabdomyosarcoma: Results of the multi-institutional trials of the Intergroup Rhabdomyosarcoma Study. Semin Surg Oncol 9:520, 1993.
16. Crist W, Gehan EA, Ragab AH, et al. The Third Intergroup Rhabdomyosarcoma Study. J Clin Oncol 13:610, 1995.
17. Hays DM, Raney RB, Wharam MD, et al. Children with vesical rhabdomyosarcoma (RMS) treated by partial cystectomy with neoadjuvant or adjuvant chemotherapy, with or without radiotherapy: A report from the Intergroup Rhabdomyosarcoma Study (IRS) committee. J Pediatr Hematol Oncol 17:46, 1995.

18. Corpron CA, Andrassy RJ, Hays DM. Conservative management of uterine pediatric rhabdomyosarcoma: A report from the Intergroup Rhabdomyosarcoma Study III and IV pilot. J Pediatr Surg 30:942, 1995.
19. Raney B, Heyn R, Hays DM, et al. Sequelae of treatment in 109 patients followed for 5 to 15 years after diagnosis of sarcoma of the bladder and prostate. Cancer 71:2387, 1993.
20. Yeung CK, Ward HC, Ransley PG, et al. Bladder and kidney function after cure of pelvic rhabdomyosarcoma in childhood. Br J Cancer 70:1000, 1994.

PART V

Eagle-Barrett Syndrome

HRAIR-GEORGE O. MESROBIAN

14

Prune-Belly Syndrome

The prune-belly syndrome, also known as the triad anomaly or the Eagle-Barrett syndrome, is very rare, occurring approximately once every 50,000 live births, with a prevalence of 3.2 per 100,000. The male-to-female ratio is 5:1, with a higher prevalence also recorded in twins and blacks.[1] The true incidence may be higher, because many patients with partial manifestations of the syndrome may not have the typical abdominal wall appearance. The prototypical patient is a boy with hydronephrosis, cryptorchidism, and absence of abdominal wall musculature. The disease can be unilateral with partial deficiency of the abdominal wall musculature, and the syndrome can go unrecognized for years, especially in girls.

The cause of prune-belly syndrome has received a great deal of attention, and two major theories of pathogenesis exist. The most widely held theory is that the syndrome arises from a major defect in the intermediate and lateral mesoderm, thus affecting the embryogenesis of the mesonephric and paramesonephric ducts in addition to the abdominal wall musculature and urinary systems.[2] Others have presented evidence of an association with urethral atresia or obstruction.[3, 4] The distinction is important and may have surgical therapeutic implications. The two theories are not mutually exclusive, and it has been well documented that urethral obstruction can occur in this syndrome secondary to telescoping or kinking of a redundant prostatic urethra in the presence of a primary mesodermal defect.[5] Therefore, the characteristics of urethral obstruction associated with prune-belly syndrome differ from those associated with other forms of urethral obstruction, including posterior urethral valves. Nevertheless, these two entities have been compared extensively in the literature with the purpose of identifying similarities and differences that might support one theory of pathogenesis over the other.[6] Of the various associated cytogenetic anomalies that have been described, the trisomies (chromosomes 13, 18, and 21) have been the most frequent.[7–9] No infectious agent or teratogen has been implicated in the pathogenesis. Furthermore, a naturally occurring animal model of the disease does not exist.

CHARACTERISTICS OF THE SYNDROME

Abdominal Wall Defect

The deficiency of the abdominal wall musculature is the most dramatic aspect of the triad. The appearance does vary between patients and in the same patient at various times of development. From the thin and lax neonatal appearance frequently revealing to the observer the waves of intestinal peristalsis, the overall appearance of the abdominal wall defect can change to the so-called "potbelly" appearance of adolescence or adulthood. Part of the reason is that the distribution of the healthy musculature varies, giving the appearance of patchy and asymmetric defects. In general, the upper rectus is healthier and more conspicuous than its lower portions. This, combined with bulging of the flanks, frequently results in the flaring of the ribs. The abdominal wall defect undoubtedly makes children with this syndrome more susceptible to the consequences of trauma, and appropriate protection is warranted during physical activity.[10] Even torsion of a renal allograft with acute infarction in a patient with this syndrome was ascribed to the abdominal wall deficiency.[11]

Cryptorchidism

Bilateral cryptorchidism is a constant finding. Most frequently, both testes are undescended and intra-abdominal, located at the level of the pelvic brim. Although this may suggest "mechanical" obstruction to the descent of the testes (because of a distended bladder or dilated ureter), histologic studies lend strong support to the theory of an intrinsic testicular anomaly. In fact, these testes are found to have significant reduction in the number of spermatogonia and Leydig cell hyperplasia compared with normal individuals, even at the fetal stage.[12] These observations have important implications for fertility because late orchidopexy (in childhood or adolescence) may be associated with infertility in sexually active men.[13] In addition, it is important to note that the anatomy of the spermatic cord and its length favor an early orchidopexy (within the first year of life), the long-term results of which promise to yield better fertility, although prostate function may remain deficient. Finally, although it was believed for a long time that these testes were not susceptible to malignancies, there are now such reports in the literature.[14, 15] Therefore, careful follow-up is indicated.

Hydronephrosis

Hydronephrosis represents the most threatening aspect of the anomaly. When associated with renal dysplasia and renal failure, it can lead to oligohydramnios, pulmonary hypoplasia, and death (Fig. 14–1). In fact, the prognosis depends on the level of renal function at birth, and dialysis and transplantation, although now available, are not curative. Infrequently, renal function can be normal with or without the presence of hydronephrosis. The latter can be secondary to vesicoureteral reflux, to obstruction, or to a large atonic urinary system. In fact, the ureter has a characteristic appearance (Fig. 14–2), and histologic studies have revealed a markedly increased ratio of collagen to smooth muscle.[16] The appearance can be asymmetric and vary markedly from a dysplastic multicystic kidney on one side to a nonobstructed hydronephrotic kidney on the other side with normal serum creatinine (Fig. 14–3). The degree of hydronephrosis is such that extreme caution should be exercised in making the diagnosis of obstruction. The usual diagnostic tools that are available may not be applicable in this setting.[17] Occasionally, when the abdominal wall defect is subtle or not present, hydronephrosis and cryptorchidism (unilateral or bilateral) coexisting in the same patient may constitute enough evidence to suspect this syndrome.

Bladder

Typically, the prune-belly bladder is very large, has a thick wall, and is irregular in shape. The thickness of the wall does not always represent hypertrophy, and the relative distribution of connective tissue to muscle fibers may determine the efficacy of ultimate function.[18] Although the syndrome is compatible with normal voiding, most patients have incomplete emptying and abnormal urodynamic parameters.[19] Straining when the abdominal musculature is deficient may not be very efficacious in the promotion of bladder emptying. In addition, straining may result in uncoordinated voiding, as has been described. In fact, voiding is variable, and, although spontaneous voiding can ultimately be achieved, 56% of patients

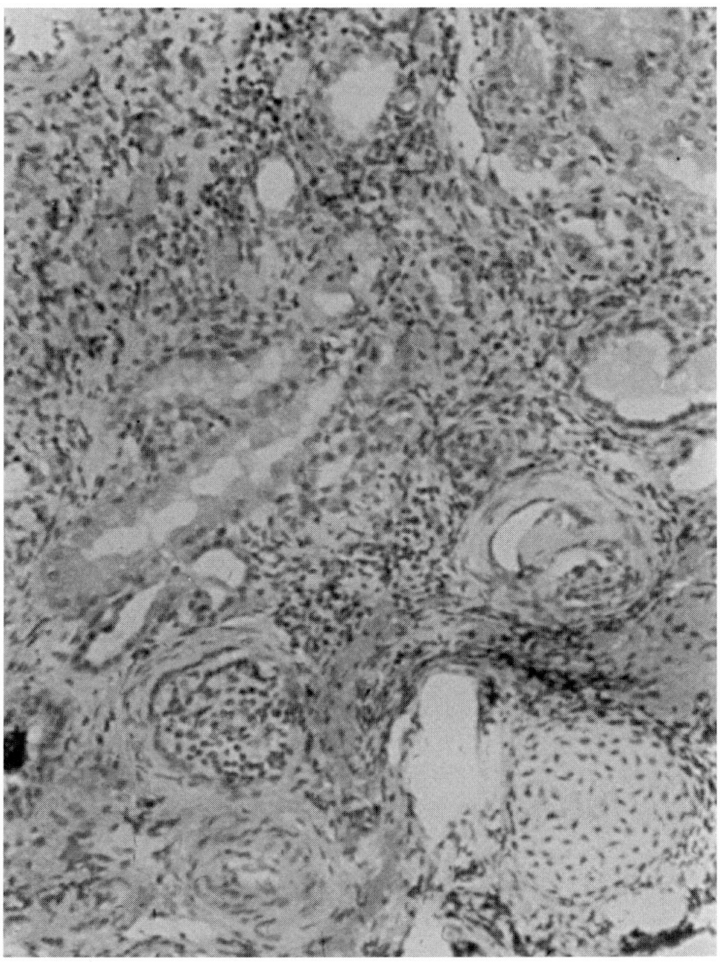

Figure 14–1 Kidney biopsy from a newborn with the prune-belly syndrome and renal failure with the hallmarks of renal dysplasia.

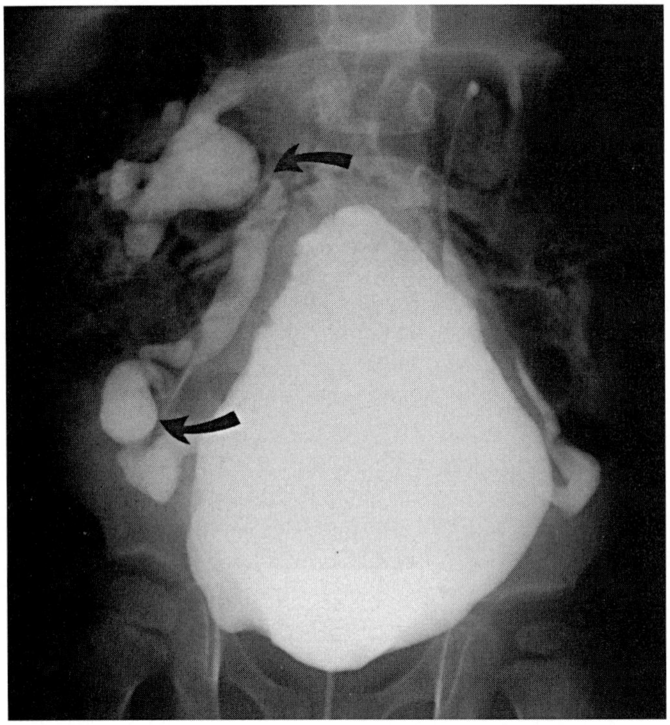

Figure 14–2 Bilateral vesicoureteral reflux in a patient with the prune-belly syndrome. Note how the ureteral caliber varies *(arrows)*.

required intermittent catheterization in one large series.[20] Radiographically, the dome of the bladder may have the appearance of a pseudodiverticulum and the bladder neck is closed but wide (Fig. 14–4). Reflux into dilated and tortuous ureters of variable caliber is the rule.

Prostate

The differential diagnosis of a wide and elongated prostatic urethra includes the prune-belly syndrome (Fig. 14–5). This appearance is secondary to prostatic hypoplasia.[5] It has been postulated that the lack of muscular support in the area of the prostatomembranous urethra results in urethral intussusception, leading to obstruction at that level early in gestation. Alternatively, the site of the narrowing at the apex of the prostatic urethra may mark the site of intrauterine obstruction. Both theories may explain why internal urethrotomy at this location may improve the voiding dynamics in selected patients.

Ureter

It is important to note that the histology of the ureter and, therefore, function varies between upper and lower portions. The upper ureter may actually have normal caliber and anatomy and peristatic ability. The lower end is almost always affected with fibrosis and deficiency in the smooth muscle component. This is associated with poor peristalsis. The differences between the upper and lower ureters are important when surgical straightening, tapering, or ureteral reimplantation is elected.

Associated Anomalies

Several reports have focused on associated anomalies, the most frequent of which are orthopedic, gastrointestinal, and, to a lesser extent, cardiac. Other anomalies that have been described include megalourethra,[21] uterine duplication with or without anorectal anomalies,[22] and ectopic vas deferens,[23] among others that are less frequent. The sequence of bladder distention with compression of the iliac vasculature resulting in lower limb deficiency is cited as evidence to support the notion of urethral obstruction occurring in utero.[24]

Gastrointestinal Anomalies. The occasional occurrence of an omphalocele or gastroschisis is regarded as further evidence for a primary mesodermal defect in this syndrome.[25] Intestinal malrotation with a universal mesentery has been well documented in the majority of patients. The occasional occurrence of imperforate anus in association with urethral atresia and the prune-belly syndrome suggests similarities with the caudal regression

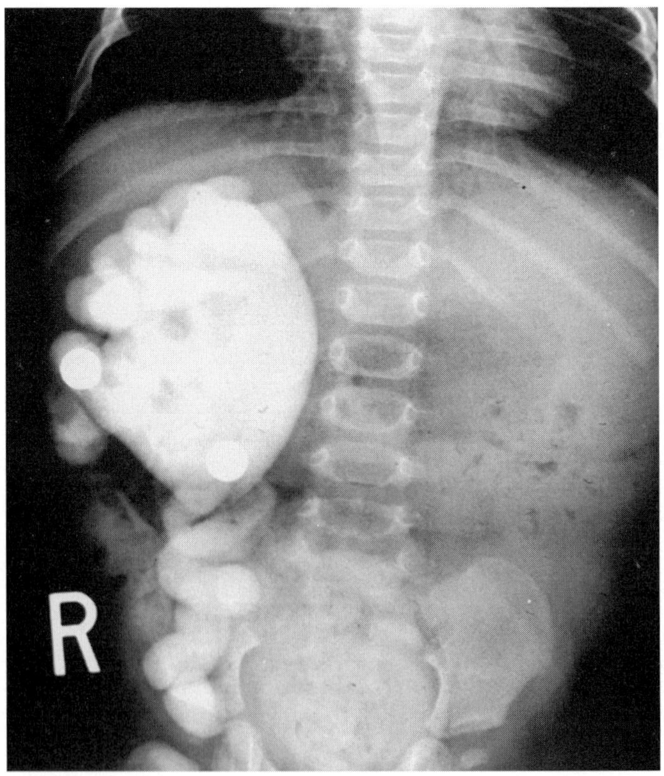

Figure 14–3 Unilateral cryptorchidism (left), multicystic dysplastic kidney (left), right hydronephrosis, and laxity of the abdominal wall in an infant who presented with a urinary tract infection.

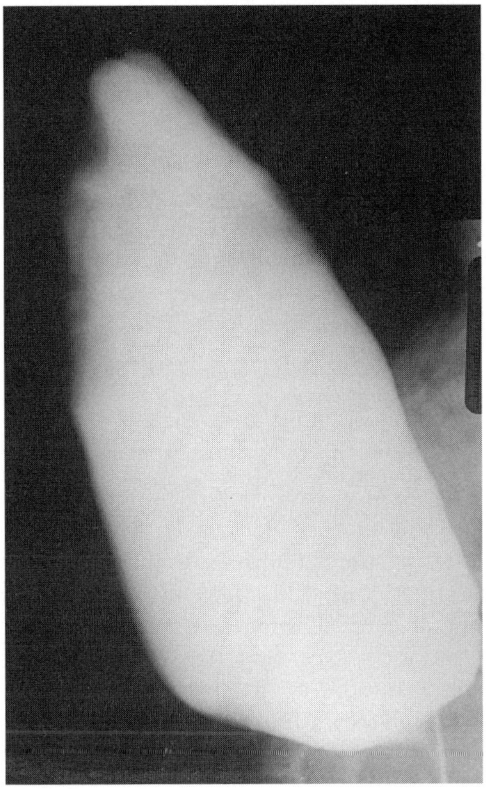

Figure 14–4 Appearance of the bladder in an adolescent with the syndrome. Note the size, shape, and appearance of the bladder with a pseudodiverticulum at the dome.

syndrome, especially in the presence of renal dysplasia.[6] Constipation may be the most frequent gastrointestinal symptom and may be very difficult to treat because of the abdominal wall deficiency. This can lead to an acquired megacolon, which can compound the urinary problems possibly by predisposing these individuals to infections. Finally, in the patients requiring a vesicostomy, it is essential to prevent constipation because excessive abdominal straining can result in bladder prolapse.

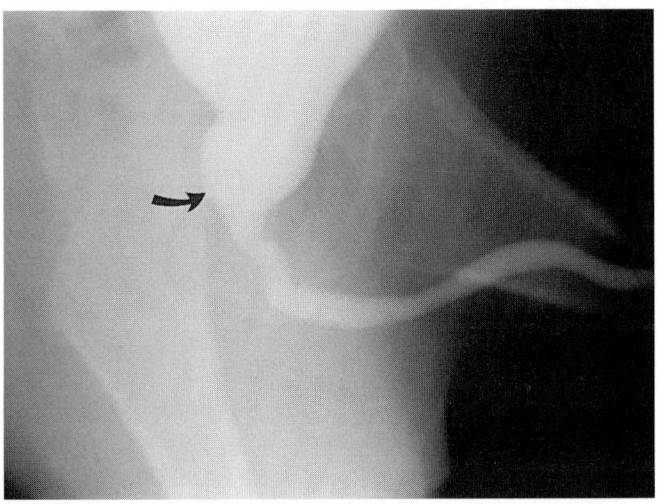

Figure 14–5 Voiding cystourethrogram in patient with the prune-belly syndrome. Note the dilated posterior urethra *(arrow)*. Cystoscopic examination did not reveal an obstructing lesion.

Musculoskeletal System. Because many children with the prune-belly syndrome now survive into adulthood, a knowledge of the musculoskeletal anomalies is useful in minimizing morbidity. The prevalence of these anomalies in this population is 45%.[26] These anomalies can be congenital (clubfoot, limb deficiencies, teratologic hip dysplasia, and vertebral malformations) or acquired (renal osteodystrophy, scoliosis, and pectus excavatum or pectus carinatum).[23] Treatment may require nonconventional approaches, and the orthopedic surgeon needs to be involved early.[27] Less significant but more frequent is the finding of a dimple on the outer aspect of the knee or elbow.

MODES OF PRESENTATION

Prenatal

The prenatal diagnosis of prune-belly syndrome hinges primarily on the detection of hydronephrosis with or without a hydroureter. A megalourethra, when present, may also be detected.[28] In addition, the presence of fetal ascites and a lax abdominal wall have been considered to suggest the presence of prune-belly syndrome. The diagnosis of hydronephrosis can be made as early as 17 weeks. However, it is very difficult to distinguish this syndrome with certainty from others prenatally. The differential diagnosis includes massive primary vesicoureteral reflux or posterior urethral valves. Intrauterine fluid aspiration for evaluation of electrolyte composition and other markers of renal dysplasia has been performed as early as 15 weeks of gestation.[29] The significance of the prenatal diagnosis resides in the opportunity for improved obstetrical and neonatal management.

Neonatal

It is relatively easy to recognize the newborn with the complete form of the syndrome. The classification proposed by Woodard and Zucker is useful (Table 14–1) and allows for prioritization of the most urgent problem for management. Class I patients have pulmonary hypoplasia and renal failure and are not likely to survive beyond the first few days of life. Class II patients have the full-blown syndrome minus the pulmonary hypoplasia and severe renal failure. Their management requires a multidisciplinary approach, including neonatologists, pediatric nephrologists, and urologists. Therefore, they are best managed at a medical center where these specialties are

Table 14–1
Spectrum of Prune-Belly Syndrome

Category	Distinguishing Characteristics
I	Oligohydramnios, pulmonary hypoplasia, or pneumothorax; may have urethral obstruction or patent urachus and club foot
II	Typical external features and uropathy of the full-blown syndrome but no immediate problem with survival; may have mild or unilateral renal dysplasia; may or may not develop urosepsis or gradual azotemia
III	External features may be mild or incomplete; uropathy is less severe and renal function stable

Modified from Woodard JR, Zucker I. Current management of the dilated urinary tract in prune belly syndrome. Urol Clin North Am 17:408, 1990. Used with permission.

well represented and supported. It is preferable to initiate this transfer before urinary tract instrumentation to minimize the chance of introducing infection. Class III patients have the incomplete or milder forms of the disease and rarely require intervention in the immediate neonatal period.

Adulthood

A few patients have been described who have presented in adulthood usually secondary to renal insufficiency, hypertension, sepsis, or infertility.[6] The incomplete forms of the syndrome are more likely to go unnoticed during infancy, especially when the abdominal wall laxity is subtle (Fig. 14–6). These patients usually will exhibit some of the internal features of the syndrome albeit in a less severe form.

RISKS ASSOCIATED WITH THE PRUNE-BELLY SYNDROME

The newborn with this syndrome is at risk for disease-specific short-term and long-term complications with the potential for considerable morbidity. In addition, there are risks associated with the surgical procedures that may become necessary; therefore, a knowledge of the potential complications is essential.

Pulmonary Complications. In patients surviving the neonatal period, pulmonary atelectasis and pneumonia may occur secondary to a weak abdominal musculature, which impedes respiratory movements and coughing. Appropriate recognition of these factors may minimize anesthetic complications. In addition, sedation should be avoided, especially in the very young. A more lethal and severe risk consists of pulmonary hypoplasia secondary to oligohydramnios, which has been well characterized and documented. The absence of amniotic fluid results in a lack of stenting of the developing fetal lung.[30] This is commonly associated with pneumothorax or pneumomediastinum, pulmonary failure, and death.

Renal Failure and Infections. The risks associated with renal failure and its treatment modalities, including dialysis and renal transplantation, are impossible to avoid when the kidneys are dysplastic from the outset. The presence of hydronephrosis per se may be well tolerated, but the introduction of infection can be quite detrimental to both renal function and the general well-being of the patient. It is, therefore, important to minimize the number of opportunities that may result in infections by minimizing the number of procedures that require entry into the urinary tract.

Infertility. The risk of infertility stems from the fact that the testes are abnormal in addition to being cryptorchid. Historically, cryptorchidism was corrected later in childhood or in adolescence, and this practice may partially explain the poor fertility.[13] It remains to be seen whether the fertility will be enhanced with early orchidopexy within the first year of life, because prostatic secretion is usually deficient.

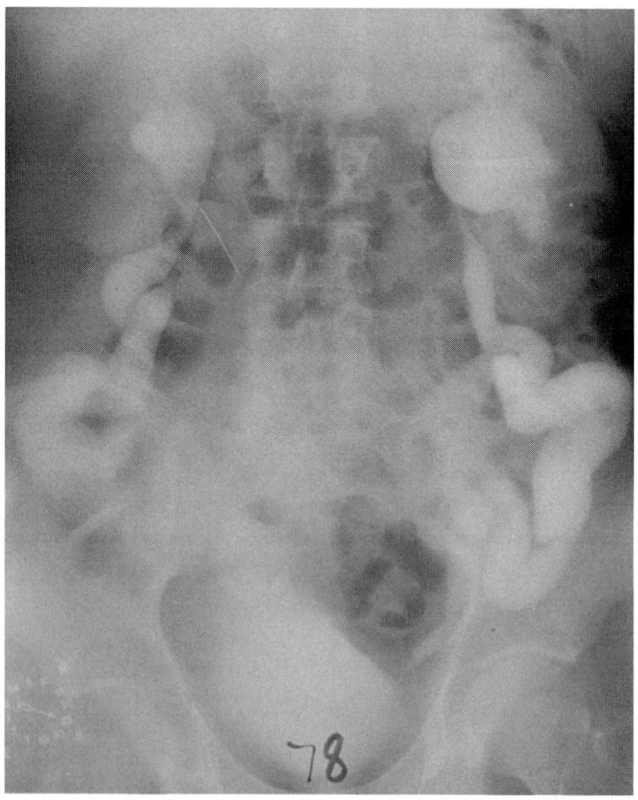

Figure 14–6 Intravenous pyelogram of 31-year-old man with the prune-belly syndrome with normal renal function and infertility.

Malignancies. In addition to the few testicular malignancies that have been reported, there has been one report of a mucinous adenocarcinoma developing in the defunctionalized bladder of a patient with the prune-belly syndrome.[31]

Trauma. The absence of abdominal wall musculature makes the viscera vulnerable to trauma.[10] Bladder rupture has occurred in these patients after relatively minor trauma, especially when the bladder is allowed to overdistend. In addition, hydronephrosis makes the kidneys vulnerable to the effects of even minor trauma.

DIAGNOSTIC EVALUATION

The external manifestations of the syndrome are self-evident and receive immediate attention; however, the internal aspects also deserve prompt evaluation. The cardiopulmonary status of the neonate requires immediate attention. In addition to pulmonary hypoplasia, the presence of a pneumomediastinum or a pneumothorax needs to be ruled out. A chest x-ray film is, therefore, mandatory. Because as many as 10% of patients may harbor a cardiac anomaly, an echocardiogram may be required in addition to the physical examination. A careful orthopedic examination, including appropriate x-ray films, is also required. The urologic evaluation must be individualized and directed by the clinical circumstances to minimize instrumentation at this early age. The serum creatinine and electrolytes are obtained serially to estimate true renal function independent of the maternal effect. A renal ultrasonogram is also obtained at this time. The presence of vesicoureteral reflux is assumed, and antimicrobial prophylaxis is initiated. Subsequent evaluation depends on the clinical course.

At some point during infancy, perhaps at 4 weeks of age (or earlier if clinically indicated), a voiding cystourethrogram and a renal scan are obtained. A treatment plan is formulated, and further urologic evaluation is dependent on the initial outcome. Subsequent periodic diagnostic urologic evaluation is individualized but should continue indefinitely.

TREATMENT, COMPLICATIONS, AND THEIR MANAGEMENT

The optimal treatment of the various aspects of this syndrome should be considered to be evolving for two major reasons: (1) the long-term results of earlier surgical approaches are just becoming known, and (2) the introduction of newer diagnostic tools are changing the way we evaluate outcome. It is safe to state that, on the one hand, the testes are best managed surgically early on and that, on the other hand, the indications for surgical reconstruction of the urinary tract are still being refined. Abdominal wall reconstruction is feasible surgically, although it has been difficult to demonstrate consistent and lasting results. Many patients do well with a nonoperative approach to the dilated urinary tract.[32] Historically, the morbidity associated with total urinary tract reconstruction has been significant.[33] Therefore, it is prudent to individualize each patient's care and formulate a rational plan of management based on the initial level of renal function and the appearance of the urinary tract as observed over a period of time. The orchidopexy can then be performed separately or in conjunction with urinary tract reconstruction and abdominoplasty. The following is a description of the various procedures that may benefit children with the prune-belly syndrome.

Urinary Diversion

Supravesical. Supravesical urinary diversion in the form of bilateral cutaneous loop ureterostomies or pyelostomies may be indicated in the small number of patients who present with very high initial serum creatinine levels or sepsis and in whom a period of catheter drainage of the bladder and antibiotic treatment does not ameliorate the clinical picture. It is important to place the ureterostomy site as lateral as possible and away from the abdomen so as not to interfere with the subsequent placement of a peritoneal dialysis catheter, if the latter becomes necessary. Because the upper ureter is more normal than the lower ureter, ureterostomy is not a popular and desirable operation for this disease. Nevertheless, it can occasionally be necessary. The long-term effect of a period of supravesical diversion and, therefore, bladder defunctionalization on ultimate bladder function is not known in this syndrome.

Vesicostomy. Vesicostomy is indicated in newborns and infants who have urinary retention with or without a progressive increase in the degree of hydronephrosis. The technical aspects of the procedure have been well described.[34] It is worth emphasizing the need to exteriorize the dome of the bladder to minimize the chance of prolapse. The abdominal straining associated with constipation predisposes to such prolapse. Because these children have normal penile and urethral sensation, intermittent catheterization is usually difficult to accept. This can delay closure of the bladder. Alternatively, these children may benefit from total urinary tract reconstruction, including a reduction cystoplasty, which may promote bladder emptying, once their upper tracts have stabilized.

Internal Urethrotomy. This can be performed to facilitate bladder emptying. Internal urethrotomy is done under direct vision at the 12 o'clock position, if an obstructing lesion can be visualized at the level of the membranous urethra. The redundancy of the prostatic urethra may predispose to this appearance. When this approach is contemplated, it is desirable to obtain objective data preoperatively for meaningful follow-up. A carefully performed urodynamic study is desirable.[35] A urinary flow rate is possibly the least invasive method of follow-up. However, this is not possible in the neonate and infant.

Orchidopexy

Of all the possible surgical procedures, orchidopexy may be the only operation needed in male patients with this syndrome. Whereas even in the recent past fears of testicular atrophy after orchidopexy hindered early referral or treatment, recent evidence suggesting that fertility may be possible in adults born with prune-belly syndrome helps to justify early surgical treatment. In addition, orchidopexy in the infant may be most successful when combined with urinary tract reconstruction and abdominoplasty by virtue of the retroperitoneal exposure obtained, which allows for extensive mobilization of the spermatic cord to the origins of the vessels.[32] When urinary tract reconstruction is not contemplated, orchidopexy alone at or about 6 months of age is indicated. In the older child, serious consideration should be given to surgical approaches that do not depend on the one-stage Fowler-Stephens approach, which carries a significant risk of postoperative atrophy.[36] These approaches include operative laparoscopic orchidopexy,[37] free transfer with microvascular anastomosis of spermatic vessels to inferior epigastric vessels,[38] and staged Fowler-Stephens orchidopexy (with open or laparoscopic first stage).

The following plan is suggested for the surgical management of the cryptorchidism:

- When urinary tract reconstruction is anticipated, orchidopexy is incorporated in that procedure. The results of transabdominal orchidopexy are excellent, especially when performed during the first year of life.
- When urinary tract reconstruction is not anticipated, orchidopexy is performed when the infant is stable and the risks of anesthesia have decreased as pulmonary function improves. Any of the surgical procedures listed previously can accomplish the desired outcome with equal success. It is far better to perform these procedures (with the exception of the microvascular approach) when the child is about 6 months of age.
- When the patient presents late and does not require urinary tract reconstruction or an abdominoplasty, the best approach may be a laparoscopic orchidopexy; this will allow extensive dissection and mobilization of the spermatic cord with less morbidity than an open procedure. Alternatively, a conventional approach can be used with conversion to a microvascular approach if standard procedures do not allow for scrotal positioning of the testis.

Urinary Tract Reconstruction

Urinary tract reconstruction consists of excision of the distal dilated and tortuous ureters, tapering and reimplantation of the more proximal ureters, excision of the dome of the bladder, and reduction cystoplasty. Depending on the clinical situation, not all of these procedures may be required in the individual patient. Traditionally, a transperitoneal route has been used to gain access to all of these anatomic parts.[39] The ureters are straightened, and their caliber is reduced after excision of the distal redundant portion.[40] Imbrication rather than excision for the purpose of tapering may minimize the chance of postoperative ureteral obstruction while correcting vesicoureteral reflux.[32] Care is taken not to interfere with the blood supply of the vas deferens during the dissection of the ureter. The ureter is stented after reimplantation into the bladder. Because the latter is capacious, any reimplantation technique can be used. It is important to obtain a long submucosal tunnel for reimplantation, especially for the bulky folded ureters. A Politano-Leadbetter or cross-trigonal technique is usually preferred.[41]

Reduction cystoplasty may be performed by overlapping the anterolateral muscle walls after excision of the mucosa on one side in a vest-over-pants fashion (Fig. 14–7). Alternatively, the bladder volume may be reduced

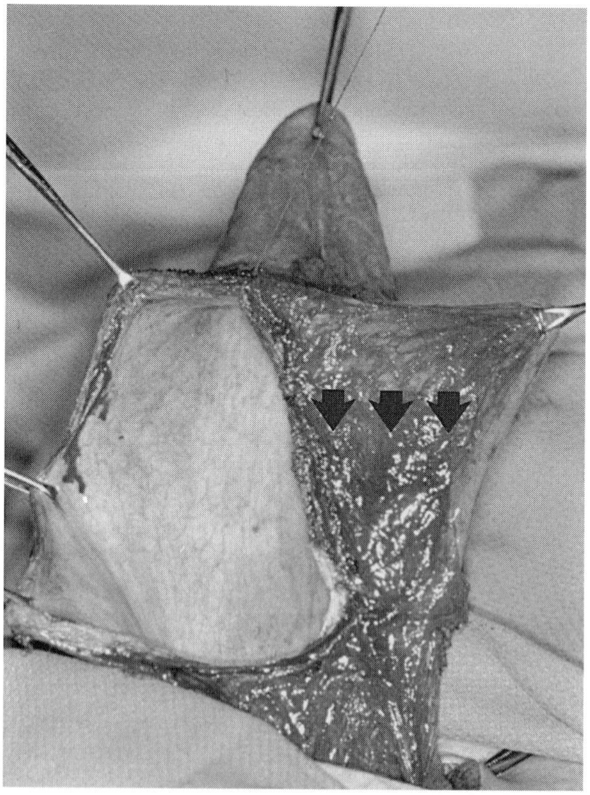

Figure 14–7 Intraoperative photograph demonstrating mucosal excision *(arrows)* in preparation for pants-over-vest closure and reduction cystoplasty. This procedure was combined with an abdominoplasty.

by excision and watertight closure. Recently, Bukowski and Perlmutter reviewed the long-term outcome of reduction cystoplasty performed in some patients as early as 1973. Six boys were older than 18 years at the time of the evaluation. The authors concluded that reduction cystoplasty did not improve voiding dynamics or decrease bladder size in the long term. However, reduction cystoplasty may have helped improve voiding and minimize infections during early childhood.[42] Other series have noted short-term improvement.[32] Double and triple voiding should be encouraged in these children, especially in those who may not appreciate the sensation of fullness.

Abdominal Wall Reconstruction

The rationale for abdominal wall reconstruction stems from cosmetic and psychological considerations and perhaps from the desire for better voiding efficiency by improving the ability to generate the intra-abdominal pressure. The surgical approach has evolved over years. Abdominal wall reconstruction initially consisted of a U-shaped incision extending from the tip of the 12th rib along the anterior iliac spine to the pubis and back to the opposite 12th rib. This was followed by excision of the redundant and lax abdominal wall and reapproximation of the presumably healthier portions to the pubic tubercles and the fascia below it.[43] This pioneering approach may not entirely remove the wrinkled appearance of the anterior abdominal wall, and laxity and persistence of the lateral bulging may recur. More recently, Montfort and colleagues devised a procedure that results in narrowing of the waist, strengthening of the abdominal wall, preservation of the umbilicus, and an improved cosmetic appearance.[44] Their excellent results were duplicated by Parrott and Woodard.[45]

The operation begins with a diamond-shaped incision anteriorly, extending from the xiphoid superiorly to the symphysis inferiorly, sparing the umbilicus, which is preserved as an island. Excision of the skin exposes the aponeurotic plate, the blood supply to which is preserved. Two lateral incisions are made in this fascial plate on either side of the excised area, exposing the intra-abdominal contents (Fig. 14–8). Any intra-abdominal procedure that is required can now be performed, including an orchidopexy. With electrocautery, the lateral peritoneum is incised, exposing the lateral musculofascial plate. Suturing of this edge to the lateral border of the midline aponeurotic plate results in a more normal waistline. The skin flaps are then trimmed and sutured together in the midline, incorporating the umbilicus in the closure (Fig. 14–9).

Other Surgical Procedures

Repair of Megalourethra. The megalourethra is usually confined to the penile portion of the urethra. Surgical treatment consists of excision of the ventral redundant urethra followed by reapproximation of the edges around a catheter of appropriate size for the age of the patient. The lack of spongy tissue in that area does not cause a functional problem. The native urethral meatus is usually normally situated.

Placement of Peritoneal Dialysis Catheter–Renal Transplantation. Occasionally, peritoneal dialysis becomes necessary, especially in infants with renal failure who are not good candidates for hemodialysis. Because of the abdominal wall deficiency, slow healing and leakage may result in complications with the program. Laparoscopically placed peritoneal catheters may circumvent the emergence of these problems.[46] Finally, renal transplantation is as successful in this group of patients as in nondiabetic renal failure patients. Graft survival and function are also similar.[47] Ironically, the laxity of the abdominal wall may allow earlier placement of an adult kidney in small infants with the syndrome whose kidneys have failed.

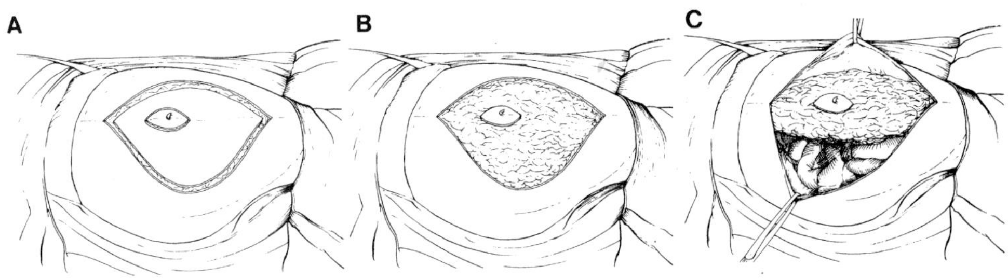

Figure 14–8 *A,* Almond-shaped incision is made on abdomen with upper end at xiphoid and lower end at symphysis pubis. *B,* Full-thickness excision of skin within parameters of incision is made, sparing umbilicus that is left in situ. *C,* Peritoneum is opened by making incision on either side of excised area. Intra-abdominal surgery can easily be performed via these lateral incisions. From Monfort G, Guys JM, Bocciardi A, et al. A novel technique for reconstruction of the abdominal wall in the prune belly syndrome. Journal of Urology 146(2):640, copyright Williams & Wilkins, 1991.

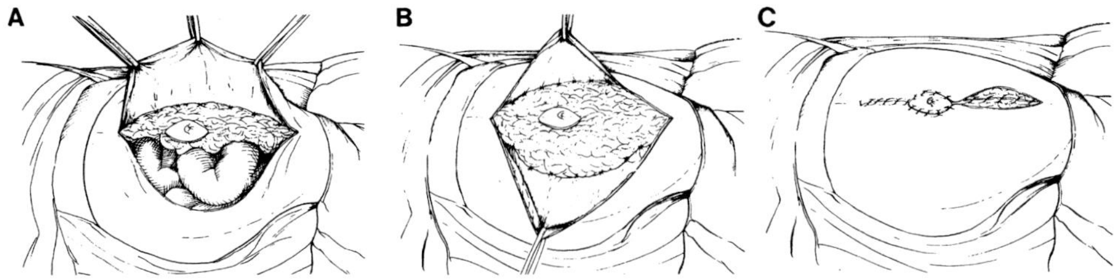

Figure 14–9 *A* and *B*, Parietal peritoneum is incised at the level necessary to achieve normal-appearing waistline. Edges of aponeurotic plate are sutured to this incision. *C*, Two lateral flaps are trimmed and sutured together at midline. Suture passes around umbilicus. From Monfort G, Guys JM, Bocciardi A, et al. A novel technique for reconstruction of the abdominal wall in the prune belly syndrome. Journal of Urology 146(2):640, copyright Williams & Wilkins, 1991.

SUMMARY

Evaluation and management of patients born with the prune-belly syndrome continue to evolve. The diagnosis can be made prenatally, especially when hydronephrosis is present. This, along with improved neonatal and urologic care, has resulted in improved survival. Each newborn with the syndrome is different, and a precise knowledge of the many and variable issues involved as described is mandatory. It remains to be seen whether early orchidopexy will enhance the fertility potential, but if any improvement is to be anticipated the early approach will have to be an essential component of the overall treatment plan. The preliminary results are very encouraging. Urinary tract reconstruction will vary and may consist of an internal urethrotomy or ureteral tailoring and reimplantation with or without a reduction cystoplasty. The improvement in voiding dynamics may not carry into adulthood and may fulfill a need in the first years of life. The prevention of infection and renal functional deterioration requires indefinite follow-up.

REFERENCES

1. Druschel CM. A descriptive study of prune belly syndrome in New York State, 1983 to 1989. Arch Pediatr Adolesc Med 149:70, 1995.
2. Stephens FD, Gupta D. Pathogenesis of the prune belly syndrome. J Urol 152:2328, 1994.
3. Reinberg Y, Chelimsky G, Gonzales R. Urethral atresia and the prune belly syndrome: Report of 6 cases. Br J Urol 72:112, 1993.
4. Manivel JC, Pettinato G, Reinberg Y, et al. Prune belly syndrome: Clinicopathologic study of 29 cases. Pediatr Pathol 9:691, 1989.
5. Hoagland MH, Hutchins GM. Obstructive lesions of the lower urinary tract in the prune-belly syndrome. Arch Pathol Lab Med 111:154, 1987.
6. Woodard JR. Prune-belly syndrome. In Walsh PC, Retik AB, Stamey TA, Vaughan ED (eds), Campbell's Urology, 6th ed. Philadelphia: WB Saunders, 1992, p 1852.
7. McKeown CM, Donnai D. Prune belly in trisomy 13. Prenatal Diagn 6:379, 1986.
8. Hoagland MH, Frank KA, Hutchins GM. Prune-belly syndrome with prostatic hypoplasia, bladder wall rupture, and massive ascites in a fetus with trisomy 18. Arch Pathol Lab Med 112:1126, 1988.
9. Amacker EA, Grass FS, Hickey DE, Hisley JC. An association of prune belly anomaly with trisomy 21. Am J Med Genet 23:919, 1986.
10. Smith DP, Jerkins GR, Noe HN. Blunt renal trauma in children with the prune-belly syndrome. J Urol 153:1960, 1995.
11. Marvin RG, Halff GA, Elshihabi I. Renal allograft torsion associated with prune-belly syndrome. Pediatr Nephrol 9:81, 1995.
12. Orvis BR, Bottles K, Kogan BA. Testicular histology in fetuses with the prune belly syndrome and posterior urethral valves. J Urol 139:335, 1988.
13. Woodhouse CR, Snyder HM III. Testicular and sexual function in adults with prune belly syndrome. J Clin Ultrasound 13:581, 1985.
14. Parra RO, Cummings JM, Palmer DC. Testicular seminoma in a long term survivor of the prune belly syndrome. Eur Urol 19:79, 1991.
15. Sayre R, Stephens R, Chonko AM. Prune belly syndrome and retroperitoneal germ cell tumor. Am J Med 81:895, 1986.
16. Gearhart JP, Lee BR, Partin AW, et al. A quantitative histological evaluation of the dilated ureter of childhood. J Urol 153:172, 1995.
17. Hunter GJ, Gordon I, Sweeney L, et al. 99mTc DTPA scanning with diuretic washout: Is it useful in the investigation of obstruction in the presence of gross renal tract dilatation? Br J Urol 59:208, 1987.
18. Workman SJ, Kogan BA. Fetal bladder histology in posterior urethral valves and the prune belly syndrome. J Urol 144:337, 1990.
19. Woodard JR. The bladder in prune belly syndrome. Dial Pediatr Urol 13:6, 1990.
20. Kinahan TJ, Churchill BM, McLorie GA, et al. The efficiency of bladder emptying in the prune belly syndrome. J Urol 148:600, 1992.
21. Mortensen PH, Johnson HW, Coleman GU, et al. Megalourethra. J Urol 134:358, 1985.
22. Reinberg Y, Shapiro E, Manivel JC, et al. Prune belly syndrome in females: A triad of abdominal musculature deficiency and anomalies of the urinary and genital systems. J Pediatr 118:395, 1991.
23. Cabral B, Majidi A, Gonzalez R. Ectopic vasa deferentia in an infant with the prune belly syndrome. J Urol (Paris) 94:223, 1988.
24. Perez-Aytes A, Graham JM, Hersh JH, et al. Urethral obstruction sequence and lower limb deficiency: Evidence of the vascular disruption hypothesis. J Pediatr 123:398, 1993.
25. Short KL, Groff DB, Cook L. The concomitant presence of gastroschisis and prune belly syndrome in a twin. J Pediatr Surg 20:186, 1985.

26. Loder RT, Guiboux JP, Bloom DA, Hensinger RN. Musculoskeletal aspects of the prune belly syndrome: Description and pathogenesis. Am J Dis Child 146:1224, 1992.
27. Brinker MR, Palutsis RS, Sarwark JF. The orthopedic manifestations of prune-belly syndrome. J Bone Joint Surg 77:251, 1995.
28. Fisk NM, Dhillon HK, Ellis CE, et al. Antenatal diagnosis of megalourethra in a fetus with the prune belly syndrome. J Clin Ultrasound 18:124, 1990.
29. Lun A, Lenz F, Priem F, et al. Biochemical diagnosis in prenatal uropathy. Clin Biochem 27:283, 1994.
30. Docimo SG, Luetic T, Crone RK, et al. Pulmonary development in the fetal lamb with severe bladder outlet obstruction and oligohydramnios: A morphometric study. J Urol 142:657, 1989.
31. Djavan B, Litwiller SE, Milchgrub S, Roehrborn CG. Mucinous adenocarcinoma in defunctionalized bladders. Urology 46:107, 1995.
32. Woodhouse CRJ, Kellett MJ, Williams DI. Minimal surgical interference in prune-belly syndrome. Br J Urol 51:475, 1979.
33. Fallat ME, Skoog SJ, Belman BA, et al. The prune-belly syndrome: A comprehensive approach to management. J Urol 802, 1989.
34. Hanna MK. Vesicostomy. In Hinman F Jr (ed), Atlas of Pediatric Urologic Surgery. Philadelphia: WB Saunders, 1994, p 356.
35. King LR. Idiopathic dilatation of the posterior urethra in boys without bladder obstruction. J Urol 102:783, 1969.
36. Gibbons MD, Cromie WJ, Duckett JW Jr. Management of the abdominal undescended testis. J Urol 122:76, 1979.
37. Docimo SG, Moore RG, Kavoussi LR. Laparoscopic orchidopexy in the prune belly syndrome: A case report and review of the literature. Urology 45:679, 1995.
38. Boddy SA, Gordon AC, Thomas DF, Browning FS. Experience with the Fowler Stephens and microvascular procedures in the management of intraabdominal testes. Br J Urol 68:199, 1991.
39. Woodard JR. The prune-belly syndrome. Urol Clin North Am 5:73, 1978.
40. Hendren WH. Functional restoration of decompensated ureters in children. Am J Surg 119:477, 1970.
41. Hinman F Jr. Ureteroneocystostomy. In Hinman F Jr (ed), Atlas of Pediatric Urology. Philadelphia: WB Saunders, 1994, p 202.
42. Bukowski TP, Perlmutter AD. Reduction cystoplasty in the prune belly syndrome: A long term followup. J Urol 152:2113, 1994.
43. Randolph J, Cavett C, Eng G. Abdominal wall reconstruction in the prune belly syndrome. J Pediatr Surg 16:960, 1981.
44. Monfort G, Guys JM, Bocciardi A, et al. A novel technique for reconstruction of the abdominal wall in the prune belly syndrome. J Urol 146:639, 1991.
45. Parrott TS, Woodard JR. The Monfort operation for abdominal wall reconstruction in the prune belly syndrome. J Urol 148:688, 1992.
46. Crompton CH, Balfe JW, Khoury A. Peritoneal dialysis in the prune belly syndrome. J Urol 14:17, 1994.
47. Reinberg Y, Manivel JC, Fryd D, et al. The outcome of renal transplantation in children with the prune belly syndrome. J Urol 142:1541, 1989.

PART VI

Genitalia

LOWELL R. KING

15

Hypospadias

More than 50 years have passed since Ormond Culp suggested it should be every boy's inalienable right to write his name in snow with urine by the time he started school. There is a lot of snow in Minnesota and, therefore, many practice opportunities. However, this act was often difficult or impossible for many hypospadias patients before techniques evolved to bring the meatus onto the glands and when chordee was released only by dissecting beneath one or two transverse incisions on the ventral aspect of the penis only, which were then closed longitudinally.

Chordee was thought to be due primarily, if not solely, to buried "scarlike" tissue on the ventral aspect of the penis. Today, however, we realize that congenital angulation of the corpora cavernosa—corporal disproportion—is the cause of most severe cases of chordee. More superficial ventral tissue may contribute, however, and milder chordee can certainly be caused by a lack of ventral skin alone. Glandular tilt is almost a separate entity and needs specific correction in many, if not most, cases.

Finally, techniques to move the meatus to the tip of the glans have gradually evolved, such that all boys should now be able to write their names in the snow. Advances in pediatric anesthesia and intraoperative monitoring have made general anesthesia safe at any age. All now recommend that operations on the genitalia be completed by the time a boy starts day care and toilet training or, in other words, starts comparing his own genitalia with that of others. Fortunately, the skin of the penis heals almost without visible scars, so after a good result is achieved a boy can grow up without knowing he had an unfinished penis. All risks of potentially catastrophic gender identity problems are avoided.[1, 2]

An "unfinished" penis has significant meaning when discussing hypospadias with parents. It is not a congenital anomaly, and one need not look all over the body for associated developmental problems. Hypospadias is usually due to the fetal testis stopping the production of male sex hormones just a little too soon to permit complete formation of the penis. In hypospadias the urethra stops short of the glans, and the foreskin does not migrate ventrally. Thus, when the meatus is on the distal penile shaft, the chordee is usually due to insufficient ventral skin, or failure of the dorsal hood to migrate. Chordee can often be corrected and the penis straightened by degloving the penis. The thin mucosa-like skin between the meatus and the glans need not be resected. It can be saved and used to form the neourethra, the back wall of the neourethra, or the distal portion of the neourethra. This skin is not "dysplastic," as was once thought by many, and grows with the child. Progressive penile elongation does not result in recurrent chordee.

However, once the penis is degloved, chordee may still be present. Commonly, the shaft is straight, but the glans is angulated ventrally. The techniques for the correction of glandular tilt and ventral corporal angulation (disproportion) are described next.

CORRECTION OF CHORDEE

To release chordee, an incision is made around the corporal sulcus. The cuff of skin left attached to the glans contracts a bit, so the incision is about 8 mm from, and parallel to, the corona laterally and dorsally. When the skin between the meatus and the corona is to be used for the neourethra, or the back of the neourethra, a strip of appropriate width is left in place, and parallel incisions are made ventrally to define this strip of preserved skin. These incisions are brought to a point behind the meatus. In hypospadias the corpora spongiosum commonly stops about 1 cm proximal to the meatus, so the urethra is very thin in this region. The penis is most safely degloved by starting laterally or dorsally. The subcutaneous tissues are divided in the lines of the incision until the corpora cavernosa is reached. The penis is then degloved in this plane, staying on Buck's fascia. This saves time, reduces bleeding, and keeps collateral circulation within the dorsal hood intact, which can be important when an onlay, transverse island flap or double-faced flap is chosen for repair.

When the corpora have been exposed dorsally and laterally, the penis is retracted rostrally and secured. Skin hooks are used to elevate the skin edges on either side of the urethra. A bougie is inserted to define the urethra and retract it dorsally. The dissecting scissors are then used to define the plane in the subcutaneous tissue above the urethra, which is then divided in the line of the skin incision. The skin and subcutaneous tissue are freed proximally from the denuded penis.

Next, an artificial erection is performed. The tourniquet is placed around the corpora, excluding the penile skin, and tightened. The corpora cavernosa are filled with normal saline. When the meatus is on the distal penile shaft, the chordee is usually corrected by degloving, and often only glandular tilt remains. However, at times, the corpora are mildly or sharply angulated ventrally, so an artificial erection is mandatory even if the meatus is at the corona or on the glans.

Complete correction when only glandular tilt remains is simple. With the tourniquet left in place, the plane between the glans and the corpora is entered dorsally. I prefer tenotomy scissors, which are blunt tipped but can be used to separate the tissues to a depth of a few millimeters. The dissection goes from the 10 to the 2 o'clock position, and then the groove is deepened by making repeated sweeps until about 1 cm of denuded glans is exposed (Fig. 15–1). I use interrupted 4-0 Vicryl, Dexon, or Monocryl sutures to sew the exposed raw surface of the glans to Buck's fascia about 1 cm proximal to the corona. Usually three sutures are sufficient: one in the midline and one on either side. The sutures are not tied until all have been placed. The artificial erection is then repeated to be sure that the glans is not angulated and that the tilt has been corrected.

When residual chordee is due to ventral angulation of the corpora cavernosa—what is now called corporal disproportion—removal of a dorsal wedge or wedges of the inner layer of Buck's fascia is necessary.[3] When the angulation is severe, two wedges are removed, one on either side of the point of greatest curvature. Generally, a single wedge is sufficient (Fig. 15–2). Although it has been shown that the glans has dual innervation, one attempts to preserve the paired dorsal nerves, arteries, and vein. This is feasible because it is relatively easy to split Buck's fascia into two layers.

The point of maximum curvature is marked. The outer layer of Buck's fascia is opened lateral and inferior to the dorsal nerve. The longitudinal incision in the outer layer of fascia is then extended to the base of the glans and proximally about 2 cm from the proposed resection point. The outer layer of Buck's fascia, containing nerves and vessels, is then teased off the inner layer. This is surprisingly easy. A counterincision is made below the dorsal nerve on the other side. When the scissors break through the septum, a vessel loop is passed to facilitate exposure of the inner fascial layer at both ends lengthwise. The artificial erection is then repeated, and the point of greatest curvature is again marked with lateral

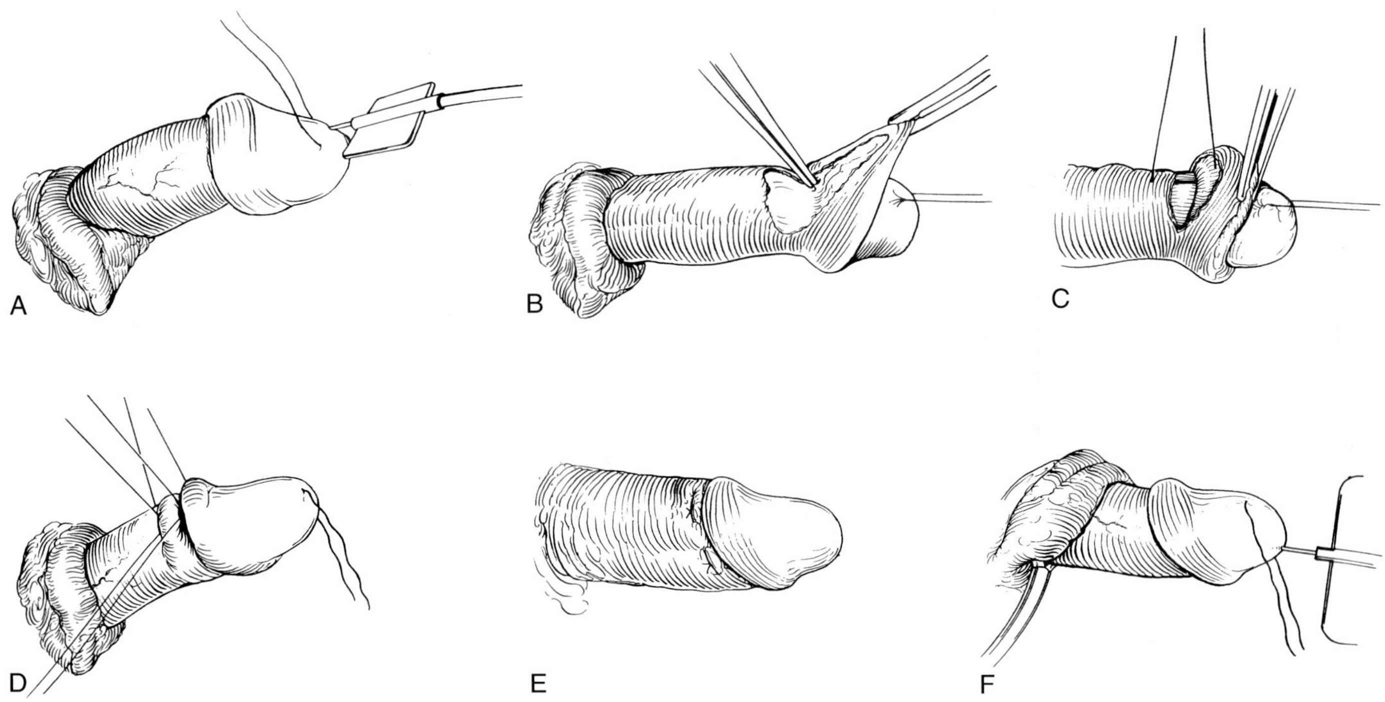

Figure 15–1 Correction of glanular tilt. *A,* An artificial erection shows residual glanular tilt after the penis has been degloved. *B,* The plane between the glans and the underlying corpora is entered dorsally. *C* and *D,* Dexon or Monocryl sutures are used to pull the dorsal glans proximally. Three such sutures are usually used. *E* and *F,* The sutures are tied, and the artificial creation is repeated.

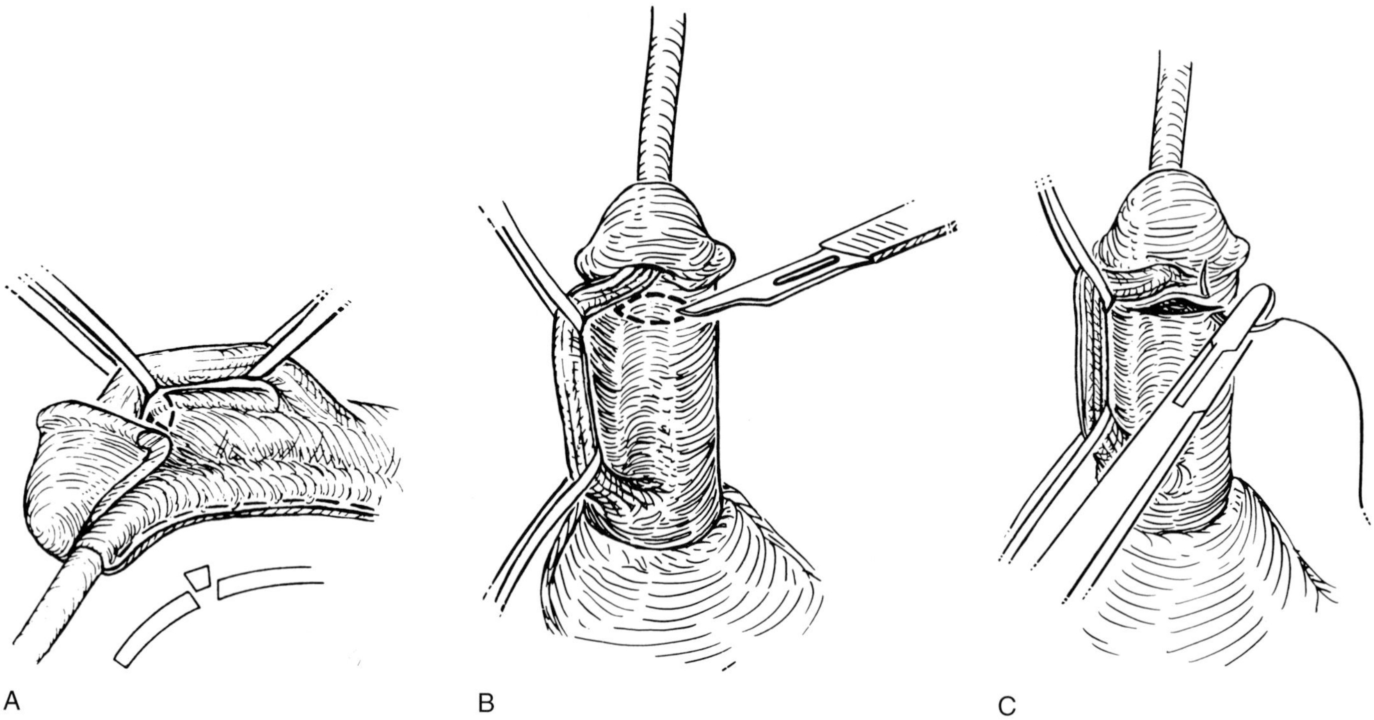

Figure 15–2 *A,* The dorsal nerves and vessels are isolated in the outer layer of Buck's fascia. *B* and *C,* A symmetric dorsal wedge of Buck's fascia is removed opposite the point of greatest curvature, and the fascia is then closed.

traction sutures. They must be exactly even, such that traction facilitates removal of a symmetric wedge. The wedge is usually 6 to 7 mm wide in the midline and tapered to the ends at the 10 and 2 o'clock positions. An effort is made to remove fascia only, not the underlying erectile tissue. The incision is closed with closely placed interrupted 3-0 chromic sutures. If artificial erection shows that the penis has been straightened, the tourniquet is released. Minor bleeding is controlled by compression, or an additional suture is placed. I have used 3-0 chromic sutures to close pediatric corporotomies for at least 15 years, and there are no long-term problems secondary to the use of absorbable sutures.

FORESKIN TRANSPOSITION

Straightening of the angulation in the penile shaft is necessary to correct chordee, but the penis will not stay straight unless healthy skin is rotated onto the ventral penile shaft to make good the lack of skin there. Fortunately, a substantial amount of this skin, rich in nerve endings and blood supply, is almost always available: the unrolled dorsal hood. Occasionally, when chordee is minimal, there is adequate skin on the ventral penile shaft, and the foreskin can simply be resected. To my eye, however, the penis usually looks best if some of the dorsal hood is transposed ventrally. This is most simply done by splitting the unrolled dorsal hood in the midline, resecting the inner layer of the foreskin, which is a poor color match and has the poorest blood supply, and bringing the shortened flaps around each side of the penis, interdigitating them ventrally to achieve a pleasing cosmetic appearance.[4]

When more skin is needed ventrally—this is not uncommon even when the meatus is near the glans—I usually prefer a van der Meulen–type foreskin transposition.[5] Van der Meulen studied the blood supply of the genitalia and found that all venous drainage of the foreskin coalesces into a single vein. Thus, when long foreskin flaps are divided in the midline, one flap usually has good venous drainage whereas the other has poor drainage. When edema occurs, the flap with less drainage is at increased risk for impaired circulation and necrosis. To avoid this problem, van der Meulen advocated transposition of the unrolled dorsal hood as a single major flap (Fig. 15–3).

The dorsal hood is unrolled. Transillumination may be used to determine which side has the best blood supply. The other side of the foreskin is then divided from the base of the foreskin laterally to the base of the foreskin in the midline. This divides the dorsal hood into major and minor flaps. A suture is placed from the corona to the apex of the incision in the foreskin at the 12 o'clock position, and the penis is checked for torsion. The minor flap is then sutured to the corona laterally. The penis is retracted rostrally, and the major flap is worked around the corona with widely spaced interrupted "trial and error" sutures. As the name implies, these sutures are adjusted as needed to prevent tension or torsion. Next, the bottom of the flap is transposed across the midline. This requires some rotation and usually a second incision in the skin at the base of the foreskin to allow enough extension of the flap. Actually, the skin incision can be carried distally to the corona, creating an island flap that can be further rotated if needed to center the flap, providing ventral coverage with pleasing symmetry. The flap has excellent blood supply so long as the pedicle remains intact. Also, this is a broad-based pedicle that lies flat and does not give the humped appearance, which is common on either side of the corona when the foreskin is simply split.

The major flap is rotated with trial and error sutures until the flap is centered ventrally and has a pleasing cosmetic appearance. Van der Meulen foreskin transpositions require a little practice but yield superior cosmetic results. The rich blood supply of the flap minimizes the risk of flap necrosis or loss. Once the surgeon is satisfied with the appearance of the penis, the skin edges are closed in two layers and a Tegaderm dressing is applied to minimize postoperative edema.

HYPOSPADIAS REPAIR

More than 300 hypospadias repairs have been described, and it has been estimated that at present about 100 are in use somewhere in the world. Obviously, selection of operation depends on the anatomy: meatus position and degree of chordee. Less obviously, personal preference is dictated by the postoperative appearance of the penis and the complication rate. In hypospadias repair, the major complication is a postoperative fistula, common enough that various repairs are often compared by quoting the fistula rate. Postoperative meatal stenosis is avoided by precisely approximating the end of the neourethra to the adjacent glandular skin, and urethral diverticula are rare after a uniform neourethra has been constructed. Strictures are uncommon but are still seen after tubularized flaps or grafts are anastomosed end to end to the native urethra. Such anastomoses should be oblique, as large in area as possible and watertight, and should probably be drained for a day or two with small suction drains.

To stent or not to stent is always the question in distal repairs, such as those using a meatus-based flap. I conclude that a stent does no harm. If the end is just inside the bladder neck, the drip tube keeps the bladder empty. If the child does not void, postoperative pain and discomfort are usually minimal. A stent also helps keep the Tegaderm dressing in place for at least a day, and this is important in preventing postoperative edema.

Glanuloplasty

When the meatus is on the ventral aspect of the glans, I seldom recommend trying to extend the urethra to the tip. On the other hand, when a dorsal hood is present,

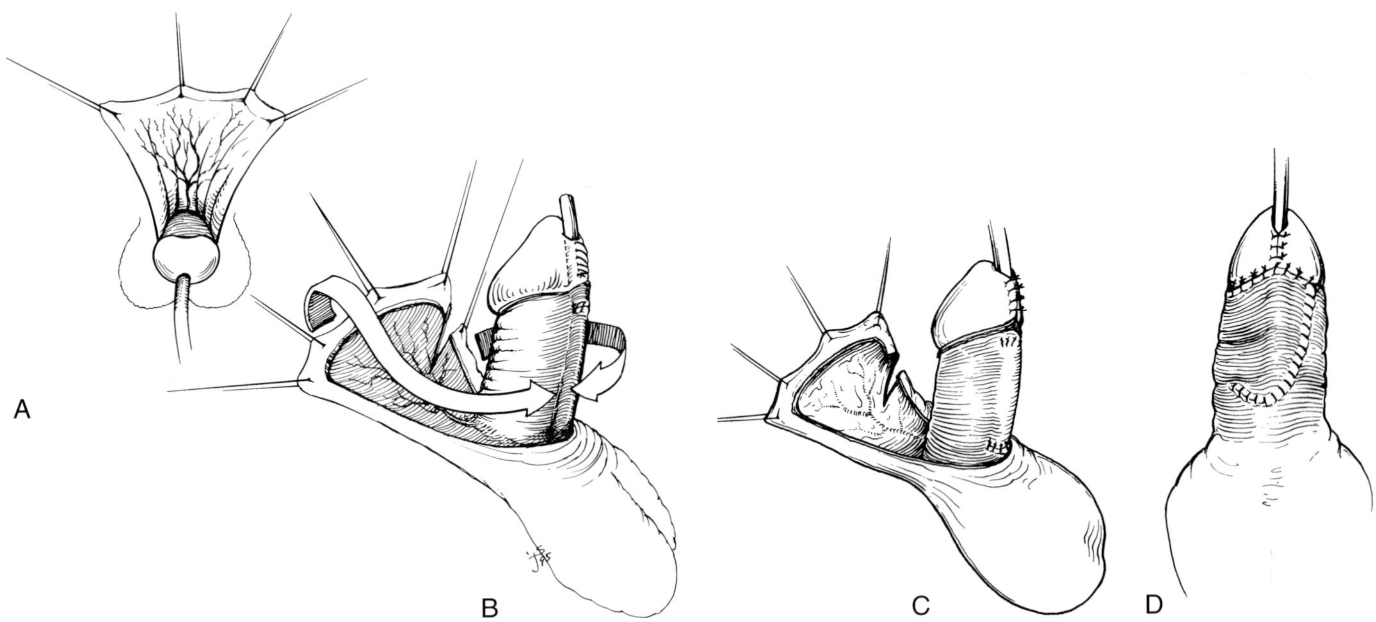

Figure 15–3 *A,* The dorsal hood is unrolled. Note that the veins coalese into a single large vein near the midline. *B,* The foreskin is divided asymmetrically so the major flap will have unimpaired venous drainage, and the foreskin is transposed *(C and D).*

with or without glandular tilt, these anomalies are quite noticeable and should be corrected. The Magpi repair is illustrated in Figure 15–4. If the meatus is very large, and the stream splatters, more of a nozzle effect should be achieved. If the foreskin is asymmetric, the penis is degloved and an artificial erection performed to assess the situation. To narrow the meatus, the tourniquet is left tightened and the inferior margin of the meatus is excised. The idea is to eliminate the epithelium between the urethra and the skin of the glans and expose some raw glandular tissue in between (Fig. 15–5). The bottom of the urethra is then closed with two or, preferably, three layers of absorbable sutures. A drip tube is inserted because urinary diversion improves the chance of healing without a fistula. Drip tubes are always sewn to the dorsal portion of the glans with two 2-0 silk sutures, one on each side. These prevent the tube from "sawing" against the glanuloplasty and pushing the edges apart. Drip tubes are generally left in place about 5 days. In infants, not yet toilet trained, the end of the tube drips into an outer diaper, which is always at least a little wet. The skin of the boy, wearing an inner diaper, remains dry.

Coronal Meatus

Patients with a coronal meatus usually require repair for cosmetic reasons. The foreskin is represented by a dorsal hood. The asymmetry that this alone produces is enough to warrant circumcision. Noticeable glandular tilt is often associated, and because an anesthetic is required it seems reasonable to move the meatus distally. The Horton-Devine glanuloplasty is illustrated in Figure 15–6.

In my view this is usually best done using a meatal-based flap, so the meatus can be brought to the tip of the glans and a nozzle effect achieved. A meatal-based flap can also be used when the meatus lies on the distal penile shaft and chordee can be corrected by degloving the penis with or without removal of a dorsal wedge. In this operation, described by Mathieu in 1932 and reinvented by Wacksman in 1981, a strip of skin and glans in the ventral midline is used for the back wall of the neourethra, and the ventrum and sides are formed from an apron of skin taken from the more proximal portion of the penis, which is left attached at the meatus.

The distance between the meatus and the tip of the penis is measured. A flap of this length is outlined below the meatus, which in boys 1 to 3 years of age is usually about 8 to 9 mm in width. The penis is degloved, leaving this flap attached to the meatus. Chordee is completely corrected. With the tourniquet in place, parallel incisions are made distal to the meatus, usually about 6 mm apart, and carried to the tip of the glans. The incisions are deepened through the proximal glans, making the sides of the glans mobile enough to close over the distal-most neourethra. The flap is then rotated distally and the free end aligned with the paired incisions in the glans. An interrupted suture is placed on each side and held, ascertaining that the meatus is symmetric. I prefer to anasto-

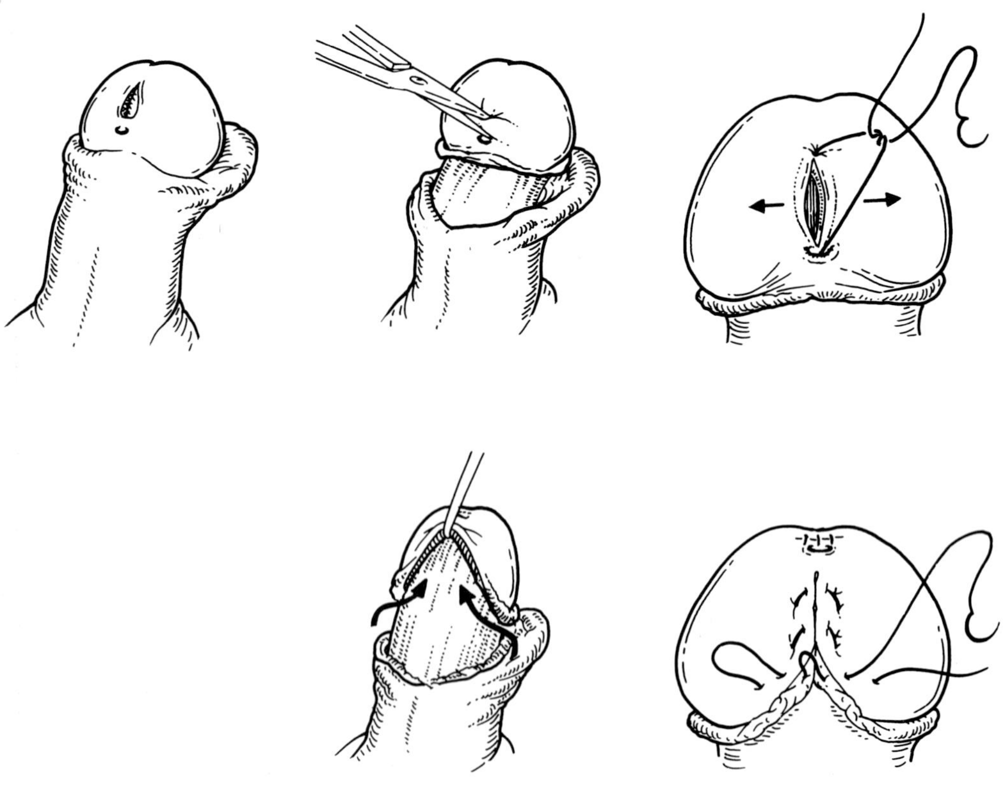

Figure 15–4 The Magpi procedure. A dorsal meatotomy connects the meatus and the groove in the glans. Three sutures are usually used to draw the back wall of the urethra distally. The edges of the glans are then approximated under the new meatus. The dorsal hood may be resected or transposed ventrally to provide needed skin to cover the ventral shaft.

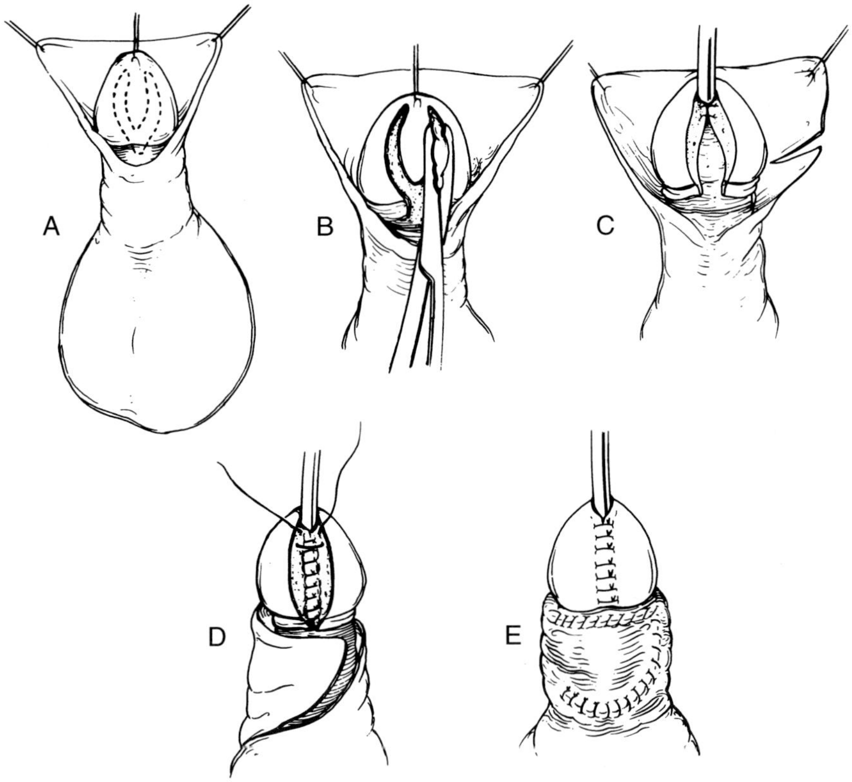

Figure 15–5 Technique of glanuloplasty when the meatus is large and near the corona. *A* and *B*, Edges of the groove in the glans are excised, outling the neourethra. *C*, The urethra is tubularized over a stent. *D*, After the urethra has been tubularized, the raw surfaces of the glans are approximated as an extra layer before the skin is closed.

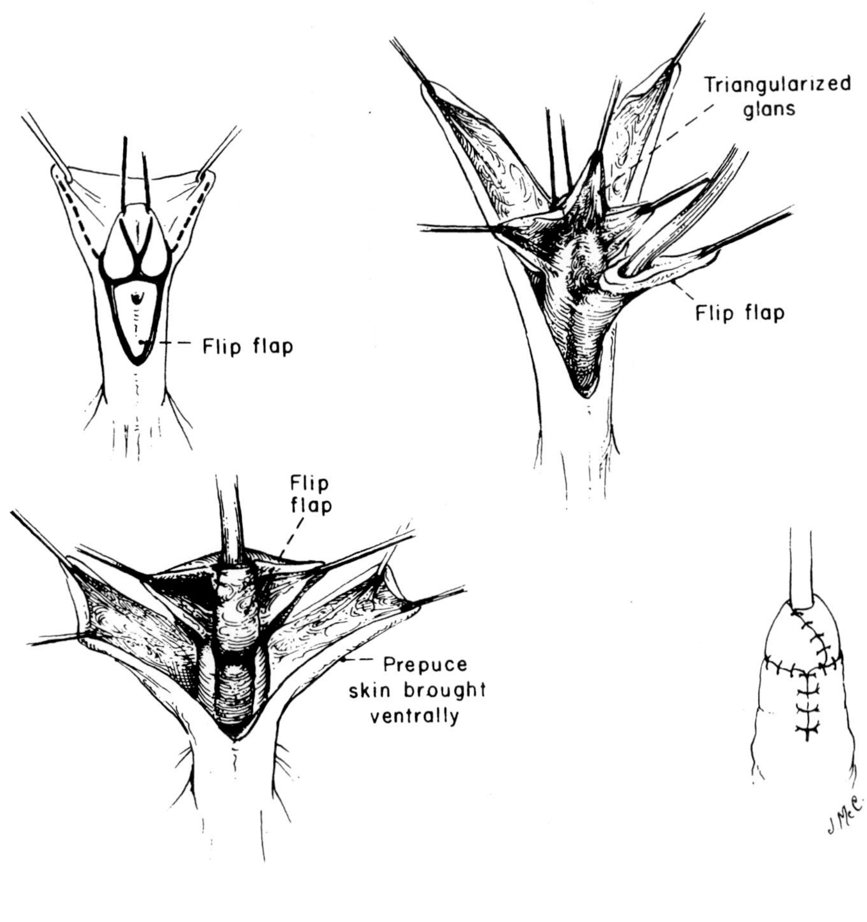

Figure 15–6 Horton and Devine's flip-flap repair for distal shaft hypospadias with or without distal chordee. From Hodgson NB. Hypospadias and urethral duplications. In Harrison JH, Gittes RF, Perlmutter AD, et al (eds), Campbell's Urology, 4th ed. Philadelphia: WB Saunders, 1978, used with permission.

mose the sides of the dorsal strip to the edge of the flap with running locked absorbable sutures, usually 5-0 chromic. A second layer is used to invert the suture line. After one side is closed, I usually insert the drip tube into the urethra and then complete the formation of the urethra. I prefer to use subcutaneous tissue attached to the outer layer of the flap for a third layer, sewn to the corpora with interrupted sutures whenever possible. Alternately, a flap of subcutaneous tissue from the proximal penile shaft may be developed and rotated distally to cover the neourethra (Fig. 15–7). Next, the glans flaps are sewn to the distal edge of the neourethra, walking these flaps around new meatus and obtaining good precise approximation there. The glans flaps are then approximated to each other below the neomeatus preferably in two layers. The glandular part of the procedure is completed by sewing the raw inside surface of the glans to the underlying corpora on either side of the urethra with an interrupted stitch to control bleeding. The tourniquet is then released. The drip tube is advanced into the bladder, and positioned just inside the bladder neck by irrigation if necessary, and sewn to the glans with 2-0 silk sutures.

The foreskin is then unrolled and transposed, usually using the van der Meulen technique. When extra foreskin is present the distal portion is excised. The flap is rotated until a pleasing appearance is achieved and skin edges are then approximated in two layers. At the corona an attempt is made to push some subcutaneous tissue forward under the glans closure and over the neourethra. If extra foreskin is present, some skin may be removed in this area, preserving the subcutaneous tissue, to buttress the closure of the outerlying skin (see Fig. 7).

A Tegaderm dressing is applied. The drip tube is left in place 4 to 6 days. The postoperative fistula rate is about 6% but as low as 1.3% in the best series.[6]

Onlay Hypospadias Repair

The onlay repair evolved when it became apparent that the thin mucosa-like skin on the ventral aspect of the penis could be preserved and tubularized to form the neourethra when chordee could be corrected by degloving the penis and, when necessary, removing a wedge from the dorsal corpora cavernosa.[7] Additionally, many have had trouble with stricture when fully tubularized transposed foreskin is anastomosed end to end to the native urethra. The onlay procedure is seen as a means of avoiding this increased risk of stricture in patients who would otherwise be candidates for a transverse island flap, in those in whom the meatus lies on the penis at midshaft or proximally, and in those in whom a reasonably long dorsal hood is present.

After the urethra is calibrated, the penis is degloved. A strip of ventral skin is left in place in the ventral midline between the meatus and the corona (Fig. 15–8).

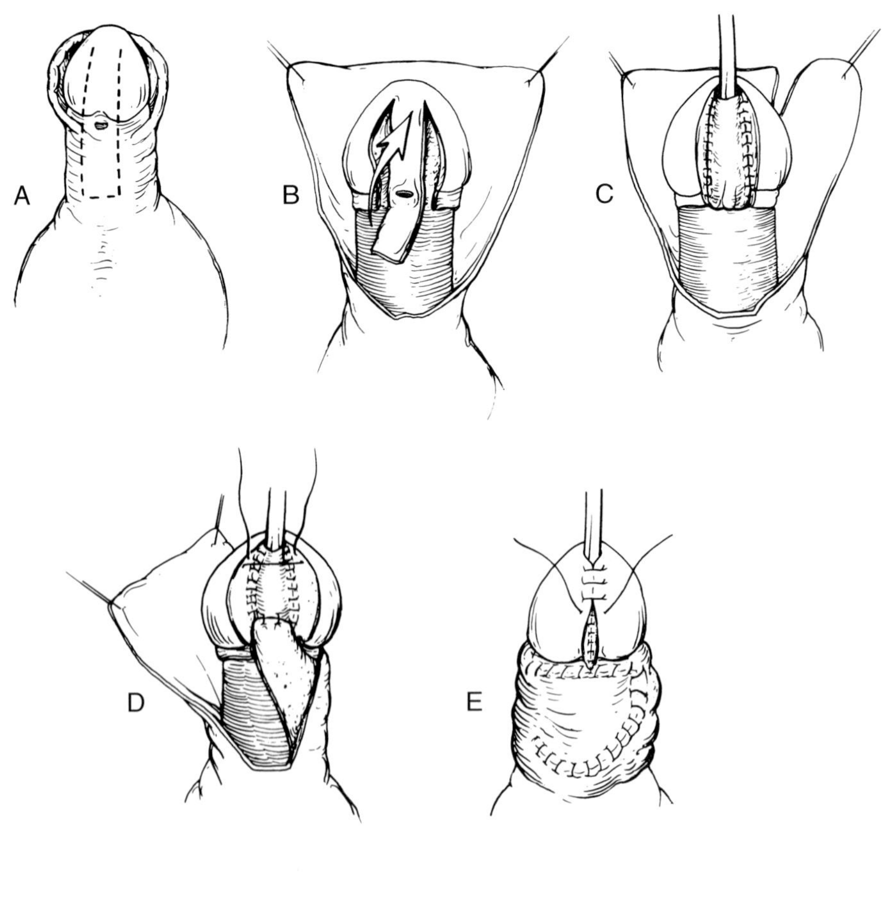

Figure 15–7 The meatal based flap is outlined (see text), and the edges of the neourethra are closed in two layers. The epithelium is removed from some of the excess distal foreskin, which is used to buttress the base of the flap *(D)*. The glanuloplasty is then completed and the dorsal hood is transposed.

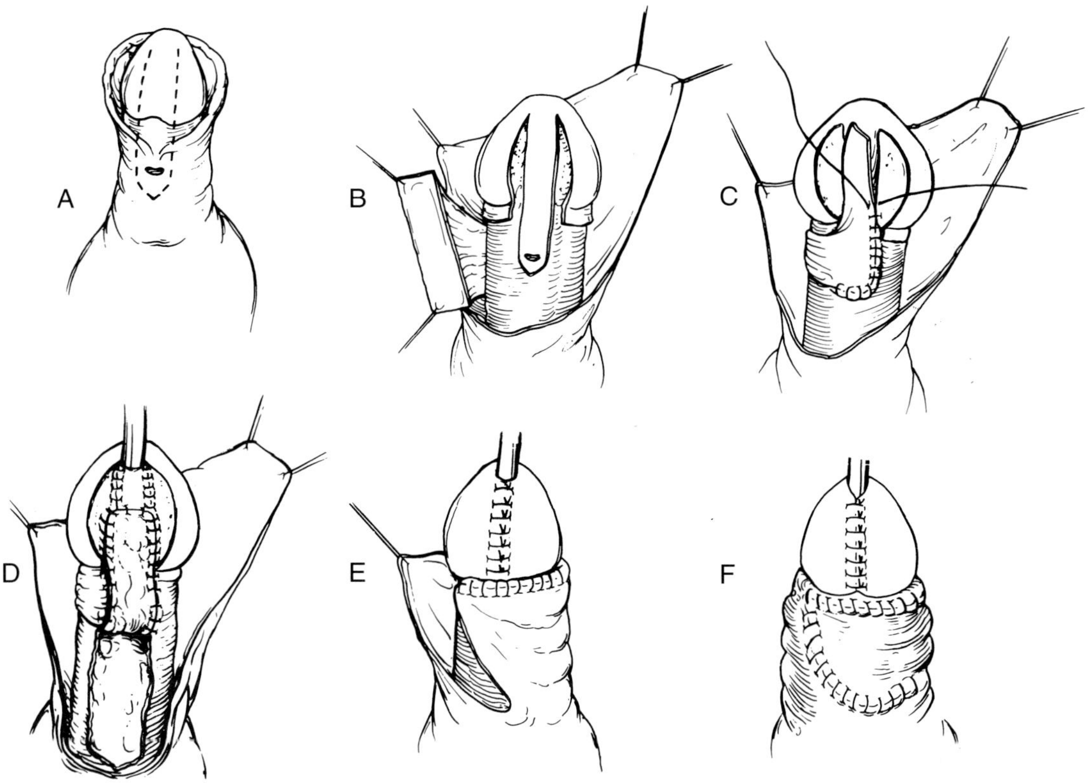

Figure 15–8 The onlay procedure (see text). In this instance, an extra layer of subcutaneous tissue is dissected away from the corpora proximally and is folded foreward (D) to cover the proximal portion of the repair.

Residual chordee and glandular tilt are corrected from behind. The rule is that when foreskin is in short supply it should be used to resurface the penis because nothing else has the appearance, texture, and innervation of penile skin. However, an onlay procedure needs only a small strip of distal-most unrolled dorsal hood tissue that is often discarded after the foreskin has been transposed.

The distance between the meatus and the tip of the erect penis is measured. Using stay sutures to manipulate the unrolled dorsal hood without trauma, a transverse strip is outlined across the distal edge. This strip should be approximately 1 cm wide at the medial end, which will become the glandular meatus, tapering to the point of a U at the lateral end. The flap is now separated from the foreskin, detaching the ends and then incising the skin only. The flap will have a separate blood supply, which is developed by separating the more proximal foreskin from the soft tissues beneath to a depth of perhaps 2 cm. The pedicle of the dorsal hood is inspected and a van der Meulen incision is made along the base of the foreskin on the wide side of the onlay flap. A suture is placed from corona to foreskin at the 12 o'clock position.

The penis is next retracted cranially and the tourniquet tightened around the base. The parallel skin incisions on the ventral aspect of the penis are extended onto the glans to the tip. The proximal glans flaps are mobilized by dissecting laterally above the corpora cavernosa. Considerable mobility of the glans is achieved in this way, allowing one to approximate the glans below the neomeatus. The onlay flap is aligned against the strip of ventral skin. Usually only one layer of running locking sutures is used to approximate the flap to the strip on the side from which the flap is based, because the pedicle of the onlay flap covers this side of the repair. A drip tube is inserted across the repair into the urethra. Two layers of running locking or horizontal mattress sutures are used on the exposed side of the neourethra. Additionally, interrupted sutures are used to bring available soft tissue over the suture line, especially at the proximal apex to buttress the closure as a third layer. Interrupted 5-0 chromic sutures are then used to obtain edge-to-edge approximation of the glans to the neomeatus and to walk the glans flaps medially. One or two small Vicryl sutures are used to approximate the raw edges of glandular tissue ventrally, and overlying chromic sutures are used to align the overlying edges precisely. Hemostatic sutures are placed between the underside of the glans and the corpora on either side of the neourethra. The tourniquet is released, and the drip tube is advanced into the bladder, positioned, and sutured to the glans.

Attention is now given to resurfacing the penis. A scrotal flap may be developed and rotated to provide skin

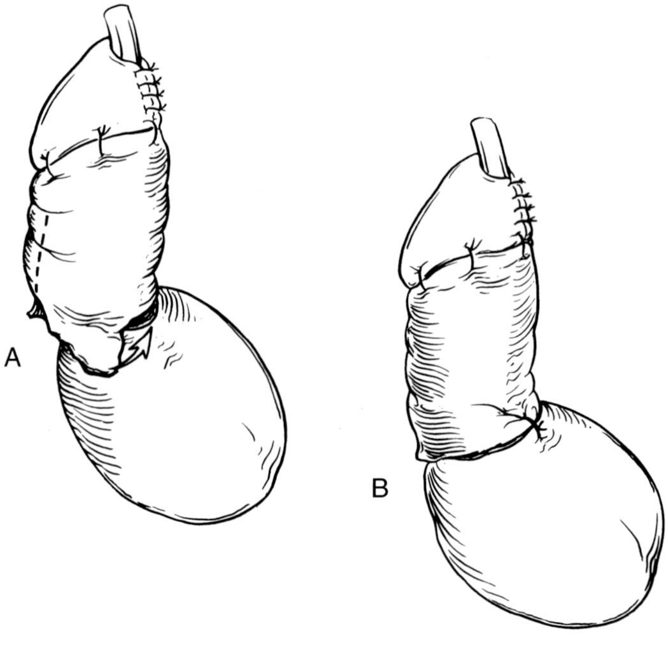

Figure 15–9 The unrolled dorsal hood is transposed with trial and error sutures but causes penile torsion. The base of the flap is then incised to permit the flap to rotate more freely (see text).

coverage at the penoscrotal junction. Such flaps look fine if they are perfectly symmetric. However, with an onlay, almost the entire dorsal hood is available for skin coverage, and scrotal flaps are seldom needed. They are discussed further as an adjunct to transverse island flap repairs.

The transposed dorsal hood is rotated toward the corona on the opposite side of the penis. Usually only the skin at the proximal base of the major flap needs to be incised transversely to permit adequate rotation to center the flap (Fig. 15–9). This skin incision may be as long as necessary to produce adequate skin mobility as long as the underlying pedicle is not disturbed. The skin edges are approximated in two layers, taking care to push some soft tissue under the glans over the neourethra. The position of the drip tube may be checked by irrigation. A Tegaderm dressing is applied.

When the Tegaderm dressing falls off or is removed, a topical antibiotic (Neosporin) is applied to the penis between diaper changes. The drip tube is usually maintained for 5 or 6 days.

Transverse Island Flap

The transverse island flap technique enables the neourethra to be formed entirely from the transposed distal dorsal hood.[8, 9] It is especially useful when the meatus is at or near the penoscrotal junction and the chordee is so severe that it is difficult to straighten the penis completely from behind after the penis is degloved, in other words, when the penile skin—the urethral "plate"—between the meatus and the corona needs to be divided to achieve a straight penis. The ventral penile skin should be saved and left attached at the corona because it may be used in forming the distal portion of the neourethra (Fig. 15–10). The most common mistake made in this operation is to use too much foreskin for the neourethra so that not enough transposable dorsal hood remains to resurface the ventral aspect of the penis. The urethral plate can also be used to cover the distal neourethra. However, skin is always in shortest supply at the penoscrotal junction, and a scrotal flap may be rotated distally to provide skin coverage there. A proximal scrotal flap looks fine when perfectly centered.

The incision is made around the corona. Ventrally, a strip of skin about 8 to 10 mm wide is left in place in the midline, as for an onlay repair. The incision is carried around the meatus proximally. The penis is degloved, and the scrotum is dissected off the urethra for a distance of about 2 cm. An artificial erection is performed. When the shaft can be straightened by one or two dorsal wedges (with or without correcting glandular tilt), an onlay repair is generally chosen if the unrolled dorsal hood is of sufficient width. To determine this, one must measure the distance between the meatus and the tip of the glans. If a strip of transposed foreskin can be used to form the floor of the neourethra, an onlay is generally chosen because it avoids the increased risk of urethral stricture often seen at the point where the tubularized island flap is anastomosed circumferentially to the native urethra.

When the penis does not straighten completely, the urethral plate is divided transversely just distal to the meatus. The skin is dissected off the underlying corpora. Scarlike tissue that lies over Buck's fascia needs to be excised or incised, often into the septum between the corpora. Further correction of corporal disproportion may be needed. If very extensive dissection is needed, the foreskin may be transposed and a staged repair per-

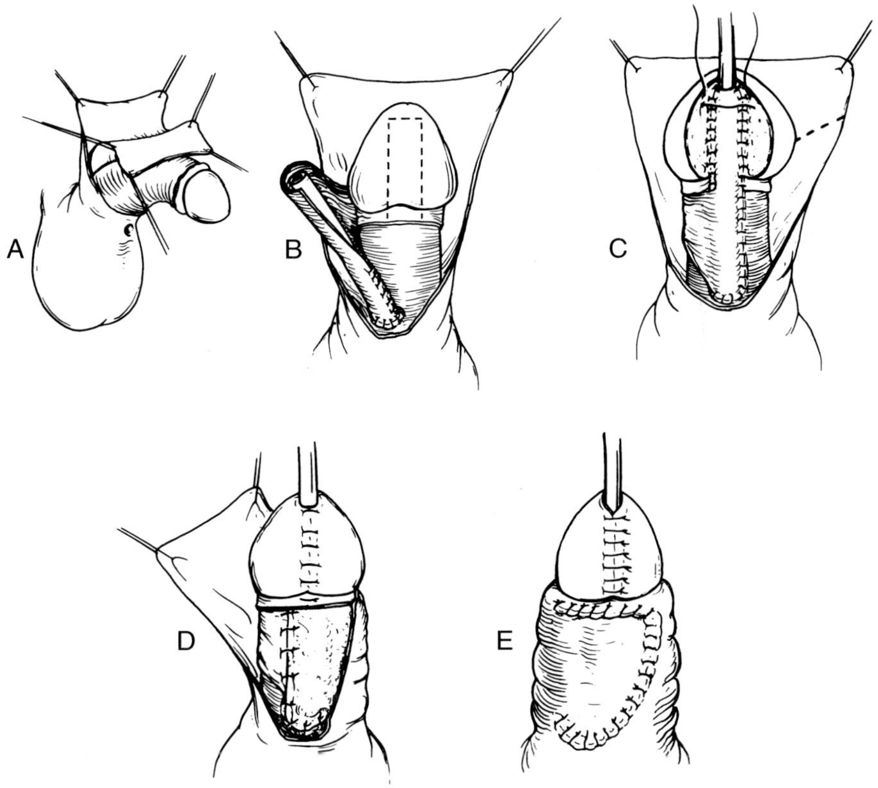

Figure 15–10 The combined transverse island flap and onlay repair (see text). Care must be taken to make a watertight urethral anastomosis, and the drip tube must be carefully positioned.

formed. In this situation, one must ensure that no transverse skinfolds are left in the ventral midline that would hamper subsequent tubularization of the ventral skin to form the urethra.

In most instances, however, one-stage repair can be performed. Enough tissue can be taken from the distal edge and sides of the unrolled dorsal hood to provide needed urethral length. The flap is outlined so that it is 5 mm longer than the distance between the meatus and the tip of the penis and 2 mm wider than the urethral caliber. The skin only is incised to begin to free the flap. Traction sutures are used liberally to minimize the need for pinching the flaps. The blood supply of the flap is separated from the more proximal foreskin by transverse incisions along the skin edge, a motion that is repeated until the vascular pedicle is defined to a depth of perhaps 2 cm. The foreskin is then transposed by making a skin incision from the base of the foreskin on one side to the base of the foreskin at the 12 o'clock position (van der Meulen) (Fig. 15–11). A suture is placed in the dorsal midline and the penis checked for torsion. The foreskin is then transposed ventrally where the island flap is tubularized over a drip tube with running, locking absorbable suture. Two layers are usually used. The suture line in the flap is oriented dorsally, and the proximal end is then anastomosed to the native urethra in precise fashion. This anastomosis should be oblique and as wide in area as possible. After the back of the anastomosis has been performed, the drip tube is advanced into the native urethra before the anastomosis is completed. Adjacent soft tissue should be drawn over the anastomosis with interrupted sutures whereever possible so that a watertight closure is achieved.

The easiest way to bring the distal end of the flap to the tip of the glans is usually to create a tunnel under the skin still attached at the corona and through the glans. A core of glans should be excised to prevent compression of the neourethra here. The tunnel should be larger in caliber than the neourethra (Fig. 15–12). The distal end of the drip tube is next drawn through the glandular tunnel. The distal end of the flap is then passed using traction sutures. The edges of the flap are then sewn to the edges of the glans in precise fashion to form the new meatus (Fig. 15–13). The remaining dorsal hood is then rotated over the neourethra and positioned with trial and error sutures until a pleasing result is achieved. The urethral plate can be used to cover the neourethra distally, or this skin may be excised and only the subcutaneous tissue preserved to provide an additional layer of coverage.

When the foreskin will not reach the penoscrotal junction without tension, a fistula is almost certain unless additional covering skin can be provided. This is obtained from the scrotum.[10] A curvilinear incision is made from the midline proximal margin of the existing incision across the base of the scrotum on one side. If only a little skin needs to be advanced, an inverted-V extension of the incision will allow scrotal skin to slide forward 1 to 1

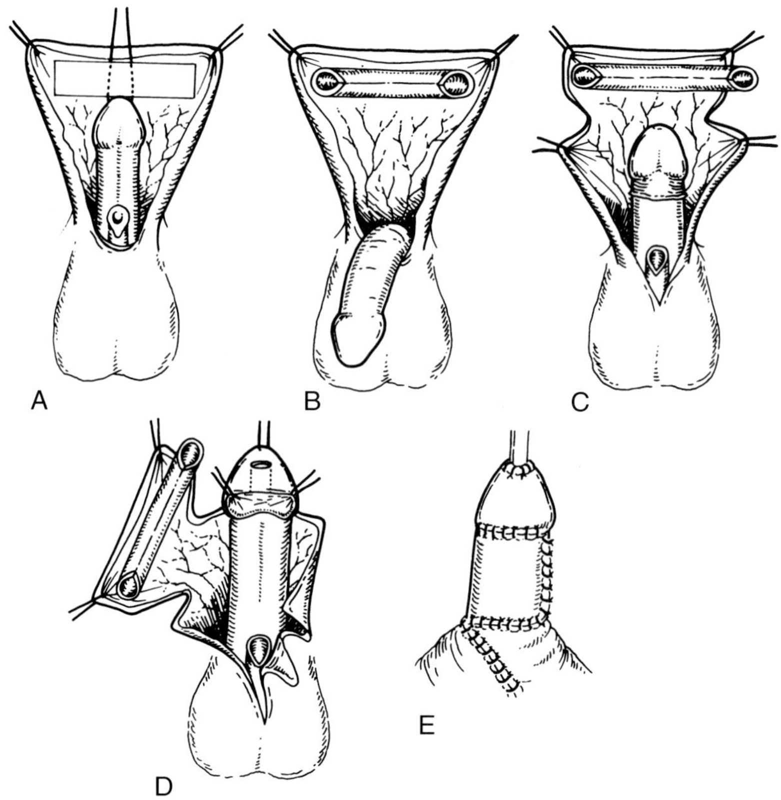

Figure 15–11 Asopa procedure as presently performed. *A,* After chordee correction, the inner layer of the prepuce is arranged as a rectangle placed transversely and is measured to the size of the urethral gap. *B,* The neourethral tube is formed with interrupted 5-0 chromic suture. *C,* The outer preputial skin is incised on both sides obliquely, leaving the central skin intact. *D,* A glans tunnel is created with scissors, and the flap is rotated around the right side. An oblique incision is then made at the penoscrotal junction on the left side. *E,* The end of the neourethra is anastomosed to the spatulated native urethra, and the distal end is brought through the glans channel and anastomosed to the opening in the glans. A Z plasty at the penoscrotal junction results in a transverse suture line at the penoscrotal area. The outer preputial skin is covering the ventral penis. From Webster GD, Kirby R, King LR, Goldwasser B (eds), Reconstructive Urology. Oxford, England: Blackwell Scientific, 1993. Used with permission.

1/2 cm. A rotational flap from one side of the scrotum is usually more secure. A flap of any length can be developed. The distal tip of the scrotal flap should be centered exactly in the midline. Sutures in several layers of scrotal tissue can be used to complete the closure over the proximal anastomosis. A small suction drain can be placed over the anastomosis, exiting through the scrotum. Such drains seldom drain, however, and may be unnecessary. The drip tube is carefully positioned and sewn to the glans. A Tegaderm dressing is placed on the penis, and a compression dressing is used to prevent scrotal edema and to immobilize the genitalia. If the compression dressing stays dry, it is left in place for 2 days. The Tegaderm dressing is removed in 4 to 6 days and the drip tube a few days later. If an obvious fistula has occurred, the drip tube can be removed sooner.

BLADDER AND BUCCAL MUCOSA GRAFTS

When penile skin is in short supply, it should be used to resurface the penis and the neourethra formed from a

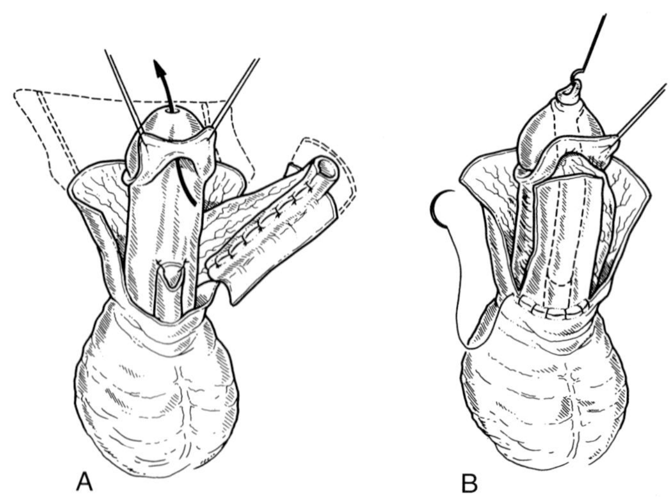

Figure 15–12 Double-faced island flap. *A,* The outer and inner preputial layers are mobilized together as an island flap. The inner layer is tubularized for the neourethra but remains completely attached to the pedicle. *B,* The urethra is channeled through the glans discarding some of the outer skin. The outer prepuce is then tailored to cover the ventral one third of the penis; the remaining penile skin covers the dorsal two thirds. From Webster GD, Kirby R, King LR, Goldwasser B (eds): Reconstruction Urology. Oxford, England: Blackwell Scientific, 1993. Used with permission.

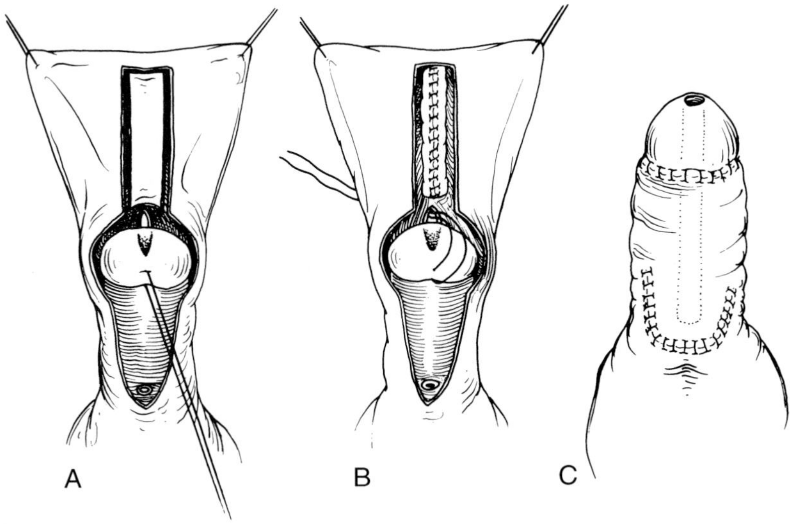

Figure 15–13 The Hodgson procedure in which the neourethra is formed from the inner foreskin and transposed as a bipedical flap. From Hodgson NB. Use of vascularized flaps in hypospadias repairs. Urol Clin North Am 8:471, 1981. Used with permission.

free graft. Split-thickness skin grafts generally contract over time, and full-thickness skin grafts from distant sites, such as the inner arm, tend to stricture. Bladder and buccal mucosa are the best tissues currently available.

Because most situations in which a free graft of non-penile skin is needed are for salvage procedures, the complication rate in reported series is generally high but is improving.[11, 12] Bladder mucosa brought to the skin at the meatus usually develops strictures repeatedly. However, tubularized bladder mucosa may be used to form the scrotal and penile portions of the neourethra when the distal-most urethra can be made from the urethral plate and glandular skin, as shown in Figure 15–14.

Buccal mucosal grafts may be used to form the entire urethra. For the graft, the subcutaneous tissue must be carefully removed because the buccal mucosa itself is relatively thick. The grafts are usually tubularized in two layers, and watertight anastomoses are important. Urinary diversion is especially important postoperatively and a suprapubic cystocatheter, as well as a drip tube in the urethra, is usually used. When feasible, the genitalia are immobilized for 3 to 4 days postoperatively before the compression dressing is removed, and urine diversion is maintained for a full 10 days.

FURTHER COMMENTS ON SURGICAL TECHNIQUE

As mentioned, it is always desirable to obtain an extra layer of tissue over the neourethra. Edges are generally closed in two layers. Additional subcutaneous tissue is

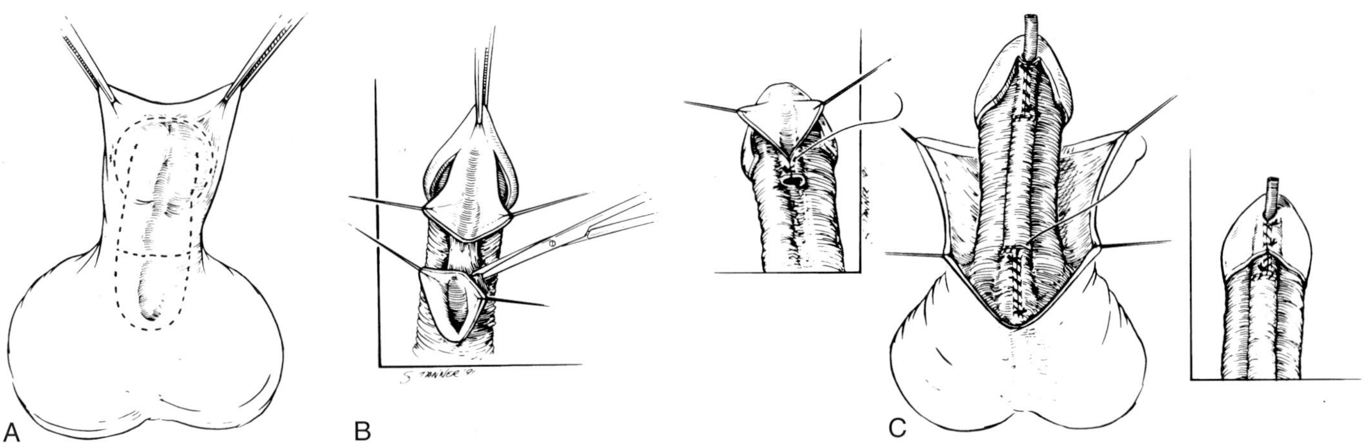

Figure 15–14 Severe hypospadias. *A* and *B*, The urethral plate is divided to permit chordee correction but left attached to the glans. *C*, The urethral plate and a strip of glans are tubularized to form the distal most neourethra, to which the tubularized graft of bladder mucosa is carefully anastomosed. The non–hair-bearing strip of skin between the two halves of the scrotum may be tubularized to form the proximal neourethra (see text).

then drawn over the neourethra whenever possible. At skin level, the Durham-Smith maneuver is valuable.[13] When a little extra skin is present, the epidermis only may be excised using repeated tangential longitudinal incisions. The denuded dermis can be sutured beneath the skin edge opposite, achieving a vest-over-pants–type closure.[14, 15]

Tunica vaginalis can be harvested from around one or both testes and transposed beneath the penoscrotal junction to cover the neourethra.[16] However, this tissue is tissue paper thin and filmy in preschool-age boys and is probably seldom of real help. Ehrlich, however, used tunica vaginalis in salvage hypospadias repair, usually in adolescents. When penile skin is lacking after chordee release, the tunica vaginalis is rotated over the denuded corpora. This serves as the vascular bed for a relatively thick, meshed, split-thickness skin graft. After healing is complete, the skin on the ventral penile shaft is tubularized and covered with the remaining tunica vaginalis. A meshed split-thickness graft is again placed over this to resurface the penis. Good results have been achieved in more than 20 patients.[17]

Chordee Without Hypospadias

This condition is usually diagnosed because, in most instances, the foreskin is present as a dorsal hood. The meatus is on the glans, but the penis is tethered ventrally and angulated when erect. Historically, chordee without hypospadias was confusing because, although at times the penis straightens after simple degloving, severe chordee may persist. It is now recognized that the residual chordee is due to congenital corporal disporportion.[18] The length of the corpora is greater dorsally than ventrally. This chordee is almost always best treated by removing a dorsal wedge or two and correcting glandular tilt. The urethra may need to be released from the underlying corpora but seldom needs to be divided. When the urethra is short and the penis does not straighten after dorsal wedges have been removed, the urethra must be divided. A transverse island flap is then interposed between the ends of the urethra. Alternately, the ends of the urethra may be placed on the skin after transposition of the dorsal hood, and the urethra reconstituted at a second operation by tubularizing the skin between.

Other Methods of Transposing the Dorsal Hood

I have emphasized the van der Meulen technique of foreskin transposition because, after a little practice, I find it the easiest way to achieve a pleasing cosmetic result. Alternative methods include those of Byars and Hodgson. In the Byars technique, the dorsal hood is unrolled and then divided in the midline to the base of the foreskin.[4] Care should be exercised to avoid major vessels near the base. A suture at the 12 o'clock position is placed, and the foreskin flaps are drawn around each side of the glans and interdigitated ventrally. As always, the flaps are repositioned until the penis looks good. Penile skin heals without much visible scar, but longitudinal suture lines are avoided to minimize the risk of recurrent chordee.

In the Hodgson transposition, a longitudinal buttonhole is made in the midline at the base of the unrolled dorsal hood. The penis is drawn through this. The foreskin is now on the ventral aspect of the penis. The buttonhole incision is deepened in the ventral midline until the foreskin will slide distally to the corona. The skin edges are then approximated in two layers. There is usually some excess foreskin laterally near the base of the penis that can be excised.

Dorsal Chordee

Dorsal chordee is an unusual congenital condition, probably related to epispadias, in which the glans and distal shaft are angulated upward on erection.[19] Treatment consists of degloving the penis and using artificial erection to identify the point of greatest curvature. Wedges of corpora are then removed ventrally on either side of the urethra, or the urethra may be mobilized to permit removal of a wedge from the 4 to the 8 o'clock position. Artificial erection is repeated to be sure that adequate tissue has been removed before closing the overlying skin and subcutaneous tissues.

Hemihypertrophy of the Corpora Cavernosa

Lateral disproportion in the corpora cavernosa is uncommon. In all but one reported case, the right corpora cavernosum was the larger.[20] Thus, the penis is angulated to the left on erection. Treatment consists of degloving the penis, performing an artificial erection, and removing wedges from the lateral aspect of the larger corpora. At least two wedges are generally needed, so these are usually taken just proximal and distal to the point of maximum curvature. I close the corpora with absorbable sutures, usually 3-0 chromic catgut, and have had no difficulties. The penis should be slightly overcorrected so that the glans is angulated about 20 degrees in the opposite direction if the penis is to remain straight after healing is complete.

Duplications of the Urethra

The dorsal channel is virtually always atretic even if orthotopic in position. Thus, repair consists of straightening the penis and then building a neourethra from the ventral meatus to the glans.[21] The dorsal channel is usually best excised. When the orifice is on or near the perineum, the repair is similar to that used for scrotal or perineal hypospadias.

Very Severe Hypospadias

When the meatus lies between the halves of a divided scrotum, chordee is usually severe in degree. All the maneuvers described previously may be needed to straighten the penis. A staged repair may be elected, using one or two strips of buccal mucosa to form the neourethra if inadequate penile skin is present.[22]

The skin in the midline between the divided scrotum is mucosa like and does not contain many hair follicles. It may be tubularized to bring the meatus to the penoscrotal junction. The repair may then be completed in one stage using the distal dorsal hood for an onlay repair or a transverse island flap when adequate skin is present. Alternately, a buccal graft may be used to form the neourethra, reserving the dorsal hood to resurface the penis. Compression dressings should be used, and urinary diversion should be maintained for 7 to 10 days until healing looks complete.

Complications

Failure of Glanuloplasty

The complication that is peculiar to modern hypospadias repair is for the glanuloplasty to unroll. This is usually due to the drip tube "sawing" through the ventral suture line in the glans. It is best prevented by securing the drip tube with sutures placed near the top of the glans on both sides of the midline and by removing the drip tube as soon as it is safe to do so.

Although one strives to place the meatus near the tip of the glans, reoperation is not always necessary. If the meatus is at the corona and the urinary stream is straight, the overall result may be quite satisfactory. This is usually so if the meatus is partially concealed by a role of transposed foreskin. On casual examination, the "dimple" in the glans then looks like the meatus.

Meatal advancement, when deemed necessary, is often most reliably accomplished using a meatus-based flap. The glans flaps can then be reapproximated in two layers over the reconstructed urethra. A drip tube is usually used postoperatively.

If using the skin beneath the meatus leaves a defect in covering skin, an inverted-V incision is made at the penoscrotal junction. The skin on the ventral penile shaft is undermined until it will slide forward to the corona. At least a two-layer skin closure must be made at the corona. The proximal incision may be closed longitudinally, because the urethra is intact in this region, or the scrotum may be advanced slightly.

Fistulas

Fistulas remain the most common complication of hypospadias repair. They occur roughly in proportion to the length of neourethra that is formed and reflect the amount of skin that is available to cover the neourethra. Fistulas are most common at the penoscrotal junction and in distal repairs near the corona. The urethra should be carefully calibrated to exclude a stricture, but a distal stricture is only occasionally the cause.

Treatment depends on the size and location of the fistula. Flaps are generally better than skin mobilization and side-to-side closure over the fistula site.[23, 24] A small fistula may be ligated. This is accomplished by circumscribing the fistula, dissecting it down to the urethra, and placing two chromic ties around the base of the fistula with fulguration of any visible skin above. The fistula site is then covered with a small flap so that the skin suture lines do not overlap the fistula. A stent may be omitted, but a Tegaderm dressing for a day or two is recommended.

Even tiny fistulas near the meatus cannot be closed without compromising the meatus. These are best dealt with by dividing the bridge of skin or glans between the fistula and the meatus and then reconstituting the distalmost urethra with a meatus-based flap and glanuloplasty. Conversely, proximal fistulas are often best closed by their excision. The urethra is closed in two layers and the overlying skin with as many layers as possible. An advanced scrotal flap is often a good solution when the fistula is at the penoscrotal junction and skin for local coverage is in short supply. A drip tube is usually used for 3 or 4 days.

Stricture

Urethral stricture are uncommon except when the neourethra is anastomosed end to end to the native meatus. Strictures are, therefore, best prevented by making such anastomoses as oblique and as large as possible and watertight. Successful treatment often depends on the age of the stricture. When the stricture is short and becomes manifest a year or more after the repair, it can often be successfully treated by direct-vision internal urethrotomy.[25] The stricture is incised in two to four places and intubated for a few days. Intermittent catheterization if tolerated can be done daily for 4 to 6 weeks to dilate the region as it heals.

Most strictures that become symptomatic within a few months after repair will be inflamed. An urethrotomy can be done, but the stricture usually recurs. It is often best to marsupialize the strictured portion of the urethra to allow the tissues to heal completely. The skin can be retubularized 4 to 6 months later with minimal chance of recurrence. The overlying skin is closed in several layers, and a drip tube or catheter is usually required for 5 or 6 days.

Diverticula

Diverticula have become uncommon after hypospadias repairs. When encountered, a distal stricture must be excluded. If the diverticulum is unsightly because it balloons with voiding or if it causes prolonged dribbling after urination, it should be excised. The penis is degloved. The diverticulum is thus exposed and is opened in the midline. Excess tissue is excised, leaving a posterior strip of proper width to be tubularized to reconstitute the urethra.

If, after opening the diverticulum, a distal stricture is found, the incision in the urethra is extended distally through the stricture. A flap is fashioned from the lateral wall of the diverticulum, which is rotated forward across the stricture to enhance the urethral caliber at that point. The remaining diverticulum is excised, and the urethra is closed in several layers. Catheter drainage or a drip tube is generally used postoperatively.

CONCLUSION

Hypospadias surgery requires creativity in design and precision in execution. The meatus is brought onto the glans in all modern techniques so after healing is complete the penis looks nearly normal. To prevent psychological damage during childhood, every attempt should be made to complete the repair by about 2 1/2 years of age, which is when boys begin to compare themselves with peers. Thus, the surgery should be done by 2 years of age so that if another operation is needed it can be accomplished 6 months later.

When the penis is small, 50 mg of testosterone can be given at 3-week intervals one to three times before the operation. This will stimulate early penile growth and cause some thickening of the penile skin, which facilitates the placement of an extra layer of skin sutures. Use of testosterone in infancy does not result in early cessation of penile growth or a phallus that is shorter than it would otherwise have been.[26]

Hypospadias surgery is demanding, but the surgeon is well rewarded when successful repair allows the boy to develop normally in every way.

REFERENCES

1. Berg G, Berg R. Castration complex: Evidence from men operated for hypospadias. Acta Psychiatr Scand 68:143, 1983.
2. Berg R, Berg G. Penile malformation, gender identify and sexual orientation. Acta Psychiatr Scand 68:154, 1983.
3. Livne PM, Gibbons MD, Gonzales ET Jr. Correction of disproportion of corpora cavernosa as cause of chordee in hypospadias. Urology 22:608, 1983.
4. Byars LT. A technique for consistently satisfactory repair of hypospadias. Surg Gynecol Obstet 100:184, 1955.
5. Van der Meulen JC. Correction of hypospadias. Br J Plast Surg 8:403, 1982.
6. Wacksman J, Sheldon C, King LR. Distal hypospadias repair. In Webster G, Kirby R, King L, Goldwasser B (eds), Reconstructive Urology. London: Blackwell Scientific, 1993, p 749.
7. Elder JS, Duckett JW, Snyder HM. Onlay island flap in the repair of mid and distal hypospadias without chordee. J Urol 138:376, 1987.
8. Asopa R, Asopa HS. One stage repair of hypospadias using double island preputial skin tube. Indian J Urol 1:42, 1984.
9. Duckett JW. The island flap technique for hypospadias repair. Urol Clin North Am 8:503, 1981.
10. Nonomura K, Koganagi T, Imanaka K, et al. One stage total repair of severe hypospadias with scrotal transposition: Experience in 18 cases. J Pediatr Surg 23:177, 1988.
11. King LR. Bladder mucosal grafts for severe hypospadias: A successful technique. J Urol 152:2338, 1994.
12. Dessanti A, Rigamont W, Merulla V, et al. Autologous buccal mucosa graft for hypospadias repair: Initial report. J Urol 147:1081, 1992.
13. Smith ED. Hypospadias. In Ashcraft KW (ed), Pediatric Urology. Philadelphia: WB Saunders, 1990, p. 353.
14. Belman AB. De-epithelialized skin flap coverage in hypospadias repair. J Urol 140:1273, 1988.
15. Retik AB, Mandell J, Bauer SB, Atala A. Meatal based hypospadias repair with use of a dorsal subcutaneous flap to prevent urethrocutaneous fistula. J Urol 152:1228, 1994.
16. Snow BW. Use of tunica vaginalis to prevent fistulas in hypospadias surgery. J Urol 136:861, 1986.
17. Ehrlich RM, Alter G. The versatility of tunica vaginalis flaps and mesh graft urethroplasty in hypospadias and stricture cripples. Paper presented at the meeting of the American Academy of Pediatrics, Section on Urology, San Francisco, October 1995.
18. Hurwitz RS, Ozersky D, Kaplan HJ. Chordee without hypospadias: Complications and management of hypoplastic urethra. J Urol 138:372, 1987.
19. Redman JF. Dorsal curvature of penis. Urology 21:479, 1983.
20. Udall DA. Correction of 3 types of congenital curvatures of the penis including the first reported case of dorsal curvature. J Urol 124:50, 1980.
21. Woodhouse CRJ, Williams DI. Duplications of the lower urinary tract in children. Br J Urol 51:481, 1979.
22. Retik AB, Bauer SB, Mandell J, et al. Management of severe hypospadias with a 2-stage repair. J Urol 152:749, 1994.
23. Walker RD. Outpatient repair of urethral fistulae. Urol Clin North Am 8:582, 1981.
24. Geltzeiler J, Belman AB. Results of closure of urethral cutaneous fistulae in children. J Urol 132:734, 1984.
25. Devine CJ Jr, Jordan GH. Strictures of the anterior urethra. AUA Update Series 2:202, 1990.
26. Levy JB, Zimmerman D, Hysmann DA. Does early androgen excess in patients with congenital advanced hyperplasia affect eventual penile size? Paper presented at the meeting of the American Academy of Pediatrics Section on Urology, San Francisco, October 1995.

LAURENCE S. BASKIN & BARRY A. KOGAN

16

Urethral Anomalies and Obstruction

POSTERIOR URETHRAL VALVES

Congenital urethral obstruction secondary to posterior urethral valves develops early in the second trimester after the remainder of the urinary tract has differentiated. The urinary tract above the congenital obstruction is subjected to abnormally high intraluminal pressures. This results in damage to the posterior urethra, the bladder, the ureters, and the kidneys. The degree of obstruction can affect each part of the urinary tract variably, resulting in the wide clinical presentation of patients with posterior urethral valves. Obstruction from the posterior urethral valve hinders the normal delivery of urine, which is required for amniotic fluid homeostasis also. In severe cases of obstruction, the lack of voided urine into the amniotic cavity can lead to oligohydramnios, which in turn can result in pulmonary hypoplasia. Renal development may be impaired and tubular injury can lead to inadequate concentrating ability. Bladder injury may result from increased pressures, leading to decreased compliance, reduced storage capacity, and abnormal bladder function, sometimes resulting in urinary incontinence.

The most common obstructing posterior urethral valve was classified by Hugh Hampton Young as type I (Fig. 16–1*A*). These can be described as a pair of leaflets passing downward and laterally from the lower border of the verumontanum (Fig. 16–1*B*) and extending around the membranous urethra to fuse anteriorly at the 12 o'clock position. Typically, the valvular leaflets are separated by a slitlike opening. Type III posterior urethral valves, which are relatively rare, are a congenital urethral membrane with a pinhole opening, typically lying below the level of the verumontanum. More recently, endoscopic inspection of posterior urethral valves before any other urethral instrumentation has visualized a filmy membrane.[1] It is hypothesized that this membrane is converted to what is known as a type I posterior urethral valve by urethral catheterization.

The embryologic explanation of posterior urethral valves has not been settled, but the most reasonable hypothesis is that the valve arises from the inferior cristal folds from the urethrovaginal folds of the urogenital sinus.[2] In the female, these structures form the anterior half of the hymenal ring. Therefore, the valvular folds in boys are analogous to an imperforate hymen in girls. Posterior urethral valves form when the ventrolateral folds of the urogenital sinus fail to regress. This process, which occurs later in embryogenesis, is to be contrasted with the presumed transient urethral obstruction occurring in the first trimester that results in prune-belly syndrome.

Diagnosis

With the advent of prenatal ultrasonography, posterior urethral valves are now most commonly diagnosed in utero. The sonographic interface between urine and tissue makes visualization of a dilated bladder, as well as hydroureteronephrosis, quite evident on routine prenatal screening ultrasonography. The high pressure created by the bladder in response to the posterior urethral valve may lead to different clinical manifestations of the disease, depending on which part of the urinary tract is affected most severely. For example, the pressure may be transmitted mostly to the bladder, resulting in a bladder diverticulum and sparing the upper tracts (Fig. 16–2*A*). Similarly, in other cases, only one ureteral orifice may be incompetent, leading to severe vesicoureteral reflux and renal dysplasia (VURD syndrome), while leaving the contralateral kidney and ureter essentially intact (Fig. 16–2*B*). Finally, the urinary tract may be spared severe injury if the patient presents with a urinoma resulting from a urinary leak from the renal sinus that may be contained in the renal capsule as a subcapsular urinoma or may rupture into the perirenal space, leading to a perirenal urinoma and subsequently urinary ascites (Fig. 16–2*C*). Once the diagnosis of posterior urethral valves is suspected, all aspects of the urinary tract should be evaluated.

Presenting Symptoms and Signs

Posterior urethral valves are now the third most commonly diagnosed urologic disorder in utero after possible

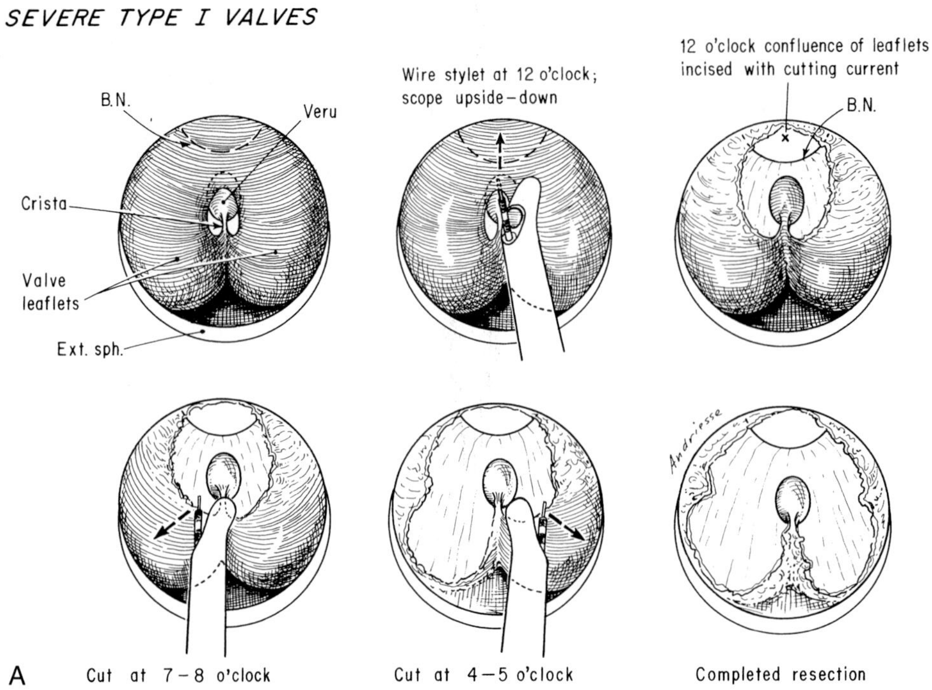

Figure 16–1 *A,* Schematic of type I posterior urethral valves demonstrating ablation with a wire stylet and ureteral catheter. (B.N., bladder neck; Ext. sph., external sphincter.) From Hendren WH. Urethral valves. In Ashcraft KW, Holder TM (eds), Pediatric Surgery, 2nd ed. Philadelphia: WB Saunders, 1993. Used with permission.

ureteropelvic junction obstruction and megaloureter. Typical antenatal findings are bilateral hydronephrosis and an enlarged bladder. Sometimes a classic "keyhole" finding showing the dilated posterior urethra is seen on ultrasonography. The prenatal diagnosis of possible posterior urethral valves should prompt a voiding cystourethrogram (VCUG) at birth. The differential diagnosis also includes prune-belly syndrome, high-grade vesicoureteral reflux, and urethral atresia. If the diagnosis is not suspected prenatally, neonates may present with respiratory distress from pulmonary hypoplasia, the result of reduced amniotic fluid. Newborns may have delayed voiding of longer than 24 hours, with a physical examination revealing a palpably distended bladder or abdominal distention resulting from ascites. Neonates may also void with a poor stream or dribbling, or "overflow" voiding, which should prompt an evaluation with ultrasonography and VCUG. The other classic presentation in the neonatal period is urinary tract infection and sepsis. Those patients with posterior urethral valves who remain uninfected may have excessive thirst and polyuria or may present with failure to thrive or dehydration.

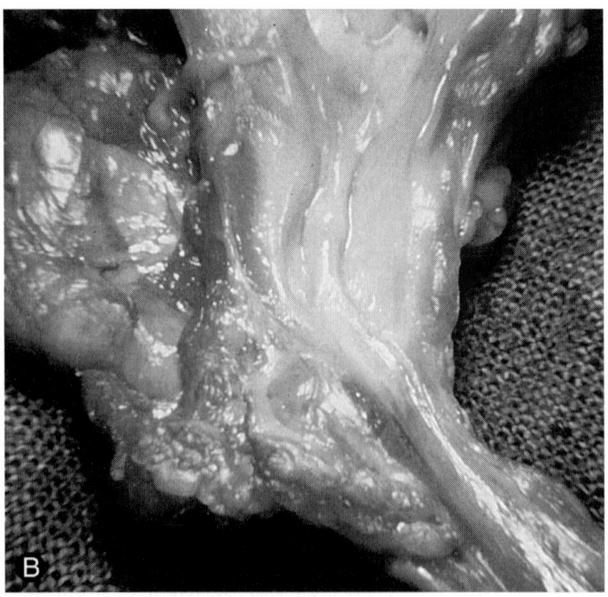

Figure 16–1 *Continued* *B,* Autopsy specimen of type 1 posterior urethral valves.

Older children with milder obstruction may present with delayed continence or even nocturnal enuresis. Patients also experience excessive thirst, polydipsia, or hematuria from mild trauma. Diagnosis in all age groups is confirmed by a VCUG and renal ultrasonography to evaluate the upper tracts.

Treatment (Fig. 16–3)

Once the diagnosis is confirmed by VCUG, continuous drainage is usually instituted with an 8 French (or in very

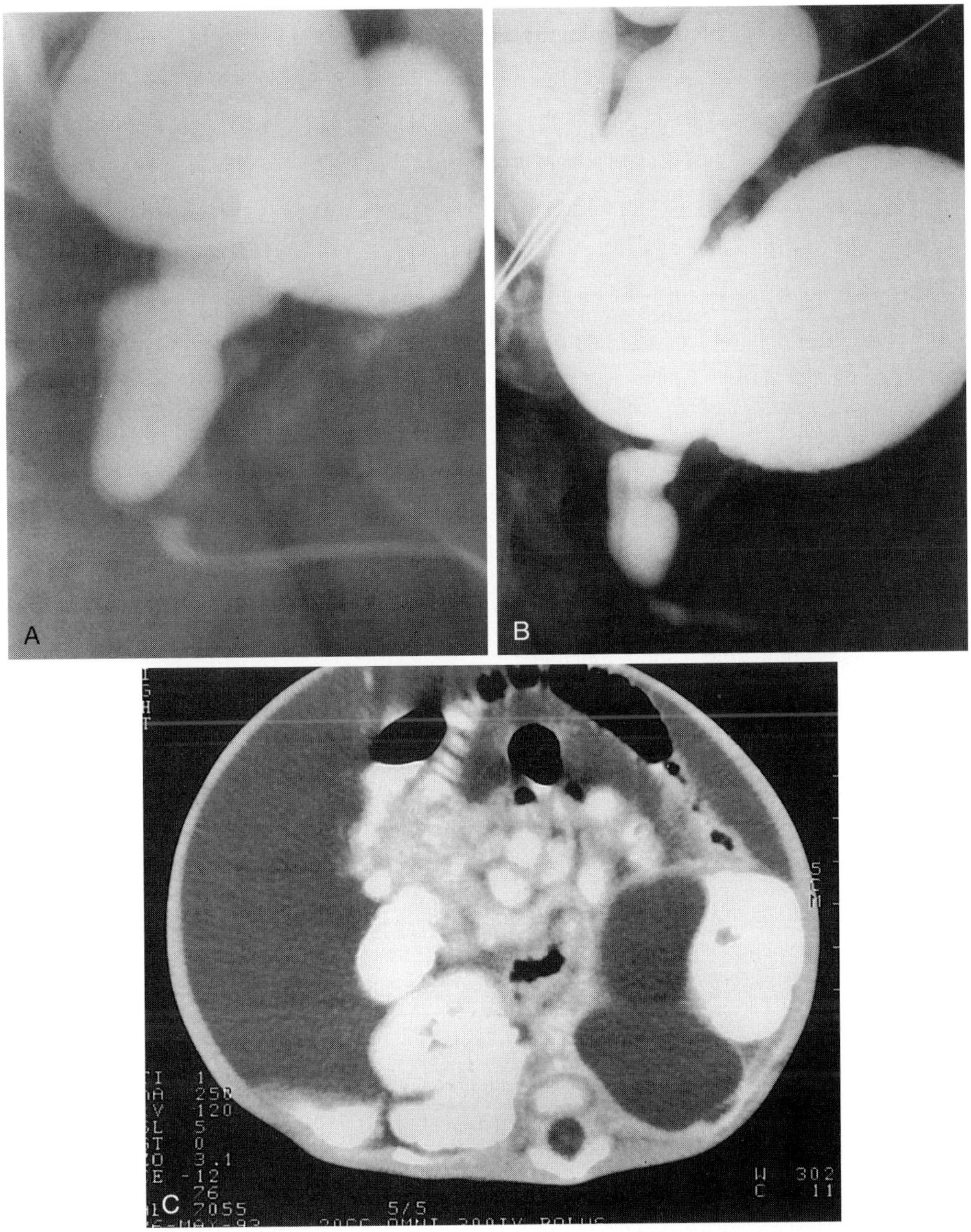

Figure 16–2 *A,* Voiding cystourethrogram: classic dilated posterior urethral and "pop-off" bladder diverticulum. *B,* Voiding cystourethrogram: classic dilated posterior urethral and "pop-off" unilateral vesicoureteral reflux. *C,* Computed tomographic scan of the abdomen: Massive urinary ascites secondary to a renal sinus leak from posterior urethral valves. Note that the kidneys are well preserved.

small infants, a 5 French) feeding tube. The catheter can be passed through the valve easily in retrograde direction, although at times the catheter may become misdirected in the dilated posterior urethra. With patience, it usually can be maneuvered through the bladder neck. However, in difficult cases a stiffer or coudé catheter will aid in passing the catheter into the bladder. Balloon-type catheters should be avoided because their intraluminal diameter tends to be much smaller than that of feeding tubes, resulting in poor drainage. In addition, spasms from the balloon may cause ureteral obstruction, preventing adequate upper tract drainage. Although catheter treatment is not associated with any urethral injury or strictures, it does allow the urinary tract to become colonized; in some cases of mild valves in a healthy child, it is reasonable to proceed to definitive treatment without prior drainage.

When it is impossible to catheterize an ill neonate, a suprapubic cystostomy may be considered; this can be

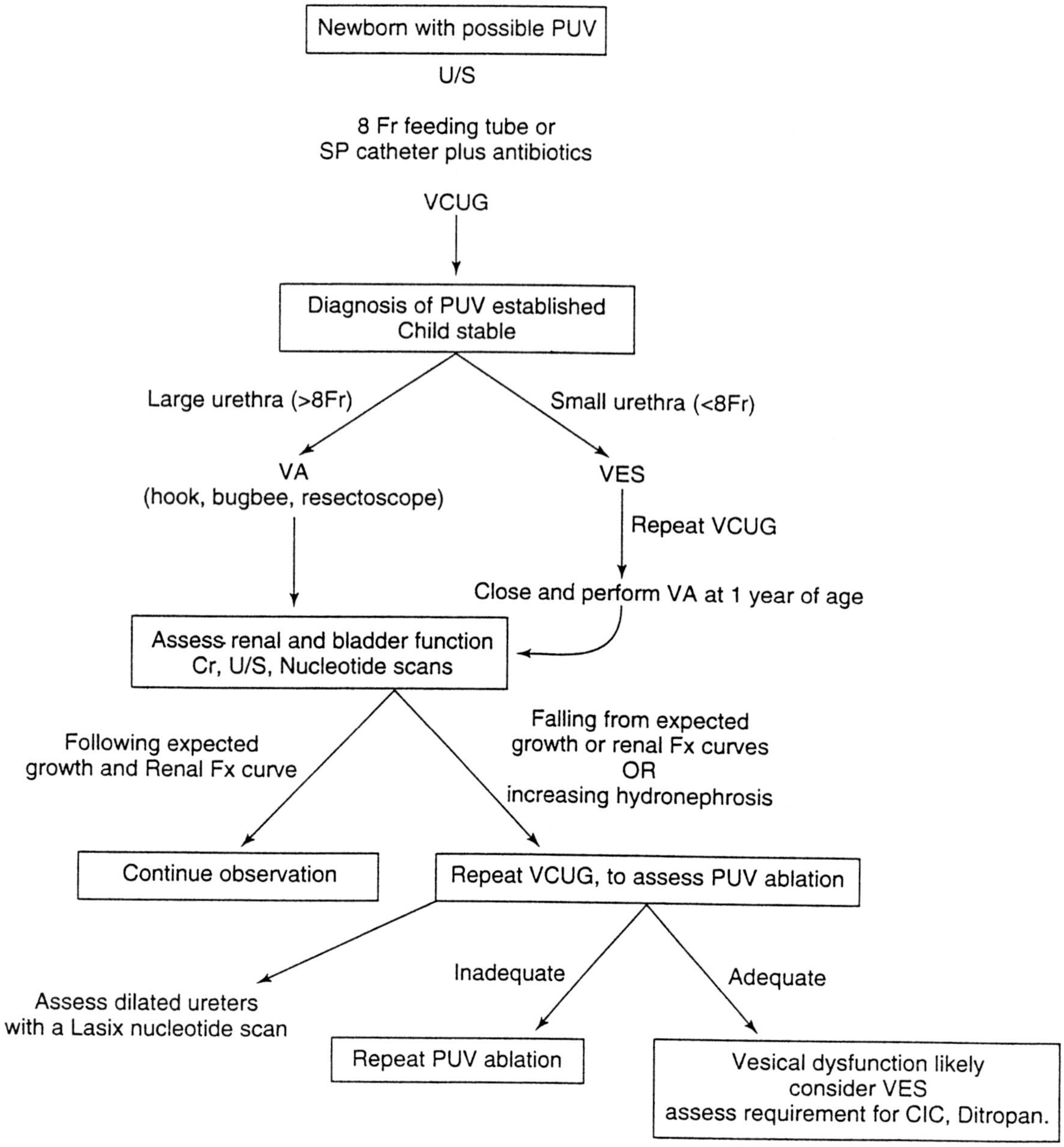

Figure 16–3 Treatment algorithm for posterior urethral valves (PUV). (U/S, ultrasound; SP, suprapubic; Fr, French; VCUG, voiding cystourethrogram; VA, valve ablation; VES, vesicostomy; Cr, creatinine; Fx, function; CIC, clean intermittent catheterization.) From Smith GH, Duckett JW. In Gillenwater JY (ed), Adult and Pediatric Urology, 3rd ed. St. Louis, MO: CV Mosby, 1996. Used with permission.

done percutaneously at the bedside in the very small infant. However, positioning of these catheters is often tenuous owing to problems with catheter fixation and the thick-walled and spastic nature of valve bladders. Hence, in a very ill infant, consideration should be given to a bedside cystostomy, which can be performed using local anesthesia.

Occasionally, anticholinergics (e.g., oxybutynin, 0.1 mg/kg three times daily) are helpful in decreasing bladder spasms when prolonged catheter drainage is needed. Bladder drainage should be followed by aggressive medical management to correct any electrolyte abnormalities and to clear infection in the case of sepsis. However, antibiotic usage should be kept to a minimum to prevent resistant organisms and fungal infections, seen particularly in neonates with stasis and catheters. A definitive operative procedure should be planned as soon as the patient is healthy enough for a general or spinal anesthetic.

Primary Valve Ablation

Primary valve ablation is usually performed endoscopically. The technique begins with calibration of the urethra.

In the past, the urethra needed to be able to accommodate an 8 French cystoscope, from which the valves could be fulgurated using a Bugbee electrode, either alongside the cystoscope or through the port. The quality of pediatric endoscopes and their miniaturization has improved, and we now routinely use a 6.9 French ureteroscope that has both a 2 and a 3 French channel enabling valve resection in smaller patients. Nonetheless, it must be emphasized that if there is any hint that the urethra is too small to adequately accept the endoscope, we would opt for an alternative, generally a primary vesicostomy. This is done on occasion in very small, premature infants, in septic infants, or in settings in which the appropriate endoscopic equipment is not available.

When viewed from the bulbous urethra, the type I posterior urethral valve leaflets come off on either side of the verumontanum (Fig. 16–4*A*–*I*). They fuse anteriorly, although this is sometimes hard to appreciate, and a significant portion of the valve is on the roof of the urethra. We first approach the valves at the 12 o'clock position using either the Bugbee electrode or, if the urethra is of adequate size, a 9.5 French resectoscope and a right-angle hook electrode. The electrode that we use has been modified by cutting off a part of the tip so that it does not protrude too far beyond the insulating sheath (the normal-sized electrode is too large for the newborn). Cutting current is used to minimize any spread into the surrounding tissue. After destroying the anterior portion of the valve at the 12 o'clock position, attention is then turned to the lateral cusps, which are easily engaged by the right-angle electrode and disrupted. When the small uretero- or cystoscope is used, the same principle is applied using a Bugbee electrode with the cutting current. No attempt is made to resect or fulgurate the bladder neck because this is not a cause of obstruction, and injury to the bladder neck may lead to incontinence. When the anatomy is visualized well, the external sphincter is untouched. If there is difficulty using the Bugbee electrode, we have also used a 3 French whistle-tip ureteral catheter with the tip cut off, attaching the cautery to the wire stylet that accompanies the catheter. The catheter itself provides the insulating sheath. By advancing the stylet just past the end of the catheter, accurate pinpoint cautery can be obtained in the same fashion as with the resectoscope.

Historically, when the urethra was too small to accept a cystoscope, perineal urethrostomy was a viable alternative, but in recent years we have gone directly to vesicostomy. Alternative techniques of valve ablation such as the Whitaker diathermy hook under fluoroscopic guidance have been described.[3] The Whitaker hook is no longer manufactured, but a similar technique using a Kohl knife valvulotome under endoscopic or fluoroscopic guidance has also been effective. Techniques for ablating valves from above should also be noted for completeness, particularly for definitive treatment after vesicostomy. However, with modern endoscopic equipment, we have been successful with retrograde primary valve ablation in patients with urethras of adequate caliber.

Vesicostomy

In premature infants with small-caliber urethras, temporary cutaneous vesicostomy has been very useful.[4] A 2-cm transverse incision is made halfway between the umbilicus and the pubis. The urachus is dissected using an extraperitoneal approach with the bladder filled (Fig. 16–5*A*). The dome of the bladder is identified and delivered into the wound with traction sutures and the cutaneous-vesical anastomosis is then created. To prevent subsequent prolapse, the fistula should be about 24 French and the most superior portion of the bladder should be used. With a proper vesicostomy, the bladder continues to cycle with voiding at low pressures through the stoma (Fig. 16–5*B*). Vesicostomy should be differentiated from continuous suprapubic cystostomy drainage, which is associated with infection, inflammation, and functional obstruction at the ureterovesical junction (refer to Hinman's *Atlas of Pediatric Urologic Surgery,* Chapter 71, for operative illustrations).

High Diversion

After adequate valve ablation or temporary cystostomy, there is generally a prompt improvement in serum creatinine.[5] When this fails to occur, we consider a high diversion. Typically, this has been after 4 to 6 weeks of observation, although others intervene earlier. High diversion, however, rarely has a significant effect on renal function and often creates a reconstructive nightmare. Many of these infants experience renal insufficiency and require peritoneal dialysis; with two draining flank stomas, this becomes even more complex. There is often massive bilateral reflux, which will eventually require both upper and lower ureteral surgery, and long-term bladder function in patients after high diversion may be very poor. Hence, our current preferred alternative to high diversion is temporary percutaneous nephrostomy to determine whether renal function will improve. If so, a high diversion may well be beneficial. If not, the nephrostomies may be removed and the reconstructive procedures averted. If ureterostomies are performed, consideration should be given to reconstruction within several months.[5]

Vesicoureteral Reflux

Vesicoureteral reflux is present in 50% of patients when they are diagnosed with posterior urethral valves.[6] Of these patients, 40% will have vesicoureteral reflux and unilateral dysplasia (VURD syndrome; see later discussion). When reflux is present, these boys should be maintained on prophylactic antibiotics, and a circumcision is

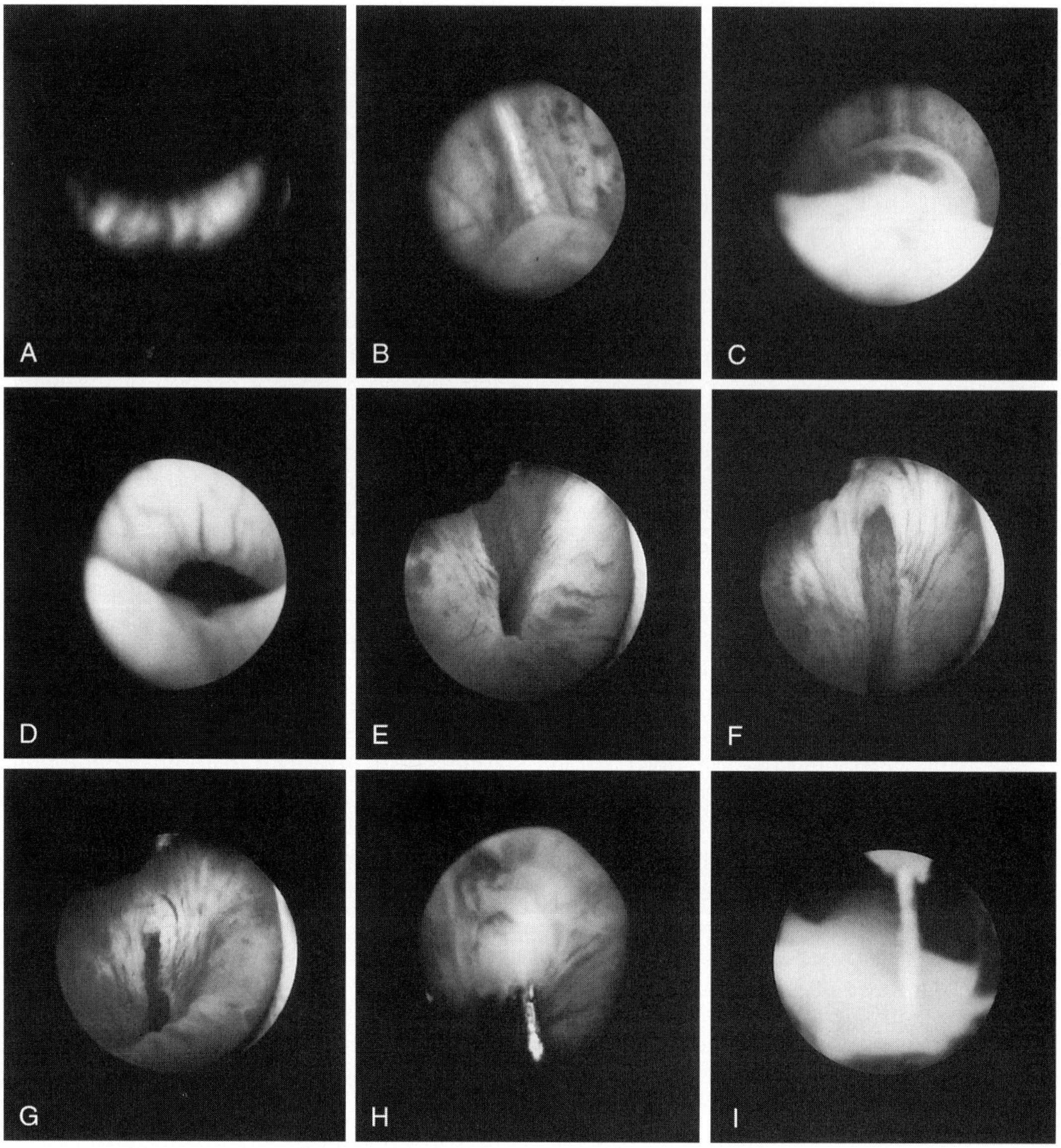

Figure 16–4 Serial endoscopic photographs of the proximal urethra in a patient with posterior urethral valves. The endoscope is being advanced distally through the urethra. *A,* View of the bladder neck and the bladder lumen in distance. *B,* Verumontanum in foreground with nonobstructing type II valves extending proximally in the posterior urethra. *C,* The valve leaflets are first seen attaching on either side of the verumontanum. *D,* The leaflets extend further distally. *E,* Moving toward the bulbous urethra, the leaflets begin to extend anteriorly, and *(F)* fuse in the 12 o'clock position. *G,* For the bulbous urethra, it is appreciated that a large portion of the "valves" is the anterior fused portion. *H,* A right-angle electrode is placed proximal to the anterior portion of the valve and pulled toward the scope. This portion of the valve is often very fibrous. *I,* The same electrode is seen behind the valve cusp at the 5 o'clock position. This portion of the valve is most likely thin. *A–G* courtesy of J. H. Johnston. *H* and *I* From Kogan BA. Treatment options for posterior urethral valves in neonates. In King LR (ed), Urological Surgery in Neonates and Young Infants. Philadelphia: WB Saunders, 1988. Used with permission.

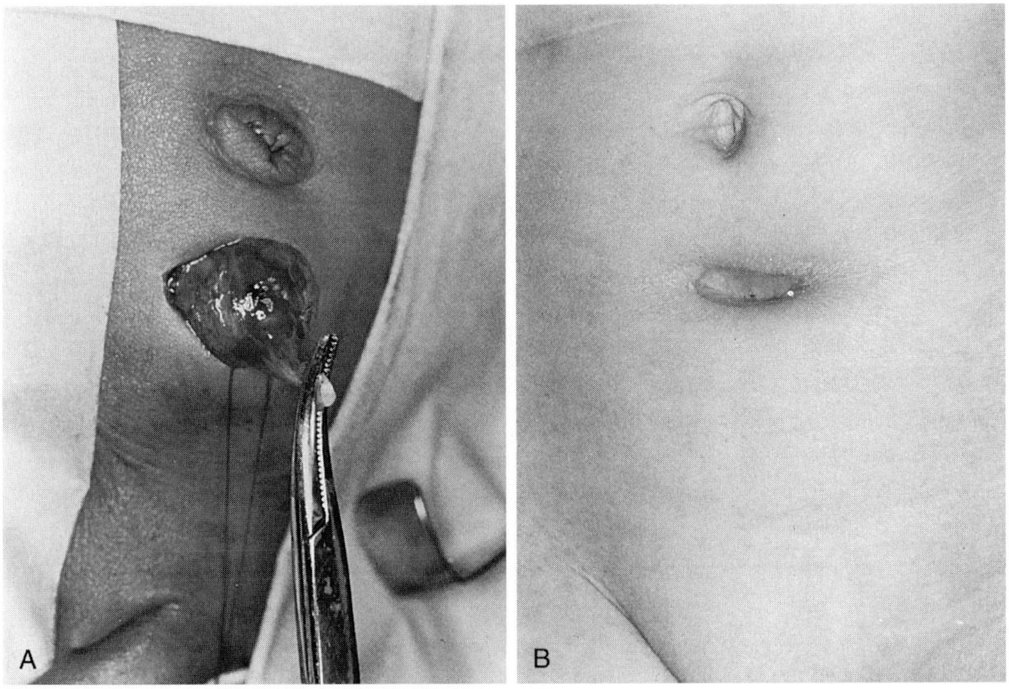

Figure 16–5 *A,* Vesicostomy incision and identification of urachal remnant to confirm location of bladder dome. *B,* Properly placed functional vesicostomy.

generally recommended because it will likely further reduce the risk of urinary tract infection.

In most of boys with posterior urethral valves and vesicoureteral reflux, the reflux will resolve spontaneously after valve ablation (and longitudinal growth). The exception is when reflux is associated with poorly functioning kidneys. Reimplantation in these instances is unlikely to improve renal function and is primarily of value if breakthrough infection occurs. It should be noted that reimplantation of markedly dilated ureters into a thick-walled, trabeculated, small valve bladder has an expected complication rate of 15 to 30%, even in expert hands. In bilateral reflux, we have used a transureteroureterostomy and a long, controlled unilateral reimplant using an extravesical, modified Paquin approach and a psoas hitch.

VURD Syndrome

Unilateral reflux into a dysplastic kidney has been termed the valves, unilateral reflux, and dysplasia (VURD) syndrome.[7–9] It remains unclear whether the reflux and high pressures are the cause of the dysplastic kidney or whether the dysplasia is the result of a coincident, severely abnormal ureteral bud. In any event, it seems that most of the in utero bladder pressure is taken by the unilateral refluxing system, which acts as a protective pop-off mechanism, usually resulting in a well-preserved contralateral kidney. Historically, it has been recommended that a nephroureterectomy be performed at approximately 1 to 2 years in these nonfunctional systems (Fig. 16–6*A* and *B*). This was to improve toilet training by removing the reflux into what has become a large "diverticulum," also preventing stasis and lowering residual urine and decreasing the risk of infection. Recently, there has been enthusiasm for preserving the dilated system and using it as augmentation material in the form of a ureterocystoplasty in case the bladder is noncompliant.[10] This decision must be individualized, however, because we have found remarkable improvement in the appearance and function of the bladder in patients with posterior urethral valves after primary fulguration alone. Thus, in most cases, it is not necessary to preserve this segment for later use.

Bladder Function

Although the exact and sequential causes are unknown, it is clear that myriad bladder abnormalities can develop, resulting in poor lower urinary tract function in many patients.[11] Clinically, this presents as recurrent urinary tract infections and urinary incontinence.[12] In fact, approximately 50% of patients with posterior urethral valves will have delayed diurnal continence.[5] Although many patients will have normal bladder function, urodynamic evaluation of these boys reveals a spectrum of abnormalities ranging from myogenic failure to hyper-reflexic or hypertonic patterns of bladder function.[13] Many of these boys will have poor concentrating ability also, and the obligatory polyuria will accentuate the bladder dysfunction. Treatment options for these patients must be individualized, but they range from timed hourly voiding and double voiding to intermittent catheterization in severe cases. Many boys benefit from anticholinergic medications, although we find that they can be extremely sensitive to them and can easily go from a hyper-reflexive

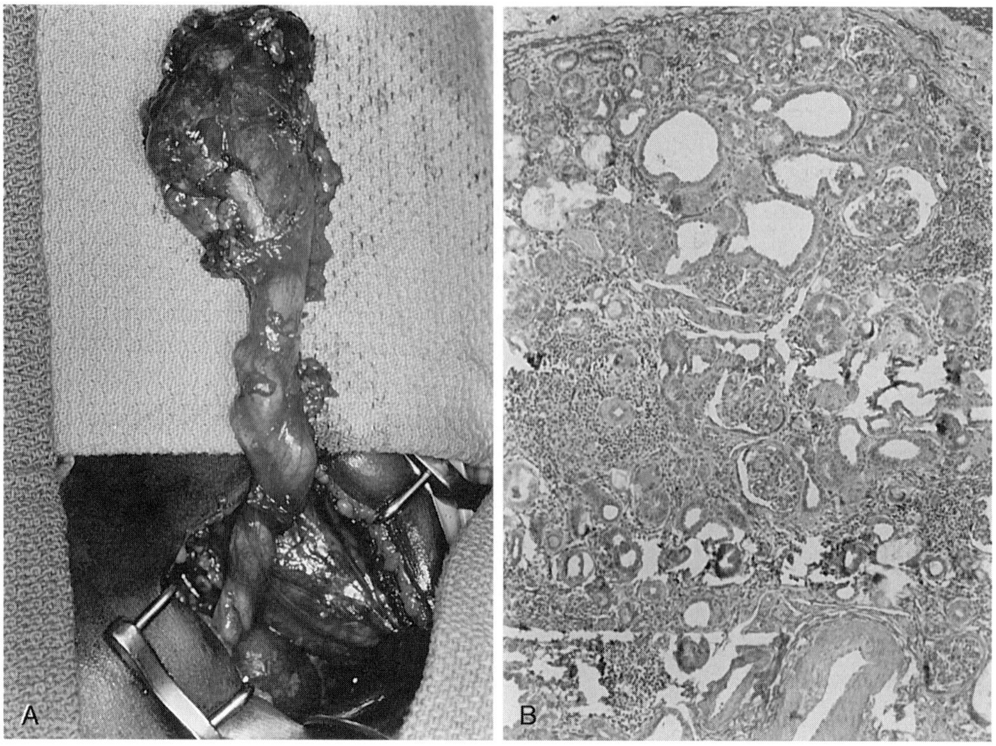

Figure 16–6 *A,* Gross specimen at the time of nephroureterectomy in a posterior urethral valve patient with unilateral reflux into a dysplastic kidney VURD (valves, unilateral reflux, and dysplasia) syndrome. *B,* Histologic renal specimen showing severe renal dysplasia.

bladder to retention. In spite of aggressive therapy, a number of children with posterior urethral valves will require treatment for end-stage renal disease. It is interesting that the majority of these will have incontinence, suggesting that bladder dysfunction may, in part, be responsible.[14] Furthermore, early reports of renal transplantation in children showed that patients with valves had the lowest long-term success, again suggesting that bladder dysfunction plays an important and continuing role. Concern that the valve bladder is responsible for continued renal deterioration and that a similar situation will result after successful renal transplantation mandates that careful bladder characterization be performed before renal transplantation. We have used the same approach in patients with neurogenic bladders secondary to spinal defects, ensuring that before renal transplantation they have both an adequate storage capacity and a means for emptying, either by voiding or intermittent catheterization. This type of policy has resulted in improved success for renal transplantation in boys with valves.

CONGENITAL URETHRAL POLYPS

Urethral polyps are benign congenital lesions located in the posterior urethra, arising from the verumontanum.[15, 16] They have a 1- to 3-cm stalk histologically consisting of fibromuscular stroma covered by transitional epithelium. The patients typically present with intermittent obstructive symptoms or may have urinary retention, hematuria, dysuria, and incontinence. The diagnosis of a urethral polyp may occasionally be made by ultrasonography (Fig. 16–7*A*) if the polyp prolapses into the bladder, but generally is made on a VCUG. This will show a filling defect that may vary in location between the bladder and anterior urethra depending on the movement of the polyp on its stalk. Treatment consists of resection. If the urethra will accept a resectoscope, an endoscopic approach is preferred (Fig. 16–7*B*). It is important to remove or fulgurate the base of the stalk, or the polyp may regrow.

COWPER'S DUCT AND DUCT CYSTS

Cowper's or the bulbourethral glands are two paired periurethral glands situated in the urogenital diaphragm and along the corpus spongiosum of the bulbar urethra.[17] Cowper's glands empty via ducts anteriorly, through the corpus spongiosum into the bulbar urethra, with small flush openings. In the female, the homologous structure is Bartholin's gland. These glands secrete clear fluid that acts as a lubricant and coagulation factor for semen during ejaculation. Reflux into a dilated duct may be seen on retrograde urethrograms in patients who have anterior urethral obstruction, usually from stricture disease. Most often, abnormalities of Cowper's ducts are asymptomatic, although they may cause hematuria, obstruction or postvoid dribbling. Rarely, a dilated Cowper's gland or duct may appear as a perineal mass. Most children do not require treatment. However, a few will benefit from transurethral marsupialization or fulguration.

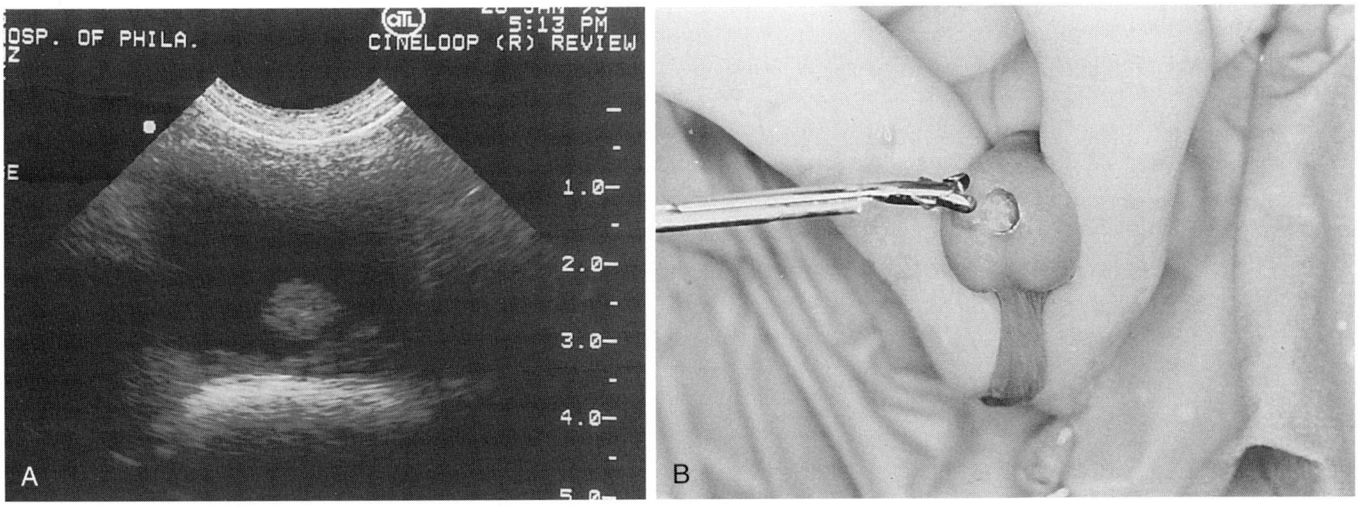

Figure 16–7 *A,* Urethral polyp diagnosed by ultrasonogram with the polyp prolapsing into the bladder. *B,* Urethral polyp being delivered at the urethral meatus after endoscopic resection.

MEGALOURETHRA

There are two types of megalourethra: scaphoid and fusiform.[18–20] The scaphoid type is associated with absence of the corpus spongiosum, and the fusiform type is associated with absence of the corpus spongiosum as well as a defective corpus cavernosum. The more common, scaphoid type acts like a urethrocele, with the urethra ballooning out ventrally during voiding. In the rare fusiform-type lesion, the whole elongated penile urethra dilates with voiding, and because there are no corporal bodies the penis is soft and flabby, consisting primarily of skin. Megalourethra is associated most often with severe abnormalities such as cloacal anomalies, prune-belly, and the VACTERL syndromes. Treatment is based on the principles of hypospadias repair. The scaphoid-type megalourethra should be opened longitudinally and redundant urethral mucosa excised. The fusiform-type lesion is most difficult to repair because there are no erectile elements, but most often these patients do not survive because of other serious anomalies.

ANTERIOR URETHRAL VALVES

Anterior urethral valves and congenital urethral diverticula are rare, with a frequency one eighth that of posterior urethral valves.[21] They can be located anywhere in the urethra; approximately 40% occur in the bulbar urethra, 30% at the penoscrotal junction, and the remaining 30% in the penile urethra. The obstruction in anterior urethral valves is usually a consequence of an associated diverticulum. During voiding, the diverticulum fills, undermining and compressing the dilated proximal urethra; the distal lip forces more urine into the diverticulum, resulting in increased obstruction.

These children present either as newborns with severe outflow obstruction or as older children with incontinence and dribbling-type micturition (or urinary tract infection). If the obstruction is distal enough, ballooning of the penile urethra and obvious penile deformity may occur with voiding.

Diagnosis is made by VCUG (catheterization may be impossible and a suprapubic tube may be necessary), and the upper tracts should be screened with ultrasonography. At least 50% of cases will have associated hydronephrosis or reflux. Therapy is usually endoscopic resection of the valve lip when possible (if the diverticulum is small); in the neonate, a two-stage urethroplasty with an initial exteriorization of the diverticulum, followed at a later date by urethroplasty, is the optimal treatment. Prognosis in this rare group of anomalies is generally good but depends on the degree of obstruction and injury to the upper tract.

URETHRAL DUPLICATION

Duplication of the urethra is a rare anomaly with numerous anatomic variations.[22–24] These fall into three main groups: (1) epispadiac, (2) hypospadiac, and (3) Y type.

Epispadias Duplication (Fig. 16–8*A–C*)

Epispadiac duplications vary widely in their severity, but are characterized by a normally positioned urethral meatus and a second meatus in the epispadiac position on the dorsal aspect of the penis (Fig. 16–8*D*). Presentation may vary depending on the completeness of the duplication. When complete, the patient is likely to void with a double stream. If this is not discovered until toilet training, the child may have a normal voiding pattern but

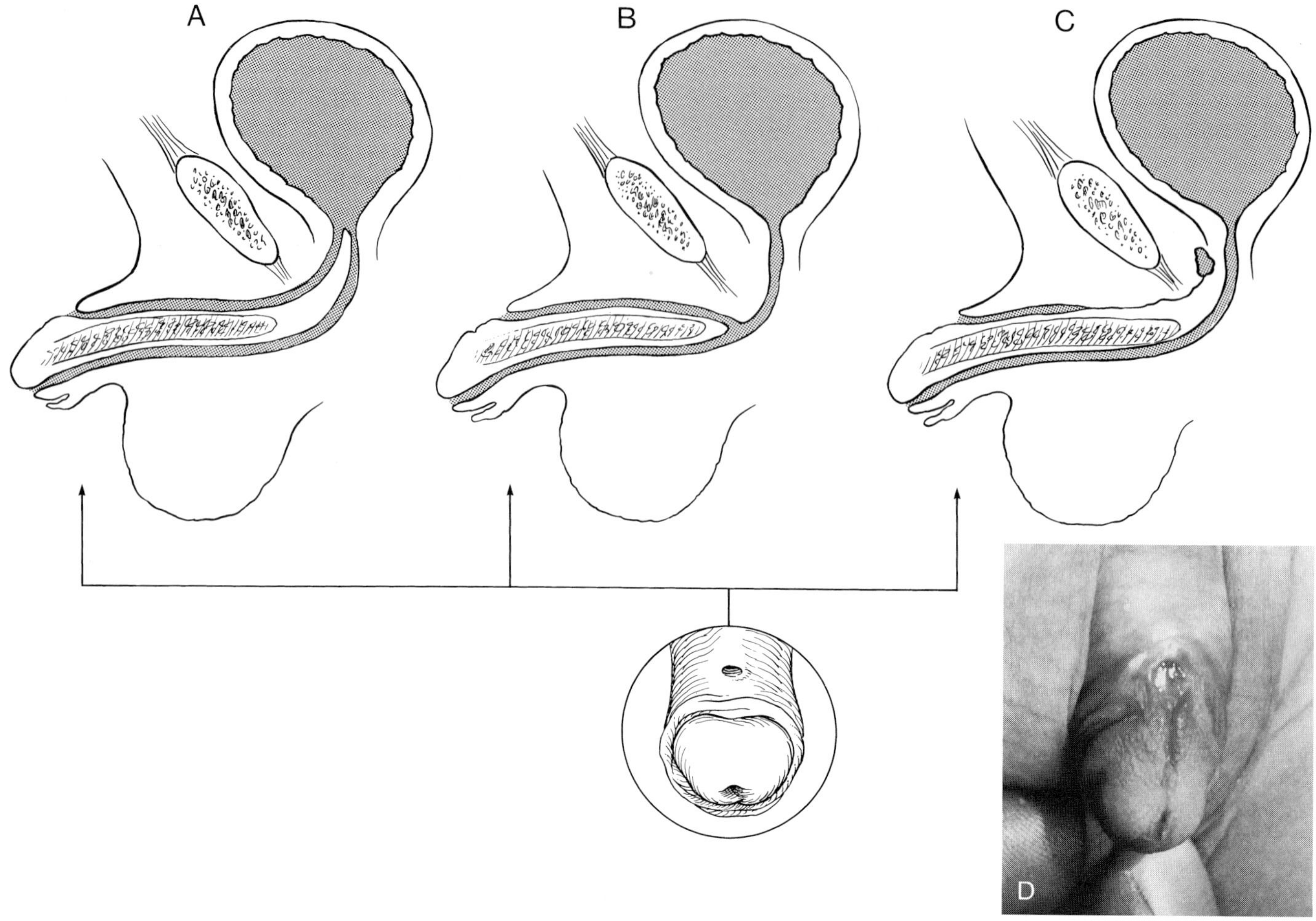

Figure 16–8 *A–C,* Variations of epispadiac duplications. Invariably the ventral urethra is the more normal one. Modified from Williams DI, Kenawi MM. Urethral duplications in the male. Eur Urol 1:209, 1975. Used with permission. *D,* Epispadiac duplication: note two urethral meatus.

constant dribbling because the dorsal urethra is in a grossly abnormal position and by-passes the urethral sphincter. Patients with an incomplete form will void with a double stream but will not have this type of incontinence. In incomplete variations, the connection of the dorsal channel to the urinary tract may be minimal, and the presenting complaint may be the abnormal appearance, although in the rare case these can present with infections. Epispadiac duplications are nearly always associated with significant dorsal curvature, and this is ultimately the major disability in most. In general, these patients do not have associated upper tract abnormalities. The diagnosis is made by physical examination and confirmed by anterograde and retrograde urethral studies.

Surgical Repair

The majority of epispadiac duplications will come to operative repair as a result of the significant dorsal penile curvature. Most cases can be approached via a circumferential coronal incision. The dorsal accessory urethra is excised as the penile skin is dissected back to the symphysis. In complete cases, the dorsal urethra disappears under the intersymphyseal ligaments, and then dissection may continue via a suprapubic approach (rarely needed). Because the symphysis is usually separated, a transpubic approach is feasible by incising the interpubic ligaments. Dissection at this point should remain strictly in the midline so as not to injure the cavernosal nerves, which enter the corporal bodies laterally. In cases of minimal urinary leakage, the dorsal urethra may be left in situ.

Artificial erection will show dorsal chordee in nearly all cases. This can be approached several ways; performing tunica albuginea plications on the ventral aspect of the penis at the point of maximum bend using an analogous approach for penile curvature associated with hypospadias is most popular. Alternatively, corporal rotation to the ventrum or even variations on the Cantwell-Ransley epispadias repair are feasible. The glans can then be repaired as needed by excising the dorsal epithelium and reapproximating glans tissue with several horizontal mattress sutures.

Hypospadiac Duplications (Fig. 16–9*A–C*)

Hypospadiac duplications occur with many different variations, but the incomplete form is by far the most common. Complete duplication may be associated with incontinence but is extremely rare. Radiographic evaluation, as in epispadiac duplication, consists of retrograde urethrography as well as VCUG. In the abortive form, the exact anatomy may be determined with the use of a metal probe at the time of surgical repair. In complete cases of hypospadiac duplication, excision all the way to the bladder is necessary; an important caveat is that nearly always the more normal urethra is the ventral one, even though the meatus of the dorsal urethra is often more normally positioned on the glans. Because complete excision of the dorsal accessory urethra is difficult without damaging the ventral urethra, an alternative approach is to incise the septum between the two urethras as the dissection proceeds distally. This is also effective in incomplete forms or in severe variations of the abortive type. Associated hypospadias can then be repaired at the same setting.

Y-Type Duplications (Fig. 16–10)

The Y-type duplication is the most common type of urethral duplication. The phallus appears grossly normal, but most of the urine passes through the perineal opening. It is this fact that usually brings the child to the physician's attention. Examination will reveal a normal meatus at the glans penis, but close inspection uncovers a second meatus deep in the perineum. Radiologic evaluation will demonstrate that only the distal 1 to 2 cm of the dorsal urethra are normal, and a catheter passed through the meatus will usually stop there. A retrograde urethrogram will show that the dorsal urethra is atretic. In contrast, the mucosa and periurethral tissue of the perineal urethra are virtually normal. A VCUG will demonstrate the atretic dorsal urethra and a normal-caliber ventral urethra. Unfortunately, the normally positioned dorsal urethra is generally unusable, whereas the ventral urethra is usually healthy and forms the basis for reconstruction. Hence, the ventral urethral channel must be separated from the anus and tunneled through the perineum into the scrotum. The remainder of the urethroplasty can be performed with a preputial island flap technique. Contami-

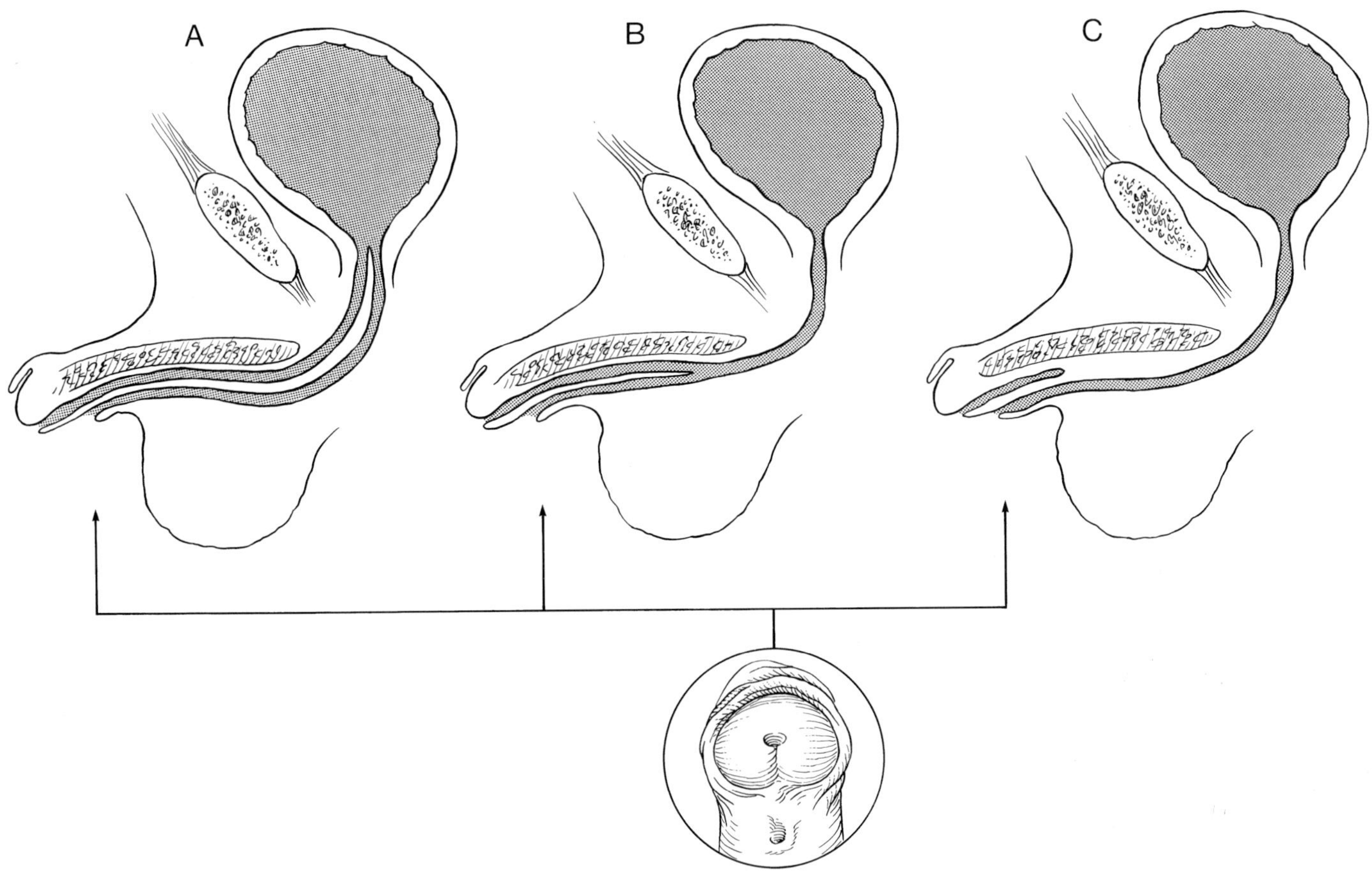

Figure 16–9 Variations of hypospadiac duplications. The abortive form (C) is the most common. The ventral urethra is the more normal one. Modified from Williams DI, Kenawi MM. Urethral duplications in the male. Eur Urol 1:209, 1975. Used with permission.

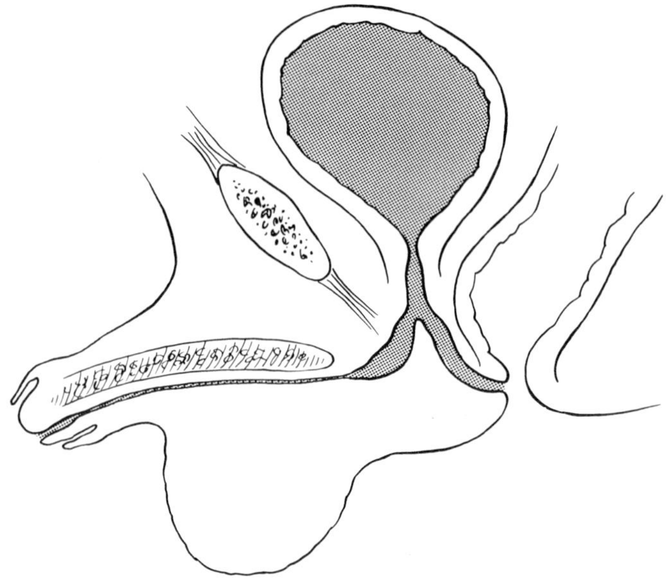

Figure 16–10 Typical anatomy in a patient with a Y-type duplication. The ventral urethra (preanal meatus) is the more normal one. Modified from Williams DI, Kenawi MM. Urethral duplications in the male. Eur Urol 1:209, 1975. Used with permission.

nation from the bowel can be reduced with good mechanical and antibiotic bowel preparation as well as the use of parenteral antibiotics at the time of surgery.

A few patients have been effectively managed with progressive dilation of the dorsal, more normally positioned, but atretic urethra (P.A.D.U.A procedure).[25] Early results show that dilation allows for a functionally normal urethra. The ventral urethra can then be safely excised. Further data are needed to substantiate these results.

Urethral Prolapse

Urethral prolapse is an uncommon event typically occurring in young girls.[26, 27] Although the cause of this condition is unclear, it occurs much more commonly in the black population. Typical symptoms are vaginal bleeding, vaginal discharge, and urinary tract infection. On examination, there is a characteristic circumferential prolapse of the mucosa (i.e., a doughnut sign) (Fig. 16–11*A*). The differential diagnosis includes urethral polyp, prolapsed ureterocele, sarcoma botryoids, periurethral abscess, and a urethral papilloma.

Initial treatment can be nonoperative with estrogen cream, sitz baths, and oral antibiotics. In most cases, the urethral prolapse will not respond to these measures, and a simple cautery excision under anesthesia with primary mucosal approximation is recommended. A urethral catheter in situ will facilitate dissection (Fig. 16–11*B*). Treatment by ligating the redundant mucosa with a suture around the catheter and allowing subsequent necrosis is

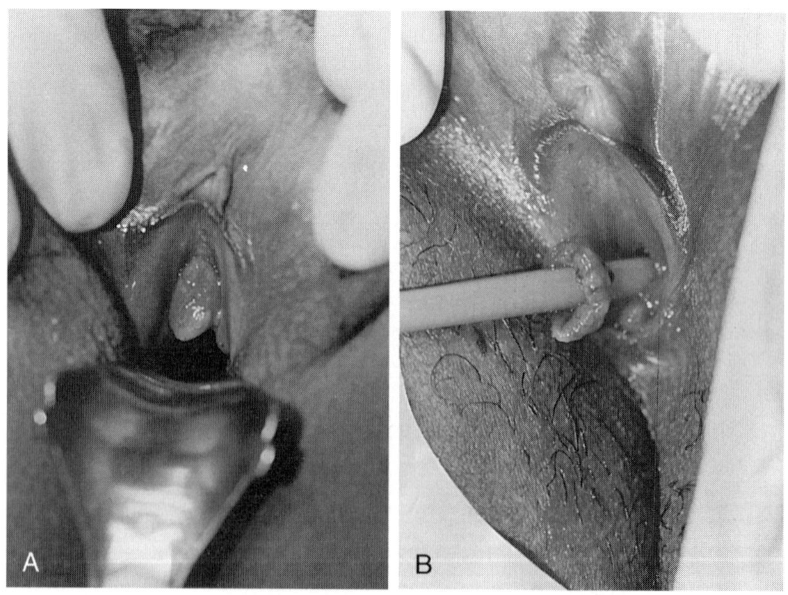

Figure 16–11 *A*, Urethral prolapse in a young black female. *B*, Surgical excision using a urethral catheter as a guide.

largely historic and should be discouraged because of the prolonged time needed.

REFERENCES

1. Dewan PA, Zappala SM, Ransley PG, Duffy PG. Endoscopic reappraisal of the morphology of congenital obstruction of the posterior urethra. Br J Urol 70:439, 1992.
2. Young B. Lower Urinary Tract Obstruction in Childhood. Philadelphia: WB Saunders, 1972.
3. Whitaker RH, Sherwood T. An improved hook for destroying posterior urethral valves. J Urol 135:531, 1986.
4. Duckett JW. Cutaneous vesicostomy in infants and children. Urol Clin North Am 1:485, 1974.
5. Smith GH, Canning D, Schulman S, et al. The long-term outcome of posterior urethral valves treated with primary valve ablation and observation. J Urol 155:1730, 1996.
6. Johnston JH. Vesicoureteric reflux with urethral valves. Br J Urol 51:100, 1979.
7. Hoover DL, Duckett JW. Posterior urethral valves, unilateral reflux and renal dysplasia: A syndrome. J Urol 128:994, 1982.
8. Rittenberg MH, Hulbert WC, Snyder H, Duckett JW. Protective factors in posterior urethral valves. J Urol 140:993, 1988.
9. Kaefer M, Keating MA, Adams MC, Rink RC. Posterior urethral valves, pressure pop-offs and bladder function. J Urol 154:708, 1995.
10. Bellinger MF. Ureterocystoplasty: A unique method for vesical augmentation in children. J Urol 149:811, 1993.
11. Parkhouse HF, Barratt TM, Dillon MJ, et al. Long-term outcome of boys with posterior urethral valves. Br J Urol 62:59, 1988.
12. Holmdahl G, Sillen U, Hanson E, et al. Bladder dysfunction in boys with posterior urethral valves before and after puberty. J Urol 155:694, 1996.
13. Peters CA, Bolkier M, Bauer SB, et al. The urodynamic consequences of posterior urethral valves. J Urol 144:122, 1990.
14. Merguerian PA, McLorie GA, Churchill BM, et al. Radiographic and serologic correlates of azotemia in patients with posterior urethral valves. J Urol 148:1499, 1992.
15. Gleason PE, Kramer SA. Genitourinary polyps in children. Urology 44:106, 1994.
16. De Castro R, Campobasso P, Belloli G, Pavanello P. Solitary polyp of posterior urethra in children: Report on seventeen cases. Eur J Pediatr Surg 3:92, 1993.
17. Maizels M, Stephens D, King L. Cowper's syringocele: A classification of dilatations of Cowper's gland duct based upon clinical characteristics of 8 boys. J Urol 129:111, 1982.
18. Stephens FD, Fortune DW. Pathogenesis of megalourethra. J Urol 149:1512, 1993.
19. Swami KS, Jurriaans E, Hammonds JC. The wider spectrum of megalourethra. Br J Urol 75:563, 1995.
20. Appel RA, Kaplan GW, Brock WA, Streit D. Megalourethra. J Urol 135:747, 1986.
21. Firlit R, Firlit C, King L. Obstructing anterior urethral valves in children. J Urol 119:819, 1978.
22. Williams D, Kenawi M. Urethral duplications in the male. Eur Urol 1:209, 1975.
23. Middleton AW Jr, Melzer RB. Duplicated urethra: An anomaly best repaired. Urology 39:538, 1992.
24. Ortolano V, Nasrallah PF. Urethral duplication. J Urol 136:909, 1986.
25. Passerini-Glazel G, Araguna F, Chiozza L, et al. The P.A.D.U.A. (progressive augmentation by dilating the urethra anterior) procedure for the treatment of severe urethral hypoplasia. J Urol 140:1247, 1988.
26. Fernandes ET, Dekermacher S, Sabadin MA, Vaz F. Urethral prolapse in children. Urology 41:240, 1993.
27. Anveden-Hertzberg L, Gauderer MW, Elder JS. Urethral prolapse: An often misdiagnosed cause of urogenital bleeding in girls. Pediatr Emerg Care 11:212, 1995.

PART VII

The Testis

17

STANLEY J. KOGAN & BHAGWANT GILL

Cryptorchidism

Although cryptorchidism has been of great interest to clinicians for many years, the diagnosis and treatment approaches continue to undergo refinement and improvement. Understanding of the pathogenesis and natural history of this condition has allowed us to formulate a rational, safe, and cost-efficient approach that optimizes treatment objectives and minimizes complications. In this chapter we have recorded the experiences gained and the lessons learned from more than 1500 orchidopexies. A rational approach to diagnosis and treatment is presented.

NORMAL AND ABNORMAL TESTIS AND DUCTAL DEVELOPMENT

To the best of our knowledge, most boys with a normal 46, XY karyotype with cryptorchidism have normal testes to begin with but suffer histologic changes subsequently that may first occur in fetal life. Besides the abnormal location, these changes are associated in some instances with hypogonadotropism, believed to adversely affect normal development of the germ cells.[1]

The main germ cell of the early fetal testis is the gonocyte. By 15 weeks' gestation transformation to Ad-spermatogonia begins. Gonocytes normally disappear in the postnatal testis by 6 months, and Ad-spermatogonia constitute the major germinal element. Failure of this transformation may be associated with subsequent increased risk of infertility and neoplasia. By 5 years of age primary spermatocytes appear in normal testes, the first cell capable of undergoing meiosis. Failure of this normal transformation process is associated with subsequent infertility. With puberty onset, primary spermatocytes undergo meiosis and progression through the normal cycle of spermatogenesis, leading to formation of mature spermatozoa. In cryptorchidism, these three major landmarks are disturbed and normal spermatogenesis does not occur.[2] Many studies have documented in detail the resultant gross alterations in germ cell development, with obvious subsequent fertility implications. In some studies, about 5% of cryptorchid testes were found to be completely devoid of germ cells by 1 year of age, increasing to about 25 to 35% thereafter.[2, 3]

Besides alteration in normal germ cell development, the other cellular elements do not develop normally in the cryptorchid testis. Leydig's cells commonly are described as atrophic, and Sertoli's cells and connective tissue abnormalities are described as well. Leydig's cell abnormalities, in particular, are believed to be directly involved in the pathogenesis of the infertility associated with cryptorchidism.[3]

Concurrent with development of the testis is the development of the ductal (excretory) system of the testis. Stimulated by local testosterone in utero, the cranial end of the wolffian duct fuses with the tubules of the rete testis, and the caudal end forms the ejaculatory duct, seminal vesicle, and vas deferens. This process often goes awry in cryptorchidism. Grossly visible abnormalities of the ductal system seen at orchidopexy occur in at least one third of cryptorchidism testes, with an increased frequency in higher undescended testes (Fig. 17–1). Germ cell counts in cryptorchid testes correlate directly with the severity of the ductal abnormality: the more severe the abnormality, the more reduced is the germ cell count, suggesting that an associated hypogonadotropism or diminished testosterone may be an underlying common factor for both.[4] Germ cell number also correlates inversely with testis location.

NORMAL AND ABNORMAL TESTIS DESCENT

Testis and epididymal descent is believed necessary for humans to produce a fertile ejaculate, because scrotal temperature is 2 to 3°C cooler than abdominal temperature. The events involving normal testicular descent in the human revolve around the gubernaculum and processus vaginalis. Sudden gubernacular swelling with extension of the processus vaginalis into the scrotum occurs after the seventh month of gestation, with rapid descent of the epididymis leading the testis. These changes may be directed or modulated by androgens, either directly or indirectly through the spinal nucleus of the genitofemoral nerve, which innervates the gubernaculum. Estrogens, müllerian inhibiting substance, or other factors may also be involved.[5] Derangements of normal descent have been

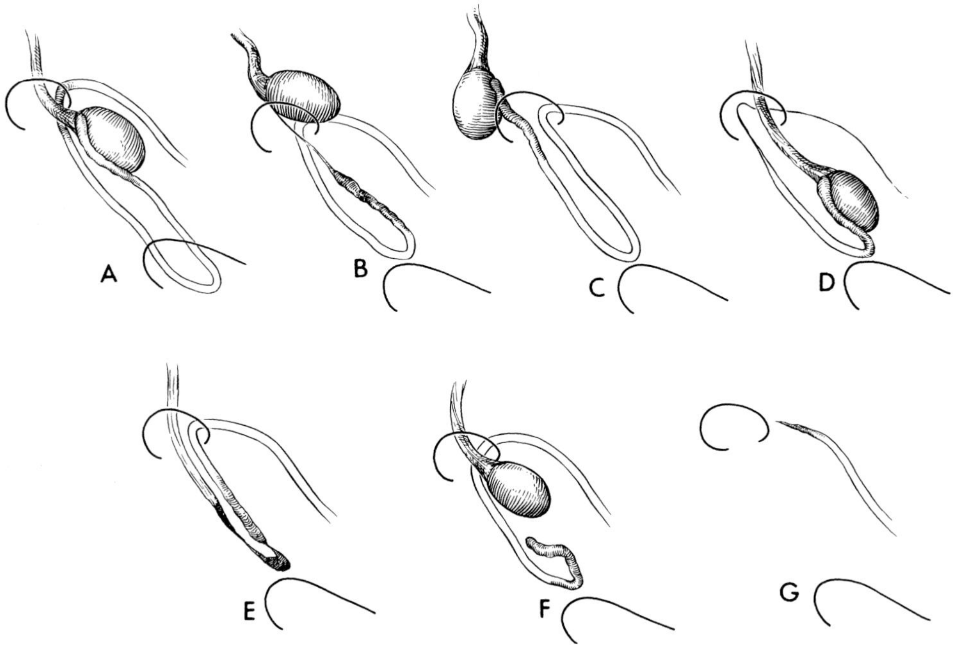

Figure 17–1 Disorders of the epididymis and vas associated with cryptorchidism. *A,* Long-loop vas. *B,* Atresia of epididymis. *C,* Long-loop vas with abdominal testis. *D,* Vasal atresia. *E,* Absent testis. *F,* Non-union of vas and testis. *G,* Atresia of distal vas and absent testis. From Kogan S. Cryptorchidism. In Kelalis PP, King LR, Belman AB (eds), Clinical Pediatric Urology, 3rd ed. Philadelphia: WB Saunders, 1992. Used with permission.

studied extensively, with a resultant range of theories and facts emerging. Because cryptorchidism is a heterogeneous disorder with a variety of causes, different mechanisms may be primarily operative in each of these differing situations.

FREQUENCY OF CRYPTORCHIDISM

The frequency of cryptorchidism at birth correlates inversely with gestational age and weight (Table 17–1), occurring in about 33% of premature boys and 3% of term boys. Two of three term boys with cryptorchidism will have descent of the testis by age 1 year, with virtually all descending during the first several months. Spontaneous descent occurs infrequently thereafter, and there is little change in the prevalence of 0.7 to 1.0% noted at 1 year and beyond.

Table 17–1
Prevalence of Cryptorchidism at Various Ages

Age	Weight (g)	Incidence (%)
Premature	451–910	100.0
	911–1810	62.0
	1811–2040	25.0
	2041–2490	17.0
Total		30.3
Full term	2491–2720	12.0
	2721–3630	3.3
	3631–5210	0.7
Total		3.4
One year		0.7–0.8
School age		0.76–0.95
Adulthood		0.7–1.0

Data from Scorer GC, Farrington GH. Congenital Deformities of the Testis and Epididymis. London: Butterworths, 1971.
From Kogan S. Cryptorchidism. In Kelalis PP, King LR, Belman AB (eds), Clinical Pediatric Urology, 3rd ed. Philadelphia: WB Saunders, 1992. Used with permission.

These observations form the basis for modern-day treatment of cryptorchidism. Because virtually all cryptorchid testes descend between birth and 6 months of age, it is reasonable to monitor boys with cryptorchid testes until that time to determine whether spontaneous descent will occur. Ultimate successful descent is influenced as well by the initial location of the testis; fewer high testes will ultimately descend than those located closer to the scrotum. Histologic deterioration occurs much earlier than previously believed, with minimal deterioration evident on biopsy at 1 year and rapid and progressive damage occurring subsequently. Orchidopexy by 1 year of age, therefore, constitutes optimal modern treatment.[6]

DIAGNOSTIC CLASSIFICATION AND NOMENCLATURE

It is important to have a working understanding of a classification of cryptorchid testes because this aids in diagnosis and treatment. A variety of classifications exist; we recommend a *functional* classification in which testis location indicates the appropriate subsequent treatment. Cryptorchid testes are classified as being either *palpable* or *impalpable* based on physical examination. Palpable undescended testes may be retractile, ectopic, or situated anywhere along the normal line of descent distal to the

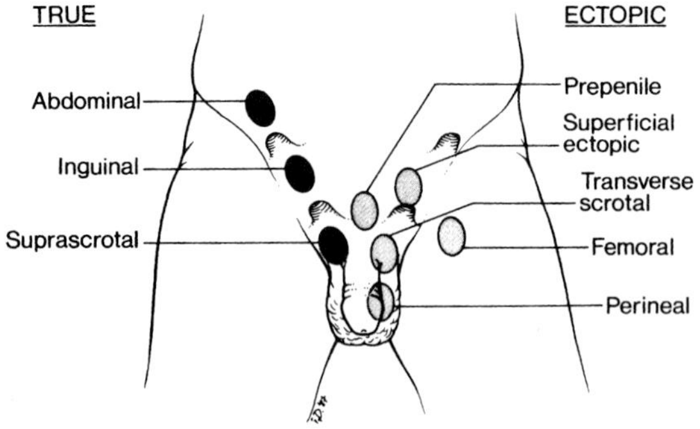

Figure 17–2 Locations of true and ectopic testes. From Kogan S. Cryptorchidism. In Kelalis PP, King LR, Belman AB (eds), Clinical Pediatric Urology, 3rd ed. Philadelphia: WB Saunders, 1992. Used with permission.

internal inguinal ring. Impalpable undescended testes may be within the inguinal canal, in the abdomen, or absent (Fig. 17–2). Overall, about 10% of cryptorchid testes are abdominal, 50 to 70% are high scrotal or ectopic, 3 to 4% are absent, and the remainder are intracanalicular. Approximately 20% of all cryptorchid testes are impalpable. When impalpable, the distribution figures change: about 50% are abdominal and approximately 33% each are inguinal or absent (these percentages varying slightly among series).

For examine, it is best to have the patient in a relaxed state in a warm room after first adjusting to the examining table. Poor patient relaxation, anxiety, obesity, and rough examiner technique all contribute to difficulties with accurate diagnosis. Diagnosis is easiest in infants because there is minimal adiposity, full relaxation, and minimally developed cremasteric reflexes. Older children may be more active and less cooperative and, especially when there is more adipose tissue, may be more difficult to examine. Distraction with puppets, toys, or music is often helpful. If the testis cannot be felt in the cooperative older child, abduction and external rotation of the hips with the knees flexed or positioning the patient in the sitting position with the legs crossed aid further in diagnosis by fully relaxing the cremasteric muscles.

Sometimes difficulty is encountered in distinguishing between boys with *retractile* and distally located truly undescended testes. Our definition of a retractile testis is one that is initially extrascrotal but remains within the scrotum without any tension once positioned and released, whereas an undescended testis will not remain in the scrotum. Another variant has been labeled as the *gliding* testis: one that lies distal to the external inguinal ring and can be manipulated into the scrotum but pulls up immediately on release. Sometimes these differential diagnoses are subtle; positioning the patient to relax the cremasteric muscles is helpful, as is a diagnostic short course of human chorionic gonadotropin (hCG) injections. This diagnosis is important and persistence is required to make these distinctions, because most retractile testes will ultimately occupy a permanent relaxed dependent scrotal position and do not require any additional treatment other than careful follow-up. In contrast, gliding testes and other undescended testes require early treatment because infertility may occur. Furthermore, testes initially thought to be retractile may ascend subsequently and on follow-up cannot be positioned in the scrotum. Reascent of a previously descended testis is a well-described phenomenon, probably occurring because of shortening of a persisting processus vaginalis or diminishing mobility of a superficial ectopic testis with increasing age. These testes are subject to the same deteriorative processes described earlier, and treatment must be provided once this diagnosis is confirmed. A high index of suspicion must be maintained, and regular testicular examinations must be done throughout puberty to ensure that a testis initially descended or thought to be retractile does not become permanently fixed in an extrascrotal location.

Impalpable cryptorchid testes give rise to further diagnostic and therapeutic problems. These testes are less likely to descend spontaneously, are associated with an increased incidence of ductal abnormalities, are usually smaller than normal testes and other more distally located cryptorchid testes, and often require additional diagnostic evaluation and special techniques of orchidopexy (see later discussion). When one testis is impalpable, laparoscopy is indicated to determine whether it is present or absent. Contralateral testicular hypertrophy (testis enlarged greater than 2 mL in volume) has been described as a useful indicator of ipsilateral testis absence when encountered at less than 2 years of age. The lack of contralateral hypertrophy does not necessarily indicate the presence of an ipsilateral testis, however.[7] When both testes are impalpable (bilateral anorchia), hormonal testing measuring the testosterone response to hCG stimulation and measurement of plasma follicle-stimulating hormone and leutinizing hormone should be done.[8] Laparoscopic confirmation of the diagnosis of bilateral anorchia may be made at the time of subsequent testicular prosthesis placement (Table 17–2).

LOCALIZATION STUDIES

Historically, a plethora of radiological tests have been used in an attempt to determine whether a testis is present or absent. It is our bias, as well as others', that none of the previously reported radiological investigations have sufficient accuracy, especially given the young ages at which current treatment is provided, to be used in the diagnosis of impalpable testes.[9] Computed tomographic (CT) scanning carries a relatively high radiation burden for the young child and is insufficiently accurate. Magnetic resonance imaging (MRI) is not cost efficient and

Table 17–2
Findings in Diagnostic Hormonal Testing for Bilateral Congenital Anorchia

	FSH, LH	Testosterone After hCG
Testes Absent		
Bilateral congenital anorchia	↑	0
Possible in prepubertal bilateral congenital anorchia (i.e., ages 3 to 9 years)	Normal	0
LHRH →	↑	0
Testes Present		
Bilateral impalpable cryptorchidism	Normal	0
Possible in hypogonadotropic hypogonadism	Low	0
Prolonged hCG →	—	↑
Possible in postpubertal bilateral hypoplastic/damaged testes present	↑	0

FSH, follicle-stimulating hormone; LH, luteinizing hormone; hCG, human chorionic gonadotropin; LHRH, luteinizing hormone–releasing hormone.
From Kogan SJ: Work-up and management of the bilateral, nonpalpable testis. In Gonzales ET Jr, Roth DR (eds), Common Problems in Pediatric Urology. Chicago: Year Book, 1991, p 302.

also falls far short of the complete accuracy needed. Ultrasonography, although noninvasive, similarly has a very high false-negative rate (testis reported as absent although it is present at exploration). We personally have had a number of boys with "absent" testes and a "negative" sonogram, only to be able to feel the testis inguinally during the physical examination! Furthermore, if a testis is located by ultrasonography, exploration is ultimately required anyway. These observations have led to our abandoning routine radiological evaluation for impalpable cryptorchid testes. Instead, laparoscopy is often used at the time of surgical exploration.

Diagnostic laparoscopy was first used in 1976 for impalpable undescended testes. Since that time, instrumentation refinements and improvements in technology as well as better understanding of the pertinent anatomy of the pelvis have led to its widespread use in this clinical setting. Issues regarding safety and diagnostic accuracy have been largely resolved. In a survey of the American Academy of Pediatrics, Urology Section, covering 5428 cases, 75% of the section members used laparoscopy for evaluating impalpable testes. The minor complication rate was about 4% and a significant complication—defined as bleeding, vascular injury, omental herniation, or bladder or bowel perforation—occurred in about 1%. With attention to detail, proper instrumentation, and skilled pediatric anesthesia, even the neonate can undergo safe and accurate laparoscopy.

The issue is whether routine use of laparoscopy (in every case) is justified or whether selective use is more rational. Proponents of the former view claim that the procedure is easy and accurate, adds little time to the overall procedure, and helps them decide incision placement and to better plan the overall approach to surgery. Furthermore, now that one- or two-stage laparoscopic orchidopexy is possible, therapy can be provided in addition to diagnosis. Advocates of the latter view suggest that routine laparoscopy is not cost effective and patient friendly because many "unnecessary" laparoscopies are done when routine inguinal exploration (with a local intraperitoneal extension when necessary) will provide the same information, making laparoscopy superfluous in most instances. Furthermore, if a testicular prosthesis is to be placed, an inguinal incision is usually used anyway. An examination of pertinent data indicates that the truth lies somewhat in between and that the surgeon's bias plays a pertinent role.

Figure 17–3 summarizes the laparoscopic findings in 432 boys with impalpable testes collated from five series. Testes were present in 241 (56%) and absent in 191 (44%). Half of the testes, when present, were located abdominally and half were located within the inguinal canal (27% and 28% of the overall group, respectively). Of those found to be surgically absent, 55% were explored and found to be inguinal "vanishing testes" (some with nubbins of remaining testicular tissue), 1% were explored and no testis or ductal tissue was identified, and 9% were intra-abdominal vanishing testes and were not explored. Of the entire group, therefore, laparoscopy was helpful only in precluding a further surgical exploration in approximately 10% (absent vas and vessels and abdominal vanishing-testis group). Exploration was required in all abdominal and inguinal testes to perform orchidopexy and to confirm the diagnosis in the inguinal vanishing-testis group.

To this simplified analysis, however, additional consideration must be given. Despite the prior analysis (which indicates that 9 of 10 laparoscopies will be unnecessary), some surgeons believe that laparoscopy often alters the choice of incision and subsequent surgery. Furthermore, for those who perform laparoscopic orchidopexy, additional benefits are obvious, because an additional 27% of patients can be treated. Routine laparoscopy, therefore, does not seem to be warranted,

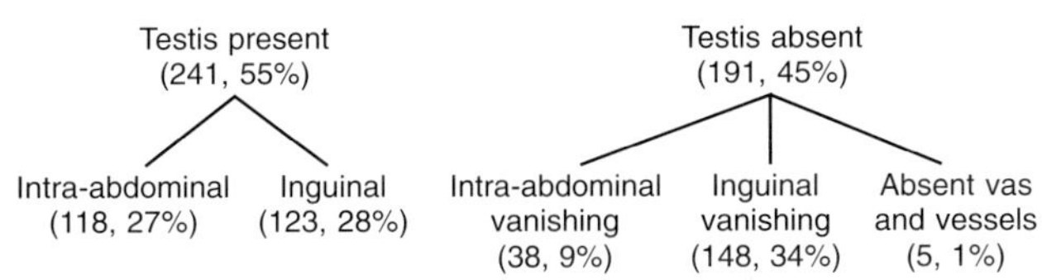

Figure 17–3 Laparoscopic findings in 432 impalpable testes: A collation of five series.

but surgical bias and preference affect the interpretation of this analysis.

Our personal preference is to practice selective laparoscopy; our experience echoes that of others in which the findings in most instances are demonstrable through a standard inguinal incision with intraperitoneal extension. In younger boys, especially in whom a hint of atrophic testicular tissue is palpable in the groin or scrotum and in whom contralateral testicular hypertrophy is present, we believe that laparoscopy is superfluous. In older obese boys with normal scrotal development in whom we suspect testes are present clinically, we similarly proceed to direct surgical exploration. We believe that laparoscopy is useful in reoperative cases, however, in which an incomplete exploration (failure to visualize spermatic vessels or explore intraperitoneally) may have occurred and for older boys in whom intraperitoneal exploration is associated with more postoperative pain and general morbidity. The decision for laparoscopy seems to rest, therefore, on the personal experience of the operator, whether a standard inguinal incision is routinely used, whether a prosthesis will be placed (necessitating an incision even if the testis is absent), and whether a laparoscopic orchidopexy will be performed if the testis is present.

Indications for Treatment

Indications for treating cryptorchid testes include (1) the potential to reduce the observed risk of diminished fertility, (2) the possible prevention of the observed increased risk of malignancy, (3) correction of the associated hernia, (4) reduction of the risk of testis torsion, and (5) alleviation of the psychological stress of an empty scrotum.

Fertility is reduced in both bilateral and unilateral cryptorchidism. Published data indicate that only about 25% of bilaterally treated cryptorchid boys will have normal sperm counts. Sterility is the rule in boys with untreated bilateral cryptorchidism. Similarly, in our extensive literature review, only about 66% of boys with unilateral cryptorchidism were found to be fertile. Failure of normal testis growth, rapid early loss of germ cells (as described previously), endocrine abnormalities associated with even infantile cryptorchidism, and congenital abnormalities of the ductal system all contribute to this reduction in fertility and may coexist.[10]

Testicular cancer also occurs more commonly in the testis that was once cryptorchid. Studies indicate that about 10% of all testis tumors occur in cryptorchid testes. Statistical calculations indicate an increased risk of cancer in cryptorchidism of 20 to 40 times[11]; patients with abdominally located testes and those with bilateral cryptorchidism have a higher risk. Controversy remains regarding whether early orchidopexy (i.e., at or by 1 year of age) will eventually prove to lessen this risk. Presently, there are no data regarding this possibility.

A more clear-cut immediate benefit of orchidopexy is treatment of the usual associated hernia. Separation and repair of the hernia sac are integral parts of the orchidopexy procedure. If a young child is encountered with a clinical hernia and undescended testis before the normal age of repair, orchidopexy should be performed earlier, at the same time as hernia repair.

The risk of testis torsion is definitely increased in cryptorchid testes. Anatomic abnormalities of the investing tunica vaginalis and epididymis are shared by cryptorchid testes as well as descended testes undergoing torsion. A painful, discolored groin mass in an infant with an empty ipsilateral scrotum should immediately raise the suspicion of torsion in an undescended testicle.

Clinicians treating older boys with an empty scrotum are impressed by the prevalence and depth of their psychopathology relating to this issue. We personally have treated several boys with absent testes who have undertaken psychotherapy because of the severe psychological unrest resulting from their condition. Peer ridicule, impairment of body image, adverse personality changes, and fear of sterility have been described.[12] These factors are preventable, in part, by placement of a testicular prosthesis at an early age.

TREATMENT

Orchidopexy is the mainstay of treatment in all but the more distally located testes, in which hormonal therapy may be considered. Choice of treatment is dependent mainly on testis location and patient age, although occasionally other factors affect this decision as well.

Hormonal Treatment

Since its introduction in the 1930s, hCG has been the mainstay of hormonal treatment. The potential for successful treatment varies with age as well as with testis location. Furthermore, success rates from individual reports vary considerably. A variety of factors are responsible for these results, including varying dosage schedules, treatment at different ages, inclusion of boys with retractile testes, and failure to segregate boys being treated who have "higher" testes from the overall group of patients treated. Several large series report a success rate of between 30 and 50%, although we believe that the higher figures pertain mostly to those boys with very distally located (i.e., gliding) testes. Significantly, in some series, early treatment (i.e., just when successful descent is most important) was associated with a much poorer success rate.

The dosage schedule recommended in 1974 by the International Health Foundation is 250 IU per dose in young infants, 500 IU per dose in children up to age 6 years, and 1000 IU per dose in older children, administered in two doses weekly for 5 weeks. Higher or more frequent doses are unhelpful and may be deleterious to the testis. Side effects include increased scrotal rugosity and pigmentation, slight penile growth, and potential for minimal pubic hair growth, which, of course, stops on discontinuation of the medication. Transient increased aggressive behavior may be noted during treatment. Premature epiphyseal closure and subsequent short stature do not occur when these short dosage schedules are used. Subsequent retraction of an initially successfully descended testis can occur in about 20% and often responds to a second brief course of hCG. The use of hCG is contraindicated when a clinical hernia is apparent, in cases with scar fixation of the testis after previous hernia or orchidopexy surgery, and in testes that are ectopically located, because these are mechanically prevented from descending into the scrotum.

Our personal experience with hCG is limited. A number of years ago, we used hCG as primary treatment in 38 prepubertal boys with bilateral cryptorchidism and 19 boys with unilateral cryptorchidism. A 6-week course of treatment (12 injections) was used in the bilateral group and three injections were given over 10 days (short course) in the unilateral group. Twenty-five percent of testes (not always both!) descended in the bilaterally cryptorchid boys and 13% descended in the unilaterally cryptorchid group. Three hernias, not present at initial examination, became clinically apparent during treatment. No other significant side effects were noted. We considered hCG to be ineffective in the unilateral group when used as primary treatment in all but those with the most distally located testes.

More recently in non–North American countries (where approval has not been given for treatment), gonadotropin-releasing hormone (GnRH) analogs have been used to induce testis descent. As with hCG, diverse success rates have been reported. Earlier reviews indicated a success rate ranging from 17 to 38% in double-blinded studies and from 13 to 78% in open studies. Critical analysis indicates that the higher success rates relate to inclusion of more distally located testes in some series, even though great efforts were made to exclude retractile testes. Besides testis location, a direct correlation existed between increasing age and success in some; in others, anatomic abnormalities identified at surgery were present in 80% of failures, which precluded their successful hormonal descent. In the hands of skilled endocrinologists, it is realistic to expect that at least 25% of inguinal cryptorchid testes and at least 66% of more distally located cryptorchid testes can be descended using GnRH.

GnRH is unavailable in the United States, however, limiting our primary treatment options to hCG or orchidopexy. In our practices, we seldom use hCG for anything other than very distal cryptorchidism, giving a short course (three injections) for unilateral cryptorchidism and a long course (6 weeks) for bilateral cryptorchidism. Parents are informed at the onset of treatment that if complete success is not achieved orchidopexy is mandatory. We have also used hCG to induce partial descent to facilitate subsequent surgery. These cases are infrequent (i.e., when additional, albeit incomplete, descent may facilitate a difficult orchidopexy because of small testis size, high position, or underdeveloped blood supply). We also use hCG as sole therapy to "assist" the descent of a borderline retractile or suprascrotal testis into the scrotum.

Surgical Treatment

The general principles of successful orchidopexy are the same as those initially described in 1899 by Bevan: adequate testis and spermatic cord mobilization, repair of the associated hernia, and adequate fixation of the testis in the scrotum. Many subsequent incisions and techniques of fixation have been described. Most investigators advocate an inguinal skin crease incision with extraperitoneal dissection of the cord and testis. An extended high retroperitoneal or intraperitoneal dissection can be done when necessary. For bilateral cases, a Pfannenstiel or midline vertical incision with retroperitoneal or transperitoneal exposure may be used. Currently, fixation of the testis is done by either passing a capsular suture through the adjacent dependent scrotal skin or suturing the tunica vaginalis adjacent to the testis to the adjacent interior of the scrotal wall. Because the choice of operation is largely determined by testicular location, procedures for palpable and impalpable testes are described separately. The procedures outlined are those that we practice and favor.

Palpable undescended testes are usually located in the superficial ectopic space or within a short distance of the external inguinal ring and are best approached by the standard inguinal skin crease incision (Fig. 17–4). Separate inguinal incisions are made when bilateral palpable undescended testes are present. Oblique groin incisions should be avoided because they do not follow Langer's lines and tend to widen, causing broad, unsightly scars. Scarpa's fascia is pierced with a hemostat, and vein retractors are used to spread this incision, exposing the external oblique aponeurosis (Fig. 17–4*A*). At this point, we utilize the useful maneuver of sliding the vein retractor above the external oblique aponeurosis down into the scrotum while lifting the inferior edge of the skin and subcutaneous fascia with the other retractor. This maneuver effortlessly exposes the entire external oblique and external inguinal ring without further dissection. The aponeurosis is then opened, avoiding the underlying ilioinguinal nerve and spermatic cord. The testis will now be evident and is grasped, elevated, and put on traction. The distal attachments to the scrotum are divided sharply by scissors or cautery but are first inspected to ensure that a long-looped vas deferens is not contained within (Fig. 17–4*B*). The spermatic cord is dissected free of the surrounding cremasteric fascia into the internal inguinal ring, carefully dividing and fulgurating the cremasteric

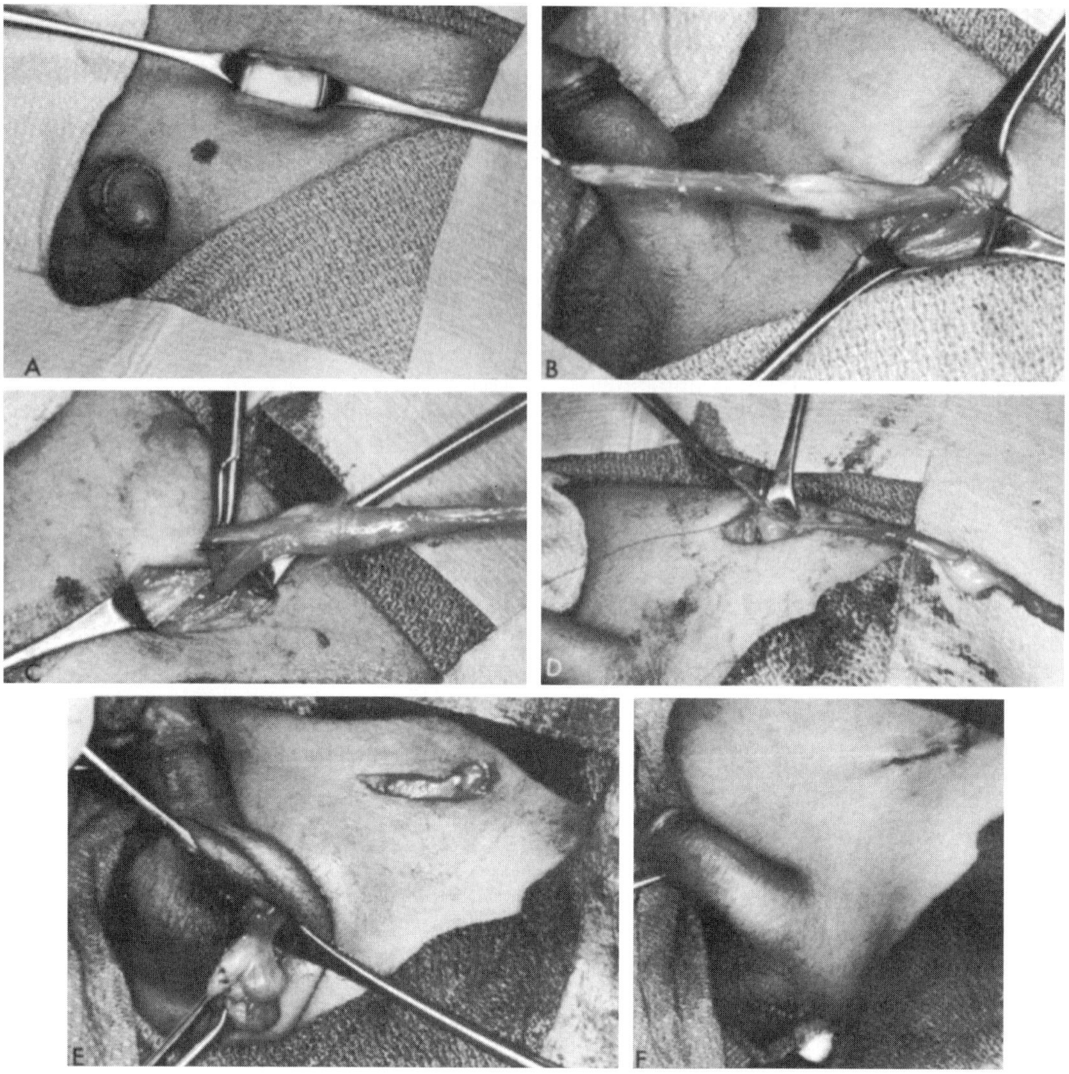

Figure 17–4 Orchidopexy techniques for palpable undescended testes. From Kogan S. Cryptorchidism. In Kelalis PP, King LR, Belman AB (eds), Clinical Pediatric Urology, 3rd ed. Philadelphia: WB Saunders, 1992. Used with permission.

vessels when necessary. A constant branch of the inferior epigastric vessels to the cremasteric fascia, the external spermatic artery and vein, often causes troublesome bleeding at this stage. This may be avoided by dividing the fascia high on the spermatic cord, allowing these vessels to drop onto the floor of the inguinal canal without bleeding. The hernia sac, lying on the anteromedial surface of the cord, is dissected free, twisted, and suture ligated with an absorbable suture (Fig. 17–4*C* and *D*). Sometimes the hernia sac may be thin walled or broad based and can be difficult to separate from the underlying cord structures. In these instances, it is often easier to deliberately open the sac and carefully apply hemostats to its edges as they are dissected free, eventually replacing all holding clamps with a single clamp across the entire sac once it is separated fully from the underlying cord. In most instances, this dissection within the inguinal canal and freeing of the hernia will provide enough length for the testis to reach the scrotum without tension. Occasionally, additional length is needed and may be obtained by dividing the tissue between the lateral abdominal wall and the spermatic cord (lateral spermatic fascia). Further length may be obtained if necessary by opening the internal inguinal ring with the cautery on its anterior surface and then dissecting the spermatic vessels off the overlying peritoneum. Dividing the transversalis fascia forming the floor of the inguinal canal may achieve a more direct path into the scrotum, gaining an additional short distance. The floor is then reconstructed over the cord, placing it in a fully retroperitoneal position and superimposing the internal on the external inguinal ring. Dissection should never be done within the cord itself because this risks damage to the testicular artery and vas deferens and does not result in any additional cord lengthening.

A pathway is then made into the adjacent hemiscrotal compartment with the dissecting finger or a clamp, and a subcutaneous scrotal pouch is fashioned for testicular fixation. A transverse incision is made in the midscrotum, and a plane is found between the overlying skin and dartos muscle and the underlying dartos fascia. A small opening is made and the testis is pulled through the opening (Fig. 17–4*E*). An absorbable suture is passed through the least vascular portion of the testis capsule, passed through the adjacent scrotal skin with a straight needle, and tied, fixing the testis in place. If a high testis is initially present or if there is any tension, the suture is passed through a gauze pledget and left for 10 days before removing (Fig. 17–4*F*). Alternatively, the adjacent covering tunica about the testis can be sutured to the interior dartos of the scrotum with absorbable sutures. Testicular biopsy is often done at this point, closing the capsular incision with a fine absorbable suture. The epididymis is placed within the upper aspect of the pouch, and the scrotal incision is closed with a running or interrupted absorbable suture. The internal inguinal ring, when dilated, is narrowed by placing absorbable sutures between the internal oblique muscle and the shelving edge of the inguinal ligament, allowing adequate room for spermatic cord mobility. The external oblique fascia and subcutaneous tissue are closed with a running absorbable suture and the skin with a fine absorbable subcuticular closure. Colloidion and tape are applied as the only dressing.

Surgical treatment of impalpable testes is much more demanding and complex. Special considerations must be given regarding choice of incision and technique of orchidopexy. Because a significant number of impalpable testes will ultimately be shown to be absent, a properly planned stepwise exploration is the key to diagnosing and confirming this finding. For some, as indicated earlier, a diagnostic laparoscopy will immediately precede any incision. For ourselves, because we practice selective use of laparoscopy in this setting, laparoscopy will be used only in the absence of clear-cut contralateral testicular hypertrophy, when bilateral impalpable cryptorchidism is present, in boys in whom a previous surgical exploration has been incomplete or older age suggests that laparoscopy may minimize morbidity, or when a laparoscopic orchidopexy or orchiectomy is contemplated to follow.

If laparoscopy is used as the "first diagnostic step," the algorithm indicated in Table 17–3 may be used. Laparoscopy may immediately localize the testis to an abdominal or nonabdominal location. If an abdominal testis is located, laparoscopic single-stage or staged orchidopexy or open abdominal orchidopexy may be accomplished. If blind-ending vas and vessels are noted, no further diagnostic exploration is needed (although a testicular prosthesis may be placed and suture fixation of the contralateral descended testis should be done). If neither vas deferens nor spermatic vessels are encountered or only a blind-ending vas is seen, either open exploration or further workup with CT scan or MRI is indicated, because a testis may be located higher (i.e., at a level between the kidney and the iliac vessels even when a blind-ending vas exists lower down in the pelvis). Testes in these locations are rare but do exist and are not visualized during routine diagnostic laparoscopy. When the vessels and vas deferens are seen entering the internal inguinal ring, open inguinal exploration is indicated.

Table 17–3
Impalpable Testis: Laparoscopic Findings and Management

Finding	Management
Abdominal testis visualized	Perform laparoscopic or open single-stage or staged orchidopexy (rarely orchiectomy).
Abdominal testis not visualized	
Spermatic vessels entering internal inguinal ring	Suggests either normal or atrophied ("vanishing") testis in inguinal canal; open inguinal exploration indicated.
Blind-ending spermatic vessels with or without vas deferens in abdomen	Testis is absent; no further exploration necessary. Contralateral scrotal orchidopexy and prosthesis are indicated.
Blind-ending vas deferens	Testis still may be present but separated from vas. Continued laparoscopic or open exploration indicated.
No spermatic vessels or vas deferens found	Testis may be present but not visualized. Perform CT or MRI or continue with higher laparoscopic or open exploration.

CT, computed tomography; MRI, magnetic resonance imaging.

When diagnostic laparoscopy is not chosen as the initial step, exploration is initiated through a standard inguinal skin crease incision. Separate skin crease incisions are used in bilateral cases unless the patient is obese, in which case a Pfannenstiel incision joining the two offers additional improved exposure. Even here some controversy exists, and some prefer a higher placed oblique extraperitoneal incision for unilateral cases or a midline extra- or intraperitoneal incision when bilateral impalpable cryptorchidism is present. We find that the standard inguinal skin crease incision does not limit exposure and can easily be extended slightly superiorly to provide wider intraperitoneal exposure when necessary.

If a testis is not encountered on opening the inguinal canal, the internal inguinal ring is immediately opened with cautery. Usually a tongue of protruding peritoneum is evident, the "harbinger" of the testis within, which will prolapse into this peritoneal sac if pressure is placed on the abdomen above. When a testis is located in this manner, it should be put on stretch along with the sac to assess its mobility to determine whether high retroperitoneal dissection and ligation of the hernia sac will provide adequate length for orchidopexy. Whereas no criteria currently exist for making this decision, with experience the surgeon learns which testes will have adequate length for this extended orchidopexy and which will require even more complex orchidopexy techniques. If local retroperitoneal exploration fails to demonstrate a testis, the peritoneum is opened without extending the retroperitoneal exploration further. Although the testis and vas deferens are truly retroperitoneal organs, they are much more easily visualized by viewing them intraperitoneally just as the ovary exists suspended on its own mesentery in an even more exaggerated "intraperitoneal" position. Packing the bowels superiorly with the patient in the Trendelenburg position facilitates this exposure. A thorough search is then made between the internal inguinal ring and the bladder, also visualizing the posterior peritoneum superiorly to the iliac artery and vein, along the usual course of the internal spermatic vessels. When bilateral cryptorchidism is present, a Pfannenstiel or midline infraumbilical transperitoneal incision may be used; we prefer the former. Figure 17–5 illustrates an algorithm that may be used for conceptualizing the approach to open surgical exploration of impalpable cryptorchid testes.

When performing these dissections, it may become apparent that a testis is absent. Monorchia occurs in about 4% of cryptorchid testes overall but in about 20 to 40% of impalpable testes. Various anatomic patterns may be found indicating the presence of monorchia: If attenuated spermatic vessels, a vas deferens, or a minispermatic cord is encountered, it is traced to its termination distally and proximally within the internal inguinal ring to the point of divergence of the vas deferens and vessels, ensuring that true spermatic vessels are present coursing up the posterior peritoneum. Identifying these vessels accurately as spermatic vessels rather than cremasteric or vasal in origin is important because blind-ending spermatic vessels signal the end of the exploration; a testis cannot exist above. If a vas deferens alone is encountered, the exploration must proceed further because wide separation of the vas and an intra-abdominal testis do occur. Similarly, if no vas or vessels are encountered, the exploration must proceed further because a more proximally

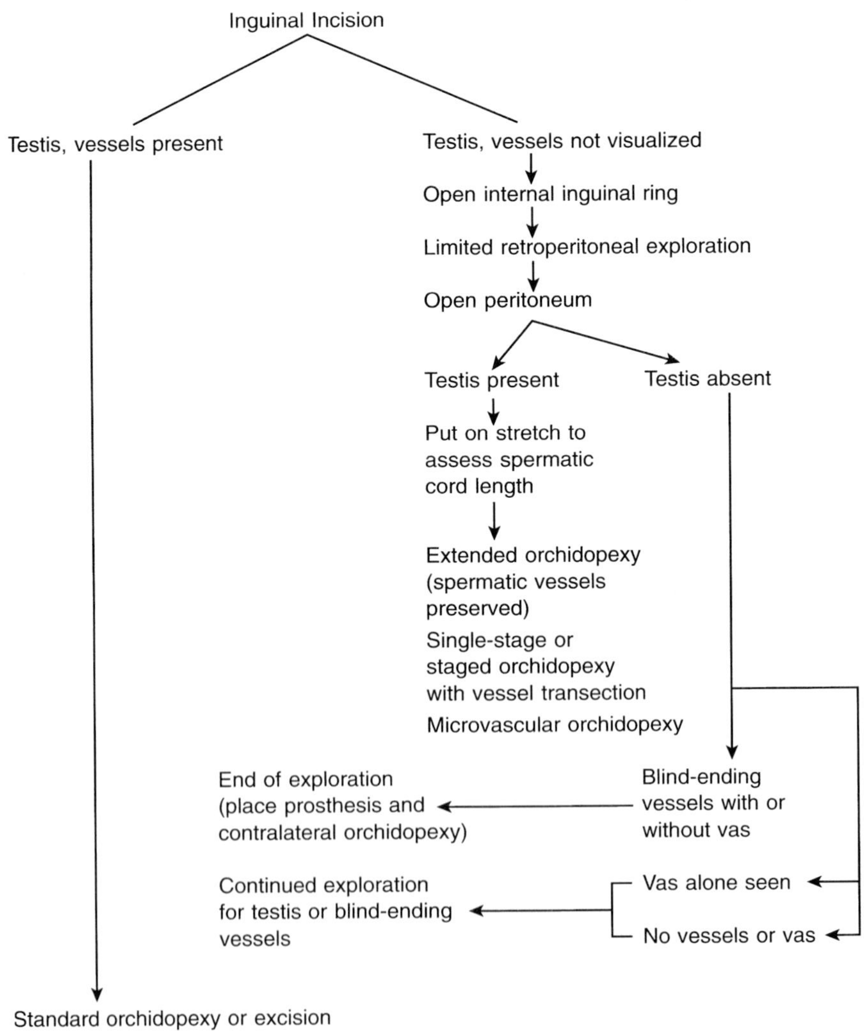

Figure 17–5 Impalpable testis: algorithm for surgical management.

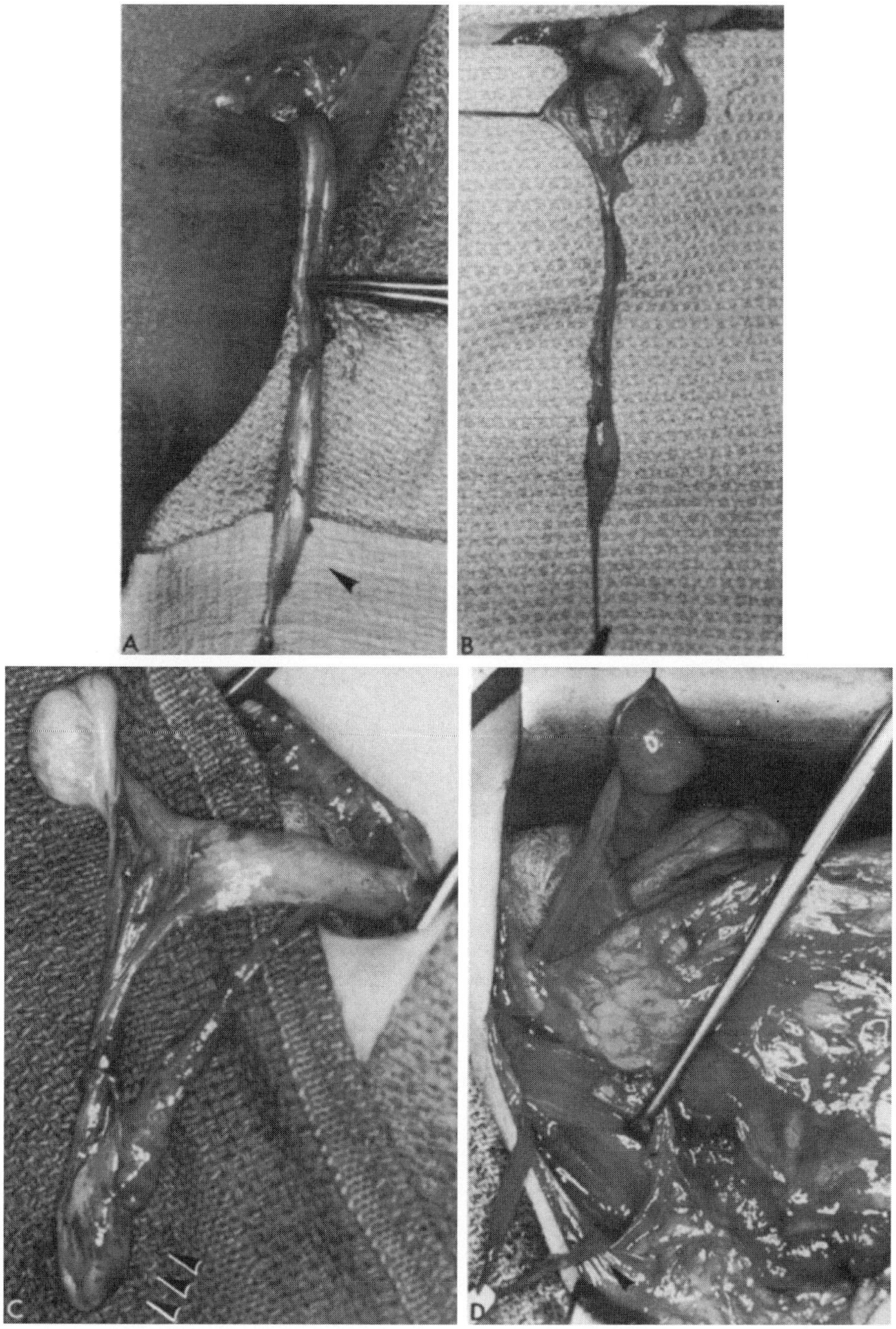

Figure 17–6 Misleading ductal structures simulating an absent testis. From Kogan S. Cryptorchidism. In Kelalis PP, King LR, Belman AB (eds), Clinical Pediatric Urology, 3rd ed. Philadelphia: WB Saunders, 1992. Used with permission.

located testis may exist above. Accurate identification of these structures is sometimes difficult and confusing, and the gross findings are easily misleading (Fig. 17–6). A looped epididymis or vas may simulate the gross appearance of a blind-ending spermatic cord or atrophic testis and may accidentally be excised, leaving an abdominal testis above. We have found testes above the level of the internal inguinal ring at re-exploration when an earlier "complete" exploration failed to include an intraperitoneal exposure. A thorough intraperitoneal exposure is mandatory with further attention to these guidelines to diagnose a testis as absent.

When monorchia occurs, we personally choose to "protect" the contralateral descended testis from any subsequent risk of torsion by performing contralateral scrotal orchidopexy. The basis for this approach is speculative in part but offers additional safety. Data indicate that almost all episodes of "absent" testes occur as a result of a previous, often prenatal, testicular torsion. Because the anatomy predisposing to torsion is often bilateral, we wish to minimize the risk of torsion ever occurring in the solitary remaining testis. A small transverse scrotal incision is made down to the underlying testis, which is everted. Two nonabsorbable sutures are taken between the testicular capsule and the adjacent dartos at the 3 and 9 o'clock positions, and the scrotum is closed. Opponents of this approach claim that the frequency of torsion in the solitary testis is minimal and that this approach potentially puts this testis at risk. We have never had a single testis become infected or suffer any visible degree of atrophy, however, from this maneuver.

Placement of a testicular prosthesis may be considered when the testis is absent. My personal experience indicates that, to some parents of younger boys and to almost all adolescent boys, a testicular prosthesis is extremely important for psychological well-being. An empty scrotum is often devastating to an adolescent, with severe effects on his body image. For these reasons, we offer a prosthesis at any age, at the same time that an absent testis is diagnosed. Controversy has existed regarding the safety of the silicone component of these testicular prostheses, citing the adverse reports of autoimmune and connective tissue diseases in women with breast prostheses with a similar filling. The initial scare regarding the safety of these silicone prostheses has to a great extent lessened as prospective, controlled studies of this problem have been done. Similar claims have not been made on any large scale for testicular prostheses. Presently, older gel-filled silicone testicular prostheses are no longer produced; the silicone elastomer models have been discontinued and saline-filled prostheses with a silicone outer shell are expected to become available in

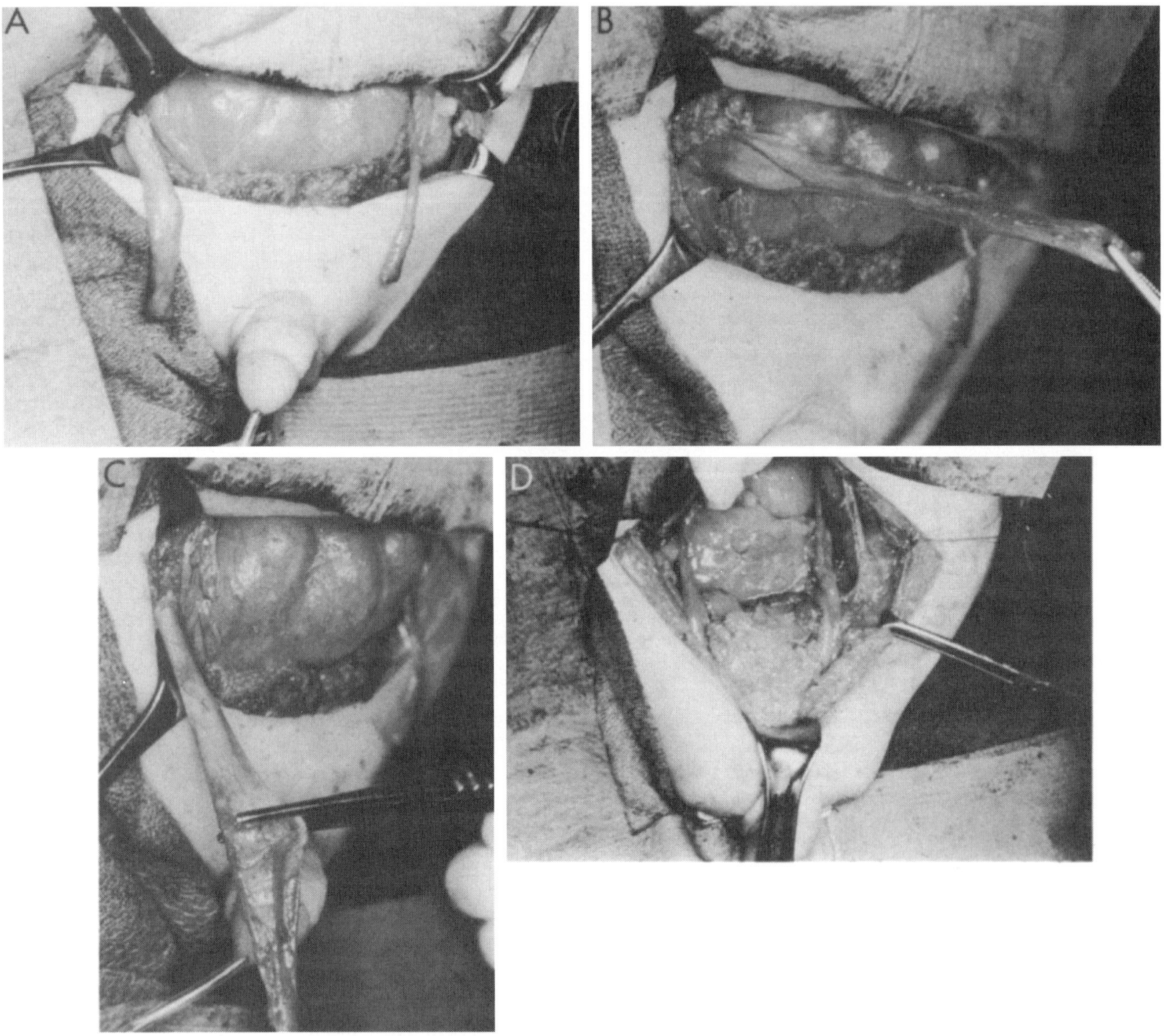

Figure 17–7 Extended orchidopexy of impalpable testes by high retroperitoneal dissection. From Gillenwater JY, Grayhack JT, Howards SS, Duckett JW (eds), Adult and Pediatric Urology, 2nd ed. Chicago: Mosby–Year Book, 1991. Used with permission.

mid-1997. Prostheses currently are available in four sizes: child, youth, and adult medium and large. An infant size will be available shortly. A small prosthesis placed in early childhood will require change for an adult size in late adolescence or young adulthood. Testicular prostheses should never be placed through a scrotal incision in childhood because there is a significant erosion rate through the thin prepubertal scrotal skin. Peri- and postoperative antibiotics are used to prevent infection for 5 days after the prosthesis is placed. We personally have never had an infected prosthesis after following these precautions.

After the testis is located, the next step is to take a holding suture through the capsule at its most avascular portion. This is an important step because, by putting gentle traction on the testis and spermatic vessel leash, the surgeon can assess the mobility of the testis and the length of the spermatic vessels. Visual inspection may indicate that a high dissection, aided by the intraperitoneal exposure, may be adequate for achieving adequate spermatic vessel length for orchidopexy (Fig. 17–7). It is surprising how many of these higher placed, even intra-abdominally located testes can be successfully descended by this technique of "extended" orchidopexy with preservation of the spermatic vessels. If this initial spermatic vessel stretch to determine mobility and length indicates, however, that the vessels seem too short, orchidopexy by spermatic vessel transection, with or without microvascular vessel reanastamosis, or staged orchidopexy is indicated. Our personal choice is to use a single-stage orchidopexy with transection of the short limiting vessels, providing the collateral blood supply is adequate (as determined by the Fowler-Stephens "test") (Fig. 17–8).

After localization of the testis as described previously, the posterior peritoneum is incised and the spermatic

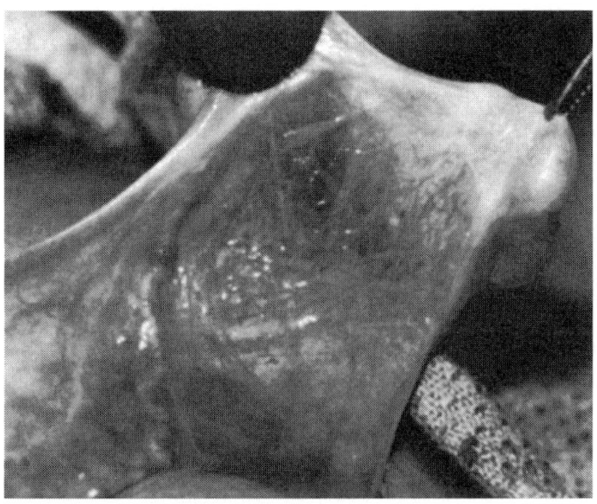

Figure 17–8 Collateral circulation between internal spermatic and vasal vessels in abdominal cryptorchidism. From Kogan S. Cryptorchidism. In Kelalis PP, King LR, Belman AB (eds), Clinical Pediatric Urology, 3rd ed. Philadelphia: WB Saunders, 1992. Used with permission.

vessels are mobilized high, in some cases to the lower pole of the kidney, an exposure which is achievable through this incision. The testis is incised after placement of a bulldog clamp high on the spermatic vessels (Fig. 17–9). If bleeding is brisk and is maintained after several minutes, we divide the spermatic vessels high away from the testis to preserve whatever collateral vessels may be present closer between the vas deferens and its collateral blood supply and the distal leash of transected spermatic vessels. A broad-based medial triangle of peritoneum is developed containing the vas deferens and preserving its blood supply and its collaterals. The testis is brought down on this pedicle, taking care to sweep all local vascular tissue with it and to align it in its most direct course into the scrotum. Usually a new entry into the scrotum is made just lateral to the pubic tubercle. The peritoneum is not closed, and a new inguinal ring is fashioned around this medially based peritoneal pedicle, carefully ensuring that no constriction occurs. Only one hernia has developed as a result of this technique through this newly created "internal-external" inguinal ring. In a previous publication, an 89% success rate in 38 of these difficult testes was achieved by using the Fowler-Stephens test to predict which testis had a viable collateral blood supply and applying meticulous attention to detail in the surgical dissection.[13] Additional essential points maximizing success have been (1) leaving a wide, medially based peritoneal strip along the vas deferens; (2) performing the procedure in a premeditated fashion, not as a salvage operation after fully mobilizing the testis as in conventional orchidopexy; (3) ligating the spermatic vessels high away from the testis; and (4) avoiding inadvertent injury to the vasal artery.[14] In our patients if the testis did not bleed adequately, single-stage orchidopexy by testicular vessel transection was not done. In two subsequent cases in which a short vas deferens was present, a staged secondary procedure was accomplished successfully, indicating that persistence is sometimes necessary in dealing with these difficult testes.

An alternative approach is planned staged orchidopexy with ligation of the spermatic vessels.[15] When the testis is exposed and is located very high, or if the collateral vessels along the vas deferens are attenuated, the spermatic vessels are ligated high away from the testis without any mobilization of the testis. An interval period of several months allows the collateral blood supply along the vas to develop, and a second-stage orchidopexy is then done. This procedure seems to be safer and more reliable, especially for the less experienced surgeon. We have used this technique selectively, especially in very small patients in whom the collateral blood supply was believed to be inadequate initially. Staged orchidopexy with initial vessel ligation also lends itself to a laparoscopic approach, with a first-stage clipping and a subsequent laparoscopic or open repair.

Microvascular orchidopexy offers an additional alter-

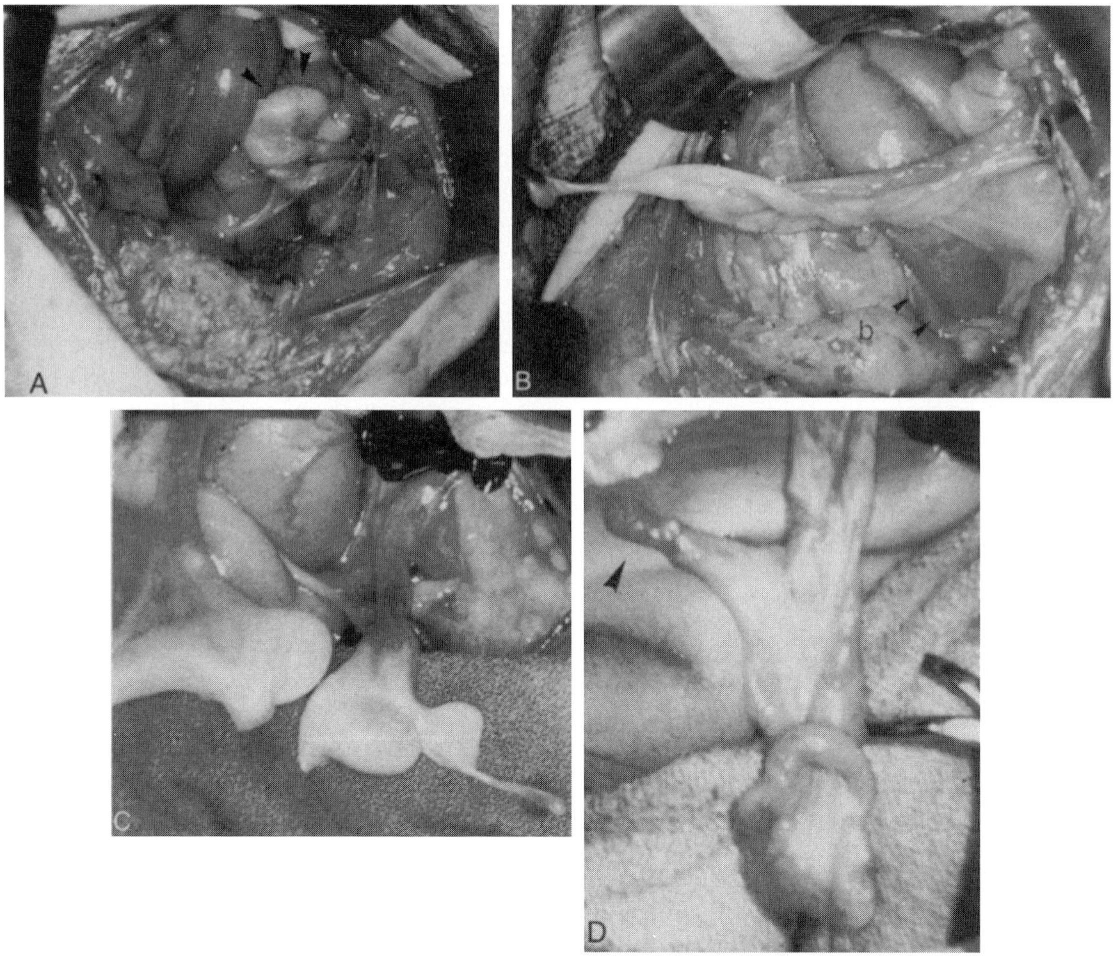

Figure 17–9 Technique of orchidopexy by spermatic vessel transection. From Kogan S. Cryptorchidism. In Kelalis PP, King LR, Belman AB (eds), Clinical Pediatric Urology, 3rd ed. Philadelphia: WB Saunders, 1992. Used with permission.

native to single-stage open repair. Re-establishment of an intact blood supply by anastomosing the internal spermatic artery to the inferior epigastric artery seems to offer additional safety beyond reliance on the collateral blood supply along the vas deferens. Because many urologists are now adept at microsurgical techniques, it is logical to expect that this procedure could come to be used more extensively, and in experienced hands the success rate with this procedure is exceptional.[16] Despite this, the operating microscope is not set up routinely for use in most cases of impalpable testes, especially for unilateral cases, and a successful result is not universally obtained in every instance. Our absolute indication for this procedure is the boy with a solitary testis. After exposure of the abdominal testis, as described previously, the spermatic vessels are dissected high, sometimes up to their junction with the aorta, vena cava, or renal vein to obtain as wide a lumen as possible. This maneuver sometimes is important because the artery often has a diameter no larger than 1 to 2 mm in the small child. The epigastric vessels are initially exposed in the floor of the inguinal canal and then dissected superiorly off the underside of the rectus muscle. Under the operating microscope, the smaller spermatic artery is anastomosed to the larger epigastric artery using an approximating microsurgical clamp and interrupted 10-0 or 11-0 nylon sutures. Controversy exists whether venous anastomosis needs to be done as well, but we have personally seen severe venous engorgement in some instances when the veins are simply ligated and prefer the venous anastomosis to be done simultaneously.

Before development of these surgical procedures, staged orchidopexy was used when the testis could not be successfully descended in one stage. Previous literature describing this procedure indicated an 80 to 90% success rate, making it a reliable technique to use with difficult impalpable cryptorchid testes. Nevertheless, the improved facility and general success with single-stage orchidopexy has made staged procedures less frequent. After maximal mobilization of the spermatic cord and testis, the testis is fixed with a nonabsorbable suture to the most dependent position obtainable without tension, usually the pubic tubercle, inguinal ligament, or upper scrotum. A second exploration and further orchidopexy are done after a 6- to 12-month interval, allowing adequate time for the spermatic cord to lengthen. These reoperations are often difficult because of scarring, with a considerable risk of vas or vessel injury.

Laparoscopic orchidopexy in either a single stage or two stages was an inevitable and logical extension of the increased use of diagnostic laparoscopy. This procedure benefits by the magnification that is obtained during laparoscopy, allowing for precise definition of the blood vessels and accurate dissection. After visualization of an abdominal testicle through an umbilical port, two additional trocars are placed under direct vision inferior to the umbilicus and lateral to the rectus muscle. The distal extent of the processus vaginalis is dissected free and transected. The peritoneal lining over the testis and vas is dissected using the transected processus for traction on the testicle. An L-type incision can be made over the internal inguinal ring, extending the longer limb proximally, lateral to the spermatic vessels. A further higher dissection may be done when necessary by mobilizing the sigmoid colon by incising the lateral peritoneal reflection. When adequate cord length is obtained, a new course is made into the scrotum immediately lateral to the pubic tubercle. A variety of techniques may be used for this procedure: initially a grasper can be tunneled into the scrotum, followed by passage of an additional trocar back into the abdomen, or graduated Teflon fascial dilators may be used retrograde in a similar fashion to enlarge the tract. Alternatively, the tunnel may be made from the outside into the abdominal cavity, with the surgeon observing under direct vision as it is made. The testis is pulled into the scrotum and fixed in a subcutaneous scrotal pouch. The abdominal cavity is inspected under reduced insufflation pressure and the trocars are removed, closing their entry points with absorbable sutures.

In evaluating the benefits of laparoscopic orchidopexy, the old adage of "just because one *can* do a procedure safely and efficiently, *should* you do it?" must be considered. Questions regarding the safety of this procedure have largely been resolved. The short-term success rate seems as good if not better than that with open orchidopexy. The procedure sometimes is of longer duration, is more costly when disposable laparoscopic instruments are used, and has been shown even at this early juncture to be overused frequently by extending it to testes that prolapse in and out of the internal inguinal ring, easily and more appropriately descended by conventional orchidopexy. Furthermore, a dangerous trend has developed demonstrating that laparoscopic orchidopexy surgeons overuse the two-stage clipping technique and perform more frequent orchiectomies.[17] The future will bring more precise definition of the indications for laparoscopic orchidopexy. Long-term follow-up studies of patients treated by laparoscopic single-stage or staged orchidopexy are needed to validate its benefit.

Regardless of the orchidopexy technique utilized, satisfactory postoperative analgesia should be provided. Local infiltration of bupivacaine 0.25% within the inguinal wound and around the ilioinguinal nerve as it exits the inguinal canal or peri- or postoperative caudal anesthesia is effective. In younger boys, simple placement of an analgesic rectal suppository is surprisingly effective as well. In older boys, I have found that nonsteroidal intravenous analgesics such as ketorolac tromethamine (Toradol) offer excellent postoperative pain relief after more extensive surgery.

RESULTS OF SURGERY AND PREVENTION OF COMPLICATIONS

Many series have attempted to analyze surgical results after orchidopexy, but most are flawed by inconsistency in locating the testis preoperatively and inconsistency in defining results. In general, about 90% of palpable testes and 60 to 80% of impalpable testes have historically had a "good" result. The most common complications noted are atrophy (2–20%) and retraction of the testis to a nondependent location (at least 10%). A 1 to 2% frequency of vasal injury is cited. A high dissection is necessary in every case to obtain adequate cord mobility for tension-free scrotal placement. Meticulous attention to detail while mobilizing the spermatic cord and preventing dissection within the cord itself, minimizing traction, and tension-free scrotal placement are all important factors in achieving optimal surgical results. Accurate identification and recognition of the entire ductal (epididymal and vasal) anatomy are essential in every case to prevent inadvertent ductal injury.

CONCLUSIONS AND RECOMMENDATIONS FOR OPTIMAL THERAPY

Ample histologic data exist confirming the detrimental effect of leaving the testis in an extrascrotal position beyond 1 year of age as well as the impact of lack of treatment on fertility. Orchidopexy, at present, is the most successful treatment for all but the most distally located testes, in which case hCG treatment may be used first. Experience also has demonstrated that, with appropriate training, surgeons can perform orchidopexy as safely and efficiently in earlier years as in the older child. Furthermore, the diagnosis of cryptorchidism is easier at this early age because the cremasteric reflex is minimally developed, and location at examination more accurately indicates true testis position at this age. Morbidity is minimized and recovery is facilitated by early treatment as well because restrictions on postoperative mobility are more easily accomplished. These factors have led to a revision of the older recommendations of the American Academy of Pediatrics regarding optimal timing of surgery for cryptorchidism. The Academy presently recommends that treatment by 1 year of age most successfully achieves these goals.[18]

REFERENCES

1. Hadziselimovic F. Cryptorchidism: Management and Implications. New York: Springer-Verlag, 1983.
2. Huff DS, Hadziselimovic F, McSnyder H, et al. Postnatal testicular development in unilateral cryptorchidism. J Urol 142:546, 1989.
3. Huff DS, Hadziselimovic F, McSnyder H, et al. Early postnatal testicular maldevelopment in cryptorchidism. J Urol 146:624, 1991.
4. Gill B, Kogan SJ, Starr S, et al. Significance of epididymal and ductal anomalies associated with testicular maldescent. J Urol 142:556, 1989.
5. Hutson JM, Beasley SW. Descent of the Testis. London: Edward Arnold, 1992.
6. Kogan SJ, Tennenbaum SZ, Gill B, et al. Efficacy of orchidopexy by patient age one year for cryptorchidism. J Urol 144:508, 1990.
7. Koff SA. Does compensatory testicular enlargement predict monorchidism? J Urol 146:632, 1991.
8. Kogan SJ. Work-up and management of the bilateral nonpalpable testis. In Gonzales ET Jr, Roth D (eds), Common Problems in Pediatric Urology. St. Louis, MO: Mosby Yearbook, 1991, p 294.
9. Hrebinko RL, Bellinger MJ. The limited role of imaging techniques in managing children with undescended testes. J Urol 150:458, 1993.
10. Kogan SJ. Fertility in cryptorchidism. An overview in 1987. Eur J Pediatr 146 (Suppl 2):S21, 1987.
11. Chilvers C, Dudley NE, Gough MH, et al. Undescended testis: The effect of treatment and subsequent risk of subfertility and malignancy. J Pediatr Surg 21:691, 1986.
12. Bell AI. Psychological implications of the scrotal sac and testes for the male child. Clin Pediatr 13:838, 1974.
13. Kogan SJ, Houman BZ, Reda EF, Levitt SB. Orchidopexy of the high undescended testis by division of the spermatic vessels. A critical review of 38 selected transections. J Urol 141:1416, 1989.
14. Gibbons MD, Cromie WJ, Duckett JW, Jr. Management of the abdominal undescended testicle. J Urol 122:76, 1979.
15. Ransley PG, Vordermark JS, Caldamone AA, Bellinger MF. Preliminary ligation of the gonadal vessels prior to orchidopexy for the intra-abdominal testicle. World J Urol 2:266, 1984.
16. Bukowski TP, Wacksman J, Billmire DA, et al. Testicular autotransplantation: A 17 year review of an effective approach to the management of the intra-abdominal testis. J Urol 154:558, 1995
17. Ferro F, Lais A, Gonzalez-Serva L. Benefits and afterthoughts of laparoscopy for the nonpalpable testis. J Urol 156:795, 1996.
18. Section on Urology, American Academy of Pediatrics. Timing of elective surgery on the genitalia of male children with reference to the risks, benefits, and psychological effects of surgery and anesthesia. Pediatrics 97:590, 1996.

ELIZABETH B. YERKES & JOHN W. BROCK III

18

Diagnosis and Management of Testicular Torsion

Early diagnosis and treatment of testicular torsion are central to the preservation of the gonad and its contribution to endocrine function and fertility. Loss of reproductive capacity and endocrine function of the ischemic gonad has been experimentally shown to occur after fewer than 12 hours of ischemia. These findings may not correlate precisely with the degree of ischemia in spontaneous torsion of human gonads but certainly lend urgency to the treatment of acute testicular torsion.[1] Diagnosis is primarily based on clinical suspicion after review of presenting symptoms and physical findings, but additional studies may be helpful in equivocal cases. Because the loss of gonadal function can occur so rapidly, surgical exploration in highly suspicious cases should never be delayed for further diagnostic studies. Testicular perfusion studies or Doppler ultrasound examinations are the best diagnostic studies currently available, but they also have some pitfalls. Exploration is the only sure diagnostic and therapeutic tool, and the decision to proceed with surgical exploration based on clinical suspicions should never be superseded by negative radiographic findings.

PATHOGENESIS

Torsion is traditionally classified as either extravaginal or intravaginal based on the anatomic relationship between the spermatic cord and the scrotal contents (Fig. 18–1). Extravaginal torsion, twisting of the spermatic cord above the level of the tunica vaginalis, occurs exclusively in the perinatal period, because the attachments between the tunica vaginalis and scrotal wall are often not established until approximately 7 to 10 days of life in full-term infants.[2] The testicle and tunica are, therefore, free to rotate as a unit about their longitudinal axis. Above-average birth weight, the stress of labor and delivery, and an overactive cremasteric reflex have been postulated to contribute to extravaginal torsion,[3] but no clear cause has been established.

Intravaginal torsion is primarily seen in older children and adolescents but has been reported in the perinatal period and in adulthood. A relatively narrow attachment of mesorchium to the testicle and an unusually high insertion of the tunica vaginalis onto the spermatic cord are the anatomic abnormalities that predispose the testicle to intravaginal torsion. Without normal support, the ovoid testicle assumes a horizontal or even an inverted position within the scrotum. The tunica vaginalis then cradles the testicle, leaving no point of contact between the posterior surface of the testicle and the scrotal wall (Fig. 18–2). This anatomic variant is often referred to as the bell-clapper deformity. The testicle can twist on its cord within the tunica, like the clapper in a bell. Individuals with this deformity are subject to torsion at any time, but the incidence increases when testicular volume increases. The already foreshortened attachment of the mesentery onto the testicle encourages twisting of the gonad on its cord. An increase in testicular volume obviously occurs at puberty but conceivably could occur acutely with trauma, severe orchitis, or growth of a testic-

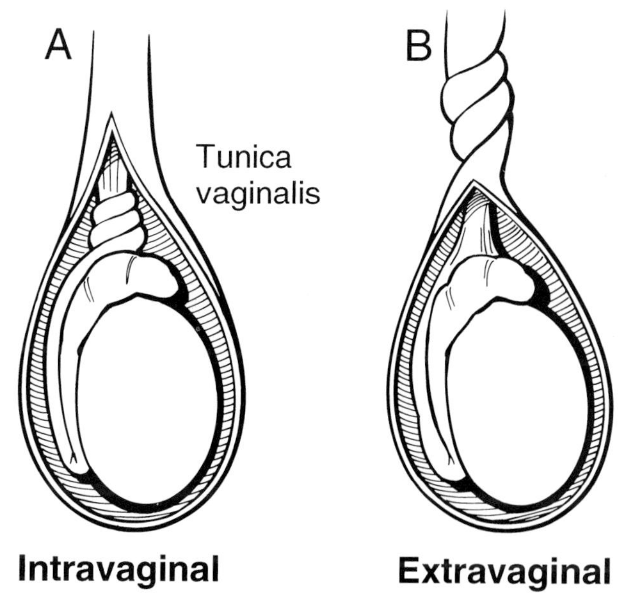

Figure 18–1 *A* and *B*, Diagrams of intravaginal and extravaginal testicular torsion.

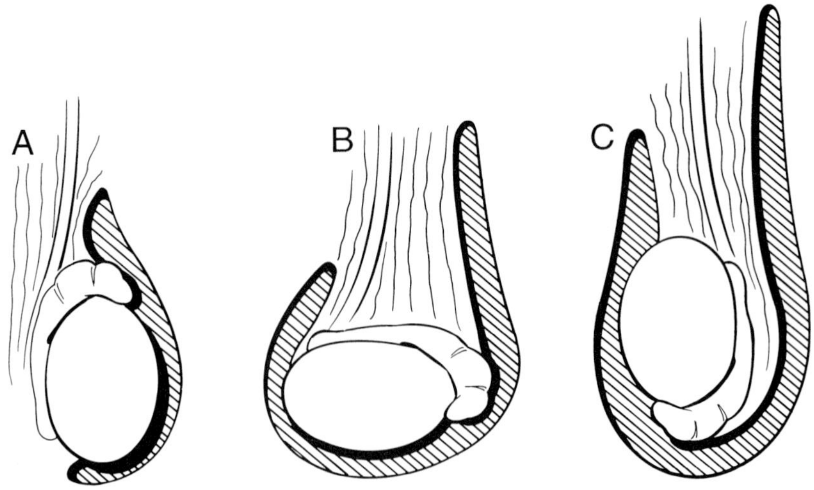

Figure 18–2 Diagram of bell-clapper deformity. *A*, Normal anatomic relationships. *B* and *C*, A high insertion of the tunica vaginalis allows the testicle to assume an abnormal lie.

ular tumor. Torsion may also occur intermittently, with pain resolving acutely as detorsion spontaneously occurs. The fleeting nature of this problem does not rule out ultimate persistent torsion. The lack of lasting findings in intermittent torsion presents special diagnostic problems. Intermittent torsion should be suspected in any male with intermittent recurrent testicular pain, even if the testicle is asymptomatic at the time of evaluation. If the patient is examined while standing, the symptomatic or contralateral testis, or both, may assume a horizontal lie suggestive of the bell-clapper deformity.[4, 5]

DIAGNOSIS

The differential diagnoses for unilateral scrotal pain, mass, or swelling vary with the age of the patient, but the urgent nature of acute testicular torsion should always place it near the top of the list. In utero torsion is a unique phenomenon in that it is generally a subacute or chronic process by the time the infant is delivered. The scrotum may be edematous with a bluish discoloration or a bruised appearance and does not transilluminate. The testicle may be enlarged and firm but appears to be nontender, with the infant in no distress. The differential diagnosis should include hydrocele, hematocele, incarcerated inguinal hernia, hematoma from birth trauma, torsion of the appendix testis or epididymis, meconium peritonitis, epididymal orchitis, ectopic viscus, or very rarely neoplasm.

Early postnatal torsion has a similar differential diagnosis, but the infant has the distinction of having a normal scrotal examination at birth. Discoloration or swelling subsequently develops, perhaps intermittently at first, and tenderness is a more prominent feature because the torsion is now occurring as an acute process.

In older children and adolescents, testicular torsion is more common and presents as acute scrotal pain, followed by erythema and edema of the scrotum and its contents (Fig. 18–3). The testicle is enlarged and tender on examination, and as edema increases, the delineation between testicle and epididymis may be impalpable. A hydrocele may be present, and the testicle often assumes a retracted and abnormal lie within the scrotum, depending on the degree of rotation about the spermatic cord. A low-grade fever may be present, but urinalysis is

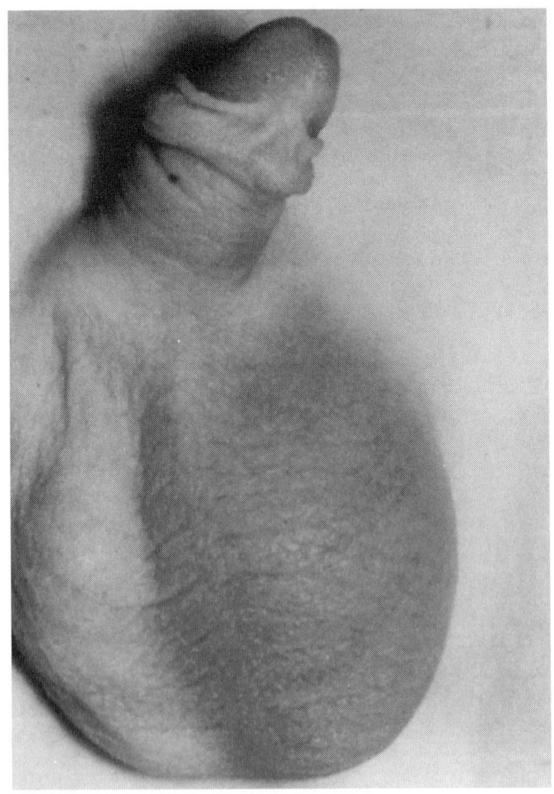

Figure 18–3 Scrotal edema and discoloration in a child with testicular torsion.

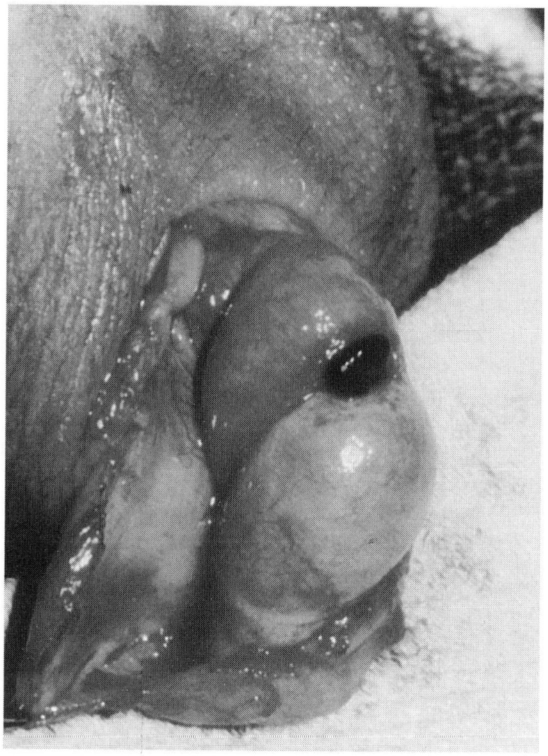

Figure 18–4 Torsion of the appendix testis.

generally clear. The physical findings or history may lead the physician to misdiagnose torsion as epididymal orchitis, torsion of testicular or epididymal appendages, idiopathic scrotal edema, trauma, or tumor. Radiographic investigation may provide helpful clarification.

Epididymal orchitis is more frequently the diagnosis in febrile patients with pyuria and among those who are sexually active, although it can occur in any age group. Torsion of one of the pedunculated peritesticular appendages presents initially with more focal pain, but the symptoms become identical to those of testicular torsion itself. If the scrotum is examined before the onset of diffuse scrotal edema, the torted and focally engorged appendix may be palpable as a discrete nodule along the superior pole of the testicle (Fig. 18–4). A subcutaneous "blue dot" may also be apparent on transillumination and is pathognomonic for torsion of the appendix testis. A torsive appendage can be managed symptomatically and nonoperatively, and symptoms can be expected to resolve spontaneously within 1 to 2 weeks. Idiopathic scrotal edema is an allergic condition producing painless swelling of the perineum and groin, most commonly in prepubertal children. Treatment includes antihistamines or observation.[6] Trauma may produce a tender scrotal mass from testicular rupture, hematoma, or hematocele. Testicular rupture also requires urgent exploration for gonadal salvage, and a severe testicular hematoma may even lead to infarction from the increased pressure within the intact tunica albuginea. Tumor requires early elective radical inguinal orchiectomy.

ADDITIONAL DIAGNOSTIC METHODS

Radiographic studies have evolved to provide supplemental information regarding both gonadal perfusion and anatomic detail. We cannot emphasize enough that findings on radiographic studies should never negate clinical suspicion of torsion, and exploration of any boy with physical or clinical findings suggestive of torsion should not be delayed to obtain further diagnostic studies. Perfusion studies should be reserved for those acute scrotal cases in which torsion is not suspected but must be ruled out and for cases in which torsion has likely been present for more than 24 to 36 hours and salvage of the testicle with even immediate intervention is unlikely.[7] Radionuclide scans were previously the gold standard for determining the presence or absence of testicular perfusion (Fig. 18–5), but in more recent years, Doppler ultrasonography has become popular because it provides equally accurate assessment of flow and also provides important anatomic cues. When these technologies are readily available and are used by *experienced* personnel, they can provide valuable additional diagnostic information in equivocal cases.

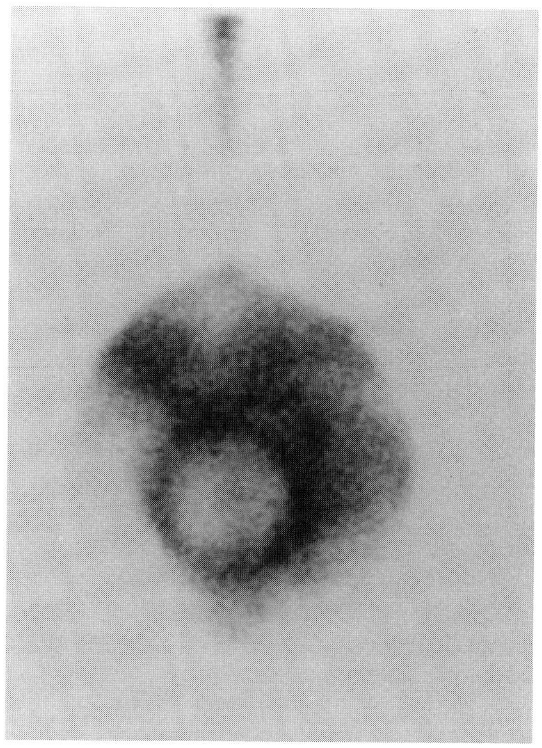

Figure 18–5 Testicular scintigraphy. Unilateral testicular torsion, with light area indicating lack of perfusion of one gonad.

Compared with testicular scintigraphy in the assessment of testicular perfusion, color Doppler sonography is a sensitive tool in most age groups. In adults, color Doppler sonography has a sensitivity of 86 to 100%, whereas scintigraphy has an 80 to 100% sensitivity. In pediatric populations, color flow sonography has a 90 to 100% sensitivity compared with nearly 100% for scintigraphic studies. Again, color Doppler sonography has the added advantage of providing anatomic correlation.[7] Color Doppler sonography and testicular scintigraphy are both limited in the diagnosis of intermittent torsion, because perfusion studies reflect flow at only one particular moment in time. Detorted testicles have return of flow and may even be associated with reactive hyperemia.[7–9]

Color Doppler sonography can be an effective adjunctive diagnostic tool in all age groups, but the examination may be more difficult in neonates and prepubertal boys. In small gonads, the intratesticular blood vessels are of a smaller caliber, and blood flows at a lower average velocity. The sensitivity of the examination becomes more dependent on the capabilities of the equipment and the experience of the examiner. As with older patients, it is important to use the contralateral asymptomatic testicle as a control.[7–9]

Real-time sonography without Doppler signals does not always provide adequate information and may lead to misdiagnosis or delay in diagnosis. The sonographic qualities of torsion and epididymal orchitis, for example, have some degree of overlap.[7, 10, 11] The sonographic appearance in torsion is in part related to the duration of torsion but may also be dependent on the degree of twisting, the amount of intragonadal hemorrhage, and the stage of testicular maturation (Fig. 18–6*A–C*).[10] Within the first few hours, the gonad maintains normal architecture, but Doppler signals are already absent. After 4 to 6 hours, the testis becomes enlarged and hypoechoic, a finding probably related to edema from early venous congestion. Arterial compromise occurs next, and the associated ischemia and hemorrhagic necrosis lead to a testicle that is enlarged and heterogenous, with cystic anechoic areas representing focal necrosis. There may be a reactive hydrocele and scrotal wall thickening as well as increased flow within the scrotal wall.[7, 12, 13] If acute testicular torsion goes undiagnosed, it will progress from the edematous acute stage to the ischemic and necrotic subacute and chronic stages. Infants born with signs of in utero testicular torsion, however, have almost always progressed to the subacute or chronic stage, and the sonographic findings are an inhomogeneously hypoechoic testicle with a brightly echogenic rim consistent with infarction.[14]

Acute torsion of a peritesticular appendage also has a distinct appearance by color Doppler sonography. The testicle itself is normal in size and echogenicity, and there is an adjacent hyperechoic mass with[15] or without[16] a hypoechoic core. As the duration of torsion increases, there may be extratesticular fluid or edematous changes in the testicle and epididymis. Epididymal orchitis, although sometimes confused with acute or subacute torsion on real-time sonography, generally has increased testicular and peritesticular flow on color Doppler sonography to distinguish it from torsion.

Overall, color Doppler sonography is currently the preferred supplemental study in the evaluation of the acute scrotum. Although scintigraphy and color Doppler sonography have comparable sensitivities in the evaluation of intratesticular flow, color Doppler sonography provides additional valuable information, is noninvasive, and can generally be obtained with less delay.

MANAGEMENT

In recent years, the management of in utero testicular torsion has been fraught with controversy. The issues hinge on the concept that in utero torsion is usually an antenatal and irreversible event. In utero torsion occurs predominantly by an extravaginal mechanism with no anatomic basis to suggest danger to the contralateral testicle after the early neonatal period. The controversies include (1) when and if the apparently torted gonad should be explored, (2) whether to remove or replace the grossly necrotic gonad, and (3) whether contralateral orchiopexy is indicated. Acute testicular torsion in the early neonatal period shares some of these controversies but obviously should always receive the emergent attention given to acute torsion in older patients.

Because in utero torsion has often progressed to subacute or even chronic torsion by the time of delivery, the testicle is rarely salvageable. Exploration need not be performed emergently but should be executed as promptly as the overall condition of the infant will safely allow. With modern pediatric anesthetic techniques and operative facilities, surgical procedures can be performed on otherwise healthy neonates with nearly no perioperative morbidity and mortality.[17, 18] Exploration can also be performed under local anesthesia in the more unstable patient with suspected acute testicular torsion.[2]

Whether torsion occurs intravaginally or extravaginally is a moot point when deciding whether or not to surgically explore an acute scrotum. Prompt exploration is critical for potential salvage of the gonad, and any delay in diagnosis or treatment may have an adverse effect on endocrine function and fertility in the long term. Donohue and Utley presented a large study of acute scrotums. On the basis of their findings, they advocated exploration of the acute scrotum in every patient younger than 18 years. Of those patients with testicular torsion, 100% of those operated on within 6 hours of onset of symptoms had normal gonads at follow-up. Seventy percent were salvaged when explored 6 to 12 hours after onset of symptoms, but only 20% were salvaged after 12

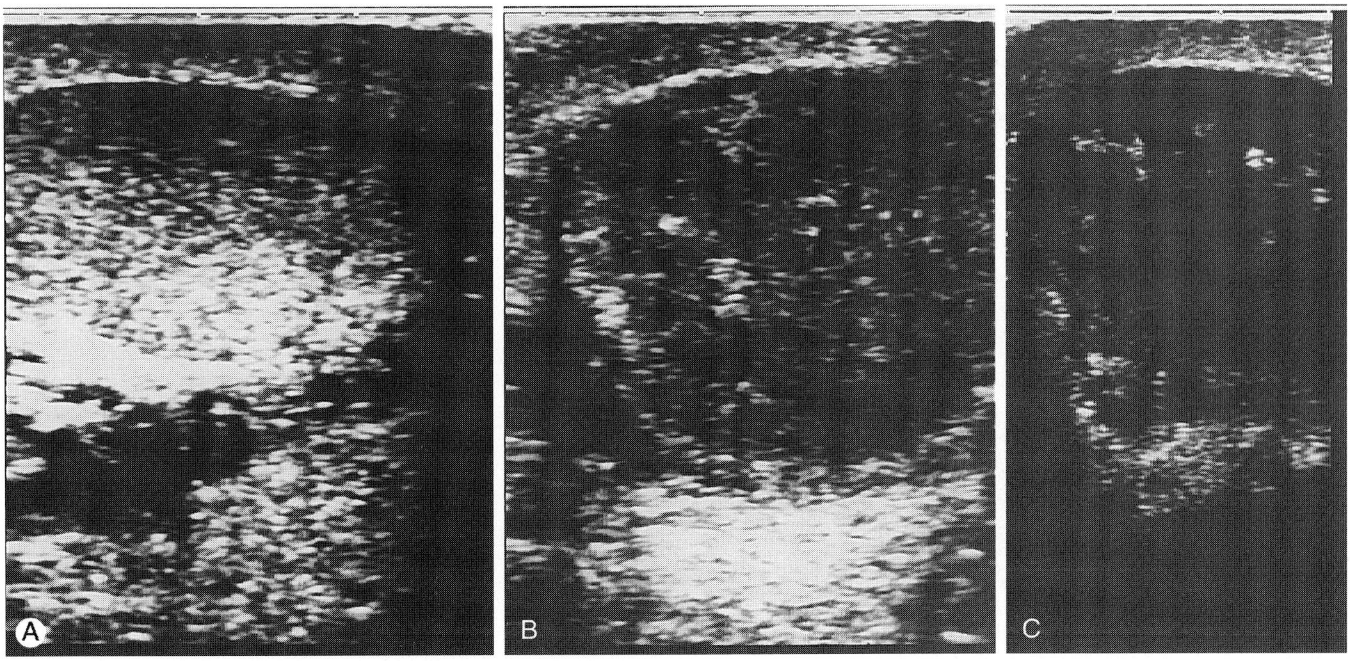

Figure 18–6 Gray-scale ultrasound images of advanced testicular torsion. *A*, Homogeneous echoes of a normal testicle. *B*, Heterogeneous appearance of subacute testicular torsion. *C*, Inhomogeneously hypoechoic gonad after chronic torsion. Note the calcifications and echogenic rim.

hours of pain and swelling.[6] Kass and colleagues, in contrast, advocated emergent color Doppler studies in all but the most obvious cases of torsion, because only 30% of all acute scrotums will ultimately require urgent operative procedures.[19]

At exploration, the gonad may be edematous and dusky or may be frankly necrotic (Fig. 18–7*A* and *B*). Bleeding with incision of the tunica albuginea may be the best prognostic sign for potential viability of the gonad. For many years, it was believed that even the grossly necrotic testicle should be replaced and fixed in the scrotum in an effort to preserve any potential endocrine and reproductive function. Experimental canine models, however, have shown that spermatogenesis is lost by 6 hours of ischemia and that Leydig's cells disappear by 10 hours of ischemia.[1] Necrotic testicles that are replaced into the scrotum and even torted testicles that are never explored at all are usually found to be absent or profoundly atrophic later on physical examination.[18, 20–22] The hypothetical ability to conserve hormone production and

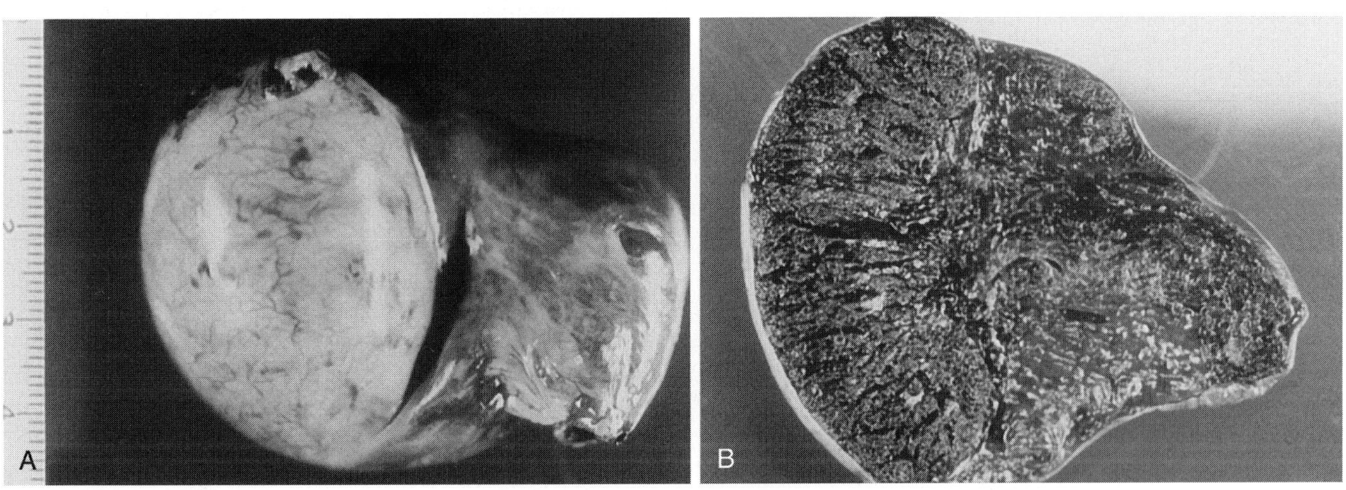

Figure 18–7 Orchiectomy specimen after exploration for torsion. *A*, Gross specimen. *B*, Cut surface.

fertility must be compared with the potential systemic toxicity of replacing necrotic material into the body. In addition, there is some speculation that testicular antigens liberated by the necrotic testicle may have adverse immunologic effects on the contralateral testicle. This seems to be the case in rodents. Early exploration with removal of obviously necrotic testicles minimizes this concern in both neonates and older patients and is the most appropriate management. One potential exception to this principle is the neonate with bilateral necrotic testicles from in utero torsion. Salvage of one of the gonads is the only potential for preservation of endocrine or reproductive function, but again the risk of toxicity must be considered.

The distinction between intravaginal and extravaginal torsion has been thought by some to be important in deciding whether or not to perform contralateral orchiopexy in patients undergoing detorsion or orchiectomy. Contralateral fixation has long been advocated in the prepubertal, pubertal, and postpubertal male with intravaginal torsion, because the anatomic predisposition (bell-clapper deformity) is often bilateral and asynchronous torsion with loss of the remaining gonad would be disastrous.

Neonatal torsion, whether in utero or in the early postnatal period, was historically believed not to be an indication for contralateral fixation, because the torsion was extravaginal and without any underlying anatomic abnormality to suggest a risk to the remaining gonad. However, not only has extravaginal torsion been reported to occur bilaterally in an asynchronous fashion,[17] but intravaginal torsion has also been noted to occur infrequently in neonates.[18, 20, 22] Furthermore, an animal model by Friedman and others revealed that, after prolonged torsion (such as in utero torsion), intravaginal torsion and extravaginal torsion were grossly indistinguishable at exploration, because the tunica and testis were heavily involved by an inflammatory and ischemic process.[23] Contralateral orchiopexy at initial exploration is recommended in all cases of unilateral torsion regardless of the age of the patient or the perceived classification of torsion as intra- or extravaginal. This procedure is minimally invasive and is not harmful to the gonad, and these few precautionary steps pay large dividends to the patient who has already lost one testicle to torsion.

SURGICAL APPROACH

In treating the neonate with presumed testicular torsion, one must consider the potential confounding differential diagnoses and remember the anatomic relationships that make scrotal contents easily accessible through an inguinal incision (Fig. 18–8*A* and *B*). Incarcerated inguinal hernia is the next most likely diagnosis, and this obviously would be better managed by an inguinal approach. In the very unlikely event that the scrotal mass is a neoplasm, choosing an inguinal incision would be prudent as well. Orchiectomy should be performed when the testicle is clearly necrotic, but the testicle may be returned to the scrotum and fixed in place if it appears viable. Contralateral trans-scrotal orchiopexy should al-

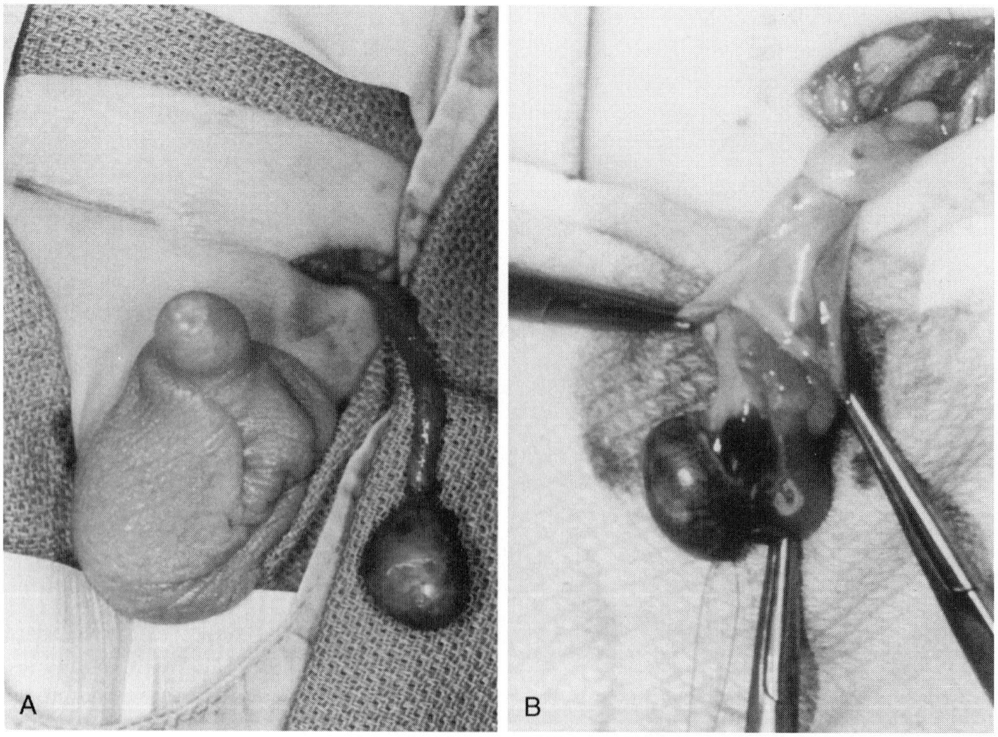

Figure 18–8 Neonatal extravaginal torsion. *A*, Inguinal approach. *B*, Opened tunica vaginalis with clearly ischemic gonad.

ways be performed at the same time. All orchiopexy procedures should consist of three-point fixation between the tunica albuginea and scrotal wall or septum using nonabsorbable suture.

Older children, adolescents, and adults are best explored trans-scrotally, unless there is some evidence to suggest the presence of a concomitant testicular tumor. The testicle should be inspected after detorsion and either removed or replaced, based on the surgeon's judgment of viability. Any testicle replaced into the scrotum, as well as the normal contralateral testicle, should be fixed in the correct anatomic position by the aforementioned technique. The lateral sulcus between testicle and epididymis is a helpful landmark for reorienting the testicle within the scrotum. Patients with presumed intermittent torsion should undergo bilateral trans-scrotal exploration and orchiopexy.

CONCLUSIONS

Loss of gonadal function may even precede gross necrosis of the testicle. Prompt diagnosis and intervention are essential if the testicle and its endocrine and reproductive functions are to be salvaged. There are no diagnostic studies that can rule torsion in or out with certainty, so the clinician must rely on the presenting complaints and physical findings to decide whether immediate surgical exploration is warranted. He or she may elect color Doppler sonography or other perfusion studies to obtain a diagnosis in more equivocal cases, but should remember that diagnostic studies may delay diagnosis or result in misdiagnosis and the loss of the gonad.

Controversy has surrounded the management of neonatal torsion. The distinction between intravaginal and extravaginal torsion is merely semantic when managing testicular torsion. All suspicious cases should be promptly explored, and the gonad should undergo detorsion or be removed. Contralateral orchiopexy must be performed in each case to protect the long-term viability of at least one testicle.

REFERENCES

1. Smith GI. Cellular changes from graded testicular ischemia. J Urol 73:355, 1955.
2. Ryken TC, Turner JW, Haynes T. Bilateral testicular torsion in a preterm neonate. J Urol 143:102, 1990.
3. Leach GE, Masih BK. Neonatal torsion of testicle. Urology 16:604, 1980.
4. Corriere JN. Horizontal lie of the testicle: A diagnostic sign in torsion of the testis. J Urol 107:616, 1972.
5. Schulsinger D, Glassberg K, Strashun A. Intermittent torsion: Association with horizontal lie of the testicle. J Urol 145:1053, 1991.
6. Donohue RE, Utley WLF. Torsion of spermatic cord. Urology 11:33, 1978.
7. Siegel MJ. Male genital tract. In Siegel M (ed), Textbook of Pediatric Sonography, 2nd ed. New York: Raven Press, 1995.
8. Patriquin HB, Yazbeck S, Trinh B, et al. Testicular torsion in infants and children: Diagnosis with Doppler sonography. Radiology 188:781, 1993.
9. Meza MP, Amundson GM, Aquilina JW, Reitelman C. Color flow imaging in children with clinically suspected testicular torsion. Pediatr Radiol 22:370, 1992.
10. Pryor JL, Watson R, Day DL, et al. Scrotal ultrasound for evaluation of subacute testicular torsion: Sonographic findings and adverse clinical implications. J Urol 151:693, 1994.
11. Bird K, Rosenfield AT, Taylor KJW. Ultrasonography in testicular torsion. Radiology 147:527, 1983.
12. Zafaranloo S, Gerard PS, Wise G. Bilateral neonatal testicular torsion: Ultrasonographic evaluation. J Urol 135:589, 1986.
13. Gross BR, Cohen HL, Schlessel JS. Perinatal diagnosis of bilateral testicular torsion. J Ultrasound Med 12:479, 1993.
14. Zerin JM, DiPietro MA, Grignon A, Shea D. Testicular infarction in the newborn: Ultrasound findings. Pediatr Radiol 20:329, 1990.
15. Cohen HL, Shapiro MA, Haller JO, Glassberg K. Torsion of the testicular appendage. J Ultrasound Med 11:81, 1992.
16. Hesser U, Rosenborg M, Gierup J, et al. Gray-scale sonography in torsion of the testicular appendages. Pediatr Radiol 23:529, 1993.
17. LaQuaglia MP, Bauer SB, Eraklis A, et al. Bilateral neonatal torsion. J Urol 138:1051, 1987.
18. Jerkins GR, Noe HN, Hollabaugh RS, Allen RG. Spermatic cord torsion in the neonate. J Urol 129:121, 1983.
19. Kass EJ, Stone KT, Cacciarelli AA, Mitchell B. Do all children with an acute scrotum require exploration? J Urol 150:667, 1993.
20. Brandt MT, Sheldon CA, Wacksman J, Matthews P. Prenatal testicular torsion: Principles of management. J Urol 147:670, 1992.
21. Weingarten JL, Garofalo FA, Cromie WJ. Bilateral synchronous neonatal torsion of spermatic cord. Urology 35:135, 1990.
22. Burge DM. Neonatal testicular torsion and infarction: Aetiology and management. Br J Urol 59:70, 1987.
23. Friedman RM, Flashner SC, Akwari OE, King LR. An experimental model of neonatal testicular torsion: Evidence against an exclusively extravaginal etiology. J Urol 150:246, 1993.

EDWARD F. IKEGUCHI & TERRY W. HENSLE

19

The Pediatric Varicocele

OVERVIEW

The testicular varicocele is a disease entity unique to human beings, unique probably because humankind's bipedal evolution has made us more susceptible to problems of venous return than our four-legged counterparts.[1] The varicocele was once considered to be of minimal significance, and it has been stated that "no other condition has offered a more lucrative field for the practice of charlatanry than varicocele."[2] Considerable research has since helped elucidate its cause, pathophysiology, and ultimate clinical consequence. Although the therapy of varicocele has evolved considerably from the "application of a suspensory bandage"[2] or the use of leeches,[3] controversies remain regarding the optimal treatment of varicocele.

Incidence and Cause

A varicocele is an ectatic and tortuous dilation of the spermatic veins. In the pediatric population, varicoceles are most frequently found in pubertal or postpubertal adolescents; they occur only occasionally in younger children. The incidence of testicular varicocele found on physical examination in adolescents is estimated to be between 2 and 11%.[4, 5]

Several theories exist regarding the cause of varicocele. Although most would agree that an increased hydrostatic pressure within the venous drainage of the testicle would ultimately lead to a varicocele,[6, 7] several studies have shown retrograde reflux of blood from the renal vein into the venous channels of the pampiniform plexus.[8] This reflux has been attributed to a failure of either venous valve mechanisms or collateral venous circulation.[9] A third theory, known as the "nutcracker" phenomenon, has been proposed. In this scenario, the left renal vein is wedged between the aorta and superior mesenteric artery, resulting in the transmission of increased hydrostatic pressure to the pampiniform plexus. Alternatively, it has also been proposed that the external spermatic veins may be affected by compression of the common iliac vein between the pelvic brim and the iliac artery.[6]

More than 90% of varicoceles occur on the left side. This predilection has been attributed to the anatomic difference between the left and right testicular venous drainage. Whereas the left testicular vein enters the left renal vein perpendicularly, the right testicular vein inserts into the inferior vena cava obliquely. Because of these differences in venous anatomy, the left testicular vein is generally longer than the right, resulting in a longer fluid column and higher hydrostatic pressures.[7] Indeed, when a patient presents with a right-sided varicocele, or any varicocele that is either sudden in onset or persistent in the supine position, a more in-depth investigation is warranted. Under these circumstances, computed tomographic scan or ultrasonography should be performed to rule out causes of venous compression such as tumors or fibrosis.

Symptoms

Varicoceles in any age group usually present asymptomatically. In adolescents, the varicocele is often detected by the patient himself or by the pediatrician during routine physical examination. When symptoms are present, they may be related to a sensation of ipsilateral testicular discomfort frequently described as a dull ache or "heavy" sensation in the scrotum.

Physical Examination

The patient should be examined in a warm examining room in the standing position. The scrotum should be first inspected for visible evidence of a varicocele. Both spermatic cords may then be palpated with and without Valsalva maneuver. A small varicocele in an initially normal-feeling spermatic cord may become palpable with venous engorgement secondary to Valsalva maneuver (grade I). Medium-sized varicoceles may only be palpable as a "bag of worms" overlying the testicle (grade II), whereas large varicoceles may be evident on mere inspection of the scrotum (grade III).[10] The patient should also be examined in the supine position to ensure that the varicocele drains appropriately.

A careful testicular examination should be performed with documentation of ipsilateral versus contralateral testicular consistency and volume. Objective size measurement may be obtained with either a caliper or an orchidometer, although testicular ultrasonography proves to be the most accurate way to measure testis volume.

Radiographic Examination

Although venography was once considered the standard of diagnosis for varicocele, this examination is invasive, technique dependent, costly, and generally no longer in use. Ultrasonography provides the advantage of being noninvasive with a high degree of sensitivity (92%) and specificity (100%).[11]

This high degree of sensitivity has led to an increasing number of asymptomatic varicoceles detected by ultrasonography.[12] What is the role of repair in varicoceles found incidentally? Should sonography be used as a screening tool for testicular varicocele?[13] In the pediatric population, there usually appears to be no need for repair of an asymptomatic varicocele found incidentally on ultrasonogram. Careful physical examination remains the foundation on which diagnosis and therapy are based.

Clinical Significance

Testicular Volume

Although no single explanation for the effect of a varicocele on the testis is universally accepted, potential theories have included scrotal hyperthermia,[14, 15] reflux of adrenal-renal metabolites,[16] and gonadal hormone imbalance.[17] The primary concern in the management of adolescent varicocele is its impact on the testicle, and multiple studies have shown its association with ipsilateral testicular growth retardation.[18–21] Furthermore, so-called catch-up growth has been consistently demonstrated in affected testes after varicocele repair.[22, 23]

Testicular Histology

In children, as in adults, the presence of a varicocele has been linked to histologic abnormalities of the testicle. Most notably, abnormalities of spermatogenesis, including maturation arrest, have been found in association with tubular hypoplasia and peritubular fibrosis.[24, 25] These histologic abnormalities have been shown to be reversible with repair of the varicocele.[26] In addition, such changes have been found not only in the ipsilateral testis but in the contralateral testis as well.[26, 27]

Semen Parameters and Fertility

An extensive literature exists pertaining to changes in semen analysis associated with varicocele in adults. The general consensus has been that the presence of a varicocele negatively impacts on certain parameters in the semen analysis, namely sperm concentration, motility, and morphology.[28, 29] This has not been as well studied in the pediatric population because the presenting complaints in children are not related to infertility per se. In addition, studies of semen parameters in children have been hindered by the difficulties in obtaining semen samples as well as the lack of established reference values for normal semen parameters in adolescents. The available reports, however, are suggestive of similar semen abnormalities to those found in adults. Haans and colleagues found a correlation between the presence of a varicocele with ipsilateral growth retardation and decreased total sperm concentration.[20]

Endocrine Abnormality

Studies evaluating serum gonadotropin and testosterone levels in patients with varicocele have generally shown no abnormality in these parameters.[20, 23] There is evidence, however, suggesting subtle alterations in the fine balance of the hypothalamic-pituitary-gonadal axis. Using the gonadotropin-releasing hormone (GnRH) stimulation test in adolescent patients with varicoceles, Kass and others in 1993 detected exaggerated responses in 31%. In addition, whereas 75% of patients with exaggerated responses to GnRH stimulation were also found to have varicocele-associated testicular growth retardation, only 50% of patients with normal GnRH stimulation tests had growth retardation.[30] Similarly, Kennedy and others found a significant physiologic improvement in testicular endocrine function in adolescents after varicocele repair as evidenced by GnRH stimulation testing.[31]

Indications for Repair

The strongest indication for the repair of a testicular varicocele in children is the presence of ipsilateral testicular growth retardation in the setting of a grade II to III varicocele. Patients who present symptomatically with complaints of testicular or scrotal discomfort should also be considered for repair once all other causes have been ruled out.

Some clinicians have suggested the repair of a varicocele in the presence of an abnormal GnRH stimulation test and have, therefore, advocated obtaining this test on all patients. This approach has not, however, been proven to be of benefit and has yet to be adopted into routine practice.[32]

Complications

The complications associated with varicocele repair vary with the treatment modality chosen. In general, early complications relate to hematoma formation and scrotal edema. Hydrocele formation has been reported after open or laparoscopic varicocele repair and averages 7%.[33] This has been attributed to the ligation of testicular lymphatics in the process of varicocele repair. Other less common complications include injury to the testicular artery and vas deferens. The most significant long-term complication has been testicular atrophy, which some investigators have attributed to testicular artery damage during the course of surgical repair. The most common long-term complication is persistence (recurrence) of the varicocele and is variable, depending on the therapeutic modality chosen.

The anesthesia risk is low in the otherwise healthy patient. Although most younger children require general anesthesia, some of the procedures may be performed under local anesthesia with mild sedation in a cooperative adolescent patient. The exception is laparoscopic varicocele repair, for which general anesthesia is required for all patients.

TREATMENT OPTIONS

In choosing a procedure for the correction of a varicocele in the pediatric patient, the surgeon must select a method that has the lowest chance of complications, poses the least surgical and anesthetic risk to the patient, and affords the shortest course of recovery. Furthermore, these considerations must be taken in conjunction with the overall cost-benefit analysis of the proposed therapy.

The current areas of controversy in the treatment of pediatric varicocele are high versus low ligation of the testicular veins, artery-sparing versus non–artery-sparing repair, and open surgery versus laparoscopic repair. There has been no conclusive, randomized trial comparing all available therapies. Patterns of practice vary widely among institutions as well as internationally. To date, however, in the United States open surgery remains standard therapy for the pediatric varicocele.

Open Surgical Techniques

High Versus Low Ligation Varicocelectomy

Open varicocele repair is performed either in the inguinal canal or cephalad to the separation of the vas deferens retroperitoneally. The rationale for high ligation came from venographic studies performed in adult varicocele patients in which more than 75% of patients were found to have either venous reflux or collaterals to the spermatic vein at its confluence with the renal vein.[6] Although these lesions would be reparable by high ligation, advocates of low (inguinal or subinguinal) ligation point out that greater than 20% of patients in those same studies had pelvic collaterals that would have been missed by retroperitoneal spermatic vein ligation. These venous collaterals generally originate from the external spermatic vessels, the vessels of the vas deferens, or the scrotum. Despite these concerns, varicocele recurrence rates with high and low ligation have been similar, ranging between 0 and 16%.[34]

Retroperitoneal Approach (Palomo)

The retroperitoneal approach to varicocele ligation was first described by Palomo in 1949.[35] Although Palomo originally described a mass ligation of all the testicular vessels above the vas deferens, the technique can be altered whereby the testicular artery is spared (modified Palomo).

Procedure: Total High Ligation. The surgeon should use loupe optical magnification (at least 3.5 power). The patient is positioned on the operating table in the supine position. Local anesthesia with sedation may be used in the compliant, older adolescent. However, younger children or those displaying excessive anxiety will require general anesthesia. A transverse skin incision of approximately 6 cm is made overlying the internal inguinal ring. The incision is carried down through the subcutaneous tissues to the level of the external oblique fascia, which is incised parallel to its fibers. A muscle-splitting technique may then be used with a curved clamp to separate the fibers of the internal oblique muscle. This will expose the transversalis fascia. Adequate exposure should be obtained with retraction of the tissues superiorly and inferiorly with hand-held right-angle retractors. The transversalis fascia may then be incised for entry into the retroperitoneum. The testicular vessels are now exposed by blunt dissection of the peritoneum medially. Localization of the testicular vessels is facilitated by placement of the patient in the reverse Trendelenburg position as well as with periodic traction on the ipsilateral testis. Once the testicular vessels are identified, they should be traced caudally to their confluence with the vas deferens to ensure that the area of dissection is clearly cephalad to the vas. The testicular vessels cephalad to the vas deferens may then be dissected free and isolated over a Penrose drain. The vascular bundle is then ligated by placing two silk ties proximally and distally and dividing between them. After the wound is irrigated and inspected for hemostasis, it may be closed in layers. The surgeon may choose to infiltrate the wound with a long-acting local anesthetic before closure.

Inguinal (Ivanissevich)

The inguinal approach to varicocele repair was described by Ivanissevich in 1960.[36] Both artery-sparing and non–artery-sparing modifications to this procedure have also been described. Although the operation described later is an artery-sparing technique, many routinely perform mass ligation of the cord above the internal ring after adequate separation of the vas deferens (Fig. 19–1). Of note, the vas deferens is dissected from the other cord

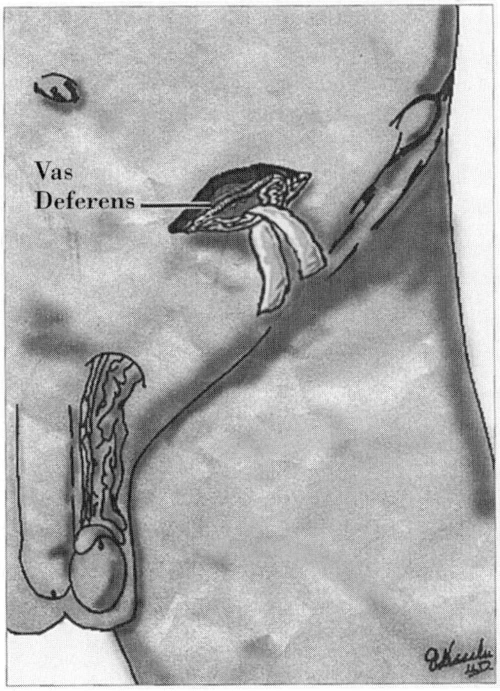

Figure 19–1 Mass ligation of the cord above the internal ring after adequate separation of the vas deferens.

structures with its adventitia intact to avoid stripping its blood supply. An inguinal approach is technically less demanding and is particularly appropriate for the obese patient in whom a retroperitoneal approach can be difficult.

Procedure. Patient positioning, preparation, and incision for the inguinal approach are identical to those for the retroperitoneal operation. Once the external ring has been identified, a small nick in the external oblique fascia is made with a no. 15 blade. Holding the fascia upward with a toothed forceps, the external oblique fascia is opened with Metzenbaum scissors. Care should be taken to avoid transection of the ilioinguinal nerve, which courses directly beneath the external oblique fascia in this area. Lifting each leaflet of the incised external oblique fascia, a peanut dissector may be used to free the spermatic cord. The surgeon may use either a Babcock clamp or a thumb and forefinger to grasp the cord structures and elevate them into the field. A Penrose drain may then be passed underneath the cord and clamped tight to the drape. The cremasteric fascia is opened next. The vas deferens should be identified first, and the surgeon should always remain conscious of its whereabouts. The dilated testicular veins at this point are usually easily teased apart with fine forceps. Placement of the patient in the reverse Trendelenburg position will accentuate venous engorgement, aiding in the identification and dissection of all varicose veins. Before ligation of the veins, the testicular artery should be identified. This may be facilitated by the use of papaverine solution dripped onto the cord. Papaverine will cause the testicular artery to dilate and allow the surgeon to visualize the arterial pulsations under loupe magnification. Once the artery is identified and the testicular veins are isolated, the surgeon may proceed to ligate the veins at the level of the internal ring. Collateral venous drainage, including cremasteric and external spermatic vessels, should be sought and ligated. Furthermore, the testis may be delivered into the operative field at which point scrotal collaterals may be identified and divided. The Penrose drain is now removed and the wound irrigated and inspected for hemostasis. The testis is then placed back into the scrotum in its original anatomic orientation. The external oblique fascia is closed using a running 4-0 absorbable suture, again taking care to avoid incorporation of the ilioinguinal nerve in the closure. In reconstructing the external ring, the surgeon should leave adequate room to avoid strangulation of the spermatic cord. The remainder of the wound is closed in layers. The surgeon may choose to infiltrate the wound with a long-acting local anesthetic before closure.

Artery-Sparing Varicocelectomy Versus Non–Artery-Sparing Varicocelectomy

Controversy exists over the issue of sparing the testicular artery during the course of varicocele repair. The argument against testicular artery ligation is that subsequent testicular atrophy may ensue. Proponents of total ligation, however, claim that the artery-sparing techniques are associated with a higher incidence of varicocele persistence or recurrence. Several comparisons between the two techniques have been made. Kass and Reitelman in 1995 reported on the outcome of their comparison between artery-sparing versus Palomo (total ligation) varicocele repair. They found a varicocele persistence rate of 11% using the artery-sparing technique compared with 1.3% with the Palomo method. Furthermore, the authors noted that no patients on follow-up examination had testicular atrophy.[37] In another study, Atassi and associates reported equivalent rates of testicular growth after Palomo mass ligation as with artery-sparing techniques.[38]

Theories explaining the higher incidence of varicocele recurrence with artery-sparing techniques generally relate to the presence of tiny venous channels in close association with the testicular artery that are missed when attempts are made at sparing the artery. In a study of pathologic specimens of testicular artery segments, two to five venous channels were found in intimate association with the artery.[33]

There appears to be a significant body of evidence in support of non–artery-sparing techniques in varicocele repair. It is generally thought that collateral arterial flow originating from the cremasteric or deferential artery affords the ability to ligate the testicular artery without significant vascular compromise to the testicle. Presumably, if ligation of the testicle did result in significant testicular ischemia, there would be a higher incidence of testicular atrophy. Bearing this in mind, it is important to note that non–artery-sparing techniques are contraindicated in patients who have undergone prior ipsilateral inguinal or scrotal surgery because arterial collaterals may have been interrupted.

Minimally Invasive Techniques

Laparoscopic Varicocelectomy

The emergence of laparoscopy has provided an alternative method of approaching many surgical diseases. Pediatric urologists have used laparoscopy in the identification of intra-abdominal testes since 1976.[39] This technology has also been applied to the treatment of varicocele, and since its introduction, a considerable experience has been gained in adults. Although there may be some benefit in regards to the level of postoperative pain experienced by the patient, as well as a quicker return to full activity,[40] there are drawbacks to the laparoscopic approach, among them the need for pneumoperitoneum, the need for general anesthesia, the prolonged operative time (approximately 120 minutes per procedure),[40] and higher cost. Varicocele persistence rates with laparoscopy have approximated those of open surgery and range from 0 to 14%.[41–43] Overall complication rates with laparoscopic varicocele ligation are low (0–4%).[44] As with all forms of laparoscopic surgery, complications include rare injuries to major vascular structures, intestinal perforation, bleeding from the inferior epigastric vessels, injury to the genitofemoral nerve, and so on. Although laparoscopic varicocele ligation has emerged as a viable option, the need for general anesthesia, the operative time, and costs incurred as well as the questionable benefit over open surgery have kept it from becoming the definitive treatment of choice.

Procedure. The patient is placed in the supine position. After general anesthesia is induced, the patient is scrubbed and a sterile paint applied from the xiphoid process to the midthighs. The patient is then placed in a Trendelenburg position. The operating staff is positioned such that the primary surgeon stands across from the varicocele, the first assistant stands on the side of the varicocele, and the scrub nurse and equipment tray are positioned ipsilateral to the varicocele. The video monitor is placed at the foot of the operating table. A cutdown technique at the inferior aspect of the umbilicus may be used to place an 11-mm video port under direct vision. The laparoscope is now inserted and the peritoneum insufflated. The laparoscope may now be directed to visualize placement of the remainder of the ports: an 11-mm suprapubic port midway between the pubis and the umbilical port and a 5-mm port midway between the umbilicus and the anterosuperior iliac spine just cephalad to the internal ring on the ipsilateral side. The primary surgeon may now manipulate the two instrument ports while the first assistant directs the laparoscope and camera.

After inspection of the abdomen, the sigmoid colon and other intestinal loops are retracted medially (for the left-sided varicocele). This may be facilitated by placement of the patient in the Trendelenburg position and by planing the operating table with the right side down. First, identify the internal ring where the testicular veins may be seen joining the vas deferens. A grasping forceps is now passed through the midline port, and the peritoneum just lateral to the spermatic vessels is retracted. Laparoscopic scissors are used through the lateral port to incise the peritoneum for approximately 5 cm parallel with the spermatic vessels. The forceps is then used to retract the medial aspect of the incised peritoneum and the scissors are used to further open the peritoneum medially over the vessels to form a T incision. The endoscopic scissors are now removed and replaced by a straight grasping instrument, which can elevate the vascular bundle from the underlying connective tissue. A curved dissector in the midline port may then be used to further separate the vascular structures into their constituents. The testicular artery may be identified by the observation of pulsations. This is facilitated by irrigating the vessels with papaverine or lidocaine. Once the testicular artery is identified, all the venous structures may be ligated. This is accomplished by the application of two clips both proximally and distally using an endoscopic clip applier. Each vein is then cut between the clips. The surgical site is irrigated and inspected for hemostasis. After all irrigant and blood have been evacuated, the abdomen is again inspected with the patient in the reverse Trendelenburg position. Each of the three instruments may now be removed with the 5-mm port first followed by the suprapubic port. After removal of each, the laparoscope should be used to inspect the site for hemostasis. Finally, the umbilical port is removed. If there is any question of adequate hemostasis at the umbilical port site, a telescope may be reintroduced with the laparoscope at the suprapubic site to inspect the umbilical site. The fascia of the umbilical and suprapubic sites is closed with a single figure-eight absorbable suture. The skin at all port sites is closed with buried sutures.

Angiographic Varicocelectomy

In an effort to minimize invasiveness, several techniques have been developed that use angiographic technology in the transvenous embolization of a varicocele. These methods use various injectable sclerosing agents as well as intraluminal placement of balloons, autologous clot, and coils[45] to obliterate the lumen of the testicular veins. Although studies in children have been limited, several report technical difficulty in the pediatric population in whom approximately 10% of attempts are unsuccessful as a result of aberrant venous anatomy, difficulty cannulating the testicular vein, extravasation of contrast during the procedure, and so on.[23, 46] These studies have generally used a retrograde technique of percutaneous sclerotherapy performed by trained radiologists. Although complications peculiar to the angiographic techniques have been described, these methods are generally not associated with testicular arterial injury or postoperative hydrocele formation.

Retrograde Sclerotherapy

Initial reports of retrograde sclerosing of varicoceles by radiologists describe success rates similar to those of operative repair.[47] Venous access in retrograde sclerotherapy is obtained via either a transfemoral or a transjugular approach. There has been limited experience in children, and most report technical difficulties in younger patients. In addition, the same studies found the incidence of varicocele persistence or recurrence to range between 6 and 15%.[23, 46, 48] In the adult literature, Bach and colleagues reported a varicocele recurrence rate of only 3.3%, although in 20% of patients the procedure could not be performed because of technical reasons.[49] Complications from these procedures have included flank pain, flank ecchymosis, thrombophlebitis of the pampiniform plexus, and vascular perforation. Rarely, instances of coil migration, renal vein thrombosis, and pulmonary embolism have been reported.[50] At present, retrograde angiographic embolization is not used as first-line therapy, although it may be considered in the management of the recurrent varicocele after laparoscopic or open surgical techniques have failed.

Anterograde Sclerotherapy

An alternative form of sclerotherapy known as anterograde sclerotherapy was described by Tauber and associates in 1988.[51] Subsequent studies using this technique report varicocele recurrence and persistence rates between 9 and 12.5%, with complications including allergic reactions, severe thrombophlebitis of the pampiniform plexus, scrotal hematoma, epididymitis, testicular atrophy, and flank erythema.[50, 52] Nonetheless, anterograde sclerotherapy has been advocated by some because of the speed, ease, and low cost of such treatments. The procedure is performed under local anesthesia and requires approximately 10 to 30 minutes per varicocele.[50, 52] Again, most of the data have been generated in adults, and the limited experience in children has shown that general anesthesia is still required because of the anxiety of the child.[52] Furthermore, at present, the use of sclerotherapy agents for anterograde injection of varicoceles has yet to obtain Food and Drug Administration approval. Therefore, although this procedure is becoming more popular abroad, in the United States there is little, if any, clinical experience. Anterograde sclerotherapy, as described by Tauber and Johnsen, is briefly summarized next.[50]

Procedure. The patient is placed in the supine position. The genitalia are scrubbed and a sterile paint is applied with the patient under conscious sedation. A 1% local anesthetic is infiltrated into the scrotal skin along the lateral border of the spermatic cord approximately 1 cm caudal to the base of the penis. A spermatic cord block may then be performed by infiltrating anesthesia deeper into the cord structures. The spermatic cord is palpated through the scrotal skin and grasped between two fingers. A 1- to 2-cm skin incision is then made along the lateral border of the cord and carried down to the level of the vas and vessels. A curved clamp is now passed beneath the spermatic cord structures and a Vesi-loop drawn through.

A dilated vein of the varicocele is then exposed and ligated with a silk suture on its distal aspect. The silk tie may then be used to apply traction while a venotomy is performed using a no. 11 blade. A 24-gauge intravenous catheter is then introduced anterograde via the venotomy site. The catheter is secured in place by a second silk tie around the proximal aspect of the vein. The catheter is then flushed with normal saline followed by 3 to 5 mL of a nonionic contrast material under fluoroscopic monitoring. This allows the surgeon to confirm anterograde flow of contrast into the spermatic vein. Sclerotherapy may now be performed. The original report by Tauber and Johnsen described the injection of the sclerosing agent by an "air block" technique whereby 1 mL of air is first injected followed by 3 mL of the sclerosing agent while the patient is performing a Valsalva maneuver.[50] The therapy is limited to a single injection; once completed the catheter is removed and the vein ligated. After checking for hemostasis, the wound is closed in layers.

Cost Analysis

In the era of managed health care, more emphasis has been placed on the concept of cost benefit. Many procedures performed by surgeons have come under intense scrutiny, particularly when multiple therapeutic options are available. This applies especially to varicocele because no single treatment has emerged as the most beneficial.

It is understood that all varicocele procedures should be able to be performed on an ambulatory basis. Most cost analyses have compared various newer techniques to open surgical repair. Retrograde percutaneous ablation has been found to cost approximately the same as open surgery. This is due to the costs of the specialty catheters, coils, and other angiographic equipment. In addition, anesthesia and radiologist fees are comparable to those of open surgery. Anterograde sclerotherapy has been reported to cost considerably less, with equipment costs estimated at $22 per procedure.[50]

Laparoscopic varicocele repair has undergone extensive cost analysis, and several studies have made cost and morbidity comparisons between laparoscopic repair and inguinal[53, 54] or subinguinal repair.[55] Factors adding considerable expense have been the need for general anesthesia, the use of costly laparoscopic equipment, and the longer operative time. Although the operating room cost of laparoscopic repair is estimated at $3500, or approximately twice that of inguinal repair, proponents of laparoscopy point out that this added expense is compensated by the savings obtained from decreased patient morbidity, including less need for analgesics and a shorter convalescence. However, when differences in these parameters were studied, no statistical difference between laparoscopy and subinguinal repair was found.[56]

REFERENCES

1. Turner TT. Varicocele: Still an enigma. J Urol 129:695, 1983.
2. Greene RH, Brooks H. Diseases of the Genito-Urinary Organs and the Kidney, 3rd ed. London: WB Saunders, 1912.
3. Cooper S. The First Lines of the Practice of Surgery. Philadelphia: DeSilver & Cowterthwaite, 1828.
4. Yerokhin AP. Classification and frequency of varicocele in children. Klin Chir 6:45, 1979.
5. Pozza D, D'Ottavio G, Masci P, et al. Left varicocele at puberty. Urology 22:271, 1983.
6. Coolsaet BL. The varicocele syndrome: Venography determining the optimal level for surgical management. J Urol 124:833, 1980.
7. Shafik A, Bedeir GA. Venous tension patterns in cord veins in normal and varicocele individuals. J Urol 123:383, 1980.
8. Ahlberg NE, Bartley O, Chidekel N. Retrograde contrast filling of the left gonadal vein. Acta Radiol Diag 3:385, 1965.
9. Ahlberg NE, Bartley O, Chidekel N, Fritjofsson A. Phlebography in varicocele scroti. Acta Radiol Diag 4:517, 1966.
10. Steeno O, Knops J, Declerck L, et al. Prevention of fertility disorders by detection and treatment of varicocele at school and college age. Andrologia 8:47, 1976.
11. Hamm B, Fobbe F, Sorensen R, Felsenberg D. Varicoceles: Combined sonography and thermography in diagnosis and post therapeutic evaluation. Radiology 160:419, 1986.
12. Eskew LA, Watson NE, Wolfman N, et al. Ultrasonographic diagnosis of varicoceles. Fertil Steril 60:693, 1993.
13. Marsman JW, Schats R. The subclinical varicocele debate. Hum Reprod 9:1, 1994.
14. Kormano M, Kahanpaa K, Svinhufvud U, Tahti E. Thermography of varicocele. Fertil Steril 21:558, 1970.
15. Lewis RW, Harrison RM. Contact scrotal thermography: Application to problems of infertility. J Urol 122:40, 1979.
16. Rodriquez-Rigau LJ, Smith K, Steinberger E. Varicocele and the morphology of spermatozoa. Fertil Steril 35:54, 1981.
17. Comhaire F, Vermeulen A. Plasma testosterone in patients with varicocele and sexual inadequacy. J Clin Endocrinol Metab 40:824, 1975.
18. Lyon RP, Marshall S, Scott MP. Varicocele in childhood and adolescence: Implications in adulthood infertility? Urology 19:641, 1982.
19. Steeno O, Knops J, DeClerck L, et al. Prevention of fertility disorders by detection and treatment of varicocele at school and college age. Andrology 8:47, 1976.
20. Haans LC, Laven JS, Mali WP, et al. Testis volumes, semen quality, and hormonal patterns in adolescents with and without a varicocele. Fertil Steril 56:731, 1991.
21. Sawczuk IS, Hensle TW, Burbige KA, Nagler HM. Varicoceles: Effect on testicular volume in prepubertal and pubertal males. Urology 41:466, 1993.
22. Okuyama A, Nakamura M, Namiki M, et al. Surgical repair of varicocele at puberty: Preventive treatment for fertility improvement. J Urol 139:562, 1988.
23. Laven JS, Haans LC, Mali WP, et al. Effects of varicocele treatment in adolescents: A randomized study. Fertil Steril 58:756, 1992.
24. Hadziselimovic F, Herzog B, Liebundgut B, et al. Testicular and vascular changes in children and adults with varicocele. J Urol 142:583, 1989.
25. Kass EJ, Chandra RS, Belman AB. Testicular histology in the adolescent with a varicocele. Pediatrics 79:996, 1987.
26. Johnsen SG, Agger P. Quantitative evaluation of testicular biopsies before and after operation for varicocele. Fertil Steril 28:58, 1978.
27. Huff D. Testicular histopathology in adolescent varicocele. Paper presented at the Symposium on Adolescent Varicocele, Society of Pediatric Urology, San Francisco, May 14, 1994.
28. Greenberg SH, Lipshultz LI, Wein AJ. Experience with 425 subfertile male patients. J Urol 119:507, 1978.
29. Baker HW, Burger HG, DeKretser DM, et al. Testicular vein ligation and fertility in men with varicoceles. BMJ 291:1678, 1985.
30. Kass EJ, Freitas JE, Salisz JA, Steinert BW. Pituitary gonadal dysfunction in adolescents with varicocele. Urology 42:179, 1993.
31. Kennedy WA II, Hensle TW, Fisch H. Improvement in testicular size and physiological endocrine function associated with varicocele repair in adolescent males. Paper presented at the Annual Meeting of the American Urologic Association, Las Vegas, NV, April 1995.
32. Kass EJ, Freitas JE, Bour JB. Adolescent varicocele: Objective indications for treatment. J Urol 142:579, 1989.
33. Hirokawa M, Matsushita K, Iwamoto T, et al. Assessment of Palomo's operative method for infertile varicocele. Andrologia 25:47, 1993.
34. Kass EJ, Marcol B. Results of varicocele surgery in adolescents: A comparison of techniques. J Urol 148:694, 1992.
35. Palomo A. Radical cure of varicocele by a new technique: Preliminary report. J Urol 61:604, 1949.
36. Ivanissevich O. Left varicocele due to reflux: Experience with 4,470 operative cases in forty-two years. J Int Coll Surg 34:742, 1960.
37. Kass EJ, Reitelman C. Adolescent varicocele. Urol Clin North Am 22:151, 1995.
38. Atassi O, Kass EJ, Steinert B. Testicular growth after successful varicocele correction in adolescents: Comparison of artery sparing techniques with the Palomo procedure. J Urol 153:482, 1995.
39. Peters CA. Laparoscopy in pediatric urology. Urology 41(Suppl):33, 1993.
40. Donovan JF, Winfield HN. Laparoscopic varix ligation. J Urol 147:77, 1992.
41. Hagood PG, Mehan DJ, Worischeck JH, et al. Laparoscopic varicocelectomy: Preliminary report of a new technique. J Urol 147:73, 1992.
42. Wuernschimmel E, Lipsky H, Noest G. Laparoscopic varicocele ligation: A recommendable standard procedure with good long-term results. Eur Urol 27:18, 1995.
43. Ralph DJ, Timoney AG, Parker C, Pryor JP. Laparoscopic varicocele ligation. Br J Urol 72:230, 1993.

44. Winfield HN, Donovan JF, See WA, et al. Urological laparoscopic surgery. J Urol 146:941, 1991.
45. Rivilla F, Casillas JG, Gallego J, Lezana AH. Percutaneous venography and embolization of the internal spermatic vein by spring coil for treatment of the left varicocele in children. J Pediatr Surg 30:523, 1995.
46. Thon WF, Gall H, Danz B, et al. Percutaneous sclerotherapy of idiopathic varicocele in childhood: A preliminary report. J Urol 141:913, 1989.
47. Gonzalez R, Narayan P, Castaneda-Zuniga WR, Amplatz K. Transvenous embolization of the internal spermatic veins for the treatment of varicocele scroti. Urol Clin North Am 9:177, 1982.
48. Porst H, Bahren W, Lenz M, Altwein JE. Percutaneous sclerotherapy of varicoceles: An alternative to conventional surgical methods. BMJ 56:73, 1984.
49. Bach D, Bahren W, Gall H, Altwein JE. Spatergebnissenach sklerotherapie der varikozele. Urologe A 23:338, 1984.
50. Tauber R, Johnsen N. Antegrade scrotal sclerotherapy for the treatment of varicocele: Technique and late results. J Urol 151:386, 1994.
51. Tauber R, Weizert P, Pfeiffer KJ, Huber R. Die antegrade sklerosierung der vena spermatica zur therapie der varicocele. In Verhandl Deutsch Gessell Urologie, 1st ed. Berlin: Springer, 1988, p 239.
52. Kuenkel MRF, Korth K. Rationale for antegrade sclerotherapy in varicoceles. Eur Urol 27:13, 1995.
53. Rashid TM, Winfield HN, Lund GO, et al. Comparative financial analysis of laparoscopic versus open varix ligation for men with clinically significant varicoceles. J Urol 151:331A, 1994.
54. Winfield HN, Donovan JF Jr, Troxel SA, Rashid TM. Laparoscopic urologic surgery: The financial realities. Surg Oncol Clin North Am 4:307, 1995.
55. Hirsch IH, Lofti AM, Moreno JG, Gomella LG. Comparison of outcome parameters in open and laparoscopic varicocele ligation. J Urol 151:332A, 1994.
56. Ross LS, Ruppman N. Varicocele vein ligation in 565 patients under local anesthesia: A long-term review of technique, results and complications in light of proposed management by laparoscopy. J Urol 149:1361, 1993.

ROBERT KAY & JONATHAN H. ROSS

20

Testis Tumors

Prepubertal testicular tumors are uncommon. They occur at an incidence of 0.5 to 2.0 per 100,000 children and represent only 1% of all pediatric solid tumors.[1] Because of the rarity of the tumors and lack of experience at any single institution, the Section of Urology of the American Academy of Pediatrics started a data base on prepubertal testicular tumors in 1980. This has allowed pediatric urologists to understand the demographics of prepubertal testis tumors and the diagnosis and also aid in their management. This information has also allowed the pediatric urologist to approach children with testicular masses in a thoughtful and rational way and then apply the information gained from this registry to manage the disease appropriately.

CLASSIFICATION

The classification of prepubertal testis tumors is based on the initial experiences of the Prepubertal Testicular Tumor Registry and the World Health Organization Classification of Adult Testis Tumors.[2] The classification recognizes that, although germ cell tumors occur prepubertally, with yolk sac carcinoma being the most common, they demonstrate a different histologic picture than in adults. Teratomas are the second most common germ cell tumors in children. It is of interest that seminomas do occur in children, albeit rare, occurring only four times in the world's literature.[3] Choriocarcinoma, a more common component of tumors in adults, does not occur in children. Mixed germ cell tumors comprise the remainder of germ cell tumors in prepubertal children. Gonadal stromal tumors occur in children, ranging from the well-defined gonadal stromal tumors, such as Leydig's cell and Sertoli's cell, to the more unusual, such as juvenile granulosa cell and undifferentiated gonadal stromal tumors. Other tumors are classified the same as in the adults, although tumor-like lesions such as epidermoid cysts and hyperplastic nodules secondary to congenital adrenal hyperplasia need to be recognized and have particular meaning in children with respect to treatment (Table 20–1).

DIAGNOSIS

The diagnosis of a testicular tumor in a child is usually not difficult. The majority of children present with a painless mass or an enlarged scrotum. In the Prepubertal Testicular Tumor Registry, 85% of all patients presented with a solid mass in the scrotum indicative of a neoplastic lesion. However, 7% of patients presented with either swelling or a hydrocele. It has been previously demonstrated that the presence of a hydrocele may hinder appreciation of a testicular tumor mass, occasionally resulting in a 6-month delay in the diagnosis of testis tumors in children.[4] Therefore, children with an unexplained hydrocele in which the testis itself cannot be clearly palpated require further evaluation, generally by sonography.

Ultrasonography is the single best imaging study to define the scrotal contents. Its accuracy is nearly 100% when distinguishing between solid testicular tumors and intrascrotal fluid collections such as hydroceles. Unusual masses such as epidermoid cysts and teratomas may show complex ultrasonographic findings suggestive of the diagnosis.[5]

Although other imaging studies such as an ultrasonogram of the retroperitoneum and computed tomographic (CT) scans may be done preoperatively to evaluate for possible metastatic lesions, sonography of the scrotum and the surgical confirmation should be done initially to define the histologic status of the tumor and the testis. Further staging should be done after the final diagnosis of a testicular tumor has been made.

Table 20–1
Pathologic Classification

Germ cell tumors	Tumor of supporting tissues
Yolk sac	Fibroma
Teratoma	Leiomyoma
Seminoma	Hemangioma
Mixed	Lymphomas and leukemias
Gonadal stromal tumors	Tumor-like lesions
Leydig's cell	Epidermoid cyst
Sertoli's cell	Hyperplastic nodule secondary to congenital adrenal hyperplasia
Juvenile granulosa cell	Secondary tumors
Mixed	Tumors of adnexa
Gonadoblastoma	

Tumor markers are critical in the diagnosis of prepubertal testicular tumors. Alpha-fetoprotein (AFP) is a serum protein produced by the embryo and the yolk sac and is elevated in nearly 90% of all yolk sac tumors.[1] Described in 1910, it is one of many fetal proteins that usually disappear after embryogenesis. It is produced by yolk sac carcinoma and, therefore, is a very specific tumor marker. It has a half-life of 5 days. An AFP level should be obtained in any scrotal mass before surgery, but exploration should not be delayed pending its results, particularly if a scrotal mass is confirmed by ultrasonographic findings. One important consideration with AFP is its normal degradation in newborns. It is well known that AFP may be elevated in infants up to 8 months of age.[6] Therefore, in infants, AFP may not be used reliably for diagnostic or initial follow-up purposes. However, it should be monitored carefully with the recognition that the persistence of an elevated AFP in the small infant may not indicate residual tumor. Despite these qualifications, AFP is an outstanding testicular tumor marker that should be obtained before surgery and monitored during the postoperative follow-up and surveillance periods.

The β subunit of human chorionic gonadotropin is a testis tumor marker monitored extensively in adults. Its half-life is 30 hours. Its usefulness in children, however, is quite limited because it is produced by the syncytiotrophoblast, which is not usually present in yolk sac tumors or the other testicular tumors of childhood.

It is important to note that a delay in diagnosis is a potential risk of prepubertal testis tumors. The initial delay may be caused by the family who denies an enlargement and awaits the routine physical exam. It also may be missed by the pediatrician or may be believed to be a simple hydrocele. When patients are seen by pediatric urologists, it is essential that any scrotal enlargement be well defined. A high index of suspicion should obviate delay in diagnosis and, it is hoped, improve both diagnostic accuracy and treatment results.

The differential diagnosis of a scrotal mass ranges from the serious, such as tumors and testicular torsion, to the benign, most commonly communicating hydroceles. It has been previously mentioned that ultrasonography differentiates fluids from solids. It should also be mentioned that AFP may not differentiate between yolk sac tumors and torsion of the testis, because AFP is often elevated in young infants.[6] If an elevated AFP is used to assume that a tumor is present and surgery is even slightly delayed, a torsion may be missed. Therefore, the clinical appearance and physical examination combined with a high index of suspicion should, in fact, dictate the appropriate treatment.

NEWBORNS

Newborn infants who present with a solid mass represent a unique group. The differential diagnosis is between torsion of the testis and testicular tumor. It is important to recognize that testicular tumors may occur in the newborn.[7] Imaging may not be of diagnostic help and AFP may be misleading. If the index of suspicion is high, then the testis should be explored and the appropriate treatment applied. The Prepubertal Testicular Tumor Registry recorded 20 patients younger than 1 month.[7] It is of interest that 6 of the newborns were found to have yolk sac tumors, 6 had undifferentiated gonadal stromal tumors, and 2 had juvenile granulosa cell tumors. Only one case of teratoma was entered into the registry. It is, therefore, important to recognize that true malignancy such as yolk sac carcinomas may present in the newborn, and treatment needs to be appropriate and timely.

MANAGEMENT

Orchiectomy

After the diagnosis of an intratesticular solid mass, surgical exploration must be performed (Fig. 20–1). The procedure of choice is a radical orchiectomy or testis-sparing surgery when deemed appropriate. Radical orchiectomy begins with a transverse inguinal incision within the skin crease. This fold is approximately halfway between the pubic tubercle and the anterosuperior iliac spine (Fig. 20–2). Electrocautery is used to divide the subcutaneous tissue to the level of the external oblique fascia, which is divided in the direction of its fibers using a pair of Metzenbaum scissors (Fig. 20–3). At this point, the spermatic cord can usually be identified, and, with a pair of nontooth forceps, the cord is grasped and elevated into the wound. The cremasteric fibers are then carefully

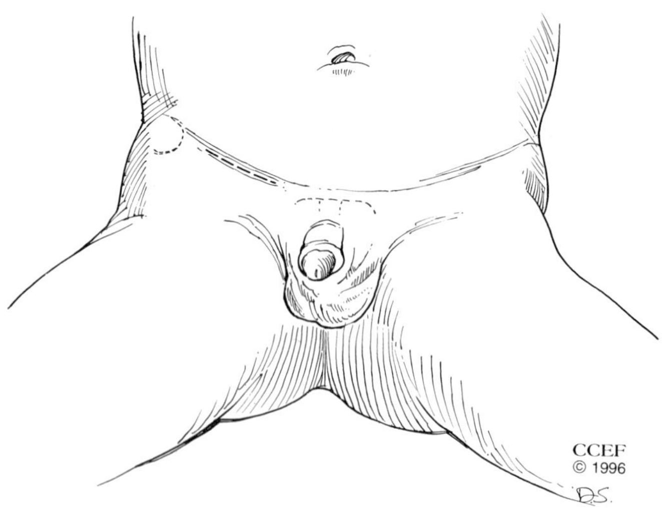

Figure 20–1 A transverse incision is made in the inguinal crease midway between the anterior superior iliac spine and the pubic tubercle.

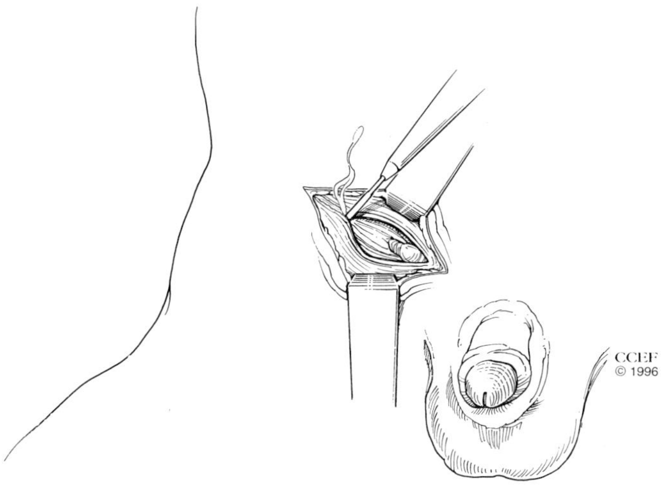

Figure 20–2 Electrocautery is used to divide Scarpa's fascia down to the level of the external oblique.

and bluntly dissected from the cord structures. At this point, a noncrushing clamp is placed across the cord structures at the level of the internal ring (Fig. 20–4). This allows manipulation of the testis while preventing migration of testicular tumor cells into the vascular system. The testis is then delivered into the wound by sharply dividing the gubernaculum using electrocautery (Fig. 20–5). This is done outside the tunica vaginalis so that there is no violation of the tunica vaginalis or the spermatic cord, or possible damage to a looped vas. If an intratesticular tumor is confirmed, the testis is then removed. This is performed by separating the cord into two portions: the vas deferens and the spermatic cord

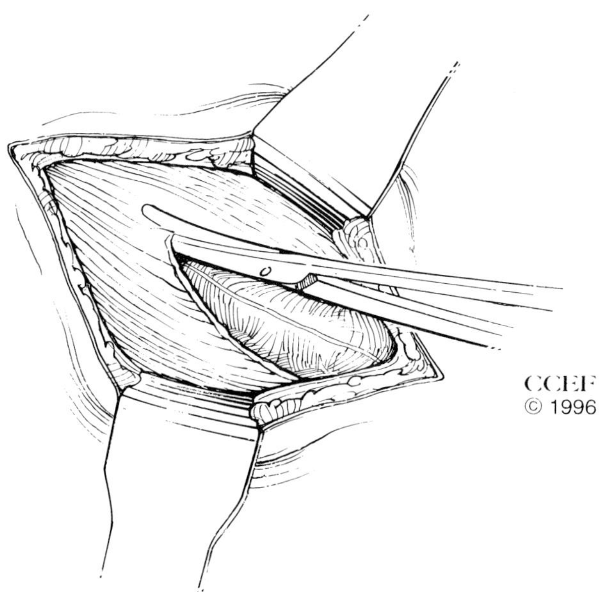

Figure 20–3 The external oblique is divided in the direction of its fibers directly over the spermatic cord.

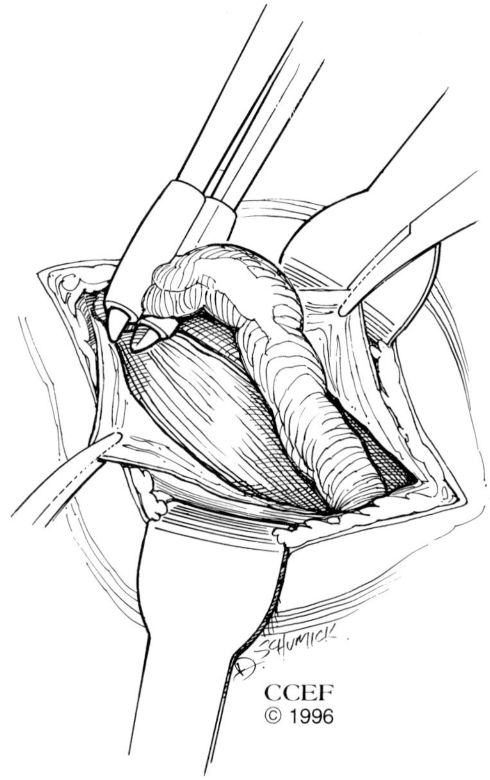

Figure 20–4 After the cord has been elevated, a noncrushing clamp is placed at the level of the internal ring.

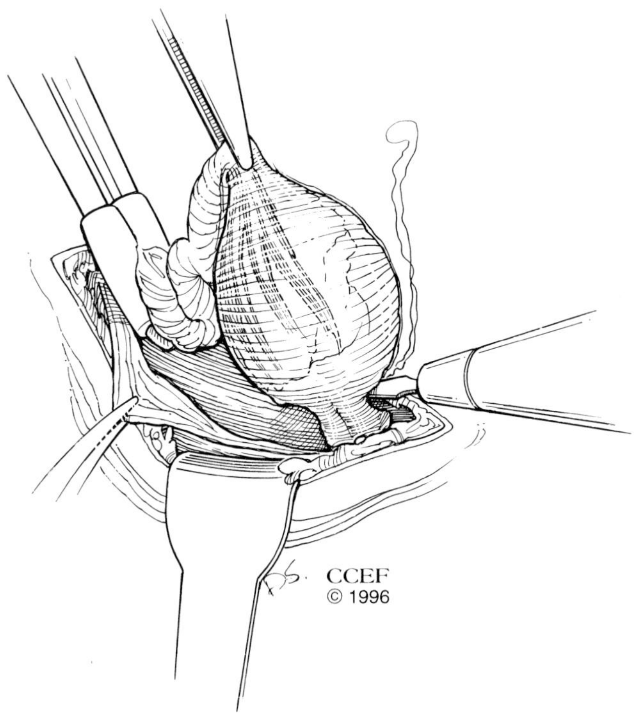

Figure 20–5 The testis is delivered into the wound, and the gubernaculum is divided sharply using electrocoagulation.

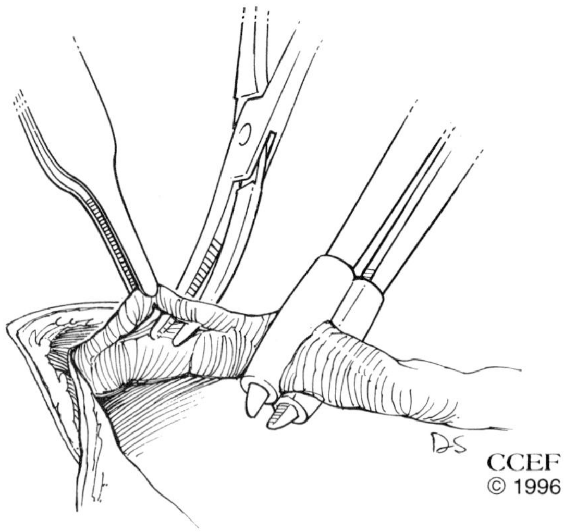

Figure 20–6 After confirmation of the intratesticular tumor, the cord is divided proximal to the crushing clamp. It is divided by isolating the vas from the spermatic vessels and dividing the vas separately.

(Fig. 20–6). Each is doubly ligated using 3-0 Vicryl, and the specimen is then removed (Fig. 20–7). The wound is then closed using a running 3-0 Vicryl for the external oblique muscle and 4-0 Vicryl for the subcutaneous tissues, including Scarpa's fascia. The skin is closed using running 4-0 or 5-0 subcuticular Vicryl. Steri-Strips are then applied, and the patient is usually discharged the same day.

No specific postoperative care is required for these patients. The procedure is usually performed on an outpatient basis, and appropriate analgesics are given. After the final pathology study has been reported, further decisions regarding management are made.

Testicle-sparing surgery does have a role in treating patients with prepubertal testis tumors.[5] Ultrasonography can be very sensitive and specific in diagnosing both teratomas and epidermoid inclusion cysts. If either of these tumors is diagnosed presumptively by sonography and negative AFP, one can feel safe in performing testis-sparing surgery. Testis-sparing surgery consists of proceeding exactly along the lines of a radical orchiectomy with delivery of both the testis and cord structures into the wound. With vascular control, using a noncrushing clamp at the internal oblique muscle, the tunica vaginalis is then opened and the testis is examined. An incision is then made into the tunica albuginea over the palpated testis mass. With a combination of both sharp and blunt dissection, the mass itself can usually be enucleated by gently teasing the seminiferous tubules from the mass. The surface of the mass serves as an excellent plane, and dissection is performed against the surface or capsule of the teratoma or epidermoid inclusion cyst. If necessary, bleeding is controlled with ligation using 4-0 chromic suture. It is important that frozen sections be performed before release of the spermatic cord. This should include frozen sections not only of the tumor but of the testis, particularly where the tumor was adherent. While awaiting the results of the frozen section, the tunica albuginea can be closed using interrupted 4-0 chromic sutures (Fig. 20–8). After the frozen section, if the diagnosis confirms a benign lesion, the spermatic cord is released and the testis is placed into the scrotum (Fig. 20–9). This can be done by gently pulling on the scrotal skin if the gubernaculum was left intact or by creating a dartos pouch if the gubernaculum had previously been divided. If the tissue examination suggests either malignancy or there is remaining tumor within the testis at the base, the testis should be excised by dividing the vas and spermatic vessels at the level of the internal ring (Fig. 20–10).

After orchiectomy, some children with testicular tumors require additional therapy. The options include

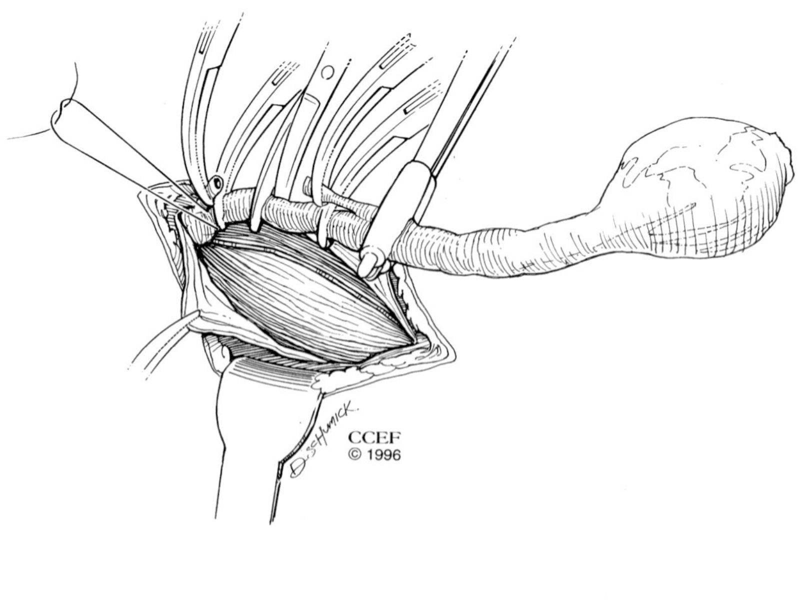

Figure 20–7 The vas has been divided, and the spermatic vessels are clamped. The cord is then sharply divided.

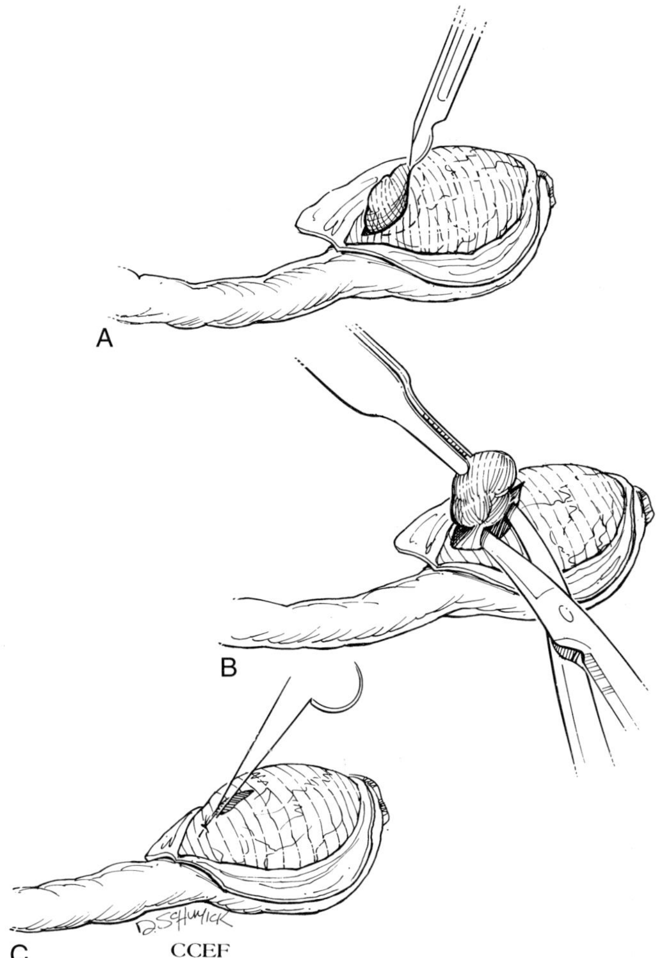

Figure 20–8 *A*, An incision is made either directly over the palpable mass or around the mass, leaving a patch of tunica albuginea, if necessary, directly on the mass. *B*, The mass is mobilized from the surrounding seminiferous tubules using sharp and blunt dissection. *C*, The tunica albuginea is closed using interrupted 4-0 chromic sutures.

chemotherapy, retroperitoneal lymph node dissection (RPLND), and radiation therapy. The type of adjunctive therapy selected will depend on the histology of the primary tumor and the results of radiographic and biochemical studies. The intensity of follow-up also depends on the malignant potential of the primary tumor.

Yolk Sac Tumor

Metastatic evaluation of yolk sac tumors includes a CT scan of the abdomen and pelvis to rule out retroperitoneal lymph node or hepatic metastases, and a chest x-ray film or chest CT scan to rule out pulmonary metastases. Bone and brain metastases are rare. Therefore, bone scans and head CT scans are obtained only when there is clinical suspicion of metastases at these sites. A serum AFP level is also measured postoperatively. Its half-life is approximately 5 days, and a persistent elevation of AFP after orchiectomy suggests the presence of metastatic disease.[15] However, AFP levels as high as 10,000 ng/mL can occur in normal infants and may not decrease to a normal range until 8 months of age.[6] Therefore, serial measurements are particularly important in small children.

Approximately 85% of children with yolk sac tumors will have stage I tumors: those limited to the testis.[8] A minority of patients will have metastatic disease. Patients with stage II tumors have a persistently elevated AFP or isolated retroperitoneal disease evident on CT scan or RPLND. Patients with hematogenous metastases, most commonly to the lungs or liver, are designated as having stage III tumors.

Historically, RPLND was the most common form of adjunctive therapy after orchiectomy for the treatment of yolk sac tumors. A standard RPLND is accomplished through a midline or transverse abdominal incision. Complete excision of all lymphatic tissue from the renal hila to 2 cm beyond the bifurcation of the common iliac arteries is accomplished. The lateral margins of dissection are the ureters, and the great vessels are completely skeletonized throughout. Modified templates limiting the contralateral dissection and nerve-sparing techniques have been described in adults in an attempt to minimize the morbidity of the dissection, particularly anejaculation. For right-sided tumors, a modified template dissection is limited medially by the anterior surface of the aorta. Below the inferior mesenteric artery (IMA), dissection is limited medially by the right common iliac artery, preserving the hypogastric plexus. The modified template for a left-sided tumor is limited medially by the anterior surface of the inferior vena cava. Below the IMA, dissection is again limited medially by the left common iliac artery. However, the efficacy of these modified techniques has not been clarified in children.

With the widespread use of AFP to detect occult metastases and improvements in multiagent chemotherapy, the reliance on RPLND to diagnose and treat metastatic disease has waned. RPLND is less beneficial for children than for adults because yolk sac tumors in children have a predilection for hematogenous spread; only a minority of metastases are limited to the retroperitoneum. A review of the Prepubertal Testis Tumor Registry found that metastases were limited to the retroperitoneum in only 32% of patients with metastatic disease, whereas metastatic disease in 46% of these patients occurred at hematogenous sites without retroperitoneal involvement.[8] The operative morbidity of RPLND in children is significant, including wound complications, bowel obstruction, and chylous ascites. Most children undergoing RPLND will be anejaculatory as adults as a result of injury to the sympathetic nerves.

Chemotherapy is very effective in treating metastatic yolk sac tumor. The most commonly used regimens in-

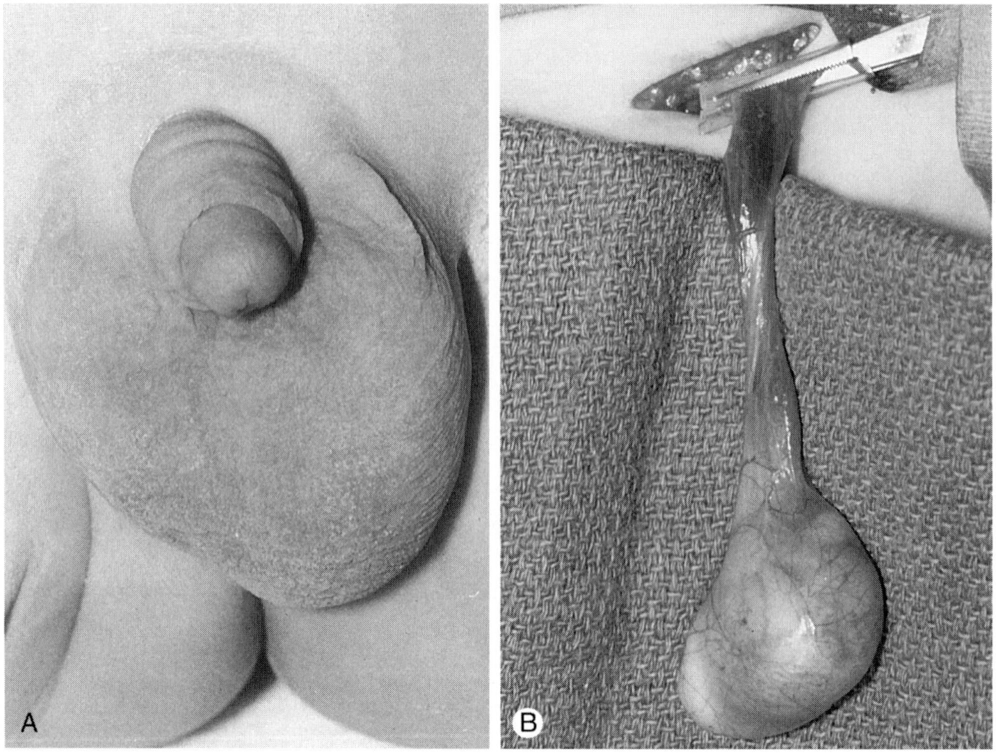

Figure 20–9 *A*, Gross photograph of 7-month-old child with left scrotal mass. *B*, Intraoperative photograph demonstrating complete mobilization of testis outside the tunica vaginalis with a rubber-shod, noncrushing clamp on the spermatic cord.

clude vincristine, actinomycin D, and cyclophosphamide and cisplatin, vinblastine, and bleomycin. Platinum-based chemotherapy is the most effective treatment. Because children with metastatic disease often have multiple sites of spread, chemotherapy (as opposed to RPLND) is particularly appropriate.

Radiation is not a standard form of treatment for metastatic yolk sac tumor. Although yolk sac tumor is radiosensitive, the doses required when radiation is used as a primary therapy are prohibitively toxic.[9] Lower doses of radiation may play a role in combination with surgery and chemotherapy for high-risk patients.

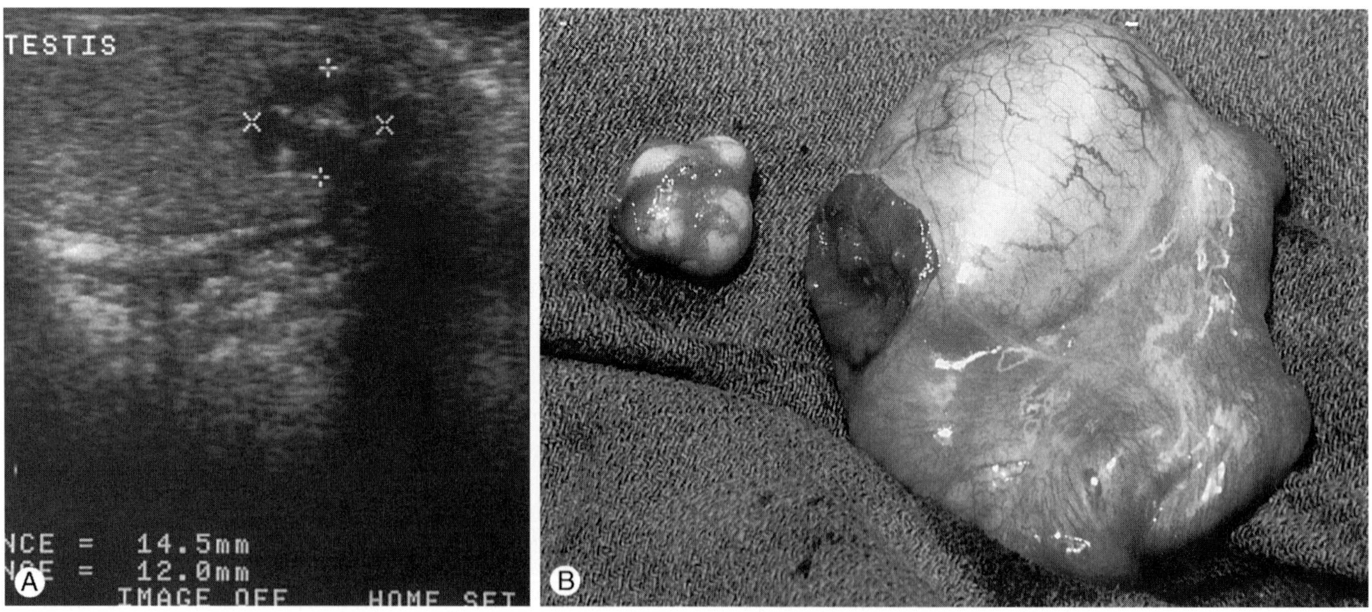

Figure 20–10 *A*, Ultrasonogram showing complex mass in lower pole of the testis. *B*, Intraoperative photograph demonstrating enucleation of epidermoid cyst in testicle-sparing operation.

As with adult germ cell tumors, the selection of adjunctive therapy for yolk sac tumor depends on the stage of the tumor. The trend in managing stage I tumors is toward observation. Most series reported in the last decade have found no survival advantage to adjuvant therapy in this group.[10–14] The recurrence rate for patients with stage I tumor managed by observation is approximately 20%, and virtually all of these patients can be salvaged with chemotherapy. Chemotherapy may be considered in high-risk patients, such as those older than 2 years or those with a normal AFP before orchiectomy who cannot be reliably monitored biochemically. However, review of the Prepubertal Testicular Tumor Registry revealed no difference in death rate based on age and only a modest increase in risk of metastatic disease for older patients (25% vs. 14%).[2]

Therefore, patients with stage I tumor are generally observed closely without adjuvant therapy. Patients are evaluated 1 month after orchiectomy with a CT scan of the abdomen and pelvis, a chest x-ray film, and a serum AFP. For 2 years the serum AFP and chest x-ray film are repeated every 6 weeks and the CT scan or sonogram every 3 months. Recurrent disease is usually treated with chemotherapy, even if it appears to be limited to the retroperitoneum. If the patient remains free of disease for 2 years, then he is almost certainly cured, and minimal follow-up is required beyond that point.[13]

Patients with a negative metastatic evaluation but a failure of the AFP to normalize are generally treated with chemotherapy. It must be remembered that a "normal" AFP in small children may be quite high.[16] Patients with positive lymph nodes on CT are also treated with chemotherapy, although consideration may be given to performing a modified RPLND in the presence of minimal retroperitoneal disease and a normal AFP. An RPLND should also be considered when retroperitoneal disease is not responding to chemotherapy.

Chemotherapy is also the mainstay of treatment for stage III disease. An RPLND should be considered for those with residual retroperitoneal disease after chemotherapy. Chemotherapy with second-line agents should be used for patients who fail to respond to standard agents. Surgical excision and radiation should also be considered for those with limited sites of metastatic disease who fail to respond to chemotherapy.

Teratoma and Epidermoid Cyst

Teratomas and epidermoid cysts are universally benign in prepubertal children. As discussed, testis-sparing surgery is a reasonable consideration for these patients. No radiographic studies or follow-up for the development of metastatic disease are thought to be required.[17]

Gonadal Stromal Tumors

Stromal testis tumors are rare in children, and there are no large series to guide their management. However, anecdotal reports and small series in the literature offer some experience on which to base therapy.

Leydig cell tumors are universally benign in children.[1] They usually present because of precocious puberty and must be distinguished from testis tumors associated with the adrenogenital syndrome. Leydig cell tumors may be treated by orchiectomy or testis-sparing excision. Persistence of androgenic effects after excision may be due to a contralateral tumor, which is rare in children.[1] Because Leydig cell tumors are sometimes difficult to detect on physical exam, an ultrasonogram may be necessary to rule out a contralateral tumor. However, even after successful removal of a solitary tumor, androgenic changes are not completely reversible, and some children may proceed through premature puberty because of activation of the hypothalamic-pituitary-gonadal axis.

Sertoli cell tumors are usually hormonally inactive in children, although they may occasionally cause gynecomastia. They generally occur in infants and small children and are benign in children younger than 5 years. There have been a few cases of malignancy in older children.[15] Orchiectomy is sufficient treatment in infants. Older children should undergo abdominal CT scan and chest x-ray film to rule out metastases. When metastatic disease is present, aggressive combination treatment, including RPLND, chemotherapy, and radiation therapy, should be considered. The large cell calcifying Sertoli cell tumor is a separate entity with a higher incidence of bilaterality and hormonal activity.[1] The treatment of this variant is the same as for other Sertoli cell tumors.

Granulosa cell tumors occur exclusively in the first months of life, most in the newborn period. Structural abnormalities of the Y chromosome and mosaicism are common.[15] These tumors are hormonally inactive and benign. Although these children should undergo chromosomal analysis, no treatment or metastatic evaluation is required beyond orchiectomy. "Mixed" or "undifferentiated" stromal tumors have an epidemiology and behavior similar to that of granulosa cell tumors. Although some of these tumors have histologic characteristics commonly associated with malignancy, their behavior is almost always benign.

REFERENCES

1. Coppes M, Rackley R, Kay R. Primary testicular and paratesticular tumors of childhood. Med Pediatr Oncol 22:329, 1994.
2. Kay R. Prepubertal testicular tumor registry. Urol Clin North Am 20:1, 1993.
3. Kay R, Kaplan GW. Testicular tumors in infants and children. Am Urol Assoc Update Series 9:114, 1992.
4. Brosnan SA. Testicular tumors in prepubertal children. Urology 13:581, 1979.
5. Ross J, Kay R, Elder J. Testis sparing surgery for pediatric epidermoid cysts in the testis. J Urol 149:353, 1993.

6. Brewer J, Tank E. Yolk sac tumors and alpha-fetoprotein in first year of life. Urology 42:79, 1993.
7. Levy D, Kay R, Elder J. Neonatal testis tumors: A review of the Prepubertal Testis Tumor Registry. J Urol 151:715, 1994.
8. Grady R, Ross JH, Kay R. Patterns of metastatic spread in prepubertal yolk sac tumor of the testis. J Urol 153:1259, 1995.
9. Griffin GC, Raney RB Jr, Snyder HM, et al. Yolk sac carcinoma of the testis in children. J Urol 137:954, 1987.
10. Fernandes E, Etcubanas E, Rao Bhaskar, et al. Two decades of experience with testicular tumors in children at St. Jude Children's Research Hospital. J Pediatr Surg 24:677, 1989.
11. Haas R, Piroska S, Gobel U, Harms D. Treatment of malignant testicular tumors in childhood: Results of the German National Study 1982–1992. Med Pediatr Oncol 23:400, 1994.
12. Huddart S, Mann J, Gornall P, et al. The UK Children's Cancer Study Group: Testicular malignant germ cell tumours 1979–1988. J Pediatr Surg 25:406, 1990.
13. Kaplan G, Cromie W, Panayotis K, et al. Genitourinary tumors. J Urol 140:1109, 1988.
14. Leonard M, Jeffs R, Leventhal B, et al. Pediatric testicular tumors: The Johns Hopkins experience. Urology 37:253, 1991.
15. Cortez J, Kaplan G. Gonadal stromal tumors, gonadoblastomas, epidermoid cysts, and secondary tumors of the testis in children. Urol Clin North Am 20:15, 1993.
16. Lange PH, Vogelzang NJ, Goldman A, et al. Marker half-life analysis as prognostic tool in testicular cancer. J Urol 128:708, 1982.
17. Manivel JC, Reinberg Y, Nifans GA. Intratubular germ cell neoplasia in testicular teratomas and epidermoid cysts. Cancer 64:715, 1989.

PART VIII

Trauma

ANTHONY J. CASALE

21

Genitourinary Trauma in Children

Trauma is the leading cause of morbidity and mortality in the pediatric age group and results in more deaths than all other causes combined. In children who suffer multiple trauma, the urinary tract is injured in frequency second only to the nervous system.[1] Of children evaluated at pediatric hospital trauma centers, 2.9% suffered significant genitourinary trauma.[2] Motor vehicle accidents, pedestrians struck by motor vehicles, sports injuries, assaults, and sexual abuse make up the litany of traumatic events in modern society that lead to genitourinary injuries. The urologist may play a number of roles in dealing with children with genitourinary injuries: primary physician, consultant, and now more often the expert in evaluating injuries that have serious legal repercussions.

Although the most important goal remains the optimal care and recovery of the injured child, the urologist must keep in mind that every physical finding and clinical symptom may be a subject of intense interest at a later date as the legal system sorts out important questions of responsibility and custody. Because of medicolegal implications, careful documentation of injuries in terms of written records, radiographs, and sometimes photographs has become not only advisable but mandatory. In cases of assault and sexual abuse, the urologist is wise to contact the local child protective agencies to delineate the physician's duty under the law.

In pediatric hospitals and most community medical centers, the initial management of acute trauma has evolved into a team approach involving multiple physicians and ancillary personnel. The urologist works best as a part of that team, which includes general surgeons and intensivists. The team is most complete in the initial evaluation and resuscitation period. Members then phase out their involvement as their skills are no longer needed. The urologist is often one of the first physicians called and, if the genitourinary tract is involved, takes responsibility as the primary physician.

EVALUATION OF CHILDREN WITH SUSPECTED GENITOURINARY TRAUMA

The circumstances of the accident or assault are invaluable in evaluating patients with suspected genitourinary injuries. The patient's history is sometimes the best account, but often the child is not able to provide information because of age or associated injuries. Parents and other witnesses, both adults and other children, may be the only reliable sources of information.

Of utmost importance are the time and mechanism of injury. If the child was in a motor vehicle accident, was he or she restrained by a car seat or seat belt? Was the child ejected from the car, and was there a loss of consciousness? How bad was the accident, and what was the extent of injuries to others involved? Details may be obtained from the emergency medical personnel who retrieved the patient from the trauma scene. In assaults, who were the assailants, how many were there, and what were their ages? If a weapon was used, what was the caliber or type, and is it available for the physician to examine? In falls, what was the height, and where did the child land? Was the surface smooth and clear, or was it irregular with rocks or tree branches? Was it hard or soft? What was the position of the child as he or she landed, and was he or she able to move? What were the child's initial complaints before he or she became unconscious or unable to speak? Did the child void before arrival at the hospital, and was there blood or pain? Too often, there is little or no history available, and the urologist must evaluate an unconsciousness child using only physical exam and radiographic studies.

Priorities of care must be observed. Although the urologist is most interested in genitourinary injuries, the first physician involved must make sure that an adequate airway is established, intravenous access is available, external bleeding is controlled, and the patient is restrained appropriately to prevent potential central nervous system and orthopedic injuries. If the urologist is not needed to perform these vital resuscitation duties, then he or she can concentrate on two goals: (1) establishing whether there are genitourinary injuries and their extent and urgency and (2) providing adequate drainage for urine.

Nothing replaces a thorough physical examination of the patient. The urologist should note abrasions or contusions of the abdomen, flank, perineum, and external genitalia. Ecchymosis of the flank may indicate a retroperitoneal hematoma. Butterfly ecchymosis of the perineum signifies bleeding within the limits of Colles' fascia as a result of genital or pelvic injury. Edema or a hematoma of the scrotum or labia may be a result of local soft tissue injury to the external genitalia or pelvic injury causing bleeding or extravasation of urine. Blood at or around the urinary meatus is important and suggests internal injuries to the urinary tract. Blood at the vaginal introitus may be a result of urethral or vaginal lacerations.

The child's abdomen must be auscultated for bowel sounds and vascular bruits. Palpation may reveal masses that might represent a hematoma surrounding a renal injury or a pelvic mass caused by a distended bladder or pelvic hematoma. Generalized abdominal distention can be due to bleeding or extravasation of urine into the peritoneal cavity. Diffuse rebound tenderness or involuntary guarding are usually a result of significant intra-abdominal injuries and resultant peritonitis. Finally, a rectal exam should reveal the presence of a pelvic hematoma or establish that the urethra, prostate, and bladder are in the proper position. In cases of assault and sexual abuse, internal examination of the rectum, urethra, and vagina should be performed under anesthesia if necessary.

Laboratory tests relevant to genitourinary trauma are the urinalysis and hemoglobin-hematocrit. The urinalysis is important because the presence of significant hematuria is a helpful, but not foolproof, indicator of injuries to the urinary tract. Although injuries to any portion of the genitourinary system can result in significant blood loss, it is extremely unlikely that these injuries will lead to life-threatening hemorrhage. The hemoglobin-hematocrit is most helpful in monitoring known injuries of the urinary tract over time and may dictate the need for operative intervention for persistent bleeding.

Radiographic evaluation of the urinary tract for trauma is usually best performed in order from the bottom to the top. The urologist first establishes that the urethra is intact with a retrograde urethrogram. This is particularly important in males with potential pelvic fractures and possible urethral disruption. Only if this study is negative can a catheter be passed into the bladder for a cystogram to rule out bladder injuries. Finally, an intravenous pyelogram (IVP) is performed to view the kidneys and ureters. Although this is still a perfectly adequate plan of study, the computed tomographic (CT) scan has dominated the acute evaluation of the injured abdomen and pelvis for the past 10 years. CT scanning has the ability to inventory all intra-abdominal injuries quickly and accurately. The CT scan, however, is not adequate to evaluate the bladder without retrograde filling through a catheter and has not replaced the retrograde urethrogram in its ability to outline urethral injuries. In patients who are not suspected of having serious genitourinary injuries but in whom isolated renal trauma is possible, renal ultrasonogram is a reasonable screening study.

Patients with multiple injuries must have their injuries prioritized. Because genitourinary injuries are seldom life threatening, injuries to the central nervous system, cardiovascular injuries, pulmonary injuries, and injuries to the abdominal viscera usually take precedence. Once the urologist has defined the extent of injury and has established adequate urinary drainage, the other services may take over primary management until the patient is stable. If exploratory laparotomy is necessary, the urologist should be available to examine any injured portions of the urinary tract and intervene if necessary.

RENAL TRAUMA

Of all blunt and penetrating abdominal injuries, 8 to 12% involve the kidneys. Of genitourinary injuries alone, the kidneys account for about 50%. Historically, in adults and children, blunt renal trauma has been much more prevalent and makes up 80 to 90% of kidney injuries.[3] In rural and suburban settings blunt trauma represents 90 to 95%, whereas in urban areas penetrating trauma resulting from violent crime is on the rise and may represent 20% of all kidney injuries.[4] Unfortunately, this is also true for the pediatric population, and the incidence of penetrating renal injuries caused by gunshot and stab wounds is increasing, particularly among inner city adolescent males.[5]

BLUNT RENAL TRAUMA

Children are more likely than adults to suffer renal injuries as a result of blunt abdominal trauma because of their different anatomy. The child's kidney is proportionally larger than the adult's, and it extends further below the protection of the rib cage. The abdominal muscles are less developed, and the entire thoracoabdominal trunk is less rigid. Children have less retroperitoneal and abdominal fat to insulate and protect the kidney. Finally, persistent fetal lobulations present in young children offer natural lines of cleavage when traumatic force is applied to the kidney.[6]

The circumstances that lead to blunt renal injuries in children are different than those in adults in that pedestrian–motor vehicle accidents are a major cause of abdominal trauma in children. Of 129 pediatric patients with blunt renal injuries, 45 (35%) were pedestrians struck by motor vehicles, 40 (31%) were passengers involved in motor vehicle accidents, 36 (28%) suffered injuries in falls, 5 (4%) were injured while playing sports, and 3 (2%) were victims of assault.[2, 7–10] Among children, about 66% of blunt renal injuries occur in boys and 33% in girls. The right kidney is involved slightly more often than the left, with a wide variation between series. Motor vehicle accidents cause 50% of renal trauma cases in the adult population, followed by vehicle pedestrian accidents

(11–18%), motorcycle accidents (11%), and assaults (9–17%).[11, 12]

Pre-existing renal anomalies in renal structure and position place the kidney at greater risk for blunt injury. The classic example of this is the hydronephrotic kidney with a ureteropelvic junction obstruction, but pelvic kidneys and hypertrophied solitary kidneys are also more susceptible to blunt trauma (Fig. 21–1). Mertz and colleagues found a pre-existing condition in 21% of patients with renal trauma.[13] When a relatively minor trauma causes unusually severe signs of renal injury, a pre-existing anomaly should be suspected.

Isolated injuries to the kidneys are rare in children because the nature of their accidents often leads to other organ injuries. In two large U.S. studies, 80% of children with all classes of blunt renal trauma suffered significant associated injuries.[2, 10] Other abdominal solid organs, namely the liver and spleen, are similar to the kidney in their resilience to injury and are only partially protected by the rib cage. The high number of pedestrian-vehicle accidents and severe falls among children is associated with head trauma and extremity injuries. In children with renal injuries, liver or spleen injuries occur in 46%, closed head injuries in 35%, and fractures in 21%.[2, 10]

The signs and symptoms of pediatric renal trauma include diffuse abdominal and flank tenderness, lower rib fractures, vertebral pedicle fractures, abdominal and flank contusions and abrasions, and hematuria. In children hematuria is a reliable sign of renal trauma; only 2.6% of all blunt renal injuries present without microscopic or gross hematuria. The majority (65.5%) of patients with *severe* renal injuries will present with gross hematuria, whereas some will have microhematuria (32.7%), and only 1.7% will have none. Ureteropelvic disruptions and traumatic renal artery occlusion have the highest incidence of the absence of hematuria, but these injuries are quite rare. Minor renal injuries such as contusions may also present with gross hematuria (31%), microhematuria (65.5%), or clear urine (3.4%).[2, 8–10, 14, 15] In most authors' experience, although the presence of hematuria is reliable, the degree of hematuria does not consistently correlate with the severity of the injury.

The definition of microhematuria is of some importance. A number of authors have tried to quantify the amount of blood in the urine that is necessary to predict renal injury accurately. Several studies have found very few renal injuries in patients with levels of microhematuria less than 20 and 50 red blood cells per high power field (RBC/HPF).[16–18]

Although the exact threshold of significant microhematuria has yet to be established, it is clear that significant renal injuries can be present with little or no blood in the urine.[19–21] The absence of hematuria cannot be used alone as a reason to omit evaluation of the urinary tract in cases of blunt abdominal trauma. Other factors that must be taken into account include the general condition of the patient, the nature and severity of the injury, and the state of consciousness when the physical examination is performed. Awake, alert, asymptomatic patients without clinical findings to suggest renal injury and less than 50 RBC/HPF may be observed or screened with sonography.

Hypotension has been relied on as a predictor of significant renal injury in adults. In a review of 1007 blunt trauma cases in adults, Mee and coworkers found that 44 had significant renal injuries (4.4%) and that each had

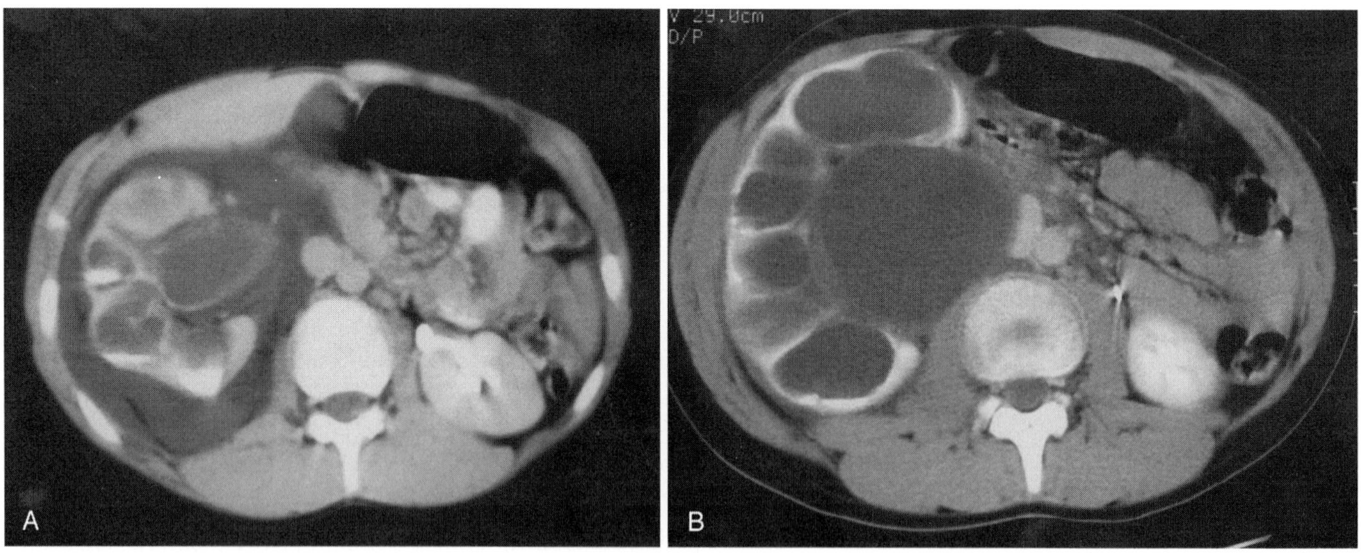

Figure 21–1 *A,* Computed tomographic scan of a 9-year-old boy injured in a fall reveals hydronephrosis, thin parenchyma, and a large perirenal hematoma. *B,* Six weeks later, the hematoma is resolved, and a hydronephrotic kidney caused by ureteropelvic junction obstruction is demonstrated.

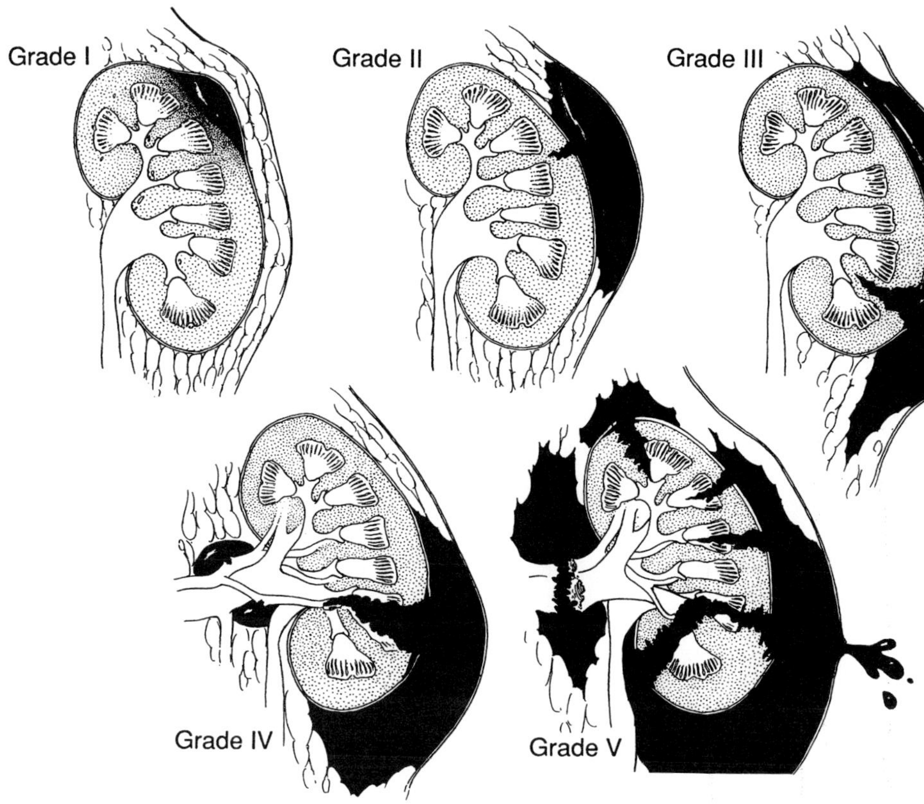

Figure 21–2 Renal injuries classified by severity. From Moore EE, et al. Organ injury scaling: Spleen, liver, and kidney. J Trauma 29:1664, 1989. Used with permission.

either gross hematuria or microscopic hematuria and shock.[22] In 812 patients who failed to meet these criteria, namely microhematuria without evidence of hypotension (diastolic blood pressure < 90 mm Hg), none had significant renal injury. Adult trauma patients with microhematuria and normal blood pressure in the absence of other clinical findings need not undergo radiographic evaluation of the urinary tract according to most authors.[23]

This does not appear to be the case with children. The incidence of hypotension in children with blunt renal trauma ranges from 5 to 46% and averages 16% in a group of 197 patients.[2, 8–10, 13, 14] Of this group, 29% have other intra-abdominal injuries that probably contributed to their hypotension. Stein and colleagues found shock absent in 16 of 17 children (94%) with microhematuria and significant renal injury.[10] Nine of the 17 had other abdominal injuries that led to imaging that diagnosed the renal injuries, but 7 of 17 (41%) had no other abdominal indications for imaging. In these children, applying the adult criteria for evaluation of the urinary tract would have resulted in significant renal injuries being missed. Our recommendation is that all children involved in significant blunt abdominal trauma regardless of hematuria should undergo imaging of the urinary tract even if normotensive. Children have an extended ability to maintain their blood pressure in the presence of hypovolemia as a result of the compliance of their vascular tree and excellent cardiac compensation mechanisms.

There are several classification systems of blunt renal injuries (Fig. 21–2). Because the mechanism of injury is blunt force, which tears renal parenchyma, the classification of injury relies on the extent of these tears or lacerations. The vast majority of blunt renal injuries are staged with CT scan, and the classification systems are based on the use of this modality. In the least severe injuries, the damage is not sufficient to cause separation of the parenchyma. If more severe force is applied to the kidney, the parenchyma tears and separates enough to be visualized on CT scan. The depth of this laceration into the kidney substance defines the next two stages of renal injury along with injury to the collecting system, which may result in urinary extravasation. Shattered kidneys and disruptions to the renal blood supply constitute the most severe injuries.

Contusions of the kidney are the least severe of all identifiable renal injuries, and they are the most common, making up 80% of total renal trauma in most series.[12, 21] Many of these minor injuries were not detectable on IVP and were only diagnosed with the development of CT scan. Contusions may be identified by an area of decreased uptake of contrast material or by a subcapsular hematoma. They may produce either microscopic or gross hematuria, and many patients have minor, if any, symptoms. Treatment consists only of bed rest until the gross hematuria resolves.

Minor lacerations limited to the superficial cortex of the kidney produce proportionally greater symptoms and are usually associated with larger hematomas. They do not enter the collecting system and, therefore, cause no extravasation of urine. These injuries are also treated with bed rest and fluid resuscitation as necessary. Hematuria and pain take several days to resolve, and, unlike simple contusions, follow-up imaging of the kidney is advisable to ensure that the hematoma does not expand and that the kidney heals.

Major lacerations of the kidney tear deep into the cortex and may enter the collecting system. These patients generally lose a significant amount of blood and develop a perirenal hematoma within Gerota's fascia. The CT scan is very sensitive in identifying extravasated contrast, which appears as a swirl of radiodense material within the hematoma (Fig. 21–3). These patients may show signs of hemodynamic instability, but the cause of hypotension is often uncertain because there is a significant incidence of associated injuries. Shock is uncommon in children with isolated renal injuries, but persistent bleeding is clearly a danger and patients should be monitored with sequential hematocrits in an intensive care unit (ICU) setting until stable. Patients with severe lacerations are at significant risk for late complications and should remain at bed rest for 7 to 10 days until hematuria clears and follow-up imaging shows stabilization of the injured kidney.

The most severe type of blunt renal injury is the shattered kidney. These kidneys have been struck so forcibly that they separate into segments (Fig. 21–4). There is always extravasation of urine and contrast along with massive bleeding, which often fills the limits of Gerota's fascial envelope. Often these segments retain their segmental blood supply and, if bleeding stops, will realign themselves and bond together to form a surprisingly

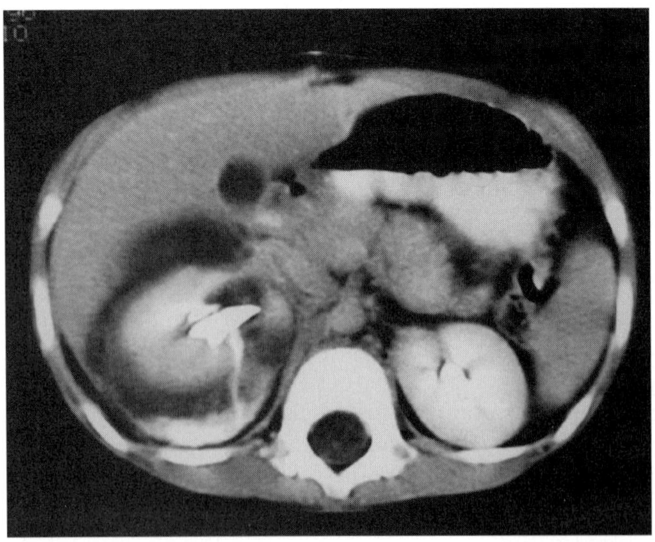

Figure 21–3 Computed tomographic scan shows a major laceration of the kidney with extravasation of contrast into the perirenal space.

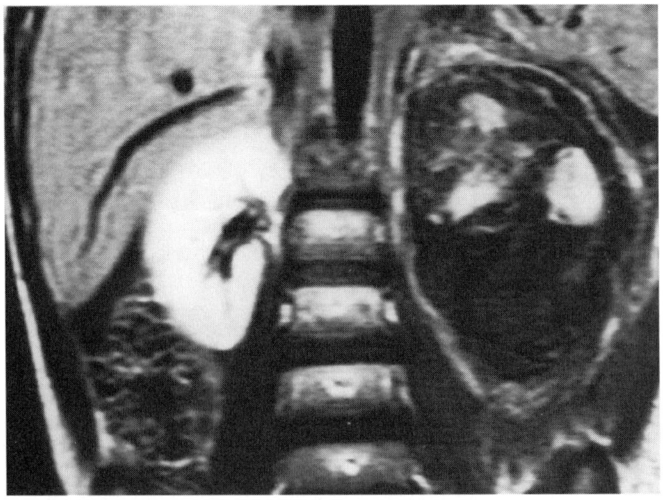

Figure 21–4 Magnetic resonance image demonstrates shattered left kidney with functioning segments separated by hematoma. Perinephric hematoma fills the entire limits of Gerota's fascia.

normal-appearing renal shape. A special case occurs when there is a significantly large, devascularized renal segment, often the lower pole. The complication rate in this instance is high, and some authors advocate early surgical repair with debridement of nonviable tissue.[24]

The initial treatment of severe lacerations and shattered kidneys has been a point of controversy over the past few years. Early surgical exploration and primary repair have yielded excellent results in some hands and still have a role in certain circumstances.[25, 26] Alternatively, conservative management with bed rest, fluid resuscitation, and close monitoring has also been successful and has the added benefit of saving the patient an emergency operation in the immediate postinjury period. Absolute indications for early surgery are signs of persistent bleeding such as an expanding or uncontained hematoma. Relative indications are massive urinary extravasation and significant (>20%) nonviable renal tissue. Using these criteria in adults in a series of 1193 patients with blunt trauma to the kidney, McAninch and colleagues found that 31 patients, or 2.6%, needed immediate exploration.[27]

A survey of 153 pediatric urologists and pediatric surgeons regarding their method of managing stable patients with blunt renal trauma defined the current patterns of care. CT scan is the uniform method of initial evaluation, although follow-up imaging of the kidneys may be done with ultrasonogram or CT scan depending on the severity of injury. The majority of patients are admitted to an ICU setting with serial monitoring of hematocrits every 4 hours and transfusion when hematocrit drops to 21. Clinical decisions for changing the level of patient activity depend on evidence that bleeding has stopped and pain and tenderness has resolved. Most

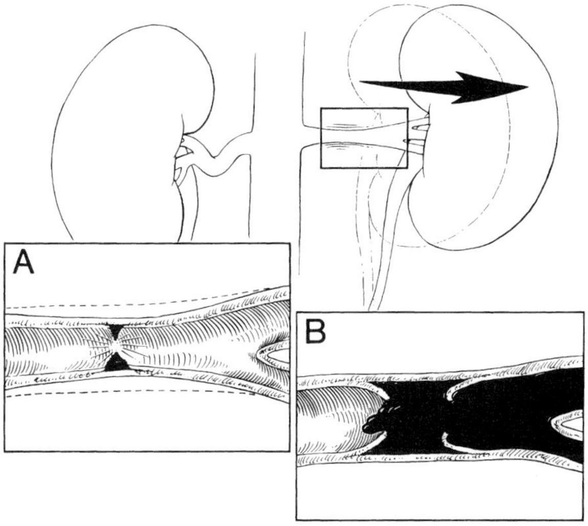

Figure 21–5 Mechanism of renal pedicle injury resulting from deceleration and stretching of the renal artery. The adventitia and muscularis layers of the artery stretch while the intima tears. Disruption of the intima allows clotting of the renal artery. From Peters PC, Bright TC III. Urol Clin North Am 4:18, 1977. Used with permission.

patients are monitored as an outpatient every 2 weeks, return to school in 2 weeks, and return to sports 3 months after discharge (AJ Casale and ME Fallet, personal communication, September 1996).

Another serious type of renal injury caused by blunt trauma is renal vascular pedicle injury, mostly involving the main renal artery. Injuries of this type have been reported in 1 to 3% of patients with blunt renal trauma.[28, 29] The mechanism of injury is believed to be the rapid deceleration of the kidney rather than a direct blow to the kidney, which occurs in other renal injuries. The patient is traveling at a high rate of speed and the body suddenly stops, as in a motor vehicle accident or fall. The kidneys are relatively mobile within the retroperitoneum and are tethered only by the short renal vessels to the nonmobile great vessels. This leads to a rapid stretching of the vessels as the kidney is pulled to a stop. The adventitia and muscularis of the artery are more elastic than the intima, and their stretching leads to disruption of the intimal lining and subsequent clotting of the artery (Fig. 21–5).

In this form of injury, hematuria is often absent and the kidney appears normal size and intact on CT scan.[30, 31] There is no hematoma in the perirenal space, but the kidney does not take up contrast, and retrograde filling of the renal vein may be observed.[32] Nonopacification of a kidney on an infused CT scan in an acute trauma setting is an indication for immediate arteriogram to establish the integrity of the renal vessels (Fig. 21–6). Because time is of the essence, some authors have suggested that arteriogram may be unnecessary and may actually be detrimental because of the 2-hour delay that it adds to the evaluation period. If an arterial injury is diagnosed and the kidney is not being perfused, then the optimal treatment is immediate surgical repair.

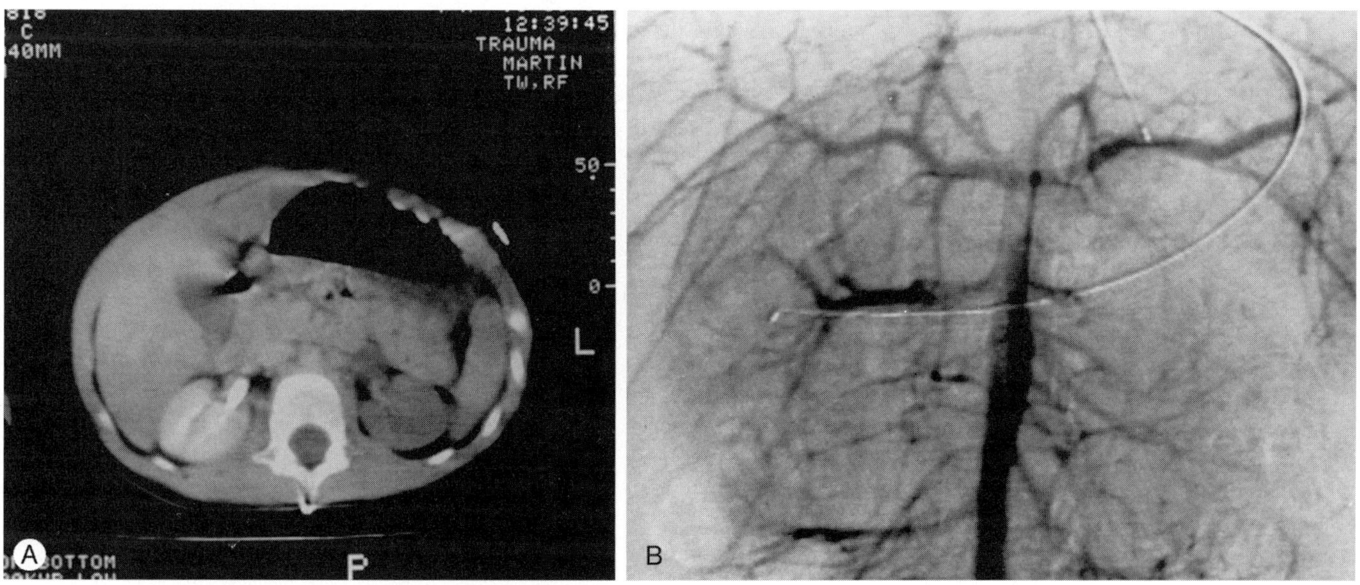

Figure 21–6 *A,* Computed tomographic scan shows normal right kidney, whereas the left kidney fails to take up contrast. The size and contour of the kidney are within normal limits. There is no perirenal hematoma. *B,* This arteriogram demonstrates complete cut off of the left renal artery due to deceleration injury.

Important considerations that affect treatment of pedicle injuries include the overall condition of the patient, the ability to tolerate surgery, the status of the contralateral kidney, and the amount of time that has lapsed since the injury. The warm ischemia time determines the survivability of the kidney, and, in general, if this time is greater than 6 hours the kidney is not salvageable, even if vascular repair is technically successful. Authors vary in their opinion on the allowable time between injury and when they would forgo surgical repair, because it is not clear whether all patients suffer complete disruption of blood flow at the time of injury. In a patient with normal contralateral renal function and who is a good surgical candidate, exploration within 12 hours of reported injury would seem reasonable.[29] Even in the best of circumstances, the salvage rate of kidneys in this situation is no more than 30%.[33, 34]

Transmural arterial and renal vein injuries are possible. They are quite rare and result in massive bleeding. Renal vein injuries are associated with vena caval injuries, are difficult to diagnose, and have a high mortality. All severe vascular injuries require immediate surgical treatment.

Initial complications of blunt renal injuries include hemorrhage, hypertension, urinoma formation, infection, and hydronephrosis (Fig. 21–7). All complications are uncommon in lesser grades of injury but occur in up to 30% of patients with severe renal lacerations and fractured kidneys.[35] Because of the risk of early complications in severe renal injuries, all patients should undergo follow-up imaging in the first week after injury. In a series of 23 patients with grade 3 and 4 injuries, Abdalati found complications in 26%, and 17% of the total required surgical treatment after initial nonsurgical management.[34] In lesser injuries clinical signs such as prolonged or increasing abdominal pain, fever, nausea, hypotension, or hypertension should dictate follow-up imaging. In the absence of clinical problems, patients with grade 1 or 2 injuries do not usually need repeated imaging studies.

The late complications of blunt renal trauma may involve delayed hemorrhage, urinoma formation, hypertension, hydronephrosis, calculi, pseudoaneurysm formation, scarring, and loss of renal function.[36] As may be expected, deep lacerations and shattered kidneys have the highest incidence of delayed complications.[37] Nearly all of these kidneys will show evidence of parenchymal scarring, and most will suffer significant loss of function. Yale-Loehr and colleagues studied five patients who suffered grade 2 or 3 renal injuries late after recovery and found that the injured kidneys contributed 30 to 45% of total renal function (mean, 38%).[38] More than half of the physicians surveyed about conservative management of

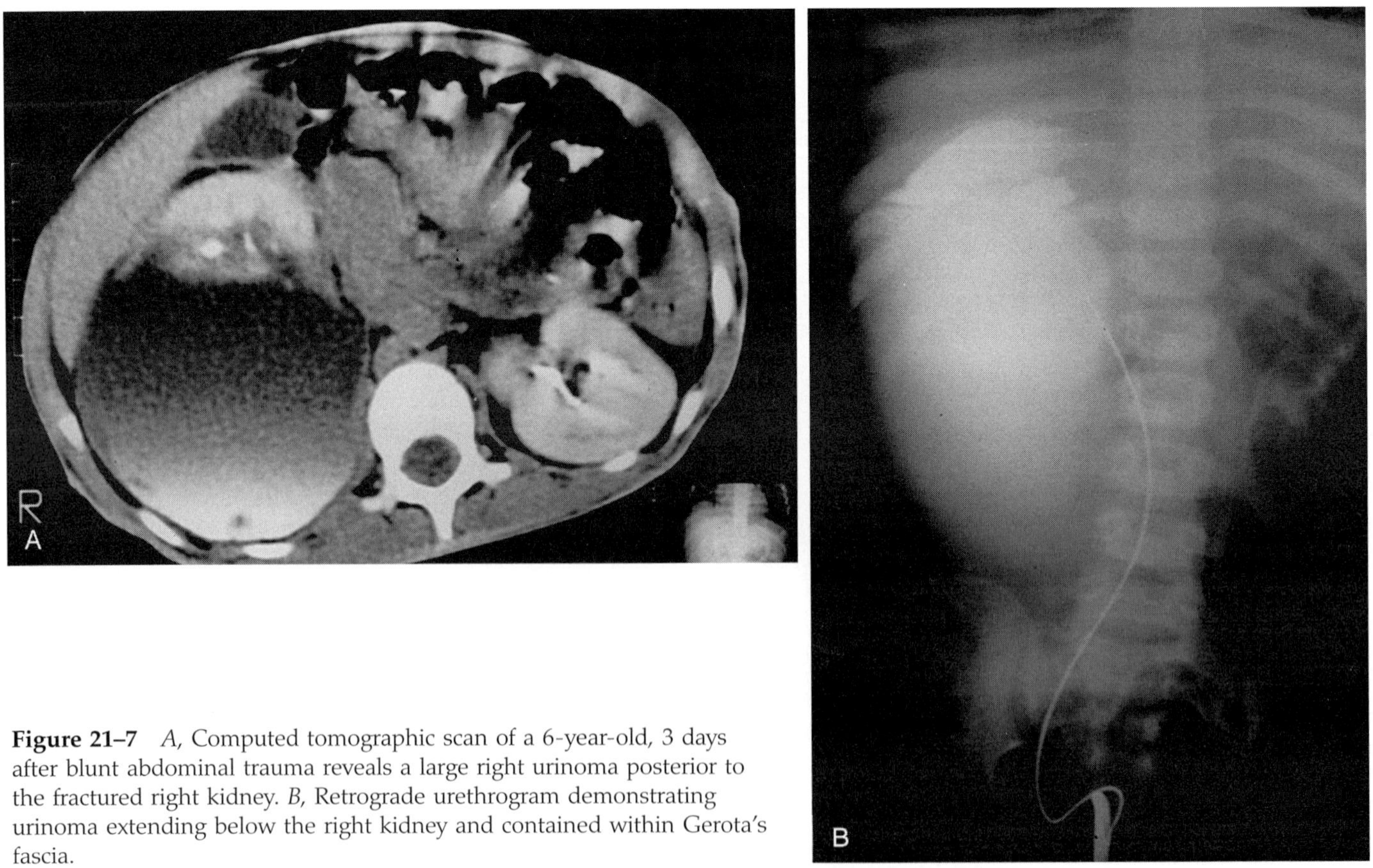

Figure 21–7 *A*, Computed tomographic scan of a 6-year-old, 3 days after blunt abdominal trauma reveals a large right urinoma posterior to the fractured right kidney. *B*, Retrograde urethrogram demonstrating urinoma extending below the right kidney and contained within Gerota's fascia.

blunt renal trauma have seen significant late complications, emphasizing the need for surveillance after injury.

In patients who suffer a renal pedicle injury and in whom surgical repair is not performed, the devascularized kidney need not always be removed. Abdalati studied six children who were treated with observation after pedicle injuries and found totally absent renal function on the affected side when imaged several months later.[34] One patient experienced sepsis and an abscess, which required nephrectomy later, but the other five recovered without complication. Delayed imaging in these patients is necessary.

PENETRATING RENAL TRAUMA

There was a time when stab and gunshot wounds in children were uncommon; however, changes in society have put children in the center of violence, particularly in urban settings.[39] Hall and colleagues at Cook County Hospital in Chicago, have termed the increase in penetrating trauma "the new epidemic in children." Over a 7-year period ending in 1993, they saw the incidence of admissions from penetrating injuries in all children rise from 20 to 36%, whereas the incidence in the 12- to 15-year age group soared from 45 to 66%. The majority of these are gunshot wounds, but stabbings have also become more frequent as street violence dominates some neighborhoods.

Of the entire group of penetrating renal injuries, stab wounds to the kidney are significantly different than gunshot wounds in their physical nature and consequences.[40] Stab wounds and some low-velocity gunshot wounds are relatively precise in causing injury at the site of penetration. As a result, the extent and severity of the injury can be established at the initial evaluation. High-velocity gunshot wounds, in contrast, cause considerable collateral damage, which may injure tissue some distance from the point of impact. Furthermore, the extent of the damaged tissue may be difficult to determine until several days after injury.

STAB WOUNDS TO THE KIDNEY

When a patient suffers a stabbing in the lateral abdomen, the flank, or the lateral back, the incidence of injury to the kidney is approximately 15%. The kidney is at greatest risk if the stabbing is in the flank (between the anterior and posterior axillary lines). Eastham and others, in a review of 244 patients stabbed in the proximity of the kidney, found that 75% of renal injuries occurred via the flank; only 12.5% occurred from stab wounds in the back and the same incidence occurred in the abdomen.[41]

More than half of the stab wounds to the kidney have been found to be minor in severity. Major renal injuries occur in 23 to 33% and vascular injuries in another 23%. In stab wounds that injure the kidney the risk of injury to intra-abdominal organs is in the range of 12 to 15%, with the colon and liver being most often involved.[42] Bernath and coworkers[43] noted that stab wounds posterior to the anterior axillary line were associated with intra-abdominal injury less than 12% of the time.

Evaluation of potential renal stab injuries depends on the location of the stab entry wound and the presence of hematuria. Hematuria occurs in 95% of patients suffering renal stab injuries. The amount of hematuria does not correlate with the severity of injury.[39] Other signs suggesting a renal injury include a flank mass, flank tenderness, and signs of significant blood loss.

Most patients suffering stab wounds have been evaluated initially with an IVP. The reliability of IVP has been established in extensive reviews. In 232 stabbing victims evaluated for potential renal injuries with IVP, there were two false-negative and seven false-positive findings for an overall accuracy of 96%.[39] In both of the false-negative cases, minor renal injuries were found at the time of exploration for other associated injuries, and neither would have needed surgical treatment itself. There has been some controversy as to the next study to obtain if the IVP is abnormal or inconclusive. Because stab injuries to the kidney seldom cause problems with extravasation of urine or cause separation of the parenchyma, CT scan is not as helpful as in blunt trauma. CT scan may also miss arterial injuries. Most authors suggest renal angiography as a secondary study because of its accuracy and potential as a therapeutic tool.[44]

Management of renal stab injuries depends on accurate staging. Eastham found 46 cases of microhematuria in a study of 244 stab wounds to the perirenal area, and 24 of these patients (52%) had renal injuries detectable on IVP. Stabbing victims with a normal IVP and no evidence of significant bleeding or intra-abdominal injury may be managed nonoperatively. All 14 patients with gross hematuria had detectable kidney injuries on IVP.[41]

Patients with minor renal stab injuries on IVP staging, namely contusions and minor lacerations, without indications of significant bleeding or associated injuries may also be managed with bed rest and monitoring. The complication rate for this conservative therapy varies from 0 to 20% depending on the sensitivity of the initial staging evaluation. Heyns and Vollenhoven found a 20% complication rate in 60 renal stab injuries managed with observation, but they admitted that a more aggressive initial evaluation with angiography would have lowered this considerably because the complications were almost exclusively vascular.[42] In fact, hemorrhage secondary to an arteriovenous fistula or pseudoaneurysm accounted for 11 of 12 complications. The other patient presented with a flank bruit from an intrarenal vascular fistula.

More serious stab injuries to the kidney with extravasation of urine, disruption of the kidney, perinephric hematoma, and nonperfused renal tissue on IVP staging should undergo immediate surgical exploration. Of 45 patients with severe renal stab injuries, a nephrectomy was performed in 4 (9%), partial nephrectomy in 7 (15%), and the other 34 (76%) underwent repair and drainage.[26] Between 37 and 45% of renal stab wounds will require surgery; the remainder may be managed nonoperatively.[26, 42]

In hemodynamically stable patients with evidence of branch renal arterial injuries or recurrent bleeding, segmental arterial embolization has been successful. Eastham found that 14 of 16 patients had prompt hemostasis after embolization.[41] Of the remaining 2 patients, both needed heminephrectomy to eventually control their bleeding. Two of the 16 suffered significant complications as a result of nontarget embolization, which led ultimately to one nephrectomy to control secondary hypertension.

GUNSHOT WOUNDS TO THE KIDNEY

Historically, renal gunshot wounds account for less than 5% of all traumatic renal injuries, but the proliferation of urban violence, including gang activities, has led to an increased incidence. There are significant differences between gunshot wounds and stabbing injuries to the kidney, among them the blast effect caused by the high-velocity missile passing through tissue, the high incidence of associated organ injuries, and the overall condition of the patient.

The most common wound site for gunshot injuries to the kidney is abdominal (54%), followed by flank (36%), chest (20%), and back (11%).[45] Physical findings are abdominal tenderness, flank tenderness, and hematuria. In a study of 87 gunshot injuries to the kidney, McAninch found gross hematuria in 50%, microhematuria in 28.6%, and no hematuria in 13.1%; 8.3% had no urinalysis.[45] The mean transfusion requirement was 3742 mL compared with 1978 mL required in 95 renal stab wounds, indicating the more severe nature of gunshot injuries.

In patients suffering renal gunshot wounds, associated organs were injured in 79 of 87 (91%). The most common associated organ injuries were as follows: small bowel, 38%; colon, 38%; liver, 33%; stomach, 30%; and spleen, 23%. The severity of renal injury was classified as minor lacerations and contusions (32%) and major injuries, including vascular injuries (68%).

Radiographic evaluation of gunshot injuries is dependent on the condition of the patient, and in 24% of cases the patient was too severely injured to obtain preoperative studies.[45] A limited IVP in the emergency department or on the operating table may be the only renal image obtainable in the majority of patients. In patients who are stable and who lack indications for immediate surgical exploration, a CT scan is the most useful modality not only to evaluate the kidney but to assess other organ injuries as well.

Because of the severity and complexity of gunshot wounds to the kidney, most patients undergo immediate surgical exploration. McAninch and colleagues explored 78.5% of their 87 patients. Of this group 11 patients had insignificant renal injuries, 12 required nephrectomy, and 46 underwent repair. Some of the removed kidneys could have been repaired technically but the patient was too unstable to undergo this procedure. There were four complications in this surgical group: one late hemorrhage and three infections.

Indications for surgery include evidence of continued renal bleeding: dropping hematocrit, expanding perirenal hematoma, or persistent gross hematuria. Urinary extravasation and nonviable renal tissue are relative indications for surgery. Those 20% of patients who do not undergo surgery are clinically stable with an IVP or CT scan that demonstrates minor renal injuries. Although the scope of early surgical exploration has been limited in blunt and stab injuries to the kidney, surgery remains the cornerstone of management in gunshot injuries. Modern management of these severely injured patients has resulted in a renal salvage rate of 86% and patient survival of 94%; no patients have died as a result of renal injuries, emphasizing the fact that renal injuries are rarely a cause of mortality.[43]

RETROPERITONEAL HEMATOMAS

The urologist is sometimes called in to evaluate a trauma patient who has undergone an exploratory laparotomy and during surgery is found to have a retroperitoneal hematoma. If a preoperative IVP or CT scan has not been obtained, a limited (one-shot) IVP can be performed on the operating table. Although not optimal to visualize the kidneys, this study can establish whether the kidneys are functioning and can rule out severe renal injuries. The decision whether to open and explore a retroperitoneal hematoma involves the characteristics of the hematoma, the presence or absence of hematuria, the findings on IVP, and the mechanism of the renal injury.[38]

All expanding or pulsatile hematomas of the retroperiteum should be explored. Stable hematomas with a normal IVP need not be opened, whereas injuries evident on IVP should be explored. The presence of gross hematuria should encourage exploration even with stable hematomas. The mechanism of injury is a consideration, and high-velocity gunshot wounds should always be explored. In cases of blunt trauma, low-velocity gunshot wounds, and stab wounds, a stable renal hematoma should be left undisturbed provided there is renal function on the IVP.

The technique of opening a retroperitoneal hematoma is somewhat controversial depending on whether the injury is blunt or penetrating. Most authors believe that control of the renal vessels should be accomplished before opening the hematoma.[46] This is done through a midline incision in the retroperitoneum, and vascular loops are first placed around the main renal artery and veins. The hematoma is then explored by reflecting the colon medially after incision of the posterior peritoneum[47] (Fig. 21–8).

Alternately, some authors have suggested that the time lost in dissecting and controlling the renal vessels is not well spent. They recommended reflecting the colon, opening Gerota's fascia, and controlling the renal vessels from a direct lateral approach.[48, 49] The criticism of this technique is that the tamponade obtained from the pressure of the hematoma within Gerota's envelope is released before vascular control is established and that

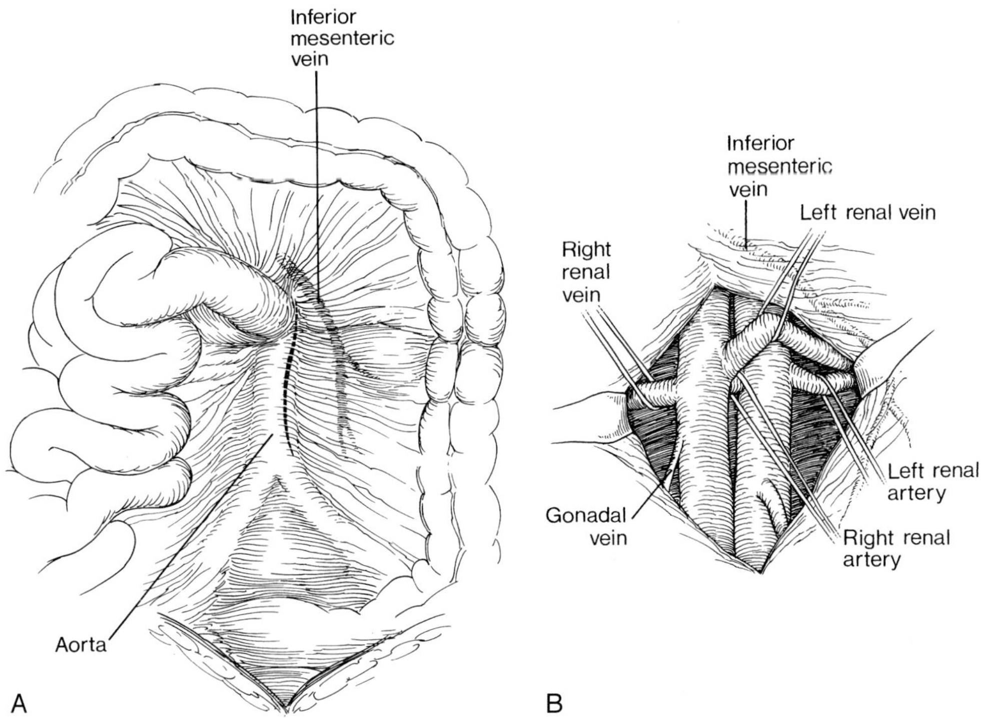

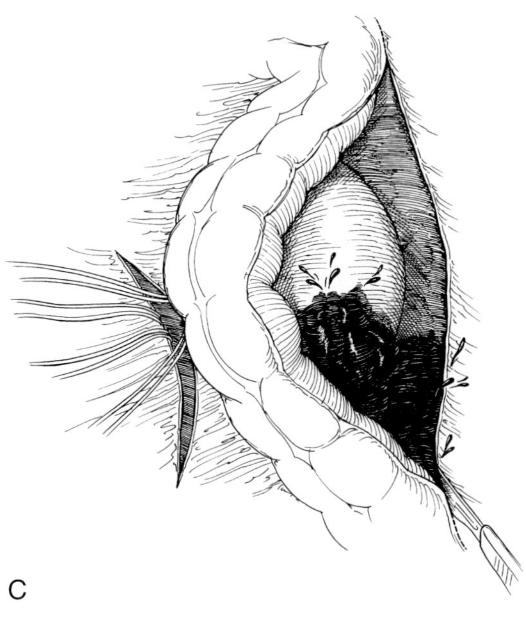

Figure 21–8 *A*, Surgical approach to the renal vessels in kidney. A retroperitoneal incision is made over the aorta. *B*, Anatomy of the renal vessels. *C*, Retroperitoneal incision lateral to the colon exposing the kidney. From McAninch JW. Surgery for renal trauma. In Novick AC, Pontes ES, Streen SB (eds), Stewart's Operative Urology, 2nd ed. Baltimore, MD: Williams & Wilkins, 1989. Used with permission.

severe bleeding may resume, making control of the vessels difficult. Either technique gives good results in the hands of those comfortable with them. However, if the patient is stable and time permits, early control of the vessels before opening the hematoma offers a more controlled surgical situation.

URETERAL INJURIES

There are two types of ureteral injuries: iatrogenic injuries resulting from pelvic surgery and traumatic ureteral injuries. Surgical trauma makes up a large proportion of adult ureteral injuries, but because nonurologic pelvic surgery is unusual in children we address only traumatic ureteral injuries.

The ureter is rarely injured. Its location along the paraspinal muscles and within the deep pelvis, along with its inherent flexibility and mobility, offers remarkable protection. The incidence of ureteral injury is reported to be less than 1% of all urologic trauma cases.[50] When injured, the ureter is more likely to suffer from penetrating rather than blunt trauma.

PENETRATING URETERAL TRAUMA

The most common cause of penetrating ureteral injury is gunshot wound, which accounts for 95% of all ureteral injuries.[51] It has been estimated that gunshot wounds to the abdomen result in ureteral injury 2.3 to 17% of the time.[52] Knife wounds are the next most common cause. Ureteral injuries are rarely isolated, and many patients suffer delay in diagnosis primarily because of the number and severity of associated injuries, absence of hematuria in 33% of patients, and a low index of suspicion.[53]

The diagnosis should be suspected in a patient who has a penetrating injury of the abdomen, retroperitoneum, or pelvis. The most reliable methods of diagnosis are surgical exploration and retrograde pyelogram. IVPs and CT scans are helpful but may miss the diagnosis in 70 to 75% of cases. Hematuria is not reliable and is present in only 23 to 45% of patients.[50]

BLUNT URETERAL TRAUMA

Blunt ureteral injury is even more rare. The most common type is avulsion of the ureter from the renal pelvis at the ureteropelvic junction.[54, 55] Several cases of blunt disruption of the proximal ureter have also been reported.[56, 57] Blunt ureteral injuries usually occur in children and are believed to be a result of body hyperextension followed by sudden deceleration and ureteral compression against

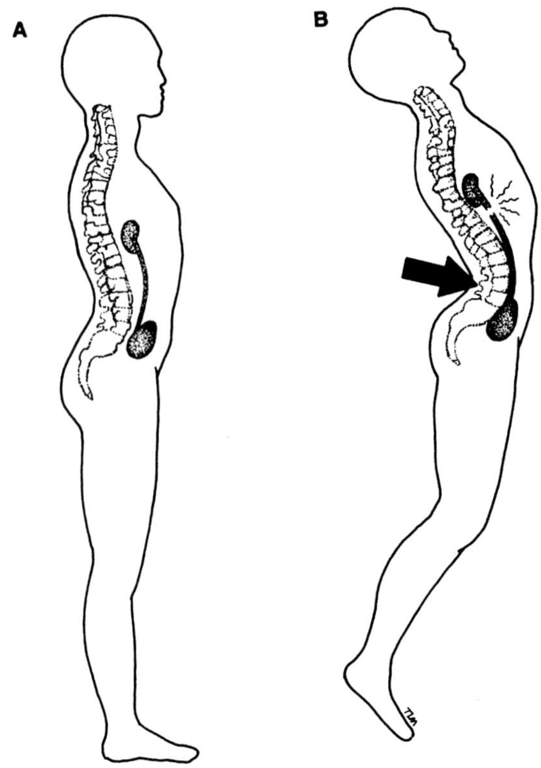

Figure 21–9 Mechanism of blunt ureteral injury in children. *A*, Normal relationship of ureter to the spine. *B*, With a sudden blow to the back the ureter is stretched against the hyperextended vertebral column and disrupts the UPJ. From Gillenwater JY. Adult and Pediatric Urology. St. Louis, MO: Mosby-Yearbook, 1996. Used with permission.

one of the vertebral bodies (Fig. 21–9). Children are believed to be more at risk for this type of ureteral injury than adults primarily because of the greater flexibility of their spinal column.

Blunt ureteral injuries occur as a result of severe trauma and are often due to pedestrian-vehicle accidents, which produce multiple injuries. Sixty percent of patients suffer a delay in diagnosis, and hematuria is absent in 31 to 66%.[48, 52] The patient eventually presents with signs of a urinoma, including flank pain, nausea, and sometimes fever. The diagnosis is usually made by CT scan with delayed imaging. IVPs with late films may also be helpful; retrograde pyelogram, however, remains the definitive imaging tool. Limited IVPs as part of the initial trauma evaluation are unreliable in diagnosing ureteral and renal-pelvic injuries. Presti found that 8 of 11 (72%) IVPs in these patients were normal or nondiagnostic. A special note is that surgical exploration in the immediate postinjury period can fail to detect a ureteropelvic disruption if the retroperitoneum is not opened with direct visualization of the kidneys.[50] A high index of suspicion and retrograde pyelography or direct visualization of the ureters and renal pelves remain the definitive method of evaluation.

TREATMENT OF URETERAL INJURIES

Once the injury is diagnosed, four considerations are important in deciding on management: site of the injury, nature of the injury, time of recognition, and associated injuries and condition.[50] The classification of traumatic ureteral injuries includes contusions, partial lacerations, complete lacerations, crush injuries, and avulsions.

Contusions may be discovered during surgical exploration and need not be treated unless the contusion is severe and ureteral necrosis is a possibility. In these cases, a ureteral stent and a periureteral Penrose drain should be placed. Partial lacerations of the ureter can be repaired primarily, stented, and drained. Partial lacerations and contusions should be treated at the time of diagnosis, and their treatment does not vary with location on the ureter.

Complete lacerations and significant crush injuries may be treated with debridement and primary reanastomosis in the upper and middle ureteral areas (Fig. 21–10). In lower ureteral injuries, ureteroneocystostomy is the best procedure. Internal stenting and periureteral drainage are indicated.

If a significant portion of distal ureter is lost, a psoas bladder hitch, Boari flap, and nephropexy may make ureteroneocystotomy possible (Fig. 21–11). If a section of the proximal or middle ureter is lost, transureteroureterostomy, autotransplantation, or ureteral replacement with bowel or appendix are options.[58, 59] In extreme cases, a temporary ureterostomy with delayed reconstruction is a wise choice. Finally, avulsion injuries at the ureteropelvic junction are managed with immediate surgery using a spatulated reanastomosis with appropriate stenting and drainage.

BLADDER TRAUMA

When full, the bladder is the largest organ in the urinary tract. In adults the bladder lies within the pelvis and is well protected by the rigid pelvic ring and thick abdominal wall muscles. In infants and children the bladder extends above the pubic rim and is more an abdominal structure. The abdominal wall in children is generally weaker and there is less intra-abdominal and pelvic fat to protect the bladder. Even in this more exposed position, the child's bladder is seldom injured without a significant bony pelvic fracture. The exception is the patient who suffers a forceful blow to the suprapubic region when the bladder is full, as in the patient wearing a lap seat belt in an automobile accident. Sivit and associates reviewed 95 children who suffered lap belt ecchymosis after trauma and found that 3 had significant bladder injuries.[60]

Blunt injury is the most common mechanism of bladder trauma. Of 111 adult bladder injuries, 86% were caused by blunt trauma and 90% were caused by motor vehicle accidents.[61] Eighty-nine percent of blunt injuries in adults were associated with pelvic fractures. The converse is not true, however, and only 10% of patients with pelvic fractures will have an injury to the bladder. Sivit identified seven children with traumatic bladder ruptures of whom four (57%) had pelvic fractures. The higher incidence of bladder ruptures not associated with pelvic fractures in children is the result of the more exposed and intraperitoneal position of the full bladder (Fig. 21–12).

Patients may complain of suprapubic pain and tenderness, inability to urinate, and hematuria. Gross hematuria occurs in 95% of cases and significant microhematuria in the other 5%.[45] Of all patients with pelvic fractures and gross hematuria, 45% will have bladder rupture.[62] The mortality associated with traumatic bladder rupture in adults is between 20 and 40% and is due to concomitant injuries such as closed head trauma, severe hemorrhage, and multisystem failure.[63]

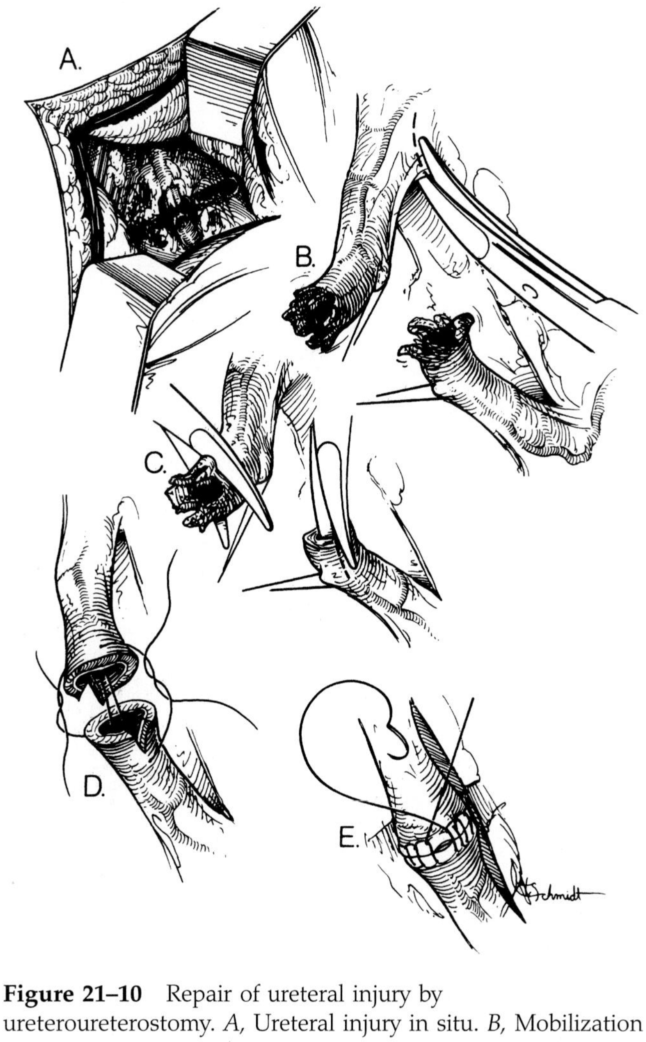

Figure 21–10 Repair of ureteral injury by ureteroureterostomy. *A*, Ureteral injury in situ. *B*, Mobilization of the ureter. *C*, Debridement and spatulation of ureter. *D*, Suturing of the ureter. *E*, Final appearance of repair. From Guerriero WG. Urologic Injuries. East Norwalk, CT: Appleton & Lange, 1984. Used with permission.

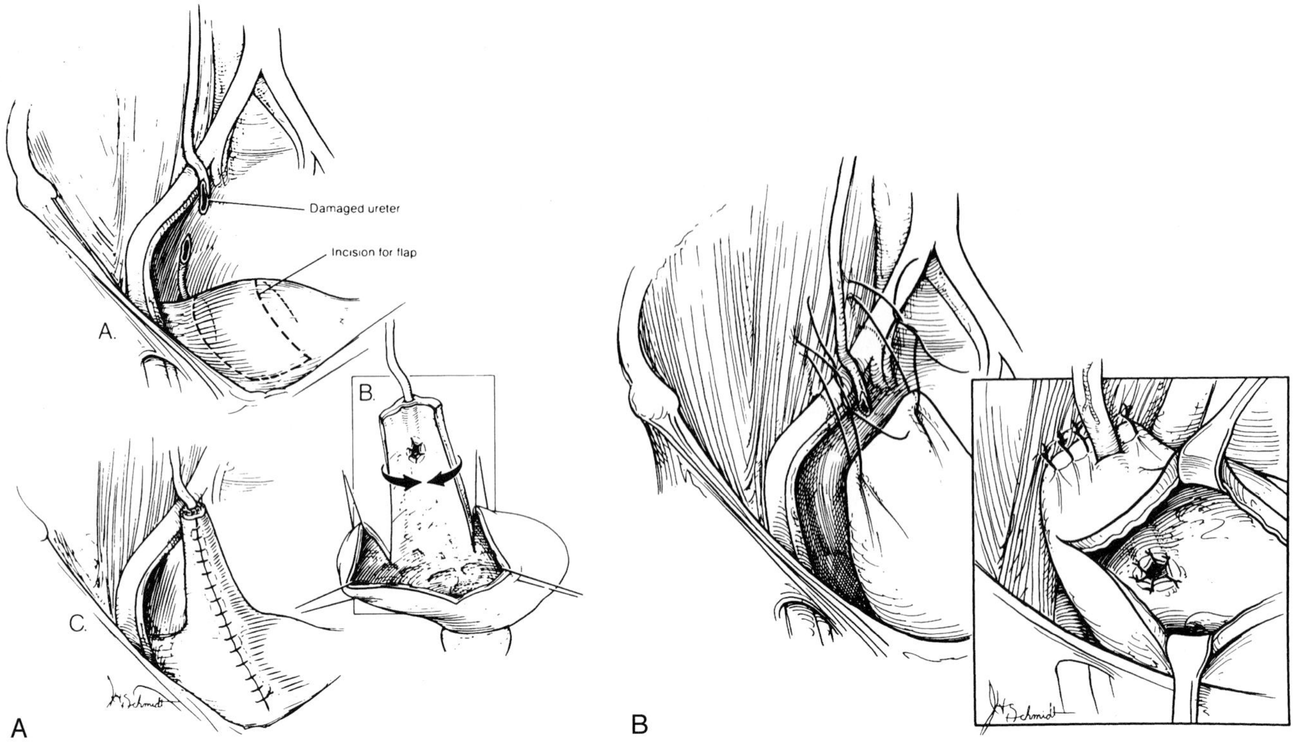

Figure 21–11 *A,* A modified Boari flap illustrating design and construction of the flap and reimplantation of the ureter. *B,* Bladder psoas hitch performed to allow primary ureteroneocystotomy. From Guerriero WG. Urologic Injuries. East Norwalk, CT: Appleton & Lange, 1984. Used with permission.

A properly done cystogram is the surest way to diagnose ruptured bladder. The bladder must be fully distended, and postdrainage films must be obtained. The appearance of the bladder on CT scan, even with a clamped Foley catheter, may not show the bladder leak because it is not forcibly distended. To make the CT scan diagnosis, the bladder must be filled retrograde through the catheter. Sivit and associates studied 1500 consecutive children with blunt abdominal trauma with a CT technique that included a delay of 20 to 30 minutes between

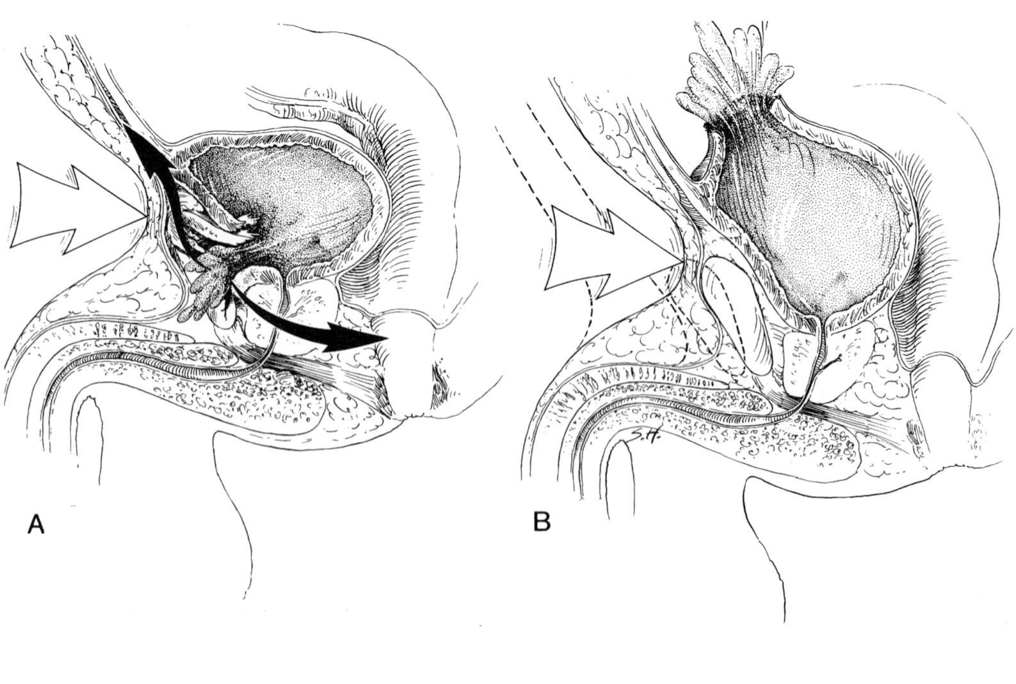

Figure 21–12 *A,* Mechanism of extraperitoneal bladder rupture associated with pelvic fracture. *B,* Mechanism intraperitoneal bladder rupture with blow-out injury of the dome. From Walsh PC, Retik AB, Stamey TA, Vaughan ED Jr. Campbell's Urology, 5th ed. Philadelphia: WB Saunders, 1986. Used with permission.

intravenous injection of contrast and scanning of the pelvis with the catheter clamped. They diagnosed seven bladder ruptures and found no clinically significant false-negative cases.[60] On the other hand, McAleer and colleagues found four children with bladder ruptures and one had a missed intraperitoneal rupture despite multiple CT scans.[2] Although the well-defined technique of delayed imaging of the bladder with CT scan may be sufficient in some hands, these studies are often performed under adverse circumstances with limited time and personnel available, making adherence to protocol difficult. In most institutions, infusion of contrast directly into the bladder remains the safest method to evaluate potential bladder trauma whether done under CT scan or fluoroscopy.

Blunt bladder injuries may be categorized as contusions, intraperitoneal ruptures, and extraperitoneal ruptures. Therapy varies depending on the nature of the injury. Bladder contusions are described as damage to the bladder mucosa or muscular wall without loss of bladder wall continuity or extravasation of urine. They account for 33% of all bladder injuries and require only catheter drainage for treatment. Most contusions may be treated with 5 days of catheter drainage or until gross hematuria has cleared. It is not necessary to obtain a second cystogram unless the patient has difficult or painful voiding when the catheter is removed.

Bladder ruptures are categorized as intraperitoneal or extraperitoneal depending on the location of the injury. Intraperitoneal rupture occurs at the dome of the bladder, which is the weakest and most mobile portion. This injury is more common in children because of the intraperitoneal position of the bladder. They account for 33% of all bladder injuries and usually result when a full bladder is rapidly compressed with blunt external force. The most common cause is a motor vehicle accident or a fall from a significant height. Intraperitoneal rupture of the bladder is diagnosed when the cystogram shows extravasation of contrast moving into the abdominal cavity, outlining loops of bowel (Fig. 21–13).

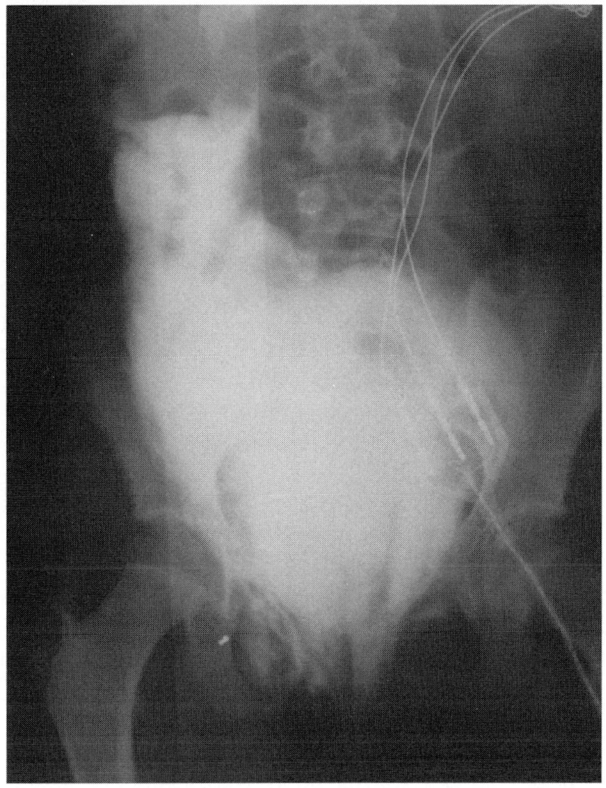

Figure 21–13 Cystogram of a 9-year-old who suffered intraperitoneal rupture of the bladder in a motor vehicle accident. Contrast extends into the right side of the abdominal cavity.

The accepted treatment of intraperitoneal bladder rupture is surgical exploration, debridement, and repair. The abdominal cavity is irrigated but not drained, and a Foley catheter is left in place for 1 week. In more severe injuries, a repeat cystogram may be obtained before removing the catheter. In cases of minor intraperitoneal rupture of the bladder, some patients have been treated with Foley catheter drainage alone.[64] They undergo drainage for 10 days, and a cystogram is performed before catheter removal to establish healing.

Extraperitoneal rupture of the bladder is seen almost exclusively with pelvic fractures. The bladder may be torn on the inferior lateral wall with disruption of the pelvic ring and occasionally will be lacerated by sharp pelvic bone fragments. On the cystogram, extravasation is confined to the perivesical soft tissues and appears as a flame-like pattern (Fig. 21–14). Most extraperitoneal ruptures can be managed with 10 days of Foley catheter drainage. More complicated injuries may require exploration, debridement, and repair. When there has been a laceration of the bladder with a penetrating segment of fractured pelvic bone it is necessary to perform an open repair, remove bone fragments, and drain the retroperitoneal space.

Although nonoperative management of extraperitoneal bladder ruptures has become the accepted norm, these patients can have significant complications. Kotkin and Koch presented a series of 29 such patients treated with catheter drainage alone.[65] Of this group, 21 (72%) healed within 10 to 14 days and another 3 (10%) healed with prolonged catheter drainage (up to 31 days). Five of the 29 (17%) had complications, including recurrent bladder calculi (1), vesicocutaneous fistulas (2), persistent extravasation with sepsis (1), and infected pelvic hematoma and subsequent death (1). The authors suggested that maintenance of adequate bladder drainage after the injury and prevention of infection with broad-spectrum antibiotic coverage will minimize complications.

Penetrating bladder injuries are rare, making up 5.5% of all bladder injuries in a review of 417 patients.[38] Gunshot wounds are the most common cause followed by

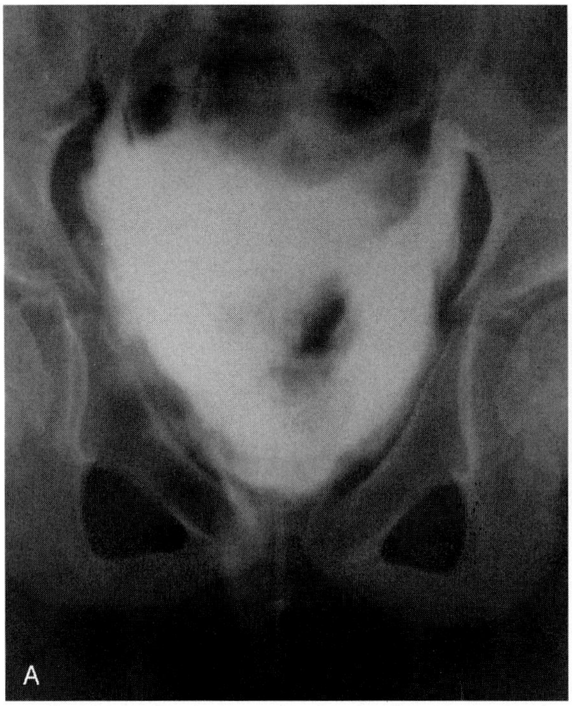

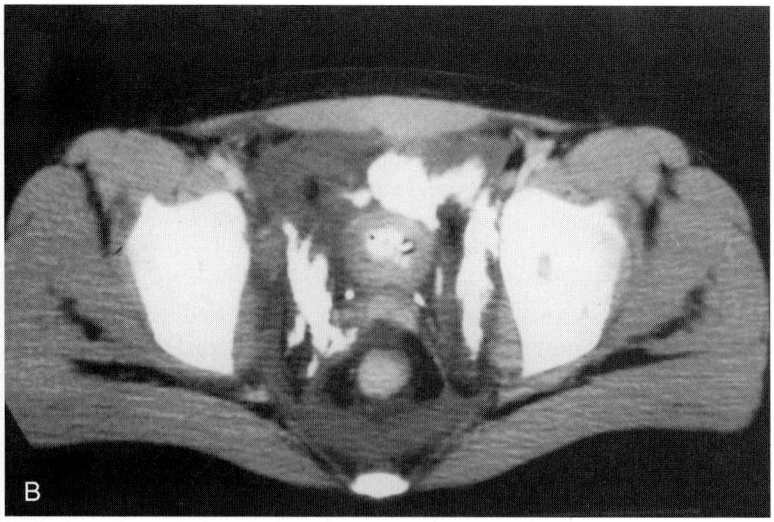

Figure 21–14 *A,* Cystogram of a patient with extraperitoneal bladder rupture. Note the flame-shaped distribution of contrast in the perivesical space. *B,* Computed tomographic scan of perivesical extravasation of urine in a patient suffering extraperitoneal bladder rupture.

stabbings. Most patients have associated nonurologic injuries, and the mortality is between 12 and 22%. The most common associated injuries involve the rectosigmoid, small bowel, and iliac vessels.

Penetrating injuries to the bladder require exploration and repair transabdominally. Debridement of nonviable bladder tissue surrounding the wound is necessary as is adequate drainage of the perivesical space and catheter drainage of the bladder. Surgical exploration is usually done in conjunction with an exploratory laparotomy to evaluate other injuries.

URETHRAL TRAUMA

The urethra, beginning at the bladder neck and extending to the base of the penis, is well protected by surrounding tissue and bone and is seldom injured. Because of its location and protection, few injuries can lead to urethral trauma, and these are consistent in both their mechanism and consequences. Injuries to the penile urethra are discussed in association with genital injuries. Injuries to the female urethra are quite rare and are discussed separately.

Posterior Urethral Injuries

Injuries to the posterior urethra are almost always associated with fractures of the bony pelvis as a result of severe blunt trauma. The urethra passes through the rigid and fixed pelvic floor. The bladder and prostatic urethra sit above the floor and the bulbar urethra below. The membranous urethra lies within the floor and is fixed in position by the floor's attachments to the bony pelvic ring. In the adult, the bladder and prostate are a structural unit made so by the bulky prostate and its wide attachment to the bladder neck. The bladder and prostate are potentially mobile within the pelvis; their position is maintained, in part, by the membranous urethra anchoring them to the pelvic floor.

When severe trauma causes a fracture of the bony pelvis, the ring that supports the pelvic floor may be disrupted, and shear forces may pull the bladder and prostate violently away from the fixed membranous urethra. The membranous and bulbar urethra remain in continuity. The incidence of urethral injury in pelvic fractures is 10%, and almost all (83%) are complete disruptions. Motor vehicle accidents cause 90% of these injuries, and falls, industrial crush accidents, and sporting accidents make up the remaining 10%.[66] Although the severity of the pelvic injury and bony deformity may vary, the site of urethral injury is constant.

The child's pelvic anatomy is different from that of the adult, and this can lead to different types of urethral injury.[67] The child's bladder is basically an intraabdominal organ, whereas in the adult the bladder lies within the pelvis. The child's immature prostate is flimsy and small, lacking both the broad attachments to the bladder and the bulk and rigidity to support and protect the prostatic urethra. The puboprostatic ligaments are also immature and weak. These differences offer alternate paths for traumatic stress within the pelvis and allow for a variety of proximal urethral injuries. Along with the classic membranous urethral disruption common in adults, children may suffer both lacerations of the true prostatic urethra and disruption of the urethra above the prostate. Boone and colleagues' series of 24 children with posterior urethral disruptions included 16 (66%) with classic prostatomembranous injury, 4 (17%) with supraprostatic urethral injury, and 4 (17%) with injuries to the prostatic urethra.[68]

Urethral disruption leads to extravasation of urine during voiding, urinary retention, and severe bleeding into the pelvic perivesical space. The bladder and proximal urethral remnant are usually forced away from the pelvic floor by the resulting hematoma, leaving a gap between the two torn urethral segments that may measure several centimeters. If the bladder neck is not involved, then the bladder will retain urine and extravasation will occur only when the patient attempts to void. If the bladder neck is torn as well, then extravasation may occur continuously and the bladder may remain small while the urinoma forms in the pelvis.

Because of the unique mechanisms that lead to most urethral injuries, the physician must suspect and evaluate the urethra for trauma in any patient who has suffered a pelvic fracture or a traumatic blow to the perineum. Blood at the urinary meatus, gross hematuria, severe pain on voiding, and urinary retention are the most common clinical findings. A butterfly hematoma of the perineum or a distended and discolored scrotum indicating hematoma or extravasated urine may be observed. Any patient suffering abdominal, pelvic, or perineal trauma should undergo a rectal examination, and, in cases of posterior urethral injury, this may reveal a pelvic hematoma or an upwardly displaced bladder and prostate.

As a result of the traumatic event, 95% of patients suffering pelvic fractures have multiple injuries, and many are in grave and unstable condition.[69] If this is the case, the urologist's initial responsibility is to document the presence of genitourinary injuries and to establish an efficient way to drain and monitor urine output. If the patient is voiding and the rectal exam is normal, a Foley catheter may be placed carefully. If the catheter does not pass easily, then the patient must be examined radiographically. In the most unstable patients, a temporary suprapubic tube may be placed either in the operating room during exploration for associated injuries or with a percutaneous technique in the emergency department.

Fortunately, most patients are not too unstable to undergo x-ray evaluation. The essential examination of the urethra is the retrograde urethrogram, which may be performed either in the radiography department or on a stretcher using a portable x-ray machine. The patient's penis is pulled upright, and if possible the patient is placed in the oblique position. A Foley catheter is placed in the distal urethra and contrast is injected under pressure for the film, which should include the penis and complete pelvis (Fig. 21–15). If the study is normal, the catheter may be advanced into the bladder and anchored in position, and the cystogram is obtained if indicated.

If a catheter is in place and the bladder is being drained at the time of the urologist's initial exam, the catheter should be left in place. If the integrity of the urethra is in question, then a small feeding tube may be placed along the Foley catheter and a retrograde injection performed to obtain an x-ray image of the urethra. This study may be delayed until the patient is stable and other more pressing problems are resolved.

The initial management of posterior urethral injuries involving the prostatic and membranous urethra remains somewhat of a controversy. At issue is whether performing immediate repair or realignment of the urethra will give better results than simply placing a suprapubic tube at the time of injury and repairing the urethra several months later. Immediate complete repair of the urethra

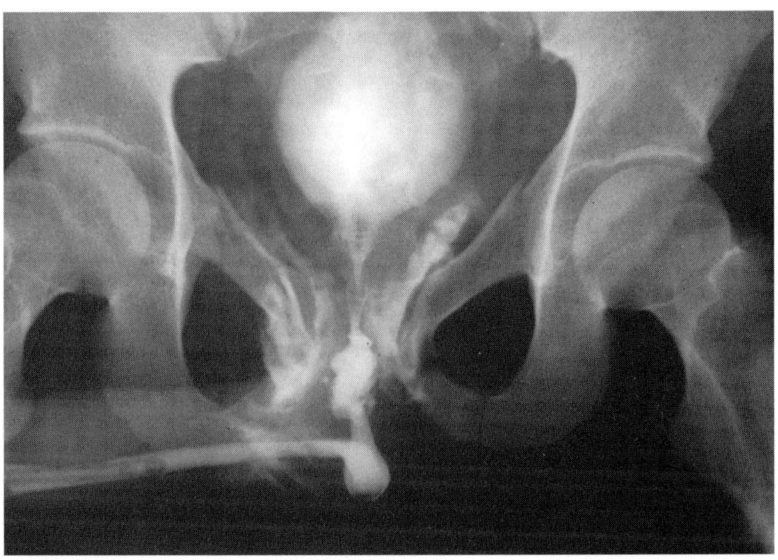

Figure 21–15 Retrograde urethrogram with prostatomembranous urethral injury. Note bilateral pubic fractures and the elevation and narrowing of the bladder contour caused by the perivesical hematoma.

in the postinjury period is not indicated because of the risk of severe pelvic bleeding and the increased incidence of long-term complications such as impotence and incontinence. Poor results of early repair led to the use of immediate suprapubic drainage and secondary urethral repair several months later. There has been a new enthusiasm for initial realignment and catheter placement (Fig. 21–16). There is no attempt to pull or sew the urethra back together.

Corriere and coworkers reported on 50 adults (mean age, 34 years) treated with immediate suprapubic drainage and delayed one-stage urethroplasty[69] (Fig. 21–17). Fifteen (30%) required at least one visual urethroplasty and 3 (6%) required dilation for urethral stricture. Thirty-eight (76%) voided normally and were continent, 7 (14%) had some mild degree of incontinence, and 5 (10%) had a neurogenic bladder and performed intermittent catheterization. At 1 year after injury, 16 (32%) were impotent. Boone and others reported on 16 children with prostatomembranous urethral injuries, 9 of whom were treated with suprapubic drainage and delayed repair.[68] Six of the 9 (67%) children had problems with strictures requiring treatment, all were continent, and 6 (67%) were impotent.

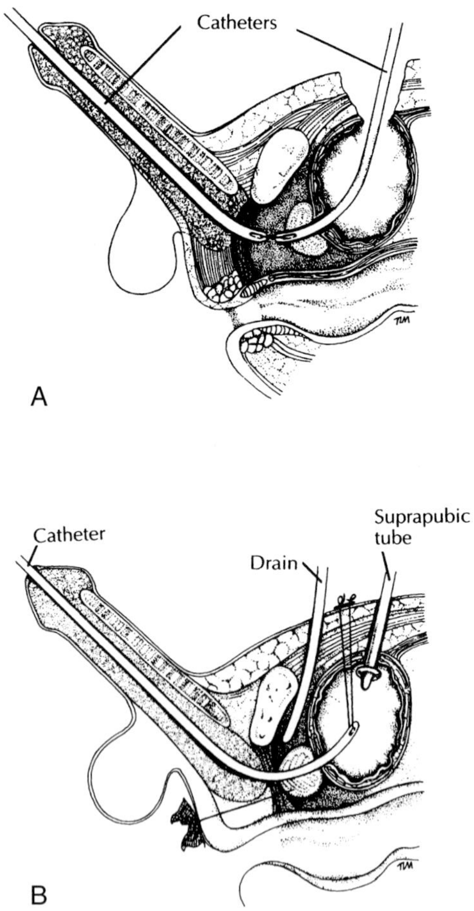

Figure 21–16 *A* and *B*, Technique for aligning a ruptured urethra using catheters for initial management of urethral disruption. From Gillenwater JY. Adult and Pediatric Urology. St. Louis, MO: Mosby-Yearbook, 1990. Used with permission.

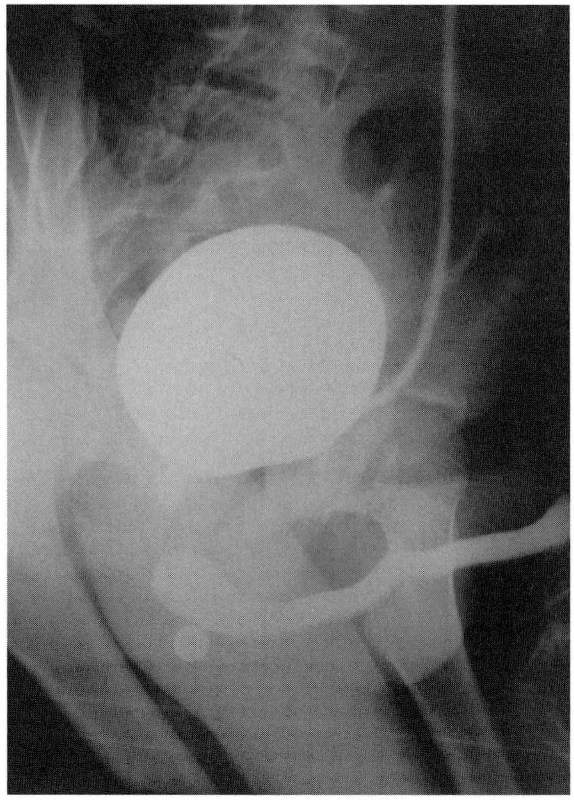

Figure 21–17 Combined retrograde urethrogram and cystogram through a suprapubic tube revealing the length of the urethral stricture after initial management of urethral injury with a suprapubic tube. The patient is ready to have delayed one-stage urethroplasty.

Follis, in contrast, reported on 20 patients treated with initial realignment of the urethra through an open cystotomy.[70] Their technique involves opening the bladder, passing a urethral sound or catheter through the urethra, and guiding it against the surgeon's finger, which is placed through the bladder neck from above. A Foley catheter is placed and secured with a suture brought out through the anterior abdominal wall and tied over a button. They emphasized that the catheter is not placed on tension nor is there significant dissection at the bladder neck. The catheter is left in place for 4 to 8 weeks. Their results showed that 7 (35%) patients required at least one urethrotomy for stricture, all were continent (2 with medication), and 4 (20%) were impotent. They also reported on 13 patients treated with delayed surgery, and these results were significantly worse. The authors admitted that some selection of favorable patients for realignment did take place. Boone and coworkers[68] included 7 children treated with primary realignment in their series. Of these

7 children, 3 (43%) had problems with strictures, all were continent, and 1 (14%) was left impotent. Patient selection may have influenced their data also.

Boone also reported on eight children with urethral injuries proximal to the membranous urethra: four with prostatic urethral trauma and four with disruption of the urethra above the urogenital diaphragm.[68] All of these patients had simultaneous bladder neck injuries, and all underwent primary immediate reconstruction. These were complicated urinary injuries and difficult operations as evidenced by the average blood loss of 2200 mL. The results were predictably poor. Six of eight patients (75%) had problems with severe strictures, and six (75%) were impotent. Two of the total were incontinent and in diapers 9 and 11 years after their injury, respectively. It is clear that these injuries are much different from the more common prostatomembranous urethral injuries in children and adults in their mechanism, severity, and outcome. Boone and coworkers suggested that bladder neck injuries must be repaired at the time of trauma but that initial repair of the urethra may not be best at this time.

The current approach in children with posterior urethral injuries depends on the patient's overall condition. If the child is taken to surgery for abdominal exploration, then the urologist may either pass a catheter per urethra or make some reasonable attempt to realign the urethra using urethral sounds or catheters with the bladder open. Dissection around the bladder neck or urethra seems unwise because of potential bleeding and risk of impotence. If attempted realignment is unsuccessful, then a suprapubic tube may be placed.

In the patient who does not need surgery for other reasons, a percutaneous suprapubic tube may be placed and its position confirmed radiographically. These tubes may be left in place for 3 weeks and replaced with a Foley catheter once the tract is mature. The Foley catheter may be changed monthly and gradually increased in size as deemed necessary. Those patients requiring a secondary repair 4 to 6 months later may undergo one of a number of techniques, including endoscopic incision of short strictures, to open transpubic or perineal reanastomosis.[65, 71]

Bulbourethral Injuries

Injuries to the bulbous urethra usually result from straddle trauma. Falls onto fixed objects such as bicycle bars, playground equipment, and fences are the most common cause. Assaults with kick injuries to the perineum can also lead to similar injuries. The blow to the perineum forces the bulbous urethra against the caudal surface of the pubis and pinches a short section of urethra. In a fall the patient's entire weight may crush the urethra and the surrounding corpus spongiosum (Fig. 21–18).

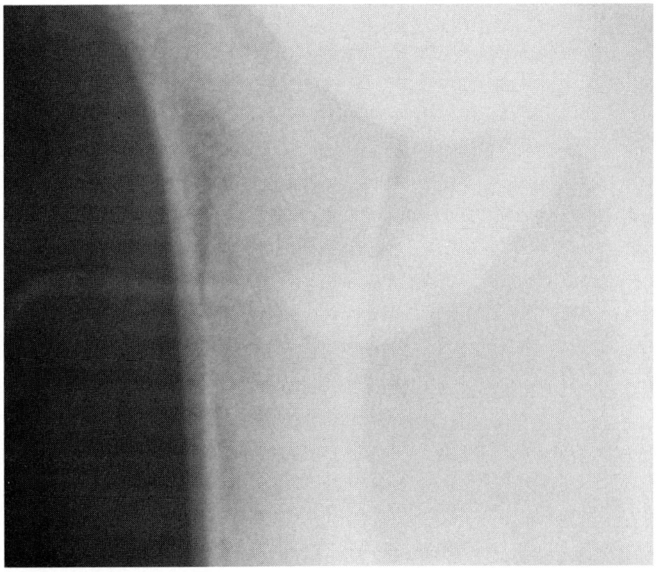

Figure 21–18 Bulbous urethral stricture after straddle injury demonstrated on voiding cystourethrogram.

Unlike injuries to the proximal urethra in pelvic fractures, straddle injuries seldom disrupt the continuity of the urethra or cause extravasation of urine. The spongiosal bleeding into the perineal spaces leads to collection of blood in a butterfly pattern within the limits of Colles' fascia (Fig. 21–19). Extravasation of urine, if it occurs, is limited to the same space. Inability to void in the immediate postinjury period usually results from edema and compression by hematoma.

Management of bulbourethral straddle injuries is conservative and involves either observation or Foley catheter drainage if the patient cannot adequately void. Pain with voiding may be considerable, and a catheter may make the patient more comfortable, help control urethral bleeding, and possibly act as a stent to facilitate healing. Many straddle injuries are relatively minor, and the patient suffers only transient dysuria and hematuria. The initial injury may be forgotten until months or years later when a stricture occurs and produces symptoms.

Injuries to the Female Urethra and Genitalia

There are two basic forms of female genital injury: (1) those associated with severe trauma and pelvic fractures and (2) injuries limited to the soft tissues of the vulva, vagina, and urethra. Both types of injury are uncommon. The low incidence of injury to the female urethra is believed to be due to three factors: the short length of the urethra, its protected location, and its greater mobility compared with that of the male.[72, 73] The mechanisms of injury and the circumstances under which they occur differ widely.

The vaginal and urethral injuries that occur in

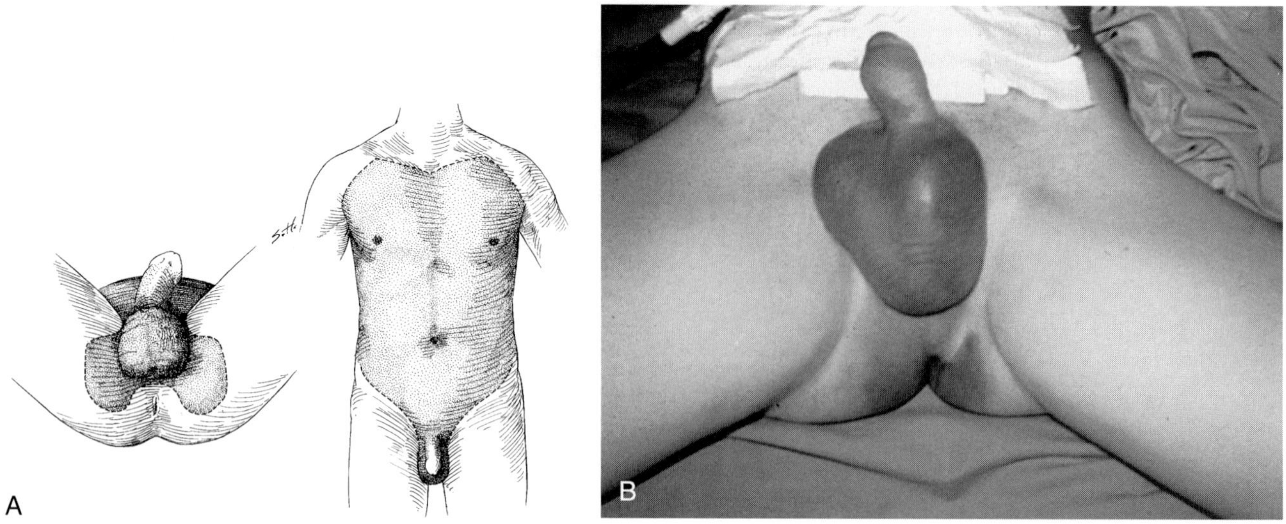

Figure 21–19 *A*, Colles' fascia attachments, which define the limits of extravasation of urine or blood from a ruptured urethra. From Walsh et al. Campbell's Urology, 5th ed. Philadelphia: WB Saunders, 1986. Used with permission. *B*, A patient with a perineal butterfly hematoma within the limits of Colles' fascia.

conjunction with pelvic fractures result from severe trauma usually associated with motor vehicles. A review of the gynecologic literature revealed a 6% incidence of urethral injuries in pelvic fractures in 2000 females.[74] Disruption of the female urethra is associated with acute violent disruption and displacement of the pubis, leading to an acute diastasis of the symphysis. Occasionally, the urethra will be lacerated by a bone spicule from the fracture. The vagina is often lacerated, as evidenced by vaginal bleeding at the time of injury in 80% of patients.[75] Labial edema and hematomas may also give evidence of these injuries.

Patients who suffered pelvic fractures and in whom it is difficult to place a urethral catheter, who have anuria after placement of a catheter, or who have vaginal bleeding should be investigated for urethral and vaginal injuries. A static cystogram may well miss such injuries if the bladder and bladder neck are intact. A voiding cystourethrogram is necessary to rule out injury. Concurrent bladder ruptures occur in 66% of urethral injuries in females.[76]

Management of injuries to the female urethra falls into three categories. If a Foley catheter can be placed into the bladder, then the urethra can be allowed to reapproximate and heal. If the urethra and bladder are severely displaced and catheterization is not possible, then a suprapubic tube may be placed and a delayed secondary repair undertaken in several months. Finally, if the injury also involves the bladder neck and threatens long-term continence, an immediate primary repair may be performed. This approach is best in injuries that involve severe lacerations of the urethra extending into the vagina, producing an acute urethrovaginal fistula. Such injuries should be irrigated, debrided, and closed in layers to promote healing and continence.[73] In all injuries to the urethra and bladder neck, a voiding study must be obtained before removing the catheter. Failure to identify persistent urethral injuries can lead to urinary extravasation and severe complications such as sepsis and necrotizing fascitis.[73]

Soft tissue injuries are due to assaults and straddle falls. These injuries cause acute bleeding and pain to a distressing degree but are not life threatening, as are the injuries associated with pelvic fractures. Straddle injuries can cause urethral injuries and large hematomas of the labia[77] (Fig. 21–20). High estrogen levels thicken and increase the distensibility of the vulvar tissues, protecting female adults and adolescent girls.[78] In a study of 32 genital injuries in prepubertal girls, Pokorny and others found that the mean patient age was 6.3 years.[78]

Girls with genital injuries should be managed initially with reassurance, ice packs, and a pressure dressing to the perineum. These measures, along with keeping the child supine and quiet, will help control bleeding and in some cases serve to gain the child's confidence and cooperation. If the child can cooperate, then a thorough external examination with lavage can be undertaken. If the child cannot cooperate, an examination under anesthesia may be necessary, including cystoscopy and vaginoscopy with a pediatric cystoscope. Any speculum regardless of size can damage the child's hymen or fragile vaginal mucosa, and the examination of the vagina with the speculum is not as good as vaginoscopy with the cystoscope.[76]

Most of the minor injuries to the external genitalia can be treated with antibiotic ointment and sitz baths.

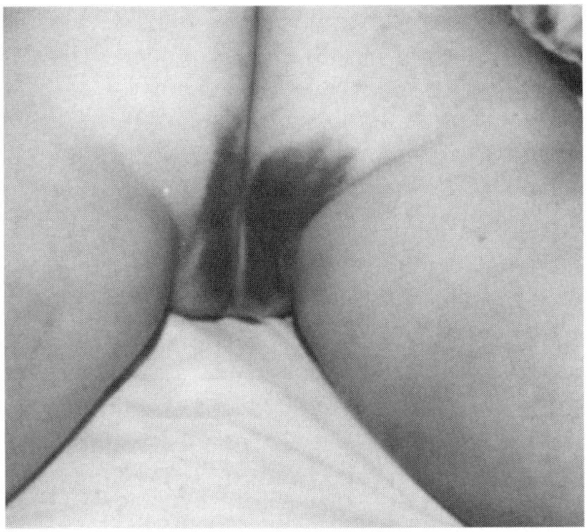

Figure 21–20 Labial hematoma resulting from a straddle injury. From Sanfilippo JS (ed). Pediatric and Adolescent Gynecology. Philadelphia: WB Saunders, 1994. Used with permission.

Cauterization of bleeding or simple sutures may be necessary. Many vaginal lacerations may be best treated with debridement, allowing the mucosa to heal with secondary intent. Occasionally, the child will form some granulation tissue at the site of injury that requires fulguration, but serious complications are rare.

One third of all genital injuries in girls may be related to sexual abuse. The features most indicative of this form of injury are a symmetric injury (indicating that the force of injury was in the midline), a transected hymen, and enlargement of the vaginal introitus.[76] In rape patients there is often a major laceration of the tissues.

At some point the child's ability to urinate must be established. It is unnecessary to catheterize or obtain a cystogram in the majority of these children. Topical viscous lidocaine applied to the periurethral area and sitz baths may allow the child to void in the emergency department. If the child cannot void, then a cystoscopy and examination under anesthesia is the best diagnostic plan.

SCROTAL AND TESTICULAR TRAUMA

Traumatic injuries to the scrotum are quite rare. The mobility, size, and location of the genitalia make them a difficult target for blunt or penetrating trauma. Blunt trauma is the more common cause of scrotal injury. The mechanism is a forceful blow to the perineum, which traps the scrotum between the pubis or thigh and some external object crushing the soft tissue in between. Straddle injuries, athletic kick injuries, and assaults are the most frequent circumstances causing blunt scrotal trauma.

Scrotal injuries may lead to intrascrotal bleeding, which may be significant in terms of producing a large hematoma but is seldom significant hemodynamically. In the event of isolated blunt scrotal injuries, the urologist must first establish that the testis is intact and viable. This may be done by physical examination, which may reveal a normal-sized, nontender testis uninvolved with the injury in minor cases. Usually, however, there is some concern about the status of the testis. The edema and tenderness of the scrotum make the testis examination difficult. In these cases a scrotal ultrasonogram may help determine the diagnosis.

Blunt trauma to the testis can result in contusions, with or without intratesticular hemorrhage, and testicular rupture if the tunica albuginea is torn. Testicular contusions require only conservative therapy and follow-up to be certain that hematomas resolve appropriately. Diagnosis is made with physical examination of a swollen, hard, tender testis and should be confirmed with Doppler ultrasonography to rule out testicular torsion and to ensure that the tunica albuginea is intact. Such trauma can result in intrascrotal hematomas, which may simulate a ruptured testis on physical examination.[79]

Testicular fracture is an injury in which a direct blow to the testis causes a tear to the tunica albuginea, allowing herniation of the seminiferous tubules and considerable bleeding within the tunica vaginalis. The injury is usually a crushing mechanism with external force trapping the testis against the pubic symphysis. The ability to salvage the testis is enhanced with early diagnosis and surgical repair.[80] Using ultrasonography, one may have difficulty differentiating between intratesticular hematoma and testicular rupture, and surgical exploration may be necessary to establish the diagnosis in some cases.[81] In the case of testicular rupture, necrotic tissue should be debrided and the tunica albuginea repaired with absorbable sutures. The scrotum should be drained adequately after thorough irrigation. Even after proper treatment, the testis may atrophy.

Penetrating testicular trauma, including stab and gunshot wounds, requires surgical exploration to obtain hemostasis, debride and clean the wound, and repair the damaged structures.[82] In the rare case of testicular amputation, the testis may be reimplanted using microsurgical techniques. The limiting factor for organ survival is warm ischemia time. Several authors have reported successful reimplantation after up to 7 hours of total ischemia.[83]

TRAUMA TO THE PENIS

Trauma to the penis is rare. In the flaccid state the penis is smaller, mobile, compressible, and protected by the thighs and pubis. When erect, it is much more susceptible to injury from blunt and penetrating trauma. The erect

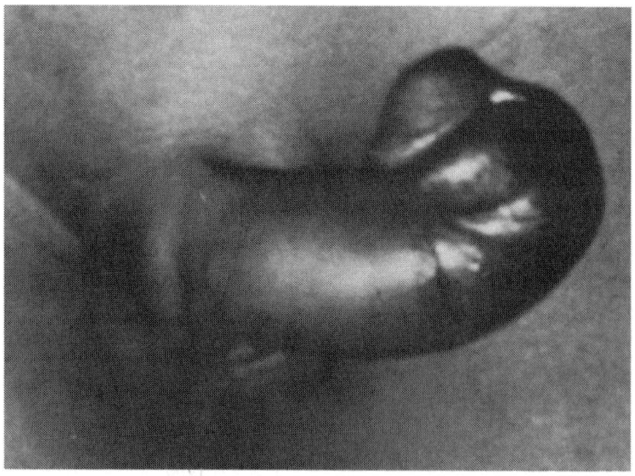

Figure 21–21 Fracture of the penis in an adolescent boy. From Belman B. Genitourinary Problems in Pediatrics. Philadelphia: WB Saunders, 1981. Used with permission.

penis is larger, rigid, and anchored to the pubis in an exposed position. Blunt injury to the penis is most uncommon, with fewer than 200 cases reported. These injuries are referred to as fractures of the penis and result when an erect penis is forcibly bent until the tunica albuginea of the corpora is torn. This results in significant local bleeding; these patients present in severe pain with a swollen, discolored, and angulated penis (Fig. 21–21). Urethral disruption occurs in approximately 10% of reported cases of penile fracture, and all but three reported cases were partial lacerations.[84]

Evaluation of the patient with suspected penile fracture involves careful palpation of the corpora, which will usually reveal the disruption in the tunica albigunea. If the hematoma is too large to adequately evaluate the corpora by palpation, then a cavernosogram may be performed.[85] The presence of blood at the meatus makes a retrograde urethrogram necessary to evaluate the patient for urethral injury.

Treatment of penile fractures involves immediate exploration and repair. The penis can be opened through a circumcision incision and degloved. The torn tunica albuginea should be minimally debrided, but the underlying erectile tissue is best preserved. This tissue may appear to be nonviable when it is contused from trauma. Debridement of the erectile tissue is unnecessary and may result in significant bleeding. The tunica can then be closed with absorbable sutures and a catheter left in place even in the absence of urethral injuries. Nonoperative management of these injuries leads to significant deformity as a result of penile curvature in 10% of patients.[86]

Penetrating wounds to the penis from gunshot or stabbing are becoming more common as a result of increasing civilian violence. Gunshot wounds to the penis are often due to a single bullet with few if any associated injuries.[80] Twenty-nine percent of patients have urethral injuries, and blood at the meatus is somewhat predictive. Sixty percent of patients with blood at the meatus will have urethral injury. Patients should have a retrograde urethrogram, and, although while extravasation does indicate urethral injury, the amount of extravasation does not correlate with the extent of injury.[87]

Penetrating wounds of the penis are treated with immediate surgery. The corpora should be repaired and debridement should be limited. Urethral injuries should be treated with urethral mobilization and a spatulated, tension-free anastomosis. Urinary diversion with a urethral catheter is acceptable in most patients. However, suprapubic diversion is preferable in severe injuries.[88]

Several forms of penile trauma are limited to children. Infants can present with penile swelling and erythema in a circumferential pattern. This may be due to a form of strangulation caused by a hair wrapped around the penis for a long period of time. The hair itself may not be visible in the emergency room. If left in place long enough, the hair may erode into the urethra or the corporal bodies or injure the neurovascular bundle.[89] Treatment involves removal of the hair and local wound care until the extent of injury can be established. Often the hair must be removed in the operating room.

Toilet seat injuries are relatively common when the raised toilet seat falls and traps the boy's penis against the toilet bowl rim. This usually causes minor contusions and abrasions and can usually be managed with local wound care and analgesics.[90] Likewise, young boys are susceptible to zipper injuries when they are in a hurry to zip their pants and trap their penis in the teeth of the zipper. This usually occurs in uncircumcised boys and the redundant foreskin is trapped. The zipper may be unlocked and separated to free the child in some cases, but a trip to the operating room may be required when the zipper has been in place for several hours.[91] Circumcision is sometimes necessary if the foreskin is damaged significantly.

REFERENCES

1. Feins NR. Multiple trauma. Pediatr Clin North Am 26:759, 1979.
2. McAleer IM, Kaplan GW, Schertz HC, et al. Genitourinary trauma in the pediatric patient. Urology 42:563, 1993.
3. Livine ML, Gonzales ET. Genitourinary trauma in children. Urol Clin North Am 12:53, 1985.
4. Kreiger JN, Algood CB, Mason JT, et al. Urologic trauma in Pacific Northwest: Etiology, distribution, management, and outcome. J Urol 132:70, 1984.
5. Sagalowsky AI, McConnell JD, Peters PC. Renal trauma requiring surgery: An analysis of 185 cases. J Trauma 23:128, 1983.
6. Hall JR, Reyes HM, Loeff DS, et al. The new epidemic in children: Penetrating injuries. J Trauma 39:487, 1995.
7. Miller RC, Sterioff S Jr, Drucker WR, et al. The incidental discovery of occult abdominal tumors in children following blunt abdominal trauma. J Trauma 6:99, 1986.
8. Smith EM, Elder JS, Spirnak JP. Major blunt renal trauma in the pediatric population: Is a nonoperative approach indicated? J Urol 149:546, 1993.

9. Levy JB, Baskin L, Ewalt DH, et al. Nonoperative management of blunt pediatric major renal trauma. Urology 42:418, 1993.
10. Stein JP, Kaji DM, Eastham J, et al. Blunt renal trauma in the pediatric population: Indications for radiographic evaluation. Urology 44:406, 1994.
11. Eastham JA, Wilson TG, Ahlering TE. Radiographic evaluation of adult patients with blunt renal trauma. J Urol 148:266, 1992.
12. McAndrew JD, Corriere JN. Radiographic evaluation of renal trauma: Evaluation of 1103 consecutive patients. Br J Urol 73:352, 1993.
13. Mertz JHO, Widhard WN, Nouse MH, et al. Injury to the kidney in children. JAMA 183:730, 1963.
14. Mayor B, Gudinchet F, Wicky S, et al. Imaging evaluation of blunt renal trauma in children: Diagnostic accuracy of intravenous pyelography and ultrasonography. Pediatr Radiol 25:214, 1995.
15. Bauman L, Greenfield SP, Aker J, et al. Nonoperative management of major blunt renal trauma in children: In-hospital morbidity and long-term follow-up. J Urol 148:691, 1992.
16. Fleisher G. Prospective evaluation of selective criteria for imaging among children with suspected blunt renal trauma. Pediatr Emerg Care 5:8, 1989.
17. Lieu TA, Fleisher GR, Mahboubi S, et al. Hematuria and clinical findings as indications for intravenous pyelography in pediatric blunt renal trauma. Pediatrics 82:216, 1988.
18. Monstrey SJM, Vander Werken C, Debruyne FMJ, et al. Rational guidelines in renal trauma assessment. Urology 31:469, 1988.
19. Mangubat EA, Eichelberger MR. Hypovolemic shock in the pediatric patient: A physiologic approach to diagnosis and treatment. In Eichelberger MR, Pratsch GL (eds), Pediatric Trauma Care. Rockville, MD: Aspen Publishers, 1988, p 69.
20. Abou-Jaoude WA, Sugarman JM, Fallat ME, et al. Indicators of genitourinary tract injury or anomaly in cases of pediatric blunt trauma. J Pediatr Surg 31:86, 1996.
21. Taylor GA, Eichelberger MR, Potter BM. Hematuria: A marker of abdominal injury in children after blunt trauma. Ann Surg 208:688, 1988.
22. Mee SL, McAninch JW, Robinson AL, et al. Radiographic assessment of renal trauma: A 10 year prospective study of patient selection. J Urol 141:1095, 1989.
23. Hardeman SW, Husmann DA, Chinn HK, et al. Blunt urinary tract trauma: Identifying those patients who require radiographic diagnostic studies. J Urol 138:99, 1987.
24. Husmann DA, Gilling PJ, Perry MO, et al. Major renal lacerations with a devitalized fragment following blunt abdominal trauma: A comparison between nonoperative (expectant) versus surgical management. J Urol 150:1774, 1993.
25. Cass AS, Luxenberg M. Conservative or immediate surgical management of blunt renal injuries. J Urol 130:11, 1983.
26. Cass AS. Renal trauma in multiple-injured child. Urology 21:487, 1983.
27. McAninch JW, Carroll PR, Klosterman PW, et al. Renal reconstruction after injury. J Urol 145:932, 1991.
28. Guerriero WG, Carlton CE Jr, Scott R Jr, et al. Renal pedicle injuries. J Trauma 11:53, 1971.
29. Lohse JR, Botham RJ, Waters RF. Traumatic bilateral renal artery thrombosis: Case report and review of literature. J Urol 127:522, 1982.
30. Cass AS, Brubrick M, Luxenberg M, et al. Renal pedicle injury in patients with multiple injuries. J Trauma 25:892, 1985.
31. Smith SD, Gardner MJ, Rowe MI. Renal artery occlusion in pediatric blunt abdominal trauma—Decreasing the delay from injury to treatment. J Trauma 35:861, 1993.
32. Cain MP, Matsumoto JM, Husmann DA. Retrograde filling of the renal vein on computerized tomography for blunt renal trauma: An indicator of renal artery injury. J Urol 153:1247, 1995.
33. Cass AS, Luxenberg M. Management of renal artery injuries from external trauma. J Urol 138:266, 1987.
34. Abdalati H, Bulas DI, Sivit CJ, et al. Blunt renal trauma in children: Healing of renal injuries and recommendations for imaging followup. Pediatr Radiol 24:573, 1994.
35. Gill B, Palmer LS, Reda E, et al. Optimal renal preservation with timely percutaneous intervention: A changing concept in the management of renal trauma in children in the 1990's. Br J Urol 74:370, 1994.
36. Teigen CL, Venbrux AC, Quinlan DM, et al. Late massive hematuria as a complication of conservative management of blunt renal trauma in children. J Urol 147:1333, 1992.
37. Surana R, Kahn A, Fitzgerald RJ. Scarring following renal trauma in children. Br J Urol 75:663, 1995.
38. Yale-Loehr AJ, Kramer SS, Quinlan DM, et al. CT of severe renal trauma in children: Evaluation and course of healing with conservative therapy. Am J Roentgenol 52:109, 1989.
39. Angus LDG, Tachmes L, Kahn S, et al. Surgical management of pediatric renal trauma: An urban experience. Am Surg 59:388, 1993.
40. Baniel J, Schein M. The management of penetrating trauma to the urinary tract. J Am Coll Surg 178:417, 1994.
41. Eastham JA, Wilson TG, Ahlering TE. Urological evaluation and management of renal-proximity stab wounds. J Urol 150:1771, 1993.
42. Heyns CF, Van Vollenhoven P. Selective surgical management of renal stab wounds. Br J Urol 69:351, 1992.
43. Bernath AS, Schutte H, Fernandez RRD, et al. Stab wounds of the kidney: Conservative management in flank penetration. J Urol 129:468, 1983.
44. Heyns CF, Van Vollenhoven P. Increasing role of angiography and segmental artery embolization in the management of renal stab wounds. J Urol 147:1231, 1992.
45. McAninch JW, Carroll PR, Armenakas NA, et al. Renal gunshot wounds: Method of salvage and reconstruction. J Trauma 35:279, 1993.
46. Carroll PR, Klosterman P, McAninch JW. Early vascular control for renal trauma: A critical review. J Urol 141:826, 1989.
47. McAninch JW, Carrol PR. Renal trauma: Kidney preservation through improved vascular control—A refined approach. J Trauma 22:285, 1992.
48. Corriere JN Jr, McAndrew JD, Benson GS. Intraoperative decision-making in renal trauma surgery. J Trauma 31:1390, 1991.
49. Atala A, Miller FB, Richardson JD. Preliminary vascular control for renal trauma. Surg Gynecol Obstet 173:386, 1991.
50. Presti JC Jr, Carroll PR, McAninch JW. Ureteral and renal pelvic injuries from external trauma: Diagnosis and management. J Trauma 29:370, 1989.
51. Corrier JN Jr. Ureteral injuries. In Gillenwater JY, Grayhack JT, Howards SS, Duckett JW (eds), Adult and Pediatric Urology, 3rd ed. St. Louis, MO: CV Mosby, 1996, p 554.
52. Brandes AB, Chelsky MJ, Buckman RF, et al. Ureteral injuries from penetrating trauma. J Trauma 36:776, 1994.
53. Campbell EW Jr, Fildreman PS, Jacobs SC. Ureteral injury due to blunt and penetrating trauma. Urology 40:216, 1992.
54. Reznichek RC, Brosman SA, Rhodes DB. Ureteral avulsion following blunt abdominal trauma. J Tenn Med Assoc 83:242, 1973.
55. Boone TB, Gilling PJ, Husmann DA. Ureteropelvic junction disruption following blunt abdominal trauma. J Urol 150:33, 1993.
56. Kotkin L, Brock JW. Isolated ureteral injury caused by blunt trauma. Urology 47:111, 1996.
57. Toporoff B, Scalea TM, Abramson D. Ureteral laceration caused by a fall from a height: Case report and review of the literature. J Trauma 34:164, 1993.
58. Fernandez AF, Ruiz SS, Martinez IG, et al. Blunt traumatic

rupture of the high right ureter, repaired with appendix interposition. Urol Int 53:97, 1993.
59. Wazzan W, Azoury B, Hemady K. Missile injury of upper ureter treated by delayed renal autotransplantation and ureteropyelostomy. Urology 42:725, 1993.
60. Sivit CJ, Cutting JP, Eichelberger MR. CT diagnosis and localization of rupture of the bladder in children with blunt abdominal trauma: Significance of contrast material extravasation in the pelvis. Am J Radiol 164:1243, 1995.
61. Corriere JN Jr, Sandler CM. Management of the ruptured bladder: 7 years experience with 111 cases. J Trauma 26:830, 1986.
62. Hochberg E, Stone NN. Bladder rupture associated with pelvic fracture due to blunt trauma. Urology 41:531, 1993.
63. Carroll PR, McAninch JW. Major bladder trauma: Mechanisms of injury and a unified method of diagnosis and repair. J Urol 132:254, 1984.
64. Mulkey AP Jr, Witherington R. Conservative management of vesical rupture. Urology 4:426, 1974.
65. Kotkin L, Koch MO. Morbidity associated with nonoperative management of extraperitoneal bladder injuries. J Trauma 38:895, 1995.
66. Cass AS, Godec CJ. Urethral injury due to external trauma. Urology 11:607, 1978.
67. Senocak ME, Ciftci AO, Buyukpamukcu N, et al. Transpubic urethroplasty in children: Report of 10 cases with review of the literature. J Pediatr Surg 30:1319, 1995.
68. Boone TB, Wilson WT, Husman DA. Postpubertal genitourinary function following posterior urethral disruptions in children. J Urol 148:1232, 1992.
69. Corriere JN, Rudy DC, Benson GS. Voiding and erectile function after delay one-stage repair of posterior urethral disruptions in 50 men with a fractured pelvis. J Trauma 37:587, 1994.
70. Follis HW, Koch MO, McDougal WS. Immediate management of prostatomembranous urethral disruptions. J Urol 147:1259, 1992.
71. Quint HJ, Stanisic TH. Above and below delayed endoscopic treatment of traumatic posterior urethral disruptions. J Urol 149:484, 1993.
72. Carter CT, Schafer N. Incidence of urethral disruption in females with traumatic pelvic fractures. Am J Emerg Med 11:218, 1993.
73. Antoci JP, Martin S Jr. Bladder and urethral injuries in patients with pelvic fractures. J Urol 128:25, 1982.
74. Orkin LA. Trauma to the bladder, ureter, and kidney. In Sciarra JJ (ed), Gynecology and Obstetrics. Philadelphia: JB Lippincott, 1991, p 1.
75. Perry MO, Husmann DA. Urethral injuries in female subjects following pelvic fractures. J Urol 47:139, 1992.
76. McAninch JW. Editorial comment. J Urol 147:143, 1992.
77. Garrett RA. Pediatric urethral and perineal injuries. Pediatr Clin North Am 22:401, 1976.
78. Pokorny SF, Pokorny WJ, Kramer W. Acute genital injury in the prepubertal girl. Am J Obstet Gynecol 166:1461, 1992.
79. Cohen HL, Shapiro ML, Haller JO, et al. Sonography of intrascrotal hematomas simulating testicular rupture in adolescents. Pediatr Radiol 22:296, 1992.
80. Stillwell T, Reading C, Leary F. Untreated rupture of the tunica albuginea. Mayo Clin Proc 61:975, 1986.
81. Cass A, Luxenberg M. Testicular injuries. Urology 37:528, 1991.
82. Brandes SB, Buckman RF, Chelsky MJ, et al. External genitalia gunshot wounds: A ten-year experience with fifty-six cases. J Trauma 39:266, 1995.
83. Shioshvils TI. A case of successful replantation of testis after autohemicastration. Eur Urol 13:285, 1987.
84. Tsang T, Demby AM. Penile fracture with urethral injury. J Urol 147:466, 1992.
85. Klein FA, Smith MJ, Miller N. Penile fracture: Diagnosis and management. J Trauma 25:1090, 1985.
86. Mears EM Jr. Traumatic rupture of the corpus cavernosum. J Urol 105:407, 1971.
87. Miles BJ, Poffenberger RJ, Farah RN, et al. Management of penile gunshot wounds. Urology 36:318, 1990.
88. Gomez RG, Castanheira ACC, McAninch JW. Gunshot wounds to the male external genitalia. J Urol 150:1147, 1993.
89. Sheinfeld J, Cos LR, Erturk E, et al. Penile tourniquet injury due to a coil of hair. J Urol 133:1042, 1985.
90. Noe HN, Jerkins GR. Genitourinary trauma. In Kelalis PP, King LR, Belman AB (eds), Clinical Pediatric Urology, 3rd ed, Philadelphia, WB Saunders, 1992, p. 1353.
91. Flowerden R, Fishman JJ, Churchill BM. Management of penile zipper injury. J Urol 117:671, 1977.

Index

Note: Page numbers in *italics* refer to illustrations; page numbers followed by the letter t refer to tables.

S

V

W

X

Y

ISBN 0-7216-6857-7

90038

9 780721 668574